Midwifery
and Childbirth
in America

Publication of this book has been supported
by a grant from The Carnegie Foundation
for the Advancement of Teaching

Midwifery and Childbirth in America

 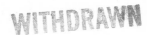

Judith Pence Rooks

Foreword by Charles S. Mahan, M.D.

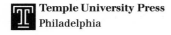 **Temple University Press**
Philadelphia

Temple University Press, Philadelphia 19122
Copyright © 1997 by Judith Pence Rooks
All rights reserved
Published 1997
Printed in the United States of America

Interior design by Anne O'Donnell

 The paper used in this publication meets the requirements of American
National Standard for Information Sciences—Permanence of Paper for
Printed Library Materials, ANSI Z39.49–1984

Library of Congress Cataloging-in-Publication Data
Rooks, Judith.
    Midwifery and childbirth in America / Judith Pence Rooks.
    Foreword by Charles S. Mahan, M.D.
    ISBN 1-56639-565-8 (cloth: alk. paper)
          p.   cm.
    Includes bibliographical references and index.
    1. Midwifery—United States.   I. Title.
RG950.R66   1997
362.1'9820233'0973—DC21   97-12790

To Charles

Contents

Chapter 8
Nurse-Midwifery in America, 1980–1995   *159*

Chapter 9
Development of Direct-Entry Midwifery, 1980–1995   *225*

Chapter 10
The Quality, Safety, and Effectiveness of Midwifery as Practiced in the United States   *295*

List of Tables

Foreword

These are hard times for American babies. More than one of every five children in our country live in poverty, and the number is steadily increasing. More families are homeless now than at any other time since the Depression. More pregnancy outcomes are being negatively affected by AIDS, drug abuse, and violence, which are epidemic in many communities. The anti-immigrant bent in some states threatens the provision of even preventive health care services to mothers and infants. Some moms are working two or three jobs to make ends meet and have to cut short breast-feeding and bonding times. Some managed care groups send new mothers home fast after delivery, with no home care follow-up and teaching. A three-pound baby born in the United States has the best chance of living compared to similar babies in other developed countries, *but* we deliver proportionally *more* three-pound babies than are born in other countries. The sad fact is that our percentage of low birth weight babies has not changed significantly in more than fifty years while other countries have enjoyed steady declines. Even though our infant mortality rate is dropping slowly, much of that decrease is a result of very expensive treatment technology, not the widespread community-friendly interventions that have served our sister countries so well and so much more effectively.

This valuable and comprehensive book documents the special gifts that the calling of midwifery has brought to the world. It exhaustively lays out the proud history and tradition of midwifery and proves the safety, quality, and cost effectiveness of such care. It shows that midwifery has, like public health, been the firm foundation of the health care pyramid for mothers and babies in most countries, except for ours. This lets the reader with even an average imagination see some of the folly of building a hierarchy of care as an inverted pyramid—with the majority of pregnant women receiving care from specialists even though most of the women are experiencing a normal physiologic event. Such is life in the U.S. health care non-system.

Well, things are changing. As one who works closely on a day-to-day basis with many of the agents of change, allow me to make some predictions about how these changes will affect the landscape of birth in America in the next decade. As the current era of cost, cutting and profit-taking comes to a close, most pregnant women will be in managed care, and capitation will rule with an even greater squeeze on profits. The answer: midwives. Payors will work to eliminate the high cost of hospitals from their birth balance sheets. The answers: birth centers run by midwives. Payors will be vexed by the rapidly escalating costs of psycho-social-medical problems such as AIDS, drug abuse, alcoholism, and family violence and their resulting effects on pregnancy. The answer: midwives. Employers will be beset by their employees for caregivers who are women, friendly, better communicators, generous with their time and who will provide high-quality, satisfying care and sit with them through the *whole* labor. The answer: midwives. Managed care groups will worry more about *primary* prevention of low birth weight in the communities they serve and will look to successful European preventive techniques such as home visiting, stress reduction and extensive maternity leave as solutions. The answer includes midwifery. Medical schools and teaching hospitals will cut faculty and residency positions and will need people interested in teaching all aspects of the management of normal prenatal care and birth to students and residents. The answer: midwives. The midwives will need expert consultation and backup services, and some—but fewer—cesarean sections and epidurals will still need to be done. The answer: obstetricians, family physicians, and anesthesiologists.

The United States in the richest nation in the history of the world. We spend more money per capita on health care than any other nation and yet end up in the bottom half of international rankings for most measures of health care outcomes. Many of our health care dollars are spent foolishly without regard for the population-based effects (or lack of them) of such expenditures or even regard for good science. As Winston Churchill once said: "Americans will always do the right thing, after they have exhausted all the other possibilities." Our time has come, Sir Winston, and midwifery is the right thing.

—Charles S. Mahan, M.D.,
    Dean of the University of South
    Florida College of Public Health

Preface

The need for a book to tell the story of childbirth and midwifery in the United States was identified by Dr. Ernest L. Boyer, president of the Carnegie Foundation for the Advancement of Teaching from 1979 until his death in December 1995. Dr. Boyer's wife, Kathryn, is a nurse-midwife. He learned about the importance of midwifery from her dedication to her work and by his presence when their daughter gave birth to their grandchild—at home, attended by Kathryn and another midwife.

Kathryn Boyer was president of the American College of Nurse-Midwives Foundation from 1984 to 1989. Under her leadership the ACNM Foundation conducted a study to identify factors that support or hinder the success of nurse-midwifery. Widespread ignorance and misinformation were identified as the most formidable barriers to greater success. When the study was completed, the foundation convened a National Advisory Panel (leaders of disciplines and institutions interested in the quality and accessibility of maternity care) to consider the findings. Dr. Boyer chaired the meeting. The panel made eleven recommendations and presented them in order of priority. The first five recommendations called for documenting the accomplishments and advantages of nurse-midwifery, educating the general public about nurse-midwifery and about the health care that is needed and is relevant to childbearing, "telling the story" of nurse-midwifery, increasing other health care professionals' understanding of nurse-midwives and the nature of midwifery, and educating the people who operate and are responsible for health care organizations and institutions about the advantages of nurse-midwifery, including cost advantages and the popularity of nurse-midwifery among consumers.

During the late 1980s the United States faced a critical shortage of physicians willing to provide care to pregnant women who were on Medicaid or had no means to pay for care. Many—eventually most—obstetricians refused to accept Medicaid-eligible women as patients. Although this problem was seen as a crisis, it was really just the culmination of long-term problems and trends. A high proportion of pregnant women are poor. Women who are poor are much more likely to have pregnancy complications and deliver babies who require very expensive intensive care. The care needed to intervene in these problems is not simple; there is no quick technological fix. Although nurse-midwives take care of a broad sprectrum of women, they have specialized in providing effective care to women who are at high risk because of poverty and other social and behavioral problems. Between 1985 and 1991 a series of prestigious committees convened by the Institute of Medicine (part of the National Academy of Sciences) and other organizations called for greater use of nurse-midwives to meet the needs of "hard-to-reach" women. But there were not enough nurse-midwives, and the annual number of new nurse-midwifery graduates was low and not increasing.

In 1989 the Carnegie Foundation responded to this crisis by convening a seminar to examine the recruitment and education of midwives. (The Carnegie Foundation, during its long history, has at times studied professional education, notably the preparation of doctors—the famous Flexner report, published in 1910—as well as lawyers, and, most recently, architects.) Dr. Boyer was especially interested in the potential impact of further development of direct-entry midwifery education on recruitment into midwifery. (Direct-entry means that students enter midwifery education directly—without the requirement of prior education in nursing.) In 1990 the Carnegie Foundation convened another seminar to explore the feasibility of establishing a single standard for professional midwifery. At the end of the second meeting Dr. Boyer encouraged creation of a work group to provide structure for continued communication between representatives of the two national midwifery organizations, one that represents

nurse-midwives and one that focuses primarily on lay and direct-entry midwives. The Carnegie Foundation helped support five meetings of this work group. Although the meetings did not produce agreement leading to the development of a single educational standard for professional midwifery, the process stimulated the lay and direct-entry midwifery community to develop the standards and processes needed to support a professional form of direct-entry midwifery.

In late 1991, Dr. Ernest Boyer asked me to write a document to tell the story of midwifery and the health care that is important for childbearing. As I began to work on it, I realized that the level of information needed required more than a report. The misunderstandings about midwifery in this country are deep. A solid base of information and analysis is needed to address them. Dr. Boyer encouraged me to take the time to write a thorough book.

Dr. Boyer asked me to undertake this task because, although I am a midwife by training, most of my career has been in public health—as an epidemiologist at the U.S. Centers for Disease Control (CDC), as an "expert" in the Office of the Surgeon General of the Public Health Service, as a project officer and public health advisor in the U.S. Agency for International Development. I was in public health first; it is my first love and my first identity. I have functioned primarily in the research arena and have not practiced midwifery since I completed my nurse-midwifery education program (at Johns Hopkins, in 1974). I wrote the book partly from inside the profession, but partly as an outside observer. My high regard for midwifery has a public health motive.

Although I believe that I look at midwifery objectively, I have been an active member of the profession. I have chaired two committees of the ACNM and served as its president from 1983 to 1985. I am an editorial consultant to the *Journal of Nurse-Midwifery* and sit on the governing board of the Fellowship of the ACNM. I was a part-time member of the faculty of the Community-based Nurse-midwifery Education Program (CNEP) of the Frontier School of Midwifery and Family Nursing from 1993 to 1995, a position from which I resigned in order to complete this book. (Although the school is based in Hyden, Kentucky, the faculty and students are located throughout the United States.)

The book is intended to help address an enormous, pervasive ignorance about midwifery and the kind of care needed by pregnant women. Although there is considerable interest in midwifery—most people have some concept of what it is and think they understand it—there is little real understanding among those who have not had experience with it and a lack of accurate, factual information about many aspects of it, even among midwives. I have attempted to provide a relatively complete compendium of relevant, accurate information, laid out clearly with authoritative references, including some data that are not available anywhere else. I tried to be accurate and objective.

The book includes some new primary research. Much of the information on direct-entry midwifery, such as the sections on educational programs and the evolution of the certification process developed by the North American Registry of Midwives (NARM), is not available elsewhere. Chapter 9 is longer than any other for that reason. Parts of Chapters 10 and 11 report original secondary analysis—new synthesis and conclusions regarding the effectiveness of midwifery care for reducing low birth weight and cesarean sections and the safety of home births.

A book of this kind is necessarily historical to some degree; several chapters are entirely historical. However, my purpose was not to provide a comprehensive historical record, and I did not do so. The individuals, institutions, and events described were included because of their singular importance or because they are characteristic of broader phenomena or trends. Thus some people

and organizations are cited, while equally important people and organizations are not.

Organization and Objectives

The book focuses on midwifery and maternal and infant health and health care in the United States between 1980 and 1995.

- Chapter 1 provides definitions and an introduction to the major concepts: What is midwifery? How does it differ from medicine?
- Chapters 2, 3, and 4 provide a brief history of midwifery and maternity care in the world and in Colonial America and the United States through the early part of the 1900s, the early development of nurse-midwifery (introduced in 1925), the effect of the social movements of the 1960s and 1970s on childbirth and nurse-midwifery, and the development of lay midwifery during the 1970s.
- Chapters 5 through 9 explain and describe the development and status of midwifery and the health problems, health care, and health-care system as it relates to meeting the needs of childbearing women in the United States from 1980 through 1995. The two main classifications of midwives—certified nurse-midwives and direct-entry midwives—differ markedly in their development, legal status, education, quality assurance processes, scope of practice, practice sites, clientele, and working relationship with physicians. All of these and other facets of both kinds of midwifery are described in Chapters 8 and 9.
- Chapters 10, 11, and 12 provide a synthesis and secondary analysis of research related to the safety, effectiveness, benefits, and costs of the care provided by midwives in the United States from 1980 through 1995. Chapter 10 also provides data that uses national birth certificate data and research findings to describe the care provided to

women during labor and delivery in most American hospitals.

- Chapter 13 provides a brief look at midwifery and maternal health care in some of our "peer" countries: Western Europe, the United Kingdom, Canada, Australia, New Zealand, and Japan.
- Chapter 14 provides an analysis of the current situation and recommendations to improve things—a summary of recommendations made by other groups, plus my recommendations based on the information laid out in the other chapters.

Most chapters begin with a summary. Factual information provided in the summary is described in greater detail later in the chapter, and the source of the information is documented there. In most cases, the source of the information is not cited in the summary.

Some information is repeated with more or less detail in more than one section or chapter. This was done to remind readers of the often complex context for information discussed in more than one part of the book.

Acknowledgments

This book is based on many sources of information and insight: my own knowledge, understanding, and experience; a vast array of written materials—from research published in leading medical journals to informal newsletters published by state midwifery organizations; in-person and telephone interviews; and constructive reviews of first drafts of every section of the book by individuals with special expertise about some aspect of the subject. Writing a book on midwifery is a communal experience. People who care about this subject were enormously responsive to requests for information and advice. After a while, I didn't even have to ask.

People I know and people I've never met knew I was writing a book on midwifery and sent me articles I would otherwise not have seen, copies of significant personal correspondence, even books and copies of entire out-of-print books. Often the exact thing I needed just arrived in my mailbox, sometimes unsolicited. I don't even know who sent some of them.

A highlight of my experience occurred in July 1996, a day or so after *The Lancet*—a leading British medical journal—published an article that reported findings from an important study conducted in Scotland. The study was a randomized, controlled trial that compared the outcomes of care managed by midwives with standard Scottish care. I don't usually read *The Lancet* and might have missed this article, but four people faxed copies to me: a medical epidemiologist from Los Angeles (part of the network of epidemiologists who have been trained and worked at the Centers for Disease Control), a nurse-midwife epidemiologist from Albuquerque (part of the American College of Nurse-Midwives network), an anthropologist from San Antonio who is part of the Midwives of North America (MANA) network (MANA is a midwifery organization that focuses primarily on direct-entry midwives), and a physician in Denmark who used to head the maternal and child health unit of the World Health Organization's office for Europe. Although I had never met him, he sent the article and volunteered to review my chapter on midwifery in other countries. Working alone in my home in Portland, Oregon, it made me feel wonderfully connected to the world— and reassured me that I would not miss anything!

The people I relied on most were nurse-midwives, especially Sally Tom, Kitty Ernst, and Liz Sharp, each of whom carefully reviewed and critiqued several chapters and provided background information, insightful interpretations, reference materials, and additional contacts for expanding my knowledge and understanding of various issues. They kept me from making many errors of fact, interpretation, omission, or tone; I am deeply indebted. Joyce Roberts, president of the ACNM and an outstanding research scientist, reviewed the section on research. Several members of the staff of the ACNM reviewed other sections for accuracy and kept me updated as things evolved; I particularly appreciated the help of Deanne Williams. Two nurse-midwife epidemiologists—Patricia Aikins Murphy and Leah Albers—reviewed and provided suggestions for Chapters 10, 11, and 12. Nancy Sullivan's work at the Oregon Health Sciences University Hospital kept me in touch with the reality of midwifery practice in an academic medical center (and reassured me that "real" midwifery can be practiced in that setting). Judy Fullerton and Kathy Camacho Carr were generous sources of reference materials and expertise. Joyce Thompson reviewed and improved the section on the International Confederation of Midwives. Elisa Morales kept me up-to-date with issues of importance to nurse-midwives who attend home births. Maggie Emory reviewed nearly every chapter.

In addition to reviewing sections or chapters that had already been drafted, nurse-midwives were the initial source of some of the information in some sections of the book. Dorothea Lang provided first-hand historical information about the role of the Maternal and Infant Care (MIC) projects in New York City. Minta Uzodinma provided information about nurse-midwifery in Mississippi during the late 1960s and early 1970s. Kate Bowland told me the story of the Birth Center of Santa Cruz. Carol Milligan gave me the history of early development of nurse-midwifery in the Indian Health Service. Johanna Borsellega, Barbara Lavery, and Ruth Payton did the same for the development of nurse-midwifery services and education in the U.S. military services. Irene Sandvold and Ann Koontz provided insight, as well as information, about the federal government's support of nurse-midwifery. Pat Burkhardt kept me abreast of the slow, painful implementation of the new Professional Midwifery Practice Act in New York State. Helen Varney Burst helped me avoid mistakes in one of the most sensitive parts of the book—the section that describes the ACNM's long process of deciding to become involved in accrediting direct-entry midwifery education programs and certifying direct-entry midwives. Some of the individuals who provided this kind of information are cited in the text of the book and are included in the list of references. Some are acknowledged here but are not referenced in the text. While reading the entire book from start to finish during the last phase of the editing process, I realized that my approach to referencing information obtained during telephone calls had changed over the several years of writing the book. Specific referencing of personal communications is much more complete in the later chapters and less complete in the earlier chapters.

I was especially grateful for and gratified by the consistent generosity and high level of help I received from members of the direct-entry midwifery community—especially Jo Anne Myers-Ciecko, executive director of the Seattle Midwifery School; Ina May Gaskin, president of MANA; Betty-Anne Daviss and Ken Johnson, a Toronto-based midwife/epidemiologist–wife/husband team who are conducting a study to describe the practices and outcomes of care provided by members of MANA and who gave me invaluable information about midwifery in Canada; Robbie Davis-Floyd, an anthropologist who is studying midwifery; and Anne Frye, who has written several textbooks for midwives (and lives in Portland). I have my own insiders' information about nurse-midwifery, but I was very dependent on members of this community for assistance in understanding this sparsely documented, rapidly changing branch of the profession. In the process I learned a lot and made some friends — outcomes that are hard to beat.

Barbara Pillsbury, my colleague at the Pacific Institute for Women's Health, helped me improve the writing of some chapters. Judy Norsigian, a founding member of the Boston Women's Health Book Collective (authors of *Our Bodies, Ourselves*) sent envelope after envelope full of information I needed. The highly competent and helpful professionals at the National Center for Health Statistics Division of Vital Statistics responded to my many queries with complete and accurate data and explanations; thanks especially to Selma Taffel and Stephanie Ventura.

I want to thank my friends, colleagues and students at CNEP—the distance-learning nurse-midwifery education program based in Hyden, Kentucky, which has students and faculty throughout the country, all keeping in touch and working together via personal computers in their homes. I learned so much from CNEP's incredibly creative faculty and students, who come to midwifery with a wonderful can-do spirit and wealth of life experience. It was very helpful to be part of that community during much of the time I was working on this book. Special thanks to Penny Armstrong, author of two wonderful books about midwifery and my colleague at CNEP, who saw that I would never finish the book unless I gave up, at least for a while, my role as teacher. Penny saw that I was stuck and, like the good midwife she is, helped me see my problem and resolve it—by leaving CNEP. Thanks also to Tekoa King; it made it easier to leave knowing that she would take responsibility for my course.

Whereas the rest of the book is based on my first-hand knowledge of midwifery and maternity care in my own country, Chapter 13—on midwifery in other industrialized countries—is based largely on information contained in published papers and documents. This is a serious limitation because it can result in bias. The journalists and journals that report trends and events related to midwifery may be more likely to report positive events and to ignore shortcomings and problems. In addition, published information is inevitably somewhat out-of-date. In order to present a realistic and current picture of midwifery in other countries I needed help from midwives and others who live in the those countries and who understand the issues confronting midwifery and maternity care in their own society. Diony Young—the editor of *Birth*, an international scientific and professional journal with wide distribution in Canada, the United Kingdom, Australia, Scandinavia, and New Zealand, as well as the United States—helped me by recommending people who might be willing to review what I had written about midwifery in their countries, and the people she referred me to often recommended others. The final version of Chapter 13 is more complete and accurate, and much more interesting thanks to the generous help of the following people: Susanne Houd (for help on the section about midwifery in Europe), Mary Renfrew (the United Kingdom), Petra ten Hoope-Bender (the Netherlands), Ulla Waldenström (Europe and Australia), Carol Thorogood and Janice Butt (Australia), Karen Guilliland (New Zealand), and Marsden Wagner (who reviewed the entire chapter). Susanne Houd coauthored a major World Health Organization study of maternity care in Europe during the late 1970s, Marsden Wagner was the physician responsible for maternal and child health at the World Health Organization Regional Office for Europe from 1978 through 1991, and Ulla Waldenström and Mary Renfrew are accomplished researchers. Margaret, Susanne, Mary, Petra, Ulla, Carol, and Karen are midwives. Karen is the national coordinator for the New Zealand College of Midwifery; all of the others are midwifery teachers and are on the faculties of universities.

The section on Canada is long because Canada, being our sister nation in North America, is especially important in the context of this book. For the accuracy and completeness of this section, I am most indebted to Betty-Anne Daviss, who reviewed the entire section, and Robbie Davis-Floyd, who organized a session at an anthropology meeting that included many papers about some aspect of midwifery in Canada and asked me to be the discussant. That gave me an opportunity to hear results from the most recent research and to meet many of the key actors in the tide of change that is affecting midwifery throughout Canada. Special thanks to Susan James (for information about midwifery in Alberta); Cecilia Benoit (for information about British Columbia); Kristine Robinson (Manitoba); Hélène Vadeboncoeur (Québec); Lesley Biggs (Saskatchewan); and Karyn Kaufman, Ivy Bourgeault, Betty-Anne Daviss, Margaret MacDonald, and Sheryl Nestel (Ontario).

I relied on several physicians to review and critique certain chapters of the book, including Mark Nichols, associate professor of obstetrics and gynecology at Oregon Health Sciences University (who is the ob-gyn representative on the board that regulates licensed direct-entry midwives in Oregon); Roger Rosenblatt, professor and vice chairman of the Department of Family Medicine at the University of Washington School of Medicine; Charles Mahan, an obstetrician-gynecologist who is dean of the College of Public Health at the University of South Florida; Lewis Mehl-Madrona, a family physician who did much of the early research on outcomes of home births in the United States; David Grimes, professor and vice chair of the Department of Obstetrics and Gynecology at the University of California at San Francisco (who is also an epidemiologist); Marsden Wagner, formerly with the World Health Organization's office for Europe; and Lawrence Pence, my father and a surgeon, who brought a long life's commitment to medicine to his review of every chapter.

I am enormously grateful for the support of the Carnegie Foundation for the Advancement of Teaching, especially Dr. Charles Glassick, interim president following the death of Dr. Boyer, who continued the Foundation's commitment to this book, and Jan Hempel, senior editor, who was my supporter and adviser in making plans for its publication. The late Dr. Ernest Boyer inspired the book and gave me the encouragement I needed, time and time again, to continue, even when the end seemed so far away. I enjoyed discussing the educational issues with him and had looked forward to working with him on the final chapter. His death was a terrible loss for the country, for the field of education, for his family and colleagues, and for me. But I thank him and his memory for his love of children, his concern about the health and well-being of mothers, and his vision for midwifery. I thank his wife, Kathryn, for being an exemplar as a midwife and a person, for her leadership of the ACNM Foundation (1984–1989), and for her constant encouragement and support to me during the long period during which this book was written.

Michael Ames, the editor-in-chief at Temple University Press, had a larger vision of the need and market for this book than even I did. His calm enthusiasm steadied and encouraged me through the early phases of the publication process. All of the staff at Temple and at Spectrum Publisher Services were a pleasure to work with.

Kitty Ernst has been a role model and mentor to me for many years and has enriched my life by drawing me into several of her many schemes to advance midwifery and improve the care of mothers. The book would not be the same without the inspiration provided by Kitty. I am also grateful for the intellectual leadership of Ruth Watson Lubic, who led the Maternity Center Association throughout most of my professional life to date, and to the wise women who established and developed the American College of Nurse-Midwives and its elegant processes for quality assurance.

The book would not have been possible without the support, loving guidance, and reliably wise counsel of my husband, Charles. Supporting me through this long haul was also an act of great generosity, for it involved much deprivation in the usual life of our household. He said that he would not have supported me at it for so long except that the book is worth it. He is a wise and utterly honest man. His belief that the result would be worth the effort gave me the courage to go on.

I enlisted and obtained the help and advice of a very large number of other people who discussed issues with me over the telephone, sent me information, or reviewed specific chapters or parts of chapters. Although I tried to keep a record of the people who responded to my myriad requests for help, the book was written over a period of six years, and I was more careful about keeping a record of who had helped me during some periods than others. I doubt my notes were complete, and I regret any omissions.

But I want to thank and acknowledge the help and contributions of the following people:

Julia Allison, Cathryn Anderson, and Joan Axelrod;

Anita Barbey, Dianne Barnes, Kate Bauer, Mary Ann Baul, Ruth Beeman, Elizabeth Berryhill, Lesley Biggs, John Boggess, Jana Borino, Lisa Bradley, Margaret Brain, Archie Brodsky, Tonya Brooks, and Sarah Brown;

Ward Cates, Justine Clegg, Nancy Wainer Cohen, Patricia Craig, Nancy Cuddihy, and Mary Ann Curry;

Kate Davidson, Eugene Declercq, Jeanne DeJoseph, Patrick DeLeon, Raymond DeVries, and Elizabeth R. Diaz;

Karen Fennell, Bruce Flamm, and Judith Flanagan;

Elizabeth Gilmore and Betsy Greulich;

Barbara Harper, Doris Haire, Susan Hodges, Victoria Holt, Diane Holzer, Carol Howe, and Sandy Huffman;

Marsha Jackson, Susan Jenkins, and Helen Jolly;

Barbara Kaye, Sheila Kitzinger, Judith Kurokawa, James Kuxhaux, and Barbara Kwast;

Miriam Labbock, Ronnie Lichtman, and Kathy Linden;

Helen Matyac, Morgaine Mehl Madrona, Teresa Marsico, Alice McCartor, Marie Meglen, Tom Mack, Laura Mann, Judith Melson, Arden Miller, and Suzy Myers;

Audry Naylor, Mark Noble, and Mike Nyland-Funk;

Deborah Oakley and Howard Ory;

Lisa Paine, Jim Papai, Vicky Penwell, and Debbie Pully;

Terra Richardson, Anne Richter, Signe Rogers, and Marilee Rush;

Carol Sakala, Alice Sammon, Karen Scheuermann, Anne Scupholme, Mary Ann Shah, Nancy Sharp, Ruth Shoemaker, Holly Sholles, Desmond Skubi, Lara Slattery, Nancy Sloan, Nancy Spencer, Peggy Spindel, Therese Stallings, Patty Starkman, and Sue Stone;

Karen Tatum, Meryl Thomas, Judith Triesman, and Jan Tritten;

Linda Walsh, and Norman Weatherby.

None of the people who reviewed and helped me with particular sections or provided information. and are acknowledged here should be blamed for any error of fact or interpretation. Most people reviewed only limited parts of the book and did not see the final version.

Chapter 1
What Is Midwifery?

This book has two subjects—childbirth and midwifery. Neither subject is understood well by most Americans, even by many professionals working in maternity care. It was written for midwives and midwifery students; for medical students and physicians, especially obstetrician–gynecologists and family physicians; for everyone who needs to have a solid understanding of midwifery and the problems and circumstances affecting the health and health care of pregnant women in the United States; and for anyone interested in learning more about the roles, lives, and health of women and the social and historical development of medicine and midwifery.

Early in this century American obstetrics became committed to a path that has led to a highly medicalized approach to the care of women during pregnancy, especially during childbirth. Prenatal care focuses on detection of pathology; labor is intensely monitored and controlled. This form of care involves the use of many unnecessary procedures and other interventions during labor and delivery. It is expensive, causes compli-

cations, results in increased use of cesarean sections, and changes the nature of the act of giving birth, robbing many women and their loved ones of a powerful, potentially life-enhancing experience. Highly medicalized pregnancy care is based on a view of pregnancy that focuses on its potential for pathology. The alternative model is midwifery; though it is a minority model in this country, it is the standard in most other developed countries. Those countries provide care that is less sophisticated technologically; they spend far less money in the process, and their results are better than ours. Virtually every year the U.S. Public Health Service announces that our infant mortality rate has decreased. The announcements fail to mention that, although lower than before, our infant mortality rate is higher than rates in almost all countries whose level of wealth, development, and medical sophistication is similar to that of the United States. The gap between our infant mortality rate and the rates in most of those countries is getting wider, and our rate would be much worse except that we lead the world in the ability to save the lives—though not always the full health and potential—of babies who are born so premature, small, or damaged that they would not survive without the most sophisticated, expensive neonatal intensive care.

This book explains the difference between midwifery and medical obstetrics—conceptual and philosophical differences and differences in history, practices, and the effects and outcomes of care. It also explains the problems that underlie the relatively high rate of infant mortality in this country—long-standing problems related to poverty, social distress, and high-risk behaviors among a large proportion of pregnant women; and persistent problems related to lack of access to maternity care for highest risk women, poor quality of maternity care for highest risk women, and care that fails to address the most serious problems.

The greatest gains in the safety of childbearing came from medical discoveries and inventions made during the first half of this century—blood transfusions, antibiotics, and medicine to treat pregnancy-induced hypertension. The ability to perform rapid, relatively safe cesarean sections was also important. These treatments arose from medicine doing what it does best—focusing on the diagnosis and treatment of disease, looking for knowledge and solutions by studying the structure and function of the human body at the level of the cells, organs, and organ systems. Medicine deserves high praise for developing these essential treatments and making them widely available. All further efforts to improve pregnancy outcomes rely on this basic level of safety. Nevertheless, much of the recent progress has come from other disciplines, including midwifery, which deal with problems and solutions that affect pregnant women and newborns at a different level. Unplanned, unwanted pregnancies; social and psychological stress; smoking, illegal drug use, domestic violence, poor nutrition, sexually transmitted infections, and poor hygiene; depression; newborn infections; inadequate nourishment and care of the infant, even physical abuse—these are the problems that need to be addressed to reduce infant morbidity and mortality further and to give American children a better start in life.

Whereas medicine focuses on the pathologic potential of pregnancy and birth, midwifery focuses on its normalcy and potential for health. Pregnancy, childbirth, and breast-feeding are normal bodily and family functions. That they are susceptible to pathology does not negate their essential normalcy and the importance of the non-medical aspects of these critical processes and events in people's lives. Midwives know about the medical risks, identify complications early, and collaborate with physicians to ensure medical care for serious problems. But attention to the medical aspects of these complex processes, although essential, is not sufficient. Midwives focus on each woman as a unique person, in the context of her family and her life. The midwife strives to support the woman in ways that empower her to achieve her own goals and hopes for her pregnancy, birth and baby, and for her role as mother. Midwives believe that women's bodies are well designed for birth and try to protect, support, and avoid interfering with the normal processes of labor, delivery, and the reuniting of the mother and newborn after their separation at birth. This is a far cry from prenatal care that focuses primarily on the uterus and fetus, the possibility of pathology, and a sequence of tests and procedures; and on childbirth care that interferes with the normal processes to such an extent that 30 percent of women cannot give birth on their own but must be assisted by cesarean sections, forceps, or vacuum equipment to pull the infant out of its mother.

The care provided by midwives reflects a deeper understanding of the needs of pregnant women and newborns and the intricacy of the natural processes of labor, birth, and breast-feeding. It also provides opportunities to address some of the problems that result in poor pregnancy outcomes. Midwifery brings benefits to all women, especially those who are most in need of support and a positive entrance into motherhood.

Medicine and midwifery are distinct professions, based on overlapping but distinct bodies of knowledge. They are inherently complementary. The competitive nature of the American health care system has accentuated the competitive aspect of the medical/midwifery relationship.

Virtually all industrialized countries experienced increasing medicalization of childbirth during the 1970s and 1980s. Dissatisfaction with that kind of care led to reforms in some countries. Studies conducted in the United Kingdom and Australia during the 1980s and early 1990s found that women wanted an opportunity to develop a relationship with an individual midwife and wanted midwives to be free to practice midwifery, not the pathology-oriented care prescribed by doctors.

The United States is unique in having two distinct kinds of midwives—certified nurse-midwives and a broad group of other midwives. At the beginning of the 1980s, most midwives who were not certified nurse-midwives were referred to as "lay midwives." As time progressed, many of the women who had become lay midwives during the 1970s became committed to developing their form of midwifery (based primarily on home births and much more independence from medicine) into a separate "direct-entry" (i.e., non-nursing) arm of the midwifery profession in this country. Although considerable efforts have been made to unify the midwifery profession, the history and position in society of certified nurse-midwives and direct-entry midwives are so different that they remain separate despite growing experience, friendships, and respect between members of the two groups and a great deal of common ground.

The proportion of births attended by midwives increased steadily during the 1980s and the first half of the 1990s. Midwives now attend the births of nearly 6 percent of the babies born in the United States. Nurse-midwives attended 90 to 95 percent of all births attended by midwives in 1994.

Etymology

The English word *midwife* is derived from *mid*, which means "with," and *wif*, which means "wife," that is, a woman. The term was used as early as 1303 (Helman et al., 1971). The literal meaning—to be "with woman" during childbirth—is the *sine qua non* of midwifery. The simplest definition of a midwife is a woman who assists other women while they are giving birth. Midwifery in that sense has existed throughout the history of mankind. Until the eighteenth century, *midwifery* referred to the care provided to women during childbirth regardless of the type of practitioner. Because most midwives were women, the term implied a female birth attendant. Male doctors who became involved in childbirth were referred to as *man-midwives*. *Sage-femme*, the French term, means "wise" or "good" woman, reflecting the larger role many midwives have played as sources of knowledge on herbal medicine, health and illness, child care, and death, as well as pregnancy and birth (Rothman, 1983). The Danish term is *jordmoder*, or "earth-mother." The focus of midwifery has been normal, that is, medically uncomplicated, pregnancies. The word *obstetrics* is derived from obstetrix, which is the Latin term for "midwife" (Cunningham et al., 1993).

The Care of Pregnant Women: Separation into Two Different Professions

As part of the normal female reproductive function and life cycle, pregnancy and childbirth across cultures have, until very recent times, been within the domain of women. Childbirth was—and is, to varying degrees—

an extreme experience, involving pain, hard labor, and the possibility of dying or losing the child; however, women had many pregnancies and childbirth was a common experience, part of everyday life. Women supported one another and shared knowledge about pregnancy and birth, as they did in other aspects of their roles as wives, homemakers, and mothers. In most communities, certain women were drawn to this special work. Women who were particularly effective at comforting and encouraging other women during childbirth and who seemed able to wrest good outcomes from frightening circumstances were esteemed among women, and their assistance was sought frequently. In this way, certain women developed skills and empirical knowledge of pregnancy and childbirth, which they passed on to younger women when additional midwives were needed. Although many midwives performed this work simply to assist the women of their extended families and communities, it became a paid occupation for some. For the most part, it was part-time work that women did from their homes.

Men were excluded from childbirth due to religion and sexual propriety and because they had no relevant expertise. Midwives in most Western societies were expected to summon a priest or other male religious authority when death of the child and/or mother seemed imminent, and midwives sometimes called a surgeon to extract and, if necessary, destroy an impacted fetus in an effort to save the woman's life. As medicine progressed, physicians' interest in pregnancy remained focused on pathology; they had little interest in pregnancies that did not involve a complication or disease. The invention of forceps in the early seventeenth century gave doctors their first technical advantage over midwives; a physician or surgeon skilled in the use of forceps could sometimes save both mother and baby in situations that previously would have resulted in the death of at least one or the other.

Medicine eventually became a learned profession, the training for which was based in universities. Medical education was available primarily to men from the wealthy and educated social elite. Most midwives, like the majority of all people, were relatively poor. When physicians began to demonstrate an advantage over midwives, first by use of forceps and later through anesthesia, wealthy women and women of the newly expanding middle class preferred to use physicians.

The history of midwifery and, to a lesser degree, obstetrics is described more thoroughly in later chapters of this book. The brief synopsis given here explains the different origins and purposes of obstetrics and midwifery and factors that led to the development of two distinct professions: One focuses on pathology and has continuously expanded the proportion of pregnancies considered pathologic. The other focuses on the healthful potential of each woman's pregnancy and tries to protect normalcy and expand the proportion of women remaining normal.

As a specialty of medicine, the main focus of obstetrics was and remains the diagnosis and treatment of pathology: complications of pregnancy and management of diseases affecting pregnant women and the fetuses they carry. Physicians became involved and increasingly dominant in maternity care through utilization of a technical innovation (forceps) that enabled greater success in overcoming a life-threatening complication. Other medical innovations—antibiotics, blood transfusions, drugs to treat pregnancy-induced hypertension, and cesarean sections—each a medical triumph over potentially lethal pathology, dramatically reduced both infant and maternal deaths. Through use of general anesthesia, systemic analgesia, "twilight sleep," and, now, epidural anesthesia, physicians have held out the promise of pain-free birth. These methods, however, cause complications and interrupt the normal powers and processes of labor, requiring use of interventions such as oxytocin and forceps. Anesthetized women are more likely to experience pathology and are, in fact, no longer having normal births. Medicine strengthened its role in maternity care by expanding the concept of obstetric pathology, using hypersensitive monitoring devices, creating constrained definitions of normal, defining variation from those definitions as pathologic, and routinizing and eventually "normalizing" childbirth characterized by a sequence of preemptive interventions. In recent years, the development of "risk assessment" (women with characteristics associated with a higher-than-average rate of poor pregnancy outcomes are defined as "high-risk") has further expanded the proportion of women considered to be in need of pathology-oriented maternity care. As in the past, many contemporary obstetricians have never witnessed a completely natural birth.

In contrast, normal pregnancy and childbearing are the primary focus of midwifery. Midwives look for early signs of pathology or other deviations from normal and involve a physician in the care of women with serious complications or diseases. But midwives' particular interest and special expertise and skills are related to the care of women with uncomplicated pregnancies. Midwives try to avoid the need for pathology-oriented interventions by giving women the information and help they need to maximize their health and prevent complications. They are critical of physicians' efforts to control labor and delivery, in part by restricting the environment and behavior of women during childbirth, and of physicians' frequent or routine use of invasive, uncomfortable procedures that limit freedom of movement and interfere with the social, emotional, and spiritual experience of giving birth. Midwives have developed and are assessing less invasive *midwifery* methods to manage some abnormal conditions successfully or to return them to normal. Whereas their primary goal is normal births, the midwife's focus is wide in time and scope. Pregnancy and labor are not the limits of her concerns, which include the sexuality from which pregnancy results, the baby with its needs, and the effects the birth and baby have on the mother and father and other children. Breast-feeding, mothercraft, and the emotional, social, cultural, spiritual, and ceremonial aspects of pregnancy and childbirth are within the scope of midwifery, in addition to the physical and biological aspects of conception, pregnancy, labor, delivery, lactation, the mother's return to a nonpregnant state, and the newborn's adaptation to extrauterine life.

Differences in the history, socialization, education and experience of physicians and midwives have led to differences in philosophy, which have led to differences in practices, and thus differences in outcomes. These are described in the following chapters. It is important to understand at the outset, however, that midwifery and obstetrics are two distinct professions—with different philosophies and overlapping but distinct bodies of knowledge.

The differences between midwifery and medicine are better understood in the British Isles and Europe than in the United States. In the United States the issues have become confounded by the development of two new kinds of health-care providers—physicians' assistants and nurse practitioners—as means to remedy a shortage and maldistribution of physicians during the 1960s. The physician assistant (PA) concept was based on the U.S. military's successful experience with paramedics. The nurse practitioner (NP) role adds specific delegated medical tasks and functions to the role of the registered nurse. Both were based on recognition that a significant proportion of health care needs arise from a limited number of common problems that can be effectively diagnosed and treated or managed by persons with less preparation than a physician. Nurse anesthetists are also part of this category. The special knowledge and functions of physician assistants and nurse anesthetists are drawn from medicine and are within its realm; their tasks are delegated to them by physicians, who supervise and retain authority over these practitioners. Physicians are also responsible for the *medical* functions of nurse practitioners. All three practice from a portion of the body of knowledge of medicine—the "midlevel" of the medical field—the entirety of which is the province of physicians.

Ever since the beginning of the development of the PA and NP concept in the mid-1960s, programs to prepare, evaluate, or support PAs and NPs have tended to group them with nurse-midwives as a category variously referred to as "physician extenders" or "midlevel" health-care providers. Although there are similarities among these categories (in amount of training and how they fit into the health-care system), they are dissimilar in their relationship to medicine. The role, functions, and body of knowledge of midwives and physicians overlap to some degree, but each profession has its own body of knowledge. Midwives are not practicing from the middle realm of obstetrics. They are practicing midwifery.

Varying Definitions and Kinds of Midwives

There are several different kinds of midwives. The word *midwife* has many overlapping but different definitions, especially in the United States, where one group of midwives is undergoing important changes.

The International Definition of a Midwife
An international definition of a midwife was developed by the World Health Organization (WHO) in 1965. A revised version was adopted by the International Confederation of Midwives (ICM) in 1972. The International Federation of Gynaecologists and Obstetricians approved and adopted ICM's definition in 1973. It was further revised by the ICM in 1990:

> A midwife is a person who, having been regularly admitted to a midwifery educational program duly recognized in the country in

which it is located, has successfully completed the prescribed course of studies in midwifery and has acquired the requisite qualifications to be registered and/or legally licensed to practice midwifery.

> She must be able to give the necessary supervision, care and advice to women during pregnancy, labour and the postpartum period, to conduct deliveries on her own responsibility, and to care for the newborn and the infant. This care includes preventative measures, the detection of abnormal conditions in mother and child, the procurement of medical assistance and the execution of emergency measures in the absence of medical help.

> She has an important task in health counseling and education, not only for the women, but also within the family and the community. The work should involve antenatal education and preparation for parenthood and extends to certain areas of gynecology, family planning and child care. She may practice in hospitals, clinics, health units, domiciliary conditions or in any other service.

How Does a Midwife Differ from a Traditional Birth Attendant?
The World Health Organization defines a traditional birth attendant (TBA) as "a person who assists the mother at childbirth and initially acquired her skills by delivering babies herself or through apprenticeship to other traditional birth attendants." Although reflecting common usage, the dictionary definition of a midwife as a woman who assists other women during childbirth* does not distinguish between midwives and TBAs, a term that is used primarily in developing countries. Although TBAs are often referred to as traditional or "indigenous" midwives, WHO tries to maintain a clear distinction between a midwife and a TBA. WHO defines a trained TBA as one who has received a short course, usually not longer than one month, through the

---

*Although most midwives are women, a small percentage of American midwives are men. However, this book uses only feminine pronouns in reference to midwives.

modern health care sector to upgrade her skills (WHO, 1992). Some ways in which midwives are different from TBAs are as follows:(1) The midwife gives care throughout the childbearing cycle (pregnancy, including labor and delivery, and the puerperium) and provides care to the newborn infant. (2) The midwife has successfully completed a recognized program of study. (3) The midwife is qualified to be registered or licensed to practice in the country where she works (Burst, 1978). These two definitions do not cover all of the possible permutations in the United States, where there are women who regularly assist other women during childbirth but do not conform to WHO's definitions of either a midwife or a TBA.

America's Many Kinds of Midwives

The history of midwifery in North America differs from that in other parts of the Western world. Due to the United States' development as a colony and country that was based primarily on immigration and was constantly extending its frontiers, for several centuries America had some immigrant midwives who had been trained in their countries of origin, but few if any good midwifery schools and little or no government regulation of midwifery practice. Under these circumstances the difference between what are now called TBAs and midwives became blurred as professionally trained immigrant midwives passed their skills and knowledge on to others without developing formal training programs. The emergence and evolution of a new kind of lay midwife during and since the 1970s has further confused the use of these terms.

Most historical studies have used *midwife* to refer to any female other than a physician who was attending births on a regular basis. As a consequence, none of the historic data on midwives and on births attended by midwives distinguishes between professional midwives and "granny" or other lay midwives. The significance of these data is further confused because some "lay midwives" approached

midwifery as a full-time or nearly full-time occupation, profession, or "calling," whereas others were pressed into service in the absence of anyone with more experience and attended the births of only their neighbors, family members, and close friends. This mixture of educated and uneducated, lay and professional midwives is also evident in the results of studies of the quality of care provided by midwives in various settings over the years.

The following subsections discuss some of the terms used to describe different kinds of American midwives, in society and in this book.

Granny and Grand Midwives. The term *TBA* is rarely used in the United States, where persons fulfilling the WHO definition of a traditional birth attendant have been referred to as *granny* or *lay midwives*. *Granny midwife* was the term used to refer to both black and white women who attended the births of women in communities throughout the southeastern United States from the founding of the country until at least the middle of the twentieth century. Women generally became granny midwives in response to a need in their communities. Some were designated by other community members to fill this role; many felt they had been "called." Their primary training was through apprenticeship to older midwives, frequently members of their family. Many of the women they cared for had little access to medical care; thus the grannies took care of complications as well as normal deliveries. Health departments in many states began efforts to train and supervise them during the early decades of the twentieth century. Although important historically, granny midwives are now virtually extinct. There has been a recent decision to refer to any American midwife who practiced under local regulation before 1965 as a Grand Midwife.

Certified Nurse-Midwives (CNMs). Certified nurse-midwives are registered nurses who have completed accredited nurse-midwifery education programs, passed a national certification examination, and met other criteria for certification by the American College of Nurse-Midwives (ACNM) or the ACNM Certification Council.* Most have master's or higher degrees, mostly in nursing. CNMs practice legally in every U.S. jurisdiction. Their practice includes independent management of the health care needed by essentially normal women and their babies during pregnancy, labor, delivery, and the postpartum/postnatal period, and providing gynecologic care, including family planning, to women who are not pregnant. Nurse-midwives practice within a health care system that provides for consultation, collaborative management, or referral as indicated by the health status of the individual woman and newborn. Although they attend births in all settings, including homes, most of the births they attend occur in hospitals. Free-standing birth centers are the next most frequent site, accounting for 3 percent of the births attended by CNMs in 1994 (Ventura et al., 1996).

CNMs work throughout the nation's diverse health care systems. Of approximately 4,000 nurse-midwives who were practicing in 1994, more than half worked for hospitals or physicians; smaller proportions worked for health maintenance organizations, health services operated by the federal government, including the Armed Services, or local health departments. Eight percent owned or worked for a private nurse-midwifery practice; 3 percent worked in a free-standing birth center (Walsh & Boggess, 1996). They play a special role in the provision of care to women who are poor.

Nurse-midwives did not enter the picture until 1925, at the apex of a vitriolic medical

campaign to disgrace and eliminate midwives of all kinds. As an embryonic profession trying to survive and gain a foothold in this milieu, nurse-midwives took care to distinguish themselves as nurses and well-educated midwives. Resulting from this history, the practice developed of grouping all American midwives into only two categories: certified nurse-midwives and lay midwives, with the latter category including all but CNMs.

Lay, Direct-Entry, and Other Midwives. *Lay midwifery* connotes domiciliary (i.e., home birth) practice and informal training that is founded in experience. *Direct-entry* implies that the person went into midwifery without first being trained as a nurse. *Other midwives* means other than a specified category, usually CNMs. The National Center for Health Statistics, which collects and summarizes birth certificate data, uses "CNMs" and "other midwives" to categorize all midwife-attended births.

In addition to the "granny midwives" of the southeastern United States, other kinds of lay midwives have included Native American midwives serving other members of their tribes, *parteras* serving Latino women in Texas and the Southwest, and informally prepared midwives serving women in communities throughout the country during most of our history.

A new kind of lay midwife emerged during the 1970s. In the beginning they had little, if any, training, developed their practices outside of the established health care system, and were truly "lay." Over time, some individuals in this category have achieved high levels of midwifery skills and knowledge. In addition, lay midwives in some areas developed more or less formal training courses and programs to assist others who wanted to become midwives. These offerings ranged from weekend workshops and correspondence courses with no clinical component to a long-standing, formally organized, state-accredited, twenty-seven-month academic and clinical midwifery educational program

---

*In 1991 the ACNM created the ACNM Certification Council as a separate organization responsible for developing and administering the examination and certifying successful candidates under agreement with the ACNM.

(the Seattle Midwifery School), with many variations in between. In practice, most lay midwives have taken advantage of or created multiple training experiences, combining short- or long-term apprenticeships with self-study and short courses. However, many were and remain "lay" in the sense of not being part of a profession that has formal educational requirements and other standards; as a consequence there has been no way to distinguish those who have achieved an adequate level of competence from those who have not. This continues to be a problem, making it seem inaccurate and inadequate to refer to them as either "professional" or "lay." In recent years, some have referred to themselves as *traditional midwives* or *independent midwives*, the latter term contrasting their independence from medicine with nurse-midwifery's self-imposed mandate for collaboration with physicians.

In Europe a direct-entry midwife is one who entered midwifery school without having attended a school of nursing (Becker et al., 1982). There are a few direct-entry midwifery schools in the United States. For awhile there was an effort to limit the *direct-entry* term to midwives other than CNMs who had completed a structured educational program that meets requirements for licensure by a state or certification by a national or local midwifery organization (Myers-Ciecko, 1988). Such usage would distinguish direct-entry midwives not only from CNMs, but also from midwives considered "lay" because they have not been held to any external standard. However, any effort to distinguish between direct-entry midwives and lay midwives is not acceptable to many people. Some people refer to all midwives who are not CNMs as lay midwives; some refer to them all as direct-entry midwives.

Lay and direct-entry midwives provide care to women during pregnancy, childbirth, and the postpartum period and give health counseling and advice regarding the use of natural and barrier methods of contraception. Most have working relationships, but not formal agreements, with one or more physicians. Lay and direct-entry midwives attend between 11,500 and 12,500 births per year. Most are home births (71 percent in 1994); most of the rest occur in free-standing birth centers (Ventura, et al., 1996). Their clients are predominantly white married women, including many Mexican and Mexican-American women who give birth in birth centers operated by midwives in El Paso and elsewhere in Texas near the Mexican border (Declercq, 1992).

Certified Professional Midwives (CPMs). Many individuals in each of these groups would like to unite under the generic term *midwife*. Although that concept is attractive, it is important to be able to distinguish between midwives who have met formal educational and other standards and those who have not. A process for examining and certifying the competence of direct-entry midwives was established in 1994. The process is controlled by the North American Registry of Midwives (NARM), which was founded by the Midwives Alliance of North America (MANA), an organization that includes all kinds of midwives but focuses primarily on issues that affect lay and direct-entry midwives. *Certified professional midwife* (CPM) is the title for a midwife who has been certified by NARM.

ACC Certified Midwives (CMs). The ACNM Certification Council (ACC) examines and certifies direct-entry midwives who successfully complete basic midwifery education programs that have been accredited by the ACNM. An ACC certified midwife has met all of the same standards as a certified nurse-midwife, but is not required to be a nurse. The first basic (i.e., direct-entry) midwifery education program to be accredited by the ACNM took its first class of students in 1996. They will graduate and take the examination in 1997.

Licensed Midwives (LMs). The term *licensed midwife* is used in the laws of some states. It designates a direct-entry midwife who is licensed by the state in which she practices. The standards vary greatly from state to state.

Birth Attendants and Doulas. A *birth attendant* or *doula* is a woman who attends births in order to support the mother and assist the primary birth attendant (whether a physician or a midwife). The term is also used by some lay and direct-entry midwives who practice in states where the practice of midwifery by anyone but a CNM or physician is illegal. *Postpartum doulas* are hired to help new mothers for a few hours each day for a week or more after the birth or after the mother and baby return home from the hospital. Short doula training courses are being established. Some experience in childbirth education is a prerequisite for admission to a doula training program.

Chapter 2
Brief History of Midwifery in the West

The development of midwifery in North America was markedly different from its development in other parts of the Western world. Yet the historical origins are the same, and midwives who had been trained in Europe and Great Britain played major roles in the early development of midwifery on this continent. As recently as the second quarter of this century, most midwives practicing in large American cities had been trained in other countries, and British midwives provided the model for American nurse-midwifery.

Antecedents: Midwifery from Earliest History Through the Middle Ages

Although husbands in some traditional cultures have assisted their wives during childbirth, experienced women have done this work in most societies. Knowledge based on observation and experience gained by attending women during childbirth was handed down from generation to generation of such women. In most cultures, men

(beginning with shamans, followed by priests or rabbis, and later by doctors or barber surgeons) were called only to deal with unusual and dangerous complications (Roush, 1979). Care of normal pregnant women was beneath the dignity of early physicians; as men, physicians were also excluded on the basis of norms regarding sexual modesty and decent behavior. Early midwives were usually uneducated peasant or working-class women who did not begin assisting other women during birth until they had borne and reared several children of their own. Until the development of organized training programs and schools, which began during different periods in different countries, most midwives learned their trade by observing and helping during their neighbors' and friends' births or by assisting an established midwife. They learned by trial and error, gaining experience with each delivery, gradually developing more effective methods to comfort women and facilitate birth, and calling physicians or more experienced midwives for help with serious complications. But childbirth was known to be dangerous; deaths of both mothers and babies were expected and accepted.

The first documented formal midwifery training program was started by Hippocrates in the fifth century B.C. The Athenians recognized two kinds of midwives—ordinary midwives, who attended normal births, and *iatpouaiai* ("doctor midwives"), who could handle complications (Roush, 1979). However, Greek midwifery was not as advanced as Greek medicine and surgery, the education for which was not accessible to women. Few midwives are mentioned in the writings of the Classical Greek period, one exception being Phaenarete, who was Socrates's mother (Roush, 1979). Despite the school started by Hippocrates, the education of midwives was halting and ineffectual during the next several centuries (Speert, 1980). During the third century B.C., an Athenian midwife named Agnodike disguised herself as a man in order to complete a course in the medical school run by Hierophilus, in Egypt. After returning to Athens, she developed a good reputation as an obstetrician, but was brought to trial on the insistence of physicians when her gender was discovered. She was acquitted on the basis of supportive testimony by leading Athenian women. Hearing of this, Hierophilus wrote what is thought to be the first book on anatomy for midwives (Withers, 1979).

The Bible's Book of Exodus tells the story of Hebrew midwives who disobeyed the Pharaoh's command to kill all sons born to Hebrew women. When brought before the Pharaoh to explain their disobedience, the savvy midwives reported that "The Hebrew women are not as the Egyptian women; for they are lively, and are delivered ere the midwives come in unto them" (Exodus, Chapter 1, verses 15–20). They were not punished; the Bible reports that "God dealt well with the midwives." Even this tyrant king respected the role and authority of midwives.

The first book on obstetrics, written by Soranus (a Greek who moved to Rome in A.D. 98), included two chapters on special qualities required of a good midwife. Although Soranus wrote that midwives should be literate "in order to comprehend the art through theory also" (Walsh, 1991), women were barred from courses in anatomy, physiology, and medicine. Nevertheless, there is evidence of some opportunity for formal training of midwives in some European cities during those early centuries. During the thirteenth century women could study nursing and midwifery at a school in Solerno, Italy (Durant, 1950).

Medicine became a profession within the context of universities, which formed during the twelfth and thirteenth centuries. Entrance was controlled by the church and was limited to upper-class males (McCool & McCool, 1989). By the end of the medieval period, medicine had begun to develop its own body of knowledge, which was preserved in Latin and thus was inaccessible even to literate midwives, and university faculties of medicine had begun to regulate and control all medical practitioners (Roush, 1979). Because pregnancy and childbirth are not illnesses, they were not usually included in the study of medicine. In addition, university-based physicians had no source of accurate knowledge of these phenomena. Physicians avoided association with midwives, who were usually of a much lower social class, and the midwives "guarded the lying-in chamber from all medical interference" (Roush, 1979). The physicians' knowledge of pregnancy was theoretical and shaped by religion. Midwives' knowledge was more accurate, but they had no systematic way to accumulate their individual experiences and knowledge and pass it on to others.

The first law to regulate European midwives was enacted in Regensburg, Germany, in 1452. It defined midwifery as a profession and ensured midwives equal rights with other craftsmen who had adopted professional codes. The Regensburg code was soon modified for use in other cities. In 1480 the midwifery code for the state of Württemberg included instructions on how a midwife could perform a cesarean section on a living woman. Before that time, cesareans had only been performed on women who had died. Historical records indicate that many women and babies survived cesarean sections performed by midwives (Scheuermann, 1995).

In 1513 Rosslin published a book on midwifery that was written in vernacular German, a language many Central European midwives could read and understand. Because of this, it was very important; ultimately it was translated into many languages. The English translation, *The Byrth of Mankynde,* was a best-seller for one hundred years. Overall, however, midwifery made little progress through the Middle Ages. Most midwives were illiterate, influenced by superstition, and of low social class. Physicians focused on illness; tended mainly to people of their own, higher social class; and left the midwives alone. Although midwives controlled maternity care, they did not organize or develop formal educational programs.

During the fifteenth and sixteenth centuries, midwives came under the control of the church and were affected by the Inquisition in some parts of Europe. Publication of *The Witchhammer* by two Dominican inquisitors in 1487 started a hunt for witches, who were believed to be the earthly companions of the devil. If a baby died, the midwife who attended its birth might be accused of having offered the baby to the devil. Midwives used herbs and many used potions and spells to assist women to give birth (DeVries, 1985). These unsanctioned rituals seemed witchlike to some priests and others, and midwives were often suspected and accused of being witches. In 1573 the Catholic church in Frankfurt enacted a law to place midwives under its authority. Midwives were required to take classes, were taught to perform emergency baptisms and take final confessions (in case a priest was not available

when a woman died), and were instructed to report abortions, irreligious conduct, children born out of wedlock, and use of contraception. Eventually they were forced to perform intrauterine baptism using a syringe filled with water that had been blessed by a priest. Because the syringes were not sterile, such injections sometimes caused infections that resulted in the mother's death. Midwives who did not comply with the code were accused of witchcraft and some were burned at the stake. About sixty thousand people were executed as "witches" between about 1450 and the mid-1700s; approximately 80 percent of them were women, more than half of whom were midwives. Fear of being accused of witchcraft drove many midwives underground, further curtailing advancement of the profession (Scheuermann, 1995; Colby, 1996).

The Catholic church's Frankfurt Midwifery Code was in effect for more than 130 years. The law that replaced it in 1703 required midwives to be able to read and write, to be married or widowed, to have given birth to at least one child of their own, to attend classes given by a physician, and to call a physician when they encountered a difficult delivery. However, the physicians' knowledge of childbirth was based entirely on theory and second-hand knowledge gained from barbers, surgeons, and midwives. This led to a deep conflict between physicians and midwives (Scheuermann, 1995).

Development of Midwifery Education in France

Although Parisian midwives came under some degree of regulation during the late 1300s, only those who wanted to attract wealthy clients applied for certification. During the sixteenth century the regulations were strengthened, and Paris became the center of secular midwifery training and knowledge (Kalisch et al., 1981). The first substantial statute concerning examination, licensure and regulation of midwives was passed in Paris in 1560 (Roush, 1979). Applicants had to provide a character witness and pass an examination conducted by two senior midwives, one physician, and two surgeons. Certified midwives pledged to report practice by uncertified midwives and to call a more experienced midwife or a physician or surgeon to help with difficult cases. There were, however, no standards for midwifery training. By the mid-1600s Paris had become the recognized European center for expertise in care of women during childbirth (Kalisch et al., 1981).

Formal education of French midwives was started as a result of the work of Louyse Bourgeois (1563–1636), a literate midwife from a propertied middle-class family who was married to a surgeon. Most French midwives of the late sixteenth century were poor, uneducated women who provided services to their neighbors on a part-time basis. Midwifery was not considered appropriate for women of Bourgeois's social standing; she went into it because of a severe financial reversal that affected her family. She prepared herself during a five-year period by reading the works of Ambroise Paré, a famous Parisian surgeon, and by assisting poor women during childbirth. Once sworn as a midwife, she developed a high reputation among Parisian aristocrats due to her education, family connections, and her skills, knowledge, and calm, resolute approach. She become midwife to the Queen of France and delivered all six heirs of King Henry IV. As she became more experienced, self-confident, and influential, her initial attitude of deference toward physicians was replaced by dismissiveness and criticism. Her career ended following the postpartum death of one of her royal clients (Kalisch et al., 1981).

Bourgeois was the first midwife to write and publish books. In her first book, Bourgeois tried to correlate her own observations and understanding of human nature with information from folk traditions and the writings of physicians. She collected information on effective procedures, added insights from her own extensive practice, and told her readers exactly when and how to use specific treatments. For example, she developed the still-used technique of dealing with an umbilical cord that is wrapped tightly around the neck of an unborn infant by tying it in two places and then severing it between the ligatures (Kalisch et al., 1981).

Bourgeois advocated a patient, nonintervening approach to childbirth, argued against the manipulations practiced by physicians, recognized the importance of the mother's emotional condition, and urged her readers to provide support, encouragement, and comfortable positions for women during labor, to treat each pregnancy as a unique and individual experience, and to respect the power and mystery of birth—advice that remains the foundation of midwifery today. Her writings included discussions about the midwife's role, duties, and ethical standards. She implored midwives to "serve the poor with the same affection as shown the rich" (Kalisch et al., 1981).

Bourgeois wanted to found a "new line of midwives, who would continue to improve themselves by learning and sharing their experiences" (Kalisch et al., 1981). During the late seventeenth and the eighteenth centuries other Parisian midwives published professional works, developed their apprenticeship system into a full-fledged midwifery educational program, and headed the lying-in wards at the Hotel-Dieu, site of the first childbirth training program for physicians. Midwifery students at the Hotel-Dieu school had to be French, Catholic, married, and able to pay tuition (Roush, 1979). In addition, the limited biographical information available on the famous Parisian midwives of that time suggests that most if not all of them were members of "Aesculapiad families"— families in which most of the men and some of the women had entered branches of the medical, surgical, or midwifery professions (Kalisch *et al.*, 1981). Thus the social class of midwives began to change in Paris. Eventually, French midwifery and medical students attended classes together at government-supported hospital schools. By the nineteenth century, experienced French midwives were teaching medical students during their obstetric training (Wertz, 1983).

Translations of Bourgeois's writings were influential throughout Europe; municipal regulation of midwives through licensure spread. By 1700, midwives in Amsterdam were required to pass a rigorous test. Midwifery programs with official ties to medical schools and hospitals were opened in Leiden in 1725, in Edinburgh in 1739, in Vienna in 1748, and in Strasbourg in 1751 (Speert, 1980). By the beginning of the twentieth century, Russia and all European countries except England had developed educational standards and government-supported midwifery schools, varying in length from six months to three years and requiring students to attend twenty to one hundred births. Schools in some countries taught suturing, manual removal of the placenta, external and internal version (turning a malpositioned fetus to the normal, head-down birth position), and delivery of babies in breech presentation (Walsh, 1992).

"Man-Midwives" and the Increasing Role of Doctors

Until the late eighteenth century, it was generally considered indecent for European men to have any role in childbirth. Doctors and barber-surgeons were called only for problems so severe that they often resulted in death of the infant, if not also the mother. As a result, early midwives and physicians had very different experiences with birth. During their careers, midwives saw hundreds of successful births; physicians saw complications unrelieved by experience with normal deliveries.

Peter Chamberlain, a British surgeon, invented forceps during the early seventeenth century. Skilled use of forceps made it possible for a surgeon to extract a live baby from an otherwise doomed labor. The invention of forceps changed the physicians' role. Chamberlain and his family did not share his invention for more than one hundred years. Based on the advantage provided by their ability to use forceps, the Chamberlains become "man-midwives" to the British royal family. Eventually other doctors bought their "secret" tool or developed similar instruments on their own. Few midwives could afford to buy them and most physicians were not willing to teach a midwife how to use them (Litoff, 1982). Instead the doctors told the midwives to call them when forceps were needed (Chaney, 1980). Many doctors wanted to develop a larger role in childbirth; when forceps gave them a way to resolve a common but serious problem, they considered themselves superior to midwives and became eager to intervene during labor (Wertz, 1983). As competition from man-midwives increased, female midwives became critical of the men's frequent use of interventions. By the end of the 1700s, obstetrics had developed into a medical specialty and was taught in medical schools.

During the late eighteenth century many European countries began to build special hospitals as places to take care of the poor and teach physicians. Prostitutes and women who were poor or unmarried were forced to deliver in these hospitals, sometimes under threat of imprisonment. In 1816 Germany's midwifery law was changed to require German midwives to receive training from physicians working in those hospitals. The new law defined birth as an illness and required midwifery students to be less than twenty-five years of age and childless (Scheuermann, 1995).

Midwifery and Obstetrics in the British Isles

Midwifery progressed more rapidly in continental Europe than in Britain, which was slower to develop government-supported midwifery training schools and effective regulations. Although religious control of midwives gave way to municipal regulation during the fifteenth century in Europe, the church controlled English midwifery until the eighteenth century (DeVries, 1985). Chamberlain championed the idea of government-supported midwifery schools and in 1616 encouraged a group of British midwives to petition the king for permission to form a society to further their profession (Walsh, 1991). Their petition was denied. A description of the "ideal" English midwife written in 1724 listed characteristics such as being grave, considerate, patient, meek, and not too fat, but made no mention of the need for special knowledge (Litoff, 1982).

Britain's first instructional manual on midwifery, written by an English midwife (Jane Sharp) in 1671, asserted basic principles such as not hurrying labor, the difficulty of a breech presentation, and the importance of sustaining the strength of women during labor (Lops, 1988). Although a needed step forward, the book focused exclusively on the practice and art of midwifery, warning midwives against an emphasis on theoretical knowledge (Litoff, 1982). In 1739 an official school of midwifery was opened in conjunction with a medical school in Edinburgh (Speert, 1980), and in 1746 Henry Deventer of London published a textbook for the purpose of teaching midwives the scientific facts he thought they needed to know. His book was written in common language and was aimed at the typical midwife of the day—if she could read. Warnings and admonitions in the book reveal concerns about the quality of midwifery practice at that time. Deventer proposed that midwives be licensed and be held liable for negligence and wrote guidelines to help husbands determine whether a particular midwife was capable or ignorant (Chaney, 1980).

William Smellie popularized the use of forceps by teaching other doctors how to use them more effectively and was one of the first physicians to record information on his maternity cases on a routine basis. After practicing in Glouster for nineteen years, he studied in France for a short period and then opened a midwifery school in London, where he held separate classes for men and for women. Clinical experience for his students was at a lying-in hospital for the poor (Chaney, 1980). The first maternity hospitals were really extensions of poor houses for homeless women (Kitzinger, 1983). The establishment of such hospitals in London during the 1740s and 1750s resulted in greatly increased opportunities for medical students to attain obstetric experience and attend some normal births (Litoff, 1982). Smellie published the first written description of deformed pelvises, made improvements in the design of forceps, and devised a machine that simulated the action of the uterus in labor for use in teaching. Although he made many important contributions to obstetrics, most midwives disliked him and ridiculed his teaching methods (Chaney, 1980).

A few other schools also offered separate courses for female midwives, most of whom would have been too embarrassed to be in a class with male students. However, most English midwives continued to have little, if any, formal training. Although they campaigned against "man-midwives" and their instruments, midwifery needed better education to survive as a profession in England (Chaney, 1980). It continued but did not advance (Roush, 1979). By the late eighteenth century, upper-class English women had come to prefer man-midwives. By the beginning of the nineteenth century, midwifery practice was confined mainly to the poor.

This downward trend began to change during the second half of the nineteenth century, as some social activists and physicians began to note negative effects from the loss of experienced midwives (Walsh, 1991). Florence Nightingale had started the first nurses' training school in London, in 1860. Until then no respectable English woman would take nursing as a career. Nightingale also proposed an institution to train midwives and "midwifery nurses" (Breckinridge, 1981). Several private hospitals began to offer midwifery courses. Although few women could afford the high tuitions, the well-to-do graduates were well positioned to improve their profession. In 1881 a small group of "gentlewomen" midwives formed the Matron's Aid Society, which later became the Midwives Institute. Its goals were to raise the status and standards of midwifery.

By 1900, midwives were attending about three-fourths of all births in England (Devitt, 1979). In 1902, after nearly twenty years of effort (and strong physician opposition), the Midwives Institute successfully supported passage of England's first national midwifery law. The Midwives Act created a physician-dominated board to regulate midwifery and prohibited unlicensed practice. Midwives were expected to remain proficient, could not leave their patients after the beginning of the second stage of labor, had to send for a doctor when abnormalities were detected during labor, and were required to report all stillbirths and deaths. Because of the risk of infection, they were prohibited from participating in care of the dead (Walsh, 1991). Some midwives opposed the law as unwarranted subjugation of midwives to physicians; others thought the rules were needed (DeVries, 1985). In 1915, an esteemed English statistician attributed the rapid decrease in maternal deaths from puerperal sepsis after 1902 to implementation of the Midwives Act. The death rate fell much more rapidly in England and Wales, where the act applied, than in Scotland and Ireland, where it did not. The infant mortality rate also fell sharply and rapidly in England and Wales, from 151 per 1,000 births in 1901, to 106 per 1,000 in 1910 (Devitt, 1979).

Most but not all English midwives were also trained as nurses. Nurses and direct-entry students were usually trained in the same midwifery schools. In 1916 the midwives' three-month training period was extended to four months for nurses and six months for other students. In 1926 the training was lengthened to six months for nurses and one year for direct-entry students. The training period was lengthened again in 1937 to one year for nurses and two years for non-nurses, and in 1981 to eighteen months for nurses and three years for direct-entry students (Robinson et al., 1983).

During the early twentieth century, British midwives were independent practitioners. They attended births in the homes and were paid by the women they served. As prenatal care was not a standard practice, they had relatively little contact with pregnant women prior to labor. In 1936 Parliament passed a law that required all local jurisdictions to establish a salaried or subsidized midwifery service (Robinson et al., 1983). Given a means for salaried employment, most midwives entered the government system (Walsh, 1991). Because nurse-midwives were favored for positions in the government, women entering the field had an incentive to become trained in nursing as well as midwifery. More than eighteen thousand midwives were practicing in England and Wales in 1968; approximately 80 percent of them were nurses (Bayes, 1968). Midwives were present at nearly all births in England in 1970, and were the senior, responsible attendant at 70 percent of the births (Arthure, 1973). Recent changes and the current status of midwifery in Britain are discussed in Chapter 13.

Midwifery in the United States: Colonial Times Through the Nineteenth Century

Midwives were responsible for the care of almost all pregnant women during the first 250 years of life in the colonies of the United States. In part, this was because few American colonists were of the educated, elite classes of Europe and Great Britain and the settlers included few university-educated physicians. In the absence of physicians, midwives were often the sole source of health care; as such, many were highly respected members of their communities (McCool & McCool, 1989). Bridget Lee Fuller, a British midwife, traveled on the *Mayflower* and probably assisted in the three births that occurred during the settlers' voyage to America (Litoff, 1982). She then settled in Plymouth, where she was paid a salary as the midwife for the town (Speert, 1980).

The midwives who came to America as colonists and later as immigrants arrived with varying degrees of preparation. A few were well trained; more were steeped in folklore. As midwifery education advanced in Europe, more of the immigrant midwives arrived with better training. Where there were no trained midwives, untrained women met the need as it arose. Given the thinness of civilization on the American frontier, the need arose in many places.

The first granny midwives came to America with the first boatloads of slaves; West African childbirth folklore, superstitions, traditions, and practices arrived with them and were handed down to a close female relative in each new generation (Robinson, 1984). Many southern plantations had their own midwives, often an older slave who assisted at the births of both black and white women. In addition to assisting during the labor and birth, granny midwives helped women bathe after giving birth, washed the bed linens, cooked, and cared for the families' other children. Black women who became midwives after emancipation often "felt they were called by the Lord to do so either through visions or dreams" (Robinson, 1984).

Most early American midwives practiced in isolation from one another, were illiterate, and did not perceive themselves to be members of a profession. Birth was viewed as a natural event for which little special knowledge was required. Midwives who had acquired training in the British Isles or Europe passed their knowledge and skills to others through apprenticeships, as did midwives whose lineage of mentors included no one

with formal training. However, they did not start schools. Observation and supervised first-hand experience were the main learning methods.

Although some colonial cities licensed midwives, most midwives practiced without any form of regulation (Rothman, 1983). Some communities gave official positions and salaries to certain midwives, whom they selected on the basis of morality and skill. The colony of New Amsterdam, for instance, appointed and paid an official "Town Midwife" to attend poor women. Childbirth, and thus midwifery, was closely associated with spiritual and religious beliefs and practices. In the Puritan society of New England there was extreme concern about witchcraft, magic, and "women's lore" (Wertz, 1983). Some midwives were accused of practicing witchcraft and were executed (Litoff, 1982). Such attacks were aberrations, however. Midwifery was a necessary, accepted part of colonial life, although it developed without formal training or standards and was not considered a profession. Many midwives were widows for whom midwifery was a way to make a living (Chaney, 1980).

The safety and efficacy of the practices of individual midwives varied greatly. This was also true of doctors, few of whom had attended medical school, of which there were none in the colonies. Most were self-taught or apprentice trained, just like midwives. There were no educational standards and few rules and regulations for either midwives, physicians, surgeons, or apothecaries during colonial times. Although in some parts of the country, anyone could claim to be a doctor, doctors could offer few effective treatments, and the drugs that were effective could be purchased from apothecaries without prescription. Many people practiced self-medication; home treatment of the family was generally the responsibility of the women of the family. It was difficult for formally trained "regular" (allopathic) doctors to prove that their treatments were different from or better than care available from "irregular" or "unorthodox" practitioners such as herbalists and homeopaths. Puritan attitudes prevented early involvement of male practitioners in normal births.

Deventer's 1746 textbook for midwives was probably widely read in the United States, which imported all of its medical knowledge from Europe and England. Although midwifery was one of the best paid female occupations, many midwives of this time were illiterate, and midwifery was considered a part-time occupation unsuitable for an educated person (Chaney, 1980). The first formal instruction of American midwives was offered in 1765 by Dr. William Shippen, Jr., a Philadelphia physician who had been trained by William Smellie in London. Breaking with the tradition of exclusively female midwifery, Shippen began attending the births of upper-class women and established a lying-in hospital for poor women, which he used as a teaching hospital, offering the first series of lectures on midwifery in America and the opportunity for both male and female midwives to take a midwifery course that included practical experience as well as theory. Only a few female midwives took advantage of this opportunity; few midwives were literate, many could not afford to attend schools, and the Puritan philosophy did not encourage education for women. Shippen soon limited his course to men (Chaney, 1980). No other midwifery schools were opened until the middle of the nineteenth century, almost a century later. In *Lying-In: A History of Childbirth in America*, sociologists Wertz and Wertz suggest that midwives' beliefs that childbirth is normal and inherently within the domain of female competence may have prevented them from seeking formal training, especially from men (Roberts, 1995b).

British doctors' increasing role in childbirth during the latter part of the eighteenth century was influential in America—one of many ideas brought home by colonial men who went to England for medical training. The concept was welcomed by American doctors, some of whom charged higher fees for deliveries than for any other service. The physician who delivered a woman's first baby often became the family's long-term, trusted doctor; obstetrics soon became the key to a successful general practice (Wertz, 1983). The same factors that were in force in Britain and Western Europe during that period worked against midwifery in America: Doctors could use forceps and opium and had the status advantage of being males with formal learning. The latter was assumed, although in fact, most American physicians were apprentice trained and had not attended a medical school (Leavitt, 1983). In contrast, most people assumed that midwives had no formal training, even though some did, and common sexist beliefs held that women were emotionally and intellectually incapable of learning and applying the new obstetric methods (Litoff, 1982). Well-to-do families, especially the urban elite, soon came to believe that physicians provided better care than was possible with female midwives and thus offered the best hope for a successful birth (Leavitt, 1983). By the end of the eighteenth century, four male-only medical schools had been established in the United States. In 1813, the medical school at the University of Pennsylvania granted obstetrics the same academic status previously reserved for medicine and surgery. It seemed that any progress that would be made in obstetrics would come from physicians.

No American midwifery schools were opened until 1848, when Samuel Gregory established the Boston Female Medical College. Gregory, who was a graduate of Yale but not a physician, was motivated by moral outrage about the growing involvement of men in the physical care of women. Twelve women were in the first class for his three-month midwifery course, which was repeated six times between 1848 and 1851. Gregory and his school were harshly criticized by the Boston Medical Society, and the school closed in 1874 (Litoff, 1982). Small, proprietary (private for-profit) midwifery schools were started in a few other Northeastern and Midwestern cities during the last half of the nineteenth century, but the instruction provided at most of them was poor.

Increased immigration during the latter part of the nineteenth century increased the number of formally trained midwives, as well as physicians who had worked with professional midwives, creating a new interest in educating midwives in this country. A few schools of higher quality were opened near the end of the nineteenth century, including the College of Midwifery of New York City (opened in 1883, with courses offered in English, German, French, and Spanish), the Playfair School of Midwifery in Chicago (opened in 1896), and the Wisconsin College of Midwifery (started by German midwives and supportive physicians in Milwaukee). All midwifery schools of that era had close ties to the medical community and relied on physicians to teach at least some of the courses (Walsh, 1992). Four midwifery schools, each offering three- to five-month courses, were opened in St. Louis, Missouri, between 1854 and 1895. The first was opened by a German midwife; after twenty years it was enlarged, incorporated under a different name, and placed under the control of physicians. Two schools were headed by medical doctors, and one was headed by a homeopathic physician. Nevertheless, of 303 midwives listed in an 1894 St. Louis Midwives' Directory, only 26 had either American or European midwifery school credentials. Although few in number, the educated midwives of St. Louis formed a professional association, arranged for continuing education, and, with help from a physician affiliated with one of the schools, published twelve issues of a monthly professional journal, *American Midwife,* which ceased publication without explanation after one year. By 1912 all four St. Louis midwifery schools had closed (Perry, 1983).

Proprietary medical, as well as midwifery schools of that period were compromised by financial instability, limited access to clinical experience for students, and lack of a sound theoretical base for the profession (Walsh, 1991). Studies conducted early in the twentieth century concluded that most of the midwifery schools had been "diploma mills" run mainly for money, usually by a physician who "received lucrative returns for a minimum outlay of time and trouble" (Litoff, 1986). A 1907 study of New York City midwives found that some had diplomas from local schools, even though they were illiterate, and concluded that midwives with diplomas were no better than those without. The study also found evidence of unethical fee-splitting by physician instructors and graduates of some midwifery schools: Midwives called a former instructor for assistance with invented complications and received a share of his fee as payment for the referral (Litoff, 1986).

Experienced midwives were among the Mormon pioneers who moved to Utah. The Latter-Day Saints Relief Society began to establish midwifery training schools in and around Salt Lake City in the middle of the nineteenth century. Because of society's opposition to polygamy, the Mormons needed to be able to rely on members of their own community for the care of pregnant women. Brigham Young's wife delivered hundreds of babies, including more than fifty born to her husband's other wives. Some Mormon midwives were trained through apprenticeships with Mormon physicians, and, beginning in 1874, some Mormon women traveled to Pennsylvania to study at the Woman's Medical College in Philadelphia. When they returned they established midwifery courses in Utah. After relatively brief training, many Mormon midwives migrated to the neighboring states of Arizona, Idaho, Nevada, and New Mexico, where they were often the only source of any kind of health care (Speert, 1980).

Availability of any quality of formal midwifery training was limited compared to the need, because there were tens of thousands of midwives at that time. Obstetric training in medical schools was also nonexistent or poor. Midwives and doctors alike relied primarily on what they learned from experience. Most midwives prepared themselves through apprenticeships with physicians or experienced midwives or self-study. Physicians in Philadelphia recruited and trained midwives to work for them. And, as always, some women began to deliver the babies of their relatives and friends with little training at all (Walsh, 1992).

Medicine became professionalized in the United States during the last half of the 1800s. The American Medical Association (AMA) was founded in 1847 and created a specialty committee on obstetrics in 1848. Obstetrics was recognized as one of the four special sections of the AMA in 1859. The American Association of Obstetricians and Gynecologists began in 1888 (Leavitt, 1986). Physicians encouraged the passage of state medical practice laws that required licensure, allowing them to control access to the profession and prevent others from practicing medicine. The definitions of medical practice built into those laws were extremely broad and usually included a provision that made it illegal for anyone not licensed as a physician to carry out any acts included in the definition (Safriet, 1992). Despite professionalization of medicine, medical education at the beginning of the twentieth century remained poor in general and in obstetrics in particular. It did not improve significantly until after publication of the Flexner report in 1910* (Starr, 1982).

Lack of Licensure and Regulation of Midwives

There was no parallel effort to license and improve the education of midwives. Unlike Europe and the British Isles, where midwifery laws were national in scope, American midwifery laws were local and varied widely. Connecticut passed a midwife licensing law in 1893 (DeVries, 1985); however, midwifery was still completely unregulated in twenty states in 1900. Midwives in most states practiced without government control until the 1920s. The few existing laws dealt mainly with moral conduct. With few midwifery schools in existence, laws requiring education could not be enforced, and with few doctors positioned or willing to attend poor women, it was not practical to outlaw midwives. The only mention of midwives in some state laws was to exempt them from the medical practice act.

It has been argued that the indifference to regulating midwives reflected lack of concern for their clientele: predominantly poor, immigrant, or Negro women and their families (Darlington, 1911). Missouri's code specified that "Nothing in this section shall be so construed as to require women practicing midwifery to obtain a license when said women do not practice midwifery as a profession, and do not make any charge for their services." Although midwifery certification was required in the affluent city of New Orleans, Louisiana's law exempted "the so-called midwife of rural districts and plantation practice who, in the sense of this act, are not considered as practicing midwifery as a profession" (Shryock, 1967; Dar-

---

*As a layman, Flexner was much more severe in his judgment than the AMA had been in its annual guides to American medical schools. "The Flexner report" (actually titled *Medical Education in the United States and Canada: A Report to the Carnegie Foundation for the Advancement of Teaching*) provided detailed documentation of the falsity of claims made in the catalogues of the many weak (mainly proprietary) schools: laboratories that did not exist, libraries with no books, faculty who were completely occupied in private practice, entrance requirements that were waived for anyone who could pay tuition. Flexner recommended that most of the schools be closed and that the better schools be improved, using the Johns Hopkins Medical School as a model. By 1915, the number of medical schools had fallen to 95—from 131 when the Flexner report was published in 1910. The AMA took on the role of accrediting medical schools, and many states enacted licensing regulations that required higher training standards for physicians (Starr, 1982; Flexner, 1910).

lington, 1911). "Granny women" without formal training were also exempt from a 1901 Missouri law that regulated the practice of professional midwives and required licensure based on an examination (Perry, 1983). Another interpretation is that these laws enabled the practice of women who were not professional midwives but, according to today's World Health Organization definitions, were actually traditional birth attendants (TBAs). No country has attempted to subject TBAs to the same types of government regulation that all countries apply to professional midwives.

Even where potentially effective midwifery laws had been enacted, the lack of professional midwifery schools made it virtually impossible to enforce the rules (Darlington, 1911). New York's 1907 law required midwives to register annually, and only those who could read and write, were "clean and moral," and had attended at least twenty labors under a physician's supervision were eligible to register. In addition to 975 midwives who were registered to practice in New York City in 1910, authorities believed that at least an equal number of unlicensed midwives were practicing in the city. Even among those who registered, the requirement of English language literacy was not enforced; many could not sign their applications. Some midwives used foreign-language newspapers published in New York City to advertise their availability to perform services (sometimes including abortions) that were prohibited by the law. In 1909, the New York City Board of Health granted a midwifery permit to a woman who had been indicted for manslaughter less than a month earlier.

By 1900 physicians were attending about half of the nation's births, including nearly all births to middle- and upper-class women. Midwives took care of women who could not afford a doctor.

Movement of Birth into Hospitals—
A Campaign to Eliminate Midwives

Due to high rates of fertility and maternal mortality, many women lost their lives, and many men their wives, to pregnancy and childbirth. By the late nineteenth century, female medical leaders and others who wanted to make childbirth safer joined elite male physicians in calling for abolition of midwifery (McCool & McCool, 1989). This culminated in a physician-led campaign to prohibit midwives from practicing, especially in areas where doctors were available and eager to provide obstetric care (Devitt, 1979). This campaign, bolstered by social and economic conditions that supported the movement of childbirth into hospitals, led to the near demise of midwifery during the first three decades of the twentieth century. The following brief paragraphs introduce some of the social and economic changes that affected midwifery at the turn of the century:

- Economic changes made families less self-sufficient. As the family shifted from being the primary unit of production to being the primary unit of consumption, women began to look beyond their local female network for assistance during birth, illness, and death—major life events that had previously been handled mainly within a network of female family and friends (Tom, 1982b).
- Scientific discoveries and the development of more effective treatments late in the nineteenth century led to increased public acceptance of the validity of allopathic medicine (Walsh, 1992).
- A rapid increase in the number of hospitals and the development of the automobile, which provided relatively fast, easy transportation to hospitals, made hospital childbirth more feasible (Litoff, 1982).
- Some large city hospitals opened special clinics to provide prenatal care to indigent women (Roberts, 1995b).
- The introduction of anesthesia for childbirth in the late 1800s and the development of "twilight sleep" in 1914 made childbirth in hospitals more attractive. Twilight sleep—a combination of morphine for relief of pain, and

scopolamine, an amnesiac that caused women to have no memories of giving birth—became popular among upper-class women, some of whom formed "Twilight Sleep Societies" to promote its use (Wertz, 1983). Women were eager for anesthesia, which became a symbol of what modern medicine had to offer (Leavitt, 1983). By the 1930s the public and doctors agreed that some form of narcotization should be used for every labor (Harper, 1994).

- As medical education and care improved, physicians organized to solidify their status and authority. The newly unified medical profession developed a structure of laws and practices to exclude other health-care practitioners and enhance its own power. New state medical practice acts defined the practice of medicine so broadly that it encompassed all forms of health care, and gave physicians sole authority to prescribe medications. Physicians also gained control of hospitals (Starr, 1982; DeVries, 1985).

- Although a large influx of immigrants between 1900 and 1920 brought many foreign-trained midwives to the large cities of America's eastern seaboard, stringent limitations on immigration during and after World War I reduced the supply of formally trained midwives and the number of foreign-born women who were the midwives' most loyal clientele.

- Economic prosperity during the 1920s increased the size of the middle class, the women of which were supposed to be wives, mothers, and "ladies," and were not expected to work for pay (Wertz, 1983). Young women who wanted careers faced social reproach. Because only lower- and working-class women worked as midwives, middle- and upper-class women could not choose a midwife from their own social strata. At the same time, physicians were becoming wealth-

ier. Well-to-do women were the first to accept the physicians' claims of superior skill (Starr, 1982). When upper- and middle-class women started to use doctors, the use of a midwife became a stigma of the lower class. Midwives became thought of as poorly trained women of low social class whose only clients were women who could not afford to use doctors. In addition, an actual decline in the number of annual births between 1921 and 1933 may have caused people to perceive births as special events that required the skills of highly trained physicians (Litoff, 1982).

The poor status of maternal and child health in the United States was discovered during the early twentieth century. The federal Children's Bureau, established in 1912, collected data that revealed a mortality rate for American infants that was higher than rates in most of Europe. One-third of the men examined for military induction during World War I were rejected as not fit. Medical experts testified that half of them would have qualified if they had received proper care as children (Tom, 1982b). Maternal mortality was also high. In 1913, at least fifteen thousand American women died from conditions related to childbirth; nearly half of the deaths were from "childbed fever" (Meigs, 1985). "Childbed fever" was the common term for puerperal fever or sepsis—postpartum infection of the mother's uterus and other pelvic organs, often due to infectious agents transmitted to the mother on the hands of the person who assisted the delivery. Midwives were attending about half of all births at the turn of the century, and a much higher proportion of the births to women who were poor. It was easy to blame the midwives, who had no formal training. In fact, doctors, who conducted autopsies and took care of patients with communicable diseases, were much more likely to be at fault. Puerperal fever was especially common among women whose babies were delivered in hospitals, an environment in which physicians often examined many patients in sequence without washing their hands.

Midwives were poorly situated to counter the campaign against them. They were women. Relatively few had formal midwifery training, and those who did were immigrants, many of whom could not speak and write English fluently, if at all. Midwives who were not recent immigrants were mainly poor, and many were black. Prejudices against the intelligence and capability of women, immigrants, black people, and poor people were used to defame midwifery. As female members of the least powerful segments of American society, midwives lacked the role models, access, experience, and resources needed to influence the institutions that wield power. Most of them were middle-aged or older, married, and had family responsibilities in addition to their time- and energy-consuming midwifery work. Married women of their social class did not have careers or enter professions. Although midwives were an exception to this rule, most worked part time and had no worksite other than their own homes and those of their clients. They made relatively little money, were not organized, and did not see themselves as professionals (Borst, 1989).

"The midwife debate" played out between about 1910 and 1935. The main themes were (1) that midwives were untrained and incompetent, (2) that pregnancy is a dangerous condition requiring complicated care available only from highly trained medical specialists, and (3) that the activities of midwives were undermining much-needed development and progress in medical obstetrics. The two "titans" of twentieth century American obstetrics—Dr. Joseph DeLee and Dr. J. Whitridge Williams—heavily influenced the debate.

The Carnegie Foundation's Flexner report on medical education in the United States and Canada, which had brought attention to the poor overall quality of medical education, singled out obstetrics as making "the very worst showing" (Flexner, 1910). Obstetric training of medical students had changed little in a century. Although the idea of "demonstrative midwifery"—teaching students by having them observe actual women during labor—had been introduced in the mid-nineteenth century, many medical schools continued to limit instruction in obstetrics to lectures, textbooks, and the use of mannequins. Thus many physicians in the early 1900s had never even seen a birth (Leavitt, 1983). The call for reform in medical education led to concern about "overcrowding" in the medical profession; the large role of midwives seemed to exacerbate that problem with regard to obstetrics. Deliveries managed by midwives and traditional birth attendants (about half of all births at that time) represented lost opportunities for training doctors. In addition, many obstetricians felt that their specialty would never gain respect as long as women without scientific training were allowed to deliver babies.

The American Association for the Study and Prevention of Infant Mortality was formed in 1910, mainly by physicians interested in raising the standards and standing of obstetrics. In 1911, Dr. J. Whitridge Williams, a professor of obstetrics at Johns Hopkins University, mailed a questionnaire to every four-year medical school in the United States and Canada to gather data for a study on behalf of the association's Committee on Midwifery. Obstetric professors at forty-three schools (half of the schools rated as acceptable by the American Medical Association, but less than 20 percent of the "unacceptable" schools) completed and returned the questionnaires. Even though the study was biased toward the better schools, one-third of the responding professors lacked any special training in obstetrics. Some were not even particularly interested in that field. Five had seen fewer than 100 deliveries; one had not observed a single birth before becoming a professor. Most of the schools were associated with hospitals in which there were fewer than 250 deliveries per year. Six schools were not affiliated with any hospital that had a maternity service. Most medical students in most of the schools saw three or fewer labors during their entire course of study (Williams, 1912).

Dr. Williams also asked the obstetrics professors to comment on the incidence of maternal mortality among women cared for by midwives in their communities as compared with that of women whose births were attended by physicians. Fifteen of the professors thought women were more likely to die of puerperal sepsis in the hands of physicians, five thought the rates were equal, and eight did not know. In addition, twenty-six thought that more women died "as the result of ignorance or of ill-judged and improperly performed operations in the hands of general practitioners as from puerperal infection in the hands of midwives." Williams was appalled by these findings, particularly because "one of the main arguments urged against the midwife is the prevalence of infection in her practice."* Although "[a]priori the replies seem to indicate that women in labor are as safe in the hands of admittedly ignorant midwives as in those of poorly educated medical men," Williams determined that "such a conclusion . . . is contrary to reason." He believed that the necessary reforms could be accomplished "more speedily by radical improvement in medical education than by attempting the almost impossible task of improving midwives." He recommended the extension of "obstetrical charities" (as sites for training young physicians), better pay for physicians providing obstetric care, and less expensive nurses. He concluded by calling for the use of obstetrically trained nurses to make home visits,

hospital care for all deliveries, and the "gradual abolition of midwives in large cities and their replacement by obstetric charities" (Williams, 1912).

Private and academic physicians publicly attacked the reputations of midwives as a group, characterizing them as being poor, black, immigrants, dirty, illiterate, untrained, ignorant, immoral, drunken, unprincipled, overconfident, superstitious, callous, rough, "relics of barbarism," and, in some cases, criminal abortionists (Devitt, 1979). The strongest contempt came from the most prestigious obstetricians. It resonated with the prejudices of the time.

The other "titan" of twentieth century obstetrics was Dr. Joseph DeLee, head of Obstetrics at Northwestern University, chair of Obstetrics and Gynecology at the University of Chicago, and author of the most frequently used obstetric textbooks. (Danforth, 1974; Leavitt, 1988). Dr. DeLee argued that childbirth is a pathologic process from which "only a small minority of women escape damage." "If the profession would realize that parturition viewed with modern eyes is no longer a normal function, but that it has imposing pathologic dignity," he wrote, "the midwife would be impossible even of mention" (DeLee, 1915). In a 1920 article promoting "prophylactic" (i.e., routine) use of forceps, DeLee wondered whether nature may have intended women, like salmon, to be "used up in the process of reproduction" (DeLee, 1920).

To avoid "laceration, prolapse and all the evils" that are "natural to labor," DeLee proposed a program of regular medical intervention: Specialist obstetricians should sedate women with scopolamine at the onset of labor, allow the cervix to dilate, give ether during the second stage, perform an episiotomy, deliver the baby with forceps, extract the placenta, give ergot to help the uterus contract, and then repair the perineum. He concluded that "instrumental delivery is safer than prolonged, hard, unassisted labor" and would save women

---

*The cause of childbed fever was discovered by Dr. Ignaz Semmelweis in the mid-1800s, who observed that the maternal mortality rate from puerperal fever was three times as high in the part of the hospital run by physicians than in the ward controlled by midwives (Roush, 1979).

from the debilitating effects of suffering, preserve the "integrity of the pelvic floor," and save babies' brains from injury (DeLee, 1920). DeLee was, of course, not the first to suggest that physicians take an active role in childbirth. Early in the nineteenth century, Walter Channing, a Harvard obstetrician, wrote that doctors must "do something" when called to the bedside of a woman in labor (Leavitt, 1988). DeLee's unique contribution was to change the focus from responding to the perception of a problem to preventing problems by directing the course of labor and delivery through a panoply of interventions (Leavitt, 1988). DeLee's article was published in the first issue of the *American Journal of Obstetrics and Gynecology*. All of the interventions he prescribed eventually became routine.

Various solutions to "the midwife problem" were proposed. Private practitioners and academic obstetricians wanted midwives to be brought under the control of doctors and to eliminate them as soon as possible. However, public health leaders and some physicians in the South recognized that it would be difficult to extend physician services to all pregnant women. Midwives were taking care of poor, working-class, immigrant, and black women, not the well-paying patients sought by private doctors. Public health-oriented leaders proposed means to educate and supervise midwives and bring them and their clients into a system that would facilitate selective referrals to medical care. Proponents of midwifery education pointed to the good pregnancy outcomes in European countries that had a highly regulated midwifery profession and state-supported schools. Most obstetricians rejected this logic, claiming that it would lead to a "double standard" in obstetrics (DeVries, 1985). In addition, the existence of midwives seemed an insult to the leading obstetricians. In 1911, DeLee complained in correspondence to Williams that "If an uneducated woman of the lowest classes may practice obstetrics, is instructed by doctors and licensed

by the State, it certainly must require little knowledge and skill—surely it cannot belong to the science and art of medicine" (Devitt, 1979). The campaign to eliminate midwives became part of obstetricians' attempts to improve their standing within medicine.

Midwifery at the Turn of the Century

Most midwives practicing in major U.S. cities between 1906 and 1924 were literate recent immigrants. Some had diplomas from midwifery schools in Europe and some had taken courses in this country (Devitt, 1979). Those in Texas were predominantly black (73 percent) or Mexican (22 percent), and only 40 percent were literate. There was great variation in the training and the quality of practice of individual midwives, circumstances reflecting the lack of both regulation and local training opportunities:

- A nurse who interviewed 500 New York City midwives in 1906 found that 40 percent had European diplomas. However, she characterized only 10 percent of them as capable and reliable. Some carried rusty scissors, old rags for use as dressings, and stiffened catheters for inducing illegal abortions (Devitt, 1979).
- Seventy percent of midwives surveyed in Chicago had been in practice for ten years or more, 30 percent had foreign diplomas, 78 percent maintained their equipment in good condition, and 72 percent had clean homes and personal appearance. But 46 percent were suspected of performing abortions, and 12 percent attended "abnormal labors" (Crowell, 1908; Devitt, 1979). (Although many European-educated midwives had been trained to manage breech and twin deliveries, births involving these complications are "abnormal" and were not considered appropriate for midwifery care [Walsh, 1992].)
- A study of midwives in Baltimore found that 28 percent had foreign diplomas,

57 percent had practiced for twenty years or more, two-thirds attended abnormal deliveries, only 30 percent carried equipment that was clean and in good condition, 32 percent were suspected of performing abortions, and only 2 percent put silver nitrate in the baby's eyes, an action that was required by law to prevent infections (Sherwood, 1909; Devitt, 1979).

- In 1914 the physician appointed to supervise midwives in Philadelphia reported that they fell into three categories: "A very small" percentage had been trained abroad and were "thoroughly competent;" about 20 percent were "useless, ignorant, and filthy;" most had "been in practice for a number of years and were anxious to learn" (Walsh, 1992).

Although the studies found many inadequacies, most urban midwives had substantial experience and many had graduated from rigorous European schools. Midwifery schools in Sweden and Italy required students to conduct one hundred deliveries under supervision (Devitt, 1979). Williams had found no American medical schools with similar requirements (Williams, 1912). A 1914 report to the New York Committee for the Prevention of Blindness concluded that "however bad the midwife is, we are sorry to have to admit that on the whole a patient is often better off in her hands than in the care of many of the physicians who compete with her. Investigations which have been made concerning the etiology of ophthalmia neonatorum and puerperal septicemia indicate that more of these cases are to be traced to physicians than to midwives" (van Blarcom, 1914).

The Children's Bureau initiated studies of maternity care in rural areas, including the practices of the rural granny midwives. A 1916–1918 study in rural Mississippi found mostly black midwives, about 90 percent of whom could neither read nor write. About 10 percent were white, but there were few differences in their practices or training. Some used no antiseptics, few knew that uncleanness could cause puerperal fever, and many adhered to an old custom of not changing the mother's bed sheets for at least three days after the birth. Only three of eighty-seven midwives interviewed said that they applied silver nitrate to the eyes of the babies they delivered. Another Children's Bureau study found that the predominantly white midwives practicing in the mountains of north Georgia also lacked some of the knowledge needed for competent attendance at births* (Litoff, 1986).

The studies found most midwives to be eager for training. A few jurisdictions developed government-supported midwifery training programs, an effort that increased during the 1920s due to the federal government's enactment of the Sheppard–Towner Maternity and Infancy Protection Act in 1921. The Sheppard–Towner act provided money to help each state develop its own plan to provide maternal and child health services. Some states used their money to train and supervise midwives (Hogan, 1975; Tom, 1982). Local studies documented the value of training and regulation:

- As a result of the 1906 investigation, the New York City Board of Health was given authority to license midwives and regulate their practice. Of 1,344 midwives included in a subsequent New York City survey, 99 percent were found to have good personal hygiene, the

---

*Despite these findings, and lack of training, lack of equipment and supplies, and lack of medical back-up for granny midwives, many of them were highly intelligent, capable women. *Listen To Me Good* tells the life story of Margaret Charles Smith, who began to practice midwifery in rural Greene County, Alabama, in 1949 and continued for several years after the 1976 passage of a law that authorized nurse-midwifery and outlawed lay midwifery in Alabama (Smith & Holmes, 1996). Mrs. Smith attended her last birth in 1981, at the age of 75. She assisted at the births of nearly 3,000 babies, never lost a mother and rarely lost an infant.

equipment of 98 percent was in satisfactory condition, and the homes of 97 percent were clean. In 1911, New York City opened a tax-supported midwifery school at Bellevue Hospital, with a curriculum based on those used in European midwifery schools. The Bellevue School of Midwifery remained in operation until 1935, when the increase in hospital maternity care facilities reduced the need for midwives, whose practice was limited to home births.

- In 1914 the city of Newark instituted a program that included conferences, lectures, and supervisory visits to the midwives' practice sites. Before the program started, Newark's maternal mortality ratio was 5.3 (maternal deaths per 1,000 live births). One year later the ratio had dropped to 3.6; after two years it had dropped to 2.2. In addition, the incidence of neonatal eye infection among babies delivered by midwives fell below the rate for babies delivered by physicians, either at home or in hospitals (Devitt, 1979).
- In 1914, the Pennsylvania Bureau of Medical Education began a program to license, supervise, and improve the practice of midwives in Philadelphia. During the 1920s, the bureau used Sheppard–Towner funds to extend the program to rural Pennsylvania. In 1932 the chief of the Division of Child Hygiene reported on 48,819 deliveries conducted by midwives between 1921 and 1931. The maternal mortality ratio for the midwives' clients was 1.8 per 1,000 births, compared with a statewide ratio of 6.6 per thousand. These positive findings were supported in a report issued by the Philadelphia County Medical Society Committee on Maternal Welfare, which concluded that "the midwife is an almost negligible factor in mortality in Philadelphia" (Walsh, 1992).

Nearly eleven thousand midwives were enrolled in federally subsidized classes in fourteen states in 1927. Twenty-nine states provided instruction or educational supervision of midwives in 1929. But the American Medical Association opposed the Sheppard–Towner act, and Congress allowed it to expire in 1929. Although the training required of midwives in New Jersey and New York was more thorough than the obstetrical training of most physicians at that time, the midwifery programs were severely underfunded, and the standards were not always met. Despite the success of the Pennsylvania program, the State Board of Medical Education and Licensure turned down a 1933 proposal to establish a nurse-midwifery education program in Philadelphia, stating that it would be dangerous to license "this class of people" (Walsh, 1992).

More states enacted laws to regulate midwifery. By 1930, all but ten states required midwives to register. The laws varied widely. In addition to registration, the main intent of most of the laws was to require midwives to conform to certain public health practices, including filling out birth certificates, washing their hands, using silver nitrate, referring complicated cases to doctors, and refraining from invasive procedures (often including vaginal examinations). Only Massachusetts, source of the most fervent opposition to midwifery, made it a crime for anyone but a doctor to attend a woman during childbirth. In contrast, Washington state's law, passed in 1917, provided for licensure of midwives with evidence of formal schooling. Midwives who had been trained in Italy, Germany, Denmark, and Japan practiced in Washington under that law until at least the 1930s (Ito, 1987).

Despite the opinions of the "titans of obstetrics," objective data from the first three decades of the twentieth century suggest that women were relatively safe in midwives' hands (Devitt, 1979):

- A paper published in 1913 reported that New York City midwives attended 40 percent of the births but only 22 percent of births to the women who later died of puerperal sepsis. Physicians accounted for 60 percent of the births and 69 percent of the deaths. In this study, deaths were ascribed to midwives if they had ever been present at the labor. In addition, the postpartum care given by midwives was found to be "infinitely superior to the aftercare given by the average doctor for the same fee." Midwives often visited the mothers and newborns for seven to ten days, doing some cooking and performing "little homely duties in addition to keeping the patient clean and caring for the baby." In contrast, the average doctor was described as arriving and leaving in a hurry, using his instruments too soon, often lacerating the perineum, and then making only one or two postpartum calls.

- Two studies conducted by the New Jersey State Department of Public Health, the first in 1915–1916 and the second in 1921, found a significantly lower incidence of neonatal and maternal mortality among births managed by midwives than among those managed by physicians. As in the New York City study, deaths were attributed to midwives if they had attended the labor at any time, "even where it appears that the result was due to unnecessary interference or negligence on the part of the doctor."

- A study to determine the causes of maternal deaths in New York City between 1930 and 1933 found that 66 percent of the deaths were preventable and that doctors were responsible for 61 percent of the preventable deaths. The patients themselves were responsible for 37 percent of the preventable deaths; midwives were responsible for 2 percent. The mortality rate for women attended by midwives at any time during labor was 1.6 per 1,000 live births, compared with 4.5 per 1,000 for women attended by physicians.

- Although a study in Akron, Ohio, found higher intrapartum stillbirth and infant mortality rates for births attended by midwives as compared with physicians, it attributed the difference to the poverty of the midwives' clients. Nearly all of the women cared for by midwives were recent immigrants, as compared with less than one-fourth of the doctors' clients, and babies of the foreign-born women had a high rate of mortality from diarrhea.

As with almost all studies that try to compare the outcomes of deliveries managed by midwives with outcomes of births managed by physicians, it is likely that physicians in these cities saw a higher concentration of complicated cases. On the other hand, most of the midwives' clients were poor. Although it is difficult to unravel the effects of these conflicting biases, an analysis of data done for the 1925 White House Conference on Child Health and Protection made a contribution. Researchers examined data from twenty-nine states to look for correlations between the percent of births attended by midwives or others (anyone but a physician) and each state's overall maternal and infant mortality rates. They found a correlation between the extent of midwifery practice and a high infant mortality rate, but no higher incidence of maternal mortality in states where midwives attended a high percentage of the births. The researchers concluded that the association between midwife deliveries and infant mortality was due to the high proportions of poor people in states with many midwives; they attributed the lack of a higher incidence of maternal deaths in those states to the care provided by the midwives. Care during childbirth is very important for preventing maternal mortality; it is only one of many factors that affect the survival of infants (Devitt, 1979).

The 1925 White House Conference on Child Health and Protection concluded that "untrained midwives approach, and trained midwives surpass, the record of physicians in normal deliveries." The conference report ascribed this record to "the fact that . . .

many physicians . . . employ procedures which are calculated to hasten delivery, but which sometimes result harmfully to mother and child. On her part, the midwife is not permitted to and does not employ such procedures. She waits patiently and lets nature take its course" (White House Conference on Child Health and Protection, 1932).

During "the midwife debate" several concerns were raised regarding problems that might occur or become worse if midwives were replaced by obstetricians (Devitt, 1979):

- It was predicted that the high fees charged by general physicians (twice those charged by midwives) and obstetricians (three times those of midwives) would make it impossible to adequately replace midwives by charity lying-in hospitals.
- Investing resources in obstetricians instead of midwives would limit the geographic availability of good maternity care, because obstetricians tend to move to cities.
- Given the autonomy and political power of physicians, it was argued that it would be much easier to regulate and improve the practices of licensed and supervised midwives than to control the quality of care provided by obstetricians.
- The success of midwives was attributed to their unwillingness to intervene in normal births. In contrast, it was pointed out, the obstetricians' beliefs that pregnancy and childbirth are fraught with danger creates a bias toward interference during labor and delivery. (At the time of the 1925 White House conference, forceps were being used in 10 to 80 percent of births in various parts of the United States, compared with only 4 percent in Scandinavia, where midwives were attending more than 80 percent of the births.)

All of the predicted problems did occur as midwifery was nearly eliminated during the first half of this century. The proportion of U.S. births attended by midwives declined from about 50 percent in 1900 to 12.5 percent in 1935 (Devitt, 1979; Jacobson, 1956). By 1932 approximately 80 percent of all midwives practicing in the United States were traditional birth attendants living in the rural south (Devitt, 1979; Jacobson, 1956).

Whenever and wherever midwifery declined, the incidence of maternal mortality and infant deaths from birth injuries increased. In the 1920s midwifery declined and maternal mortality rose in Newark and Cleveland, whereas an increase in midwifery in Pittsburgh was accompanied by a decrease in the ratio. Midwives delivered 10 percent of babies born in the District of Columbia in 1915, and the maternal mortality ratio was 6.6 per 1,000 live births. By 1923 the midwives' share of D.C. births had fallen to 4 percent and the maternal mortality ratio had risen to 10.1. When Massachusetts made midwifery illegal in 1907 the state's maternal mortality ratio was 4.7; it rose to 5.6 in 1913 and 7.4 in 1920. Throughout the nation, infant deaths from birth injuries rose by 44 percent between 1918 and 1925, as the overall practice of midwifery declined (Devitt, 1979).

The National Negro Health Movement, established in 1930, joined with other groups in calling for elimination of the granny midwife, whom many black people considered to be unclean and dangerous (Robinson, 1984).

The Real Causes of High Maternal and Infant Mortality Rates

Recent retrospective studies of the reduction in maternal and infant mortality between 1800 and 1950 have thrown more light on the relative importance of various factors. Early in this century, levels of both infant and maternal mortality in the United States were as high as they are in many developing countries now (Maine, 1991). Maternal mortality plateaued at a high level

(600 to 700 deaths per 100,000 births) between 1900 and the mid-1930s and then began a steep decline coincident with the availability of antibiotics, blood transfusions, and drugs to treat pregnancy-induced hypertension (Maine, 1991; Loudon, 1992; AbouZahr & Royston, 1991). The most important contributing factor was the sudden availability of antibiotics. Sulfonamide drugs were being used for obstetric infections by the late 1930s. Penicillin became available to the civilian population at the end of World War II. The number of infection-related maternal deaths fell from 3,719 in 1937 to 392 in 1954 (Maine, 1991).

Similar drops in maternal mortality occurred throughout the Western industrialized world. The U.S., the Netherlands, and Britain experienced dramatic reductions in maternal mortality starting in the mid-1930s but had very different forms of maternity care: In the United States obstetricians delivered most of the babies in hospitals. In the Netherlands professional midwives delivered most of the babies in homes. Britain had both home and hospital births and used midwives, general practitioners, and specialist obstetricians. These differences had no apparent effect on the rate of maternal mortality (Maine, 1991). Unlike infant mortality, which is closely linked with the general socioeconomic well-being of populations, maternal mortality is relatively insensitive to socioeconomic factors except insofar as these determine the availability of qualified birth attendants. Based on intensive study of maternal mortality in many countries between 1800 and 1950, Loudon (1992) concluded that poor obstetric care "could either consist of ignorance of basic procedures (judged by the standards of the time), or it could consist of dangerous and unwarranted interference by trained personnel. . . . High maternal risk could be associated with cheap untrained midwives or expensive over-zealous and unskilled doctors. Sound obstetric practice by well-trained midwives could produce a low level of maternal mortality even in populations which were socially and economically deprived."

Contraception and abortion also play important roles. Illegal abortion is a major cause of maternal mortality whenever there is poor access to effective contraception and legal abortion.

Infant mortality declined more or less steadily in all Western countries during the first half of the twentieth century. Most of that decline was in postneonatal mortality—deaths of infants who have reached at least twenty-eight days of age. Neonatal deaths (those occurring prior to twenty-eight days of age), are usually caused by conditions arising during the pregnancy or birth, whereas postneonatal deaths usually result from causes related to the environment and parenting, including lack of adequate breast-feeding. A large part of the high U.S. infant mortality rates of the early 1900s was due to the generally poor social and economic conditions of both the urban and rural poor of that period of time. Improvements in standards of living and nutrition and public health measures that resulted in better water, housing, and sanitation led to reductions in infant mortality that were independent of changes in medical and midwifery care. Although obstetrics made a contribution, it was a double-edged sword. In the United States, a large increase in infant mortality from birth injuries was associated with what medical historians have described as an "orgy" of obstetrical interference in birth (Devitt, 1979; Loudon, 1992).

Development of Obstetric Nursing

While midwifery was receding to a minimal, almost invisible role in the United States during the early twentieth century, nursing was developing from its start during the Civil War. Florence Nightingale founded the first school of nursing in England in 1860. Several American schools had opened by the early 1870s. The predecessor to the American Nurses' Association was established in 1896. As American medical care became more complex, nursing required more scientific background and the American Nurses' Association began to promote baccalaureate and graduate education for nurses.

Although Florence Nightingale considered midwifery to be a branch of nursing, most early American nursing leaders considered midwifery part of medicine. In a description of American nursing education prepared for the Third International Congress of Nurses in 1901, Lavina Doc was proud to report that "The midwife question, so distracting in other countries, does not exist here as a complication to nurses, and is consequently a question that we may leave to the medical profession to settle" (Roberts, 1995b). In 1909 the American Society of Superintendents of Training Schools for Nurses directed that obstetrical training for nurses should be limited to emergencies, observing and reporting symptoms and problems, and general nursing care, such as bathing the mother and infant and making the bed. The Society did, however, support the idea of "suitable training, registration, licensure, supervision and control of women engaged in the practice of midwifery" (Roberts, 1995b). The lack of means to ensure the quality of midwifery services was widely seen as contributing to the health problems of mothers and babies.

Even if early nursing leaders had wanted to train nurses as midwives, it would have been difficult to do so within the new hospital-based nursing schools, because most normal births occurred in private homes. When nurses did become involved in maternity care (to "supervise" the midwives), the task fell to public health nurses working in residential communities, which is where the care of pregnant women and babies took place (Roberts, 1995b).

When childbirth moved into hospitals it became necessary to prepare nurses to provide care to women during labor, delivery, and the early postpartum period, and to take care of newborns while their mothers were in the hospital. These subjects were incorporated into the curricula of most basic nursing schools. Subsequently, certain maternity hospitals became leaders in the new field of obstetric nursing education. By the mid-1900s, at least twenty-five hospitals with university affiliations were offering graduate programs to prepare experienced maternal and child health nurses for positions in teaching, administration, and public health (Speert,1980). Some of these programs began to prepare maternity nurses to carry out some of the functions of obstetricians, especially to provide the care needed during labor until the time of the actual birth. Thereafter, management of the labor of most women who give birth in American hospitals has been primarily in the hands of nurses, who follow routines and "standing orders" established by physicians and are responsible for recognizing abnormal labor patterns or other complications and bringing them to the attention of the woman's doctor. Obstetric nurses are expected to notify each patient's physician in time for him or her to come to the maternity unit to deliver the baby. Most of the nurses who carry these responsibilities learn this role mainly through mentoring and other informal on-the-job training. Midwifery training has never been included in regular nursing education programs.

The Natural Childbirth and Breast-Feeding Movements Begin

During the 1930s Grantly Dick-Read, an English obstetrician who had observed women giving birth without assistance, published a book in which he asserted that much of the pain of labor and delivery results from tension induced by fear. He believed that women who were confident in their own health and believed that pregnancy and birth are normal processes could experience childbirth without fear. His book, *Childbirth Without Fear: The Principles and Practices of Natural Childbirth,* was published at a time when administration of analgesia and anesthesia was part of the routine care of nearly all women giving birth in hospitals in England (Dick-Read, 1959). His theory was considered radical, and he was accused of "abusing" women (Harper, 1994).

Dick-Read's book was not published in the United States until 1944. When it was, it stimulated the beginning of a small "natural childbirth movement" and childbirth education classes for pregnant women. Dick-Read believed that women needed to understand the physiology of labor and be prepared to be active participants. His book described exercises to help women strengthen the voluntary muscles that augment the force of labor and breathing techniques to help them relax during contractions (Dick-Read, 1959). Margaret Gamper, a pioneer childbirth educator from Chicago, combined Dick-Read's breathing methods with her own massage techniques. She, in turn, influenced Dr. Robert Bradley of Denver, who, with his nurse, Rhondda Hartman, developed the Bradley method of "husband-coached childbirth" (Harper, 1994).

In 1951 two French obstetricians went to Russia to observe childbirth methods based on Pavlovian principles; their goal was to eliminate fear responses by teaching women to use active breathing techniques to control pain during contractions. When they returned to Paris, the French physicians began to train women in these methods. An Ameri-can woman, Marjorie Karmel, who had gone to France seeking support for a natural birth experience, met one of them—Dr. Ferdinand Lamaze—by chance, and told him about Dick-Read's method for "childbirth without fear." Dr. Lamaze told her that he could help her have childbirth without pain. Karmel trained with Lamaze and his nurse and gave birth to her first child in a French hospital in 1956. After using Lamaze's techniques for another birth, she wrote her story, the now-famous book, *Thank You, Dr. Lamaze,* published in 1959 (Harper, 1994).

The International LaLeche League was founded by seven Chicago-area women in 1956. The women had breast-fed their babies despite lack of any support or encouragement from their doctors or the nurses in the hospitals where they had delivered their babies. The group thought it strange and wrong that women who bottle-fed their babies were given help, but those who wanted to breast-feed were advised to give it up. Although doctors initially objected to the distribution of "professional medical information" by lay women, the women persisted in informing others through small support-group classes. They also researched and produced educational materials regarding the effects of formula and early introduction of solid foods on infants, and the emotional aspects of breast-feeding (Harper, 1994).

Chapter 3
The Beginning of Nurse-Midwifery

As the granny midwife was becoming obsolete, the seed of professional midwifery was sown in the United States. In 1911 the commissioner of health for New York City criticized the United States as "the only civilized country in the world in which the health as well as the life and future well-being of mothers and infants is not safeguarded so far as possible through the training and control of midwives." (His statement wasn't entirely accurate; the same situation existed in Canada.) The first publicly funded midwifery training program was started at Bellevue Hospital that same year (Speert, 1980). In 1912 the general superintendent of Nurses' Training Schools in New York's Bellevue and Allied Hospitals predicted gradual elimination of "the old familiar type of midwife" and her replacement by "trained and certified midwives, working under visiting nurse or charitable organizations . . . whether as the midwife pure and simple, or as a further development of the nurses' work" (Walsh, 1992).

Studies conducted by the federal Children's Bureau after its establishment in 1912 provided more information than had previously been available on the health problems of American mothers and babies, some of the circumstances leading to those problems, and the fact that maternal and infant mortality rates were higher in this country than in most countries of Western Europe. This expanding base of information led many to conclude that a substantial proportion of maternal and infant deaths might be prevented by providing care and advice to pregnant women. This was the beginning of a now long-standing public health interest in prenatal care. Poor and rural women, who had the most problems, were likely to rely on granny midwives for any pregnancy care and advice, but most grannies had no formal training and they functioned outside the formal health care system. Public health nurses, who worked in communities but were part of the system, were seen as a way to link granny midwives and their clients with physicians and public health agencies. In 1917 the Children's Bureau drew up a plan that called for efforts to instruct pregnant women in nutrition and other aspects of self-care and recommended that public health nurses begin to provide such instruction (Hogan, 1975). The bureau also recommended that public health nurses should teach principles of hygiene and prenatal care to granny midwives.

Findings from the Children's Bureau's early studies also led to enactment, in 1921, of the Sheppard–Towner Maternity and Infancy Protection Act, a federal law that encouraged states to make their own plans to improve maternal and child health and provided funds to train the people who would be needed to implement the plans. Plans submitted by many southern states called for programs in which public health nurses would teach and supervise granny midwives.

Articles published in several respected journals during this period went a step further by advocating the actual training of nurses to be midwives (Tom, 1982). In a speech at the annual meeting of the National Organization of Public Health Nursing in 1914, Dr. Frederick Taussig, a physician from St. Louis, introduced the idea of "nurse-midwives" (a new term) as an alternative solution to the "midwife question" and suggested the development of midwifery schools for the further training of graduate nurses (Perry, 1983). He thought midwifery education would be more efficient this way, since nurses were already knowledgeable about anatomy, basic hygiene, and nutrition (Speert, 1980). The idea was implemented in 1925, when Mary Breckinridge imported British nurse-midwives to establish the Frontier Nursing Service (FNS) in Leslie County, Kentucky.

Mary Breckinridge and the Frontier Nursing Service

Mary Breckinridge, born in 1881, was a well-educated and widely traveled woman from a prominent Southern family (Ernst, 1979).

Her grandfather served as vice president of the United States under President Buchanan; her father was an American ambassador to Russia. Her first contact with midwives was at her brother's birth in Russia, when she was fourteen years old. Although two doctors stood by, the young Breckinridge was impressed by the midwife who managed the birth. Widowed at age twenty-five, she studied nursing in New York City, where she experienced the coarse and inadequate conditions in which most poor women gave birth. She remarried, but divorced and, after both of her young children died in rapid succession, determined to use her life to improve conditions for children. While awaiting a position with the Red Cross in the war-ravaged parts of France, Breckinridge completed three assignments in the United States: traveling throughout the country to gather information for the Children's Bureau, working as a volunteer in the battle against the 1918 influenza epidemic in the District of Columbia, and studying public health nursing in the Boston slums (Breckinridge, 1981).

Then, in France, she imported goats to supply milk for starving mothers and babies; fought epidemics of scarlet fever, diphtheria, and dysentery; and created the first Child Hygiene and Visiting Nurses Service in that country. While there, she realized that to help children, one must help their mothers first. Although she admired the excellent care provided by French midwives, she thought it odd that they had no background in nursing—just the opposite of the situation in America, where nurses were not trained as midwives. Through the Red Cross she also encountered British nurse-midwives. The combination of nursing and midwifery was what she thought was needed to deal with the conditions and health problems of poor mothers and their children in rural, medically underserved parts of the United States. After three years in France, Breckinridge wanted to return to her own country to do something for its children.

In 1923 she returned to the United States and went to Leslie County, a remote, mountainous, doctorless county in eastern Kentucky, where she had family ties. The Kentucky health department officials with whom she consulted recommended that she begin by surveying all families in the county to determine their conditions and produce accurate data on births and maternal and infant deaths. Thus she spent the summer riding horses and mules alone over the creeks and up the "hollers" of the county, asking the people about their health problems and what health care they used, and staying with them in their humble but hospitable homes. Then, knowing of their problems, she prepared herself to establish a nursing and midwifery service in Leslie County. That fall she went to England, where she completed a four-month midwifery training program, worked as a district midwife in a London slum, took a short course for midwifery teachers, observed nurse-midwives working out of a district nursing center in rural Scotland, and recruited two British nurse-midwives to help her start a decentralized public health nursing and midwifery service in Kentucky (Ernst, 1979).

Mary Breckinridge founded the Frontier Nursing Service (FNS) in Leslie County, Kentucky, in 1925. One of her first actions was to recruit a medical director and write protocols establishing the clinical relationship between nurse-midwives and physicians. FNS established its first nursing outpost in 1926 and another in 1927. By the end of 1928 it had built a twenty-five-bed, twelve-bassinet hospital and health center in the town of Hyden and had a medical advisory committee (Tom, 1982; *Nation's Health*, May 1975).

The doctors and nurse-midwives worked together to develop FNS medical directives. By 1933 the hospital and physicians were "backing-up" eleven district nursing centers located throughout the county. Nurse-midwives residing at the district centers provided both midwifery and nursing care to the people of the area, traveling by horseback to attend births or provide care during emergencies. Home births were the norm for the first twenty-five to thirty years, but de-

clined rapidly during the 1950s, belatedly following the national trend (Ernst & Gordon, 1979).

Because of the initial survey and meticulous record keeping, FNS was able to document its remarkable success. Dr. Louis Dublin of the Metropolitan Life Insurance Company studied the first 1,000 deliveries. He was very impressed that there had been no maternal deaths. "The study shows conclusively," he wrote, " . . . that the type of service rendered by the Frontier nurses safeguards the life of mother and babe. If such service were available to the women of the country generally, there would be a saving of 10,000 mothers' lives a year in the United States. There would be 30,000 less stillbirths and 30,000 more children alive at the end of the first month of life" (Tom, 1982). Perinatal and neonatal mortality in Leslie Country dropped dramatically from a level that had been among the highest in the country. These accomplishments were particularly remarkable because FNS served a low-income, poorly nourished and thus high-risk population (Browne & Isaacs, 1976; Frontier Nursing Service, 1958; Steele, 1941).

FNS was originally staffed with British midwives and American public health nurses whom Breckinridge had sent to England for midwifery training. They provided public health nursing as well as midwifery. In addition, FNS became one of the first organized health services in the world to provide birth control pills and other modern family planning methods. Mary Breckinridge was brilliant, well connected, articulate, and completely committed to this work. As such, she was an effective fund-raiser who recruited and inspired the first generation of American nurse-midwifery leaders.

The Maternity Center Association: Beginnings of Nurse-Midwifery Education

In 1915 the health commissioner of New York City named three physicians to a committee to analyze obstetric conditions in

Manhattan. The committee recommended that the city be divided into ten maternity care zones and that a maternity center be established in each zone. In response to this recommendation, the Women's City Club developed a program to provide prenatal care and education in one zone of the city. In 1918 the City Club program became incorporated as the Maternity Center Association (MCA), a not-for-profit voluntary health agency based in Manhattan (Lubic, 1988). By 1920 MCA was supervising thirty neighborhood centers in and from which public health nurses working under the direction of physicians provided prenatal care and education to pregnant women and their families; much of the care was provided to women in their own homes. MCA's board soon realized that the nurses were not well enough prepared. They studied how maternity care was being provided in the countries with the world's lowest maternal and infant mortality rates, concluded that there was a need to prepare nurses to do normal obstetrics, and discussed opening a school of nurse-midwifery (Varney, 1987).

In 1921, MCA decided to concentrate on a single demonstration center that could provide complete maternity care. In 1923, MCA tried to arrange for the Bellevue School for Midwives to instruct its public health nurses in midwifery. The plan was rejected by a city commissioner. In 1930, a group of MCA board members and others, including Mary Breckinridge, incorporated themselves as the Association for the Promotion and Standardization of Midwifery. After much work, the two affiliated organizations opened the Lobenstine Clinic, the nation's second nurse-midwifery service and, in 1931, the Lobenstine Midwifery School, the nation's first nurse-midwifery educational program, in New York City. The objectives specified that nurse-midwives prepared through the program would "accept responsibility for the care of normal maternity patients delegated by the obstetrician after a complete physical examination had been done," would not be in private practice "but would function as part of a team where medical and other consultation services would be available" (Beck, 1972), and would serve "as instructors and supervisors for the untrained midwives and for nurses with only an elementary, deficient training in obstetric nursing" (Hemschemeyer, 1962). Despite such modest objectives, the plans for a midwifery service and school drew harsh opposition from many physicians, and several obstetricians resigned from the MCA Medical Board (Hsia, 1982). The service was established in a part of New York City that had poor housing, poverty, and high birth and infant death rates (Tom, 1982).

Mary Breckinridge sent an FNS nurse-midwife to start the school at the Lobenstine Clinic (Sharp, 1983). Selection of its first class of six students gave priority to public health nurses from states with high infant mortality and many untrained granny midwives (Hogan, 1975). The first four months of the ten-month curriculum were instruction in public health nursing; this part of the program was supervised by faculty of the Department of Nursing Education of Columbia University's Teachers College. The last six months were devoted to midwifery. Although this included observation and instruction in maternity hospitals, it was based primarily on home births and services provided at the clinic. The school established high standards at the outset. Most of the first students had already graduated from college, and many held master's degrees (Speert, 1980). In 1934 the first class of students graduated and the MCA assumed responsibility for the school. Although the original reason for starting the school was to prepare public health nurses to supervise untrained midwives, the emphasis evolved toward training nurse-midwives to provide direct midwifery care to women. During its twenty-six years of operation from 1932 to 1958, midwives of the Lobenstine/MCA program attended 7,099 births, most in the mother's home (Varney, 1978). The maternal mortality rate for MCA births was 0.9 per 1,000 live births; the national average during the same period was 10.4 per 1,000—more than ten times higher (Roberts, 1995b).

The Frontier Nursing Service hoped to establish a school of midwifery in conjunction with the University of Kentucky but was unable to raise enough money (Breckinridge, 1981). When the onset of World War II made it impossible to continue to recruit enough British nurse-midwives to meet its needs, FNS opened its own school—the country's second nurse-midwifery education program—in 1939. The Lobenstine and FNS schools were both based on adaptations of the British nurse-midwifery curriculum.

In 1941 a third school, the Tuskegee School of Nurse-Midwifery, was opened in Alabama with support provided by federal, state, and county funds. The purpose was to prepare nurse-midwives to provide maternity care to poor black women living in isolated parts of Alabama. Its students were black public health nurses. It closed in 1946 due to problems arising from racism. Although it graduated only twenty-five nurse-midwives, the program had a dramatic positive effect on the health of mothers and infants in the county in which it was based (Walsh, 1992). The fourth school to open was another short-lived program to train black nurse-midwives; the Flint-Goodridge School of Nurse-Midwifery opened in New Orleans in 1942 but graduated only two students and closed in 1943. It was a joint project of the Flint-Goodridge Hospital and Millard University (Tom, 1982).

The fifth nurse-midwifery education program was the Catholic Maternity Institute (CMI) School of Nurse-Midwifery, which was opened by MCA graduates who were members of the Medical Missionary Sisters of Philadelphia, a Roman Catholic order, in Santa Fe, New Mexico, in 1944. It was started in conjunction with a service that provided maternity care to Spanish-speaking women in the area around Sante Fe. This led to the opening of the first master's degree program for nurse-midwives, established in the nursing school of the Catholic University of America, in Washington, D.C., in 1947. Students could earn a nurse-midwifery certificate in the six-month program in Sante Fe (lengthened to one-year in 1954), or continue on to earn a master of science in nursing (MSN) degree from Catholic University. The nurse-midwifery certificate was issued by MCI, but the degree was issued by Catholic University (Roberts, 1995b).

All of the first five schools were developed in association with midwifery services designed to meet the needs of special populations—people cut off from other sources of care by geography, poverty, language barriers, or cultural and racial isolation. Although some were based in leading academic schools of nursing, none of these programs was associated with the mainstream of American health care. The founding of nurse-midwifery education by public health nurses and its location in poor, medically underserved communities led to the development of its particular long-standing and continuing emphasis on family-oriented health care, awareness of cultural and environmental factors, and collaboration with other disciplines (Walsh, 1992; Roberts, 1995b).

Twenty years after it opened the first nurse-midwifery education program, the Maternity Center Association published a monograph to share its experiences and thoughts about the future. The development of nurse-midwifery between 1933 and 1955 had been slow, in part, because of "connotations of untaught, non-professional midwifery." Recommendations for the future included that nurse-midwifery education should result in the granting of a diploma from a recognized university, development of standardized requirements for admission to any nurse-midwifery education program, and standardization of the curriculum (Sharp, 1983). MCA's commitment to basing nurse-midwifery education in university graduate schools led to the opening of a program in maternal and newborn health nursing within the graduate department of Yale University's School of Nursing in 1956 (Nickel *et al.*, 1992).

A workshop on nurse-midwifery education was held in Baltimore in 1958, by which time there were six nurse-midwifery programs, three that awarded certificates and three that offered master's degrees in addition to nurse-midwifery certificates (Roberts, 1995b). The workshop participants agreed that nurse-midwifery was a clinical nursing specialty. Although preparation at the master's level was considered desirable, they recognized that nondegree (certificate) programs would need to be continued and that faculty from both types of programs would need to develop joint educational standards. They discussed the need for a process to evaluate and accredit nurse-midwifery educational programs that would be separate or in addition to accreditation by the National League for Nursing. They also recognized the need to document nurse-midwifery practice so that the educational programs could be made compatible with the actual needs of the practitioner (Sharp, 1983).

The Work of the First Nurse-Midwives

The graduates of these programs were nurses as well as midwives; they were accustomed to working in organized health care programs. Except for graduates of the schools in Alabama and New Orleans, they were mainly white, native-born citizens—young, unmarried members of the middle class. Nurse-midwifery was new and different, blessed with the inspirational leadership of Mary Breckinridge, and challenged by a unifying commitment to improve the lives of poor mothers and their babies. Most nurse-midwives were imbued with a sense of midwifery as a social mission. Some were Catholic nuns. Unlike the foreign-trained midwives who preceded them, they did not set up private practices. They could not, even if they had wanted to because the laws of most states were extremely restrictive. Instead the new nurse-midwives worked for the Frontier Nursing Service in the rugged and isolated mountains of Kentucky or the Maternity Center Association in the slums of New York City, provided care to Hispanic families in New Mexico, served poor black families in Alabama, or joined missionary organizations and went to work in other countries. Some fulfilled MCA's expectation that they would work for the public health departments of states with many granny midwives. Most were public health nurses to begin with; many became leaders in that field. Others taught maternal and newborn nursing, were obstetric nursing supervisors or staff nurses, or worked in research or parent education (Thomas, 1965). Although nurse-midwives were in demand for these other roles, they were allowed to attend births only in rural areas where there were few if any doctors, or in inner-city areas such as Harlem, where few doctors chose to work.

Despite few opportunities for clinical midwifery practice, the early nurse-midwives planted many important, though slow-to-grow seeds of change in the rapidly expanding business of hospital childbirth. In 1947 the Maternity Center Association invited Grantly Dick-Read, the English obstetrician who had started the "natural childbirth movement" in Europe, to visit the United States. One consequence was a project developed jointly by MCA and the School of Medicine and School of Nursing at Yale University to prepare women for childbirth through education and exercise and to integrate childbirth education into maternity care (Nickel *et al.*, 1992). Nurse-midwives at Yale also played central roles in developing the concept and implementing a model for mother/baby "rooming-in" and studied the effects of childbirth education and unanesthetized labor and delivery on women and their births (Varney, 1987). Sister Mary Stella introduced the concept of "family-centered maternity care" in Evanston, Indiana, during the 1950s (Young, 1992). Ernestine Wiedenback, a renowned nursing educator who was one of the first to develop a cogent theory of professional nursing practice, became a nurse-midwife at the age of forty-six. After five years of nurse-midwifery practice at MCA in New York City, she went to Yale, where she eventually accepted a position as maternity nursing instructor for undergraduate nursing students. In addition to promoting nurse-midwifery education at Yale, Wiedenback authored the first nursing textbook with an emphasis on family-centered maternity nursing (Nickel *et al.*, 1992).

In 1955 the Columbia-Presbyterian-Sloan Hospital in New York City became the first mainstream medical institution to open its doors to nurse-midwives (Roush, 1979). Shortly thereafter, two nurse-midwives accepted positions as "obstetric assistants" in the Department of Obstetrics at Johns Hopkins. The evasive title was recommended by the physicians supporting the nurse-midwifery service because, in the words of Dr. Nicholson Eastman, "to the vast majority of obstetricians the very word midwife is anathema, whether or not it is coupled with the term nurse," and because "obstetric assistant" was thought to be more accurate in connoting "the main function which we would envisage for such nurses, namely, the rendering of skilled assistance to obstetricians" (Roberts, 1995b). Nevertheless, Dr. Eastman described the raison d'être of the nurse-midwife as "bringing a *quality* to maternity care that greatly enhanced its effects" (Beebe, 1979).

In 1959 MCA convened a meeting of groups and individuals interested in childbirth reform. It was attended by members of local childbirth education parent groups from throughout the country and resulted in the founding of the International Childbirth Education Association (Newton, 1986).

The Origins and First Work of the American College of Nurse-Midwives

Sixteen nurse-midwives in Kentucky formed the first American nurse-midwifery organiza-

tion. They incorporated it as the Kentucky State Association of Midwives in 1929. Although the name was later changed to the American Association of Nurse-Midwives (AANM), it was primarily an organization of graduates of the FNS (Tom, 1982).

In 1944 the National Organization for Public Health Nursing (NOPHN) established a section for nurse-midwives. Committees organized within the Midwifery Section of the NOPHN prepared a roster of all nurse-midwives in the United States, defined the practice of nurse-midwifery, and maintained data on nurse-midwives, the nurse-midwifery schools in existence at that time, and their curricula. By 1952 the Midwifery Section had developed a philosophy that emphasized pregnancy and childbearing as a normal process "and an important event in family growth and development." It also helped to develop, interpret, and popularize the concept of family-centered maternity care (Tom, 1982).

The NOPHN was dissolved in 1952, during the formation of the American Nurses' Association (ANA) and the National League for Nursing (NLN). Although nurse-midwives were elected to leadership positions in the Maternal and Child Health Council of the NLN, they found themselves combined with nurses involved in pediatrics, orthopedics, school nursing, and the care of children with physical disabilities, as well as nurses involved in maternity care (Hogan, 1975). In addition, although individual nurse-midwives were recognized as authorities in maternal and child health, many of their colleagues did not know that they were midwives. This lack of recognition was unacceptable to nurse-midwives, who were fighting for recognition of their profession. Sister Theophane Shoemaker (then director of the Catholic Maternity Institute in Santa Fe, New Mexico) wrote to the presidents of both of the ANA and the NLN, seeking a specific niche for nurse-midwives within one of the new nursing organizations. The responses were not encouraging; officers of both organizations felt that nurse-midwifery was really part of medicine, and thus did not belong in an organization for nurses or nursing* (Tom, 1980).

The twenty nurse-midwives who attended the ANA's convention in 1954 formed a Committee on Organization. In May 1955 the Committee on Organization voted unanimously to form the American College of Nurse-Midwifery (ACNM), which held its first annual meeting the following November (Varney, 1978). Its initial goals were to study, develop, and evaluate standards for nurse-midwifery education; to support and assist in the development of nurse-midwifery services and education programs, in association with allied professional groups; to evaluate and approve nurse-midwifery education programs and services; to sponsor nurse-midwifery research; to develop relationships with medicine, nursing, and midwives in other countries; and to participate in the International Confederation of Midwives (Sharp, 1983; Walsh, 1991). The professional journal began with the first *Nurse-Midwife Bulletin*, dated December 1955, which was mimeographed and mailed to 468 nurse-midwives. A Committee on Curriculum and Accreditation was formed in 1957. In 1968 the American College of Nurse-Midwifery merged with the Kentucky-based American Association of Nurse-Midwives and changed its name to the American College of Nurse-Midwives. The *Nurse-Midwife Bulletin* became the *Journal of Nurse-Midwifery* in 1974 (Shah, 1975).

The Move into University Medical Centers and High-Volume Charity Hospitals

When the Frontier Nursing Service and the Maternity Center Association schools were founded, most American births took place in homes. During the 1930s the place of birth began to shift to hospitals—a shift that accelerated at the end of World War II. Advances in medical technology during the war enhanced the role of hospitals in American health care. Shortly after the war ended, Congress approved the Hill-Burton program, which provided large amounts of federal and state money for constructing hospitals. Whereas hospitals accounted for only 37 percent of births in 1935, 88 percent of all U.S. births occurred in hospitals in 1950, and 97 percent were in hospitals in 1960. Nurse-midwives were not welcome in hospitals, which were physicians' turf. For thirty years FNS's small hospital in Hyden, Kentucky, was the only American hospital in which nurse-midwives attended births.

The first hospital-based nurse-midwifery services were established within the obstetric services of medical school-affiliated, publicly funded hospitals that cared for the urban poor. Columbia University's graduate program in maternal nursing, started in 1955, was the first nurse-midwifery educational program to provide clinical training in an academic medical center. It was a cooperative program involving the Department of Nursing and the School of Public Health and Administrative Medicine of Columbia University, the obstetrics and gynecology departments of the Presbyterian-Sloan Hospital and the Kings County Hospital, and the Maternity Center Association (MCA). Graduates received master of science degrees in nursing and nurse-midwifery certificates. MCA was instrumental in starting similar educational programs at Johns Hopkins Hospital and at the Yale University School of Nursing in 1956. In 1958, MCA moved its own program, which had been in operation since 1932, to the State University of New York Downstate Medical Center.

The medical schools' interest in nurse-midwives derived in part from the need to provide better clinical experience for physicians who were training to be obstetrician–gynecologists (Hellman, 1975). Although

---

*The American Nurses' Association did not recognize nurse-midwifery as a specialty within nursing until 1968 (Roberts, 1995b).

earlier academic obstetricians had opposed midwives in part to increase the supply of obstetric patients for training physicians, the postwar "baby boom" reversed the problem from too few obstetric patients to too many. City- and county-supported hospitals provided the main clinical experience for medical students, interns, and residents at most of the country's best medical schools. In return, the schools assumed responsibility for all medical care provided in those hospitals. Obstetric residency training programs became overwhelmed by the huge numbers of poor women who were going to those hospitals to have their babies. Although most of them had normal pregnancies, the large number of deliveries left little time and energy for the young doctors to learn and the professors to develop the nascent but needed subspecialties of gynecology and high-risk obstetrics. Heads of some academic obstetrics and gynecology departments began to view nurse-midwives as a potential source of relief (Hellman, 1975).

These programs created opportunities for nurse-midwives to practice in hospitals. However, nurse-midwifery practice had to change when its largest services and educational programs moved into hospitals and came under the authority of academic obstetricians. In hospitals it was possible for nurse-midwives to take care of women with complications that would have made them ineligible for midwifery care at home. In addition, it was difficult for, a few nurse-midwives to affect policies and practices in a hospital. This was a significant departure from nurse-midwifery practice in homes or maternity centers, where the nurse-midwife had control (Sharp, 1980). Thus negative as well as positive effects resulted from these new opportunities—attenuation of nurse-midwives' control over their practice, including the need to incorporate procedures such as frequent use of episiotomies; greater medical influence on their educational programs; and loss of home birth experience for their students.

Chapter 4
Midwifery Amid
the Social Movements of
the 1960s and 1970s

The nation entered the 1960s having been forced by Martin Luther King, Jr., and the civil rights movement to face the realities of poverty and racial injustice and acknowledge their moral and social costs. The country was ready to move beyond the self-satisfaction that followed our victory in World War II; change was in the air. John Kennedy declared his presidency to be symbolic of the passing of responsibility to a new generation and challenged all Americans to ask what they could do for their country. America was prosperous, and more and more young people were going to college. The birth control pill became available in 1960. We started a space program and asserted our intention to send an American to the moon. There was a sense that we could not only face but solve our problems, in part through federal laws and government programs. When President Kennedy was killed, President Johnson undertook an even more ambitious legislative agenda, signing new national civil rights leg-

islation and declaring a "War on Poverty." But more leaders were gunned down, and we became deeply enmeshed in an unpopular, unwinnable war in Southeast Asia. Ultimately much of the energy and optimism of this period was focused in new directions. Young women began to meet to "raise their consciousness" about gender discrimination and their sense of their own potential power. Many young people wanted and took more freedom and were more emotionally and educationally able to question or defy traditional sources of authority. Some simply turned their backs on "establishment" society, creating their own "counterculture."

The effects of the energy and turmoil of this period permeated society and created new conditions for midwifery: growing recognition of societal responsibility for the well-being of children and the importance of the quality of childbearing; federal initiatives and programs to finance and provide health care, especially obstetric care and family planning, to indigent women; the training of new kinds of health care professionals, who were needed to meet the expanded demand for health care created by the new federal programs; women who were better informed, more critical health care consumers; growing use of sophisticated technology as part of routine obstetric care; an "epidemic" of teenage pregnancies, and an antiauthority culture of sexually active young people who were critical of obstetricians and needed someone to help them birth their babies.

In 1963 the Children's Bureau sponsored the first national survey of nurse-midwives in the United States. Of 535 nurse-midwives living in the country at that time, only 34 (6.4 percent) were providing direct clinical midwifery care that included management of labor and delivery. Most of the practicing nurse-midwives worked in Kentucky, New Mexico, or New York City—the only three jurisdictions with laws that clearly sanctioned their practice. A few worked in Georgia, Maryland, and South Carolina, where nurse-midwives could practice under laws intended for granny midwives. Two worked under a temporary legal arrangement developed for a special demonstration project in Madera County, California (Thomas, 1965). The Children's Bureau survey was conducted thirty-eight years after the Frontier Nursing Service was established; its findings documented the slow and tenuous beginnings of nurse-midwifery.

During the 1970s the social changes that began during the 1960s propelled nurse-midwifery into a period of rapid growth. By 1976, nurse-midwifery practice was legal in all but a few midwestern states and nurse-midwives were practicing in every region of the country (Forman & Cooper, 1976). The number of educational programs increased from seven in 1960 to nineteen in 1979 (Adams, 1984). The number of babies delivered by certified nurse-midwives in hospitals more than doubled between 1975 and 1979. Most nurse-midwives practicing in 1979 worked in services that provided care to low-

income women. A few had established private practices, and nurse-midwives were playing an important role in the health care programs run by the Indian Health Service, the military services, and some health maintenance organizations. In addition, although granny midwives had become nearly extinct, a new kind of lay midwife emerged and gained prominence in response to a widening interest in home births.

Support for Nurse-Midwives as Health Care Providers for the Poor

The need to provide effective care to poor and medically underserved pregnant women had motivated the importation of nurse-midwifery to America. The Frontier Nursing Service and the Catholic Maternity Institute were started to help poor mothers and children in rural Kentucky and New Mexico. The Maternity Center Association and the programs it helped to start were developed to serve poor inner-city families in New York and other cities of the U. S. eastern seaboard. By 1960, the medical literature contained several articles that reported reductions in maternal and infant mortality and morbidity in such populations after the introduction of nurse-midwifery care:

- In 1955 the *American Journal of Obstetrics and Gynecology* published an article that reported the outcomes of the care provided to 5,765 pregnant women during the Maternity Center Association's first twenty years of operation (1931–1951). MCA nurse-midwives had delivered 87 percent of the women in their own homes. Their maternal mortality ratio of 8.8 per 10,000 live births was far lower than the national ratio, which was 31.7 per 10,000 at the midpoint of that period (1941). MCA obtained these good outcomes despite a high incidence of poor nutrition, poor home conditions, low income, unmarried mothers, and high parity among the women served by the nurse-midwives (Laird, 1955).

• The Frontier Nursing Service kept careful statistics and evaluated its progress after every thousand births. All maternal and infant outcome statistics for FNS's first thirty years of operation (1925–1954) were better than for the country as a whole, despite extreme poverty in the area and a high proportion of pregnancies carried by women at the extremes of the childbearing age span and by women of very high parity. The biggest differences were in the maternal mortality rate (9.1 per 10,000 births for FNS, compared with 34 per 10,000 for the United States as a whole) and low birth weight (3.8 percent for FNS, compared with 7.6 percent for the country) (Browne & Isaacs, 1976). In 1958 the Metropolitan Life Insurance Company of New York published a report which estimated that national implementation of services like those of the FNS would prevent at least 60,000 perinatal deaths each year (Metropolitan Life Insurance Company, 1958).

These positive findings encouraged the development of other nurse-midwifery services, including a demonstration project that was started in Madera County, California, in 1960. Although midwifery was illegal in California, a special law allowed nurse-midwives (referred to as "nurse obstetrical assistants") to practice in a state-supported project designed to alleviate chronic physician shortages in a rural hospital that served the entire population of Madera County. Although the project documented improved pregnancy outcomes associated with the introduction of nurse-midwifery care, the special law was rescinded and the project was terminated in 1963. In 1968 a team of researchers conducted a retrospective study of maternity care and outcomes in Madera County before, during, and after the project (Levy *et al.*, 1971). They found a significant increase in attendance at prenatal clinics and large reductions in both prematurity (from 11.0 to 6.4 percent of all births) and neonatal deaths (from 23.9 to

10.3 per 1,000 live births) during the three-year project and reversal of these improvements after the midwives left. Even though additional physicians moved into the area and were providing services after the project ended, loss of the nurse-midwifery service was associated with a rebound in the incidence of prematurity (to 9.8 percent) and neonatal deaths (to 32.1 per 1,000 live births).

In 1968, the Josiah Macy, Jr., Foundation convened a conference on "The Midwife in the United States." The conferees were asked to address problems in the provision of maternal and child health care. Dr. George Silver, then deputy assistant secretary of the Department of Health, Education and Welfare (now the Department of Health and Human Services, DHHS), opened the conference with a discussion of the country's "failure to cope adequately with the maternal and child health needs of our people. Despite our affluence, our abundance of resources, our (comparatively) ample supply of professional people, our enormous expenditures over thirty years on maternal and child health programs," Silver reported, "infant mortality in the United States stands at 24.8 compared with Sweden's 14.2." He went on to describe the "shameful and humiliating circumstances" under which care was being provided to women who were poor, black, or members of other minority groups in "our great public hospital clinics": "50 to 100 women who wait to be examined, in a two and a half hour clinic session, by a busy resident who ordinarily is called away to a delivery before 10 per cent of the patients have been seen." Silver blamed these conditions for the fact that many women never came for prenatal care (Silver, 1968).

Everyone acknowledged the need for more people to take care of the large numbers of women having babies in inner-city municipal hospitals. Many speakers, however, went beyond concern about the *quantitative* problem and spoke of the *qualitative benefits* of nurse-midwifery care. Dr. Donald Swartz, professor of obstetrics and gynecology at Columbia University College of Physicians and Surgeons, explained his decision to start a nurse-midwifery service at Harlem Hospital, where, he said, the "conditions and attitudes of callousness . . . almost defy description." During his residency training at Johns Hopkins he had been impressed with "the interest, competence, and indeed dedication which the nurse-midwife brought to the problems of obstetric care." He knew of the long-standing emphasis of the Maternity Center Association and the American College of Nurse-Midwives on patient-centered and family-centered maternity care and felt that "the introduction of staff with these attitudes and emphases would reinforce greatly all other effort to produce a more humanitarian quality of service" (Swartz, 1968).

Despite these accolades, there was wide agreement that nurse-midwives should be restricted to hospitals and caring for the poor. Dr. Silver warned that "without careful and effective preventive measures, we may be faced with a new profession in private entrepreneurial practice, a development which must be avoided at all costs." The director of gynecology and obstetrics at Johns Hopkins University made the same point in presenting his vision of the nurse-midwife as someone who "will function in a medical center, where adequate physician consultation is available and where she will be a member of the team concentrating on total maternity care—antepartum, intrapartum, postpartum, family planning and so forth. She will most certainly not go into private practice by herself, nor will she move towards a return to domiciliary care" (Barnes, 1968). As long as nurse-midwives remained salaried hospital employees, they were not seen as a threat to the authority of physicians (Hsia, 1984).

In addition to certain academic obstetric leaders, support for nurse-midwifery came primarily from those with responsibility for public health, as illustrated in the following examples:

- In 1968 the New York City Department of Health began a program to recruit nurse-midwives and facilitate their employment at twelve hospitals affiliated with its Maternal and Infant Care (MIC) projects (Harris *et al.*, 1971). Because of the immense need in New York City, the MIC program could offer a clinical service position to almost all graduates of the increasing number of nurse-midwifery education programs. In addition, New York's MIC program drew attention, becoming a model for MIC programs in many other cities (Lang, 1995). The use of certified nurse-midwives (CNMs) has since became a permanent attribute of many New York City hospitals.

- Senator Robert Kennedy's 1965 visit through the Mississippi Delta country resulted in a federally funded County Health Improvement Program for Holmes County, Mississippi, which was started in 1969. To prepare nurse-midwives for this project, the federal Division of Nursing provided funds to begin a post-baccalaureate nurse-midwifery education program based in the Department of Obstetrics and Gynecology at the University of Mississippi School of Medicine. The education program began to receive support through grants from the federal Maternal and Child Health Service in 1971. Although the original plan required students entering the program to be nurses with bachelor's degrees, this criterion made most Mississippi nurses ineligibile for the program, and few applied. In response to this situation, the University of Mississippi also began to offer a certificate nurse-midwifery education program that would accept nurses without degrees. Large numbers of nurses from throughout the southeastern region, as well as other parts of the country, applied (Yzodinma, 1995). The infant mortality rate in Holmes County declined from 42.5 to 21.8 per 1,000 births during the first three years of the nurse-midwifery project (Meglen & Burst, 1974).

In 1972 another component of the Department of Health, Education and Welfare provided funds to enable the University of Mississippi to expand the nurse-midwifery education program, making it able to accept much larger numbers of students. The purpose of the expansion was to prepare nurse-midwives to work in Alabama, Florida, Georgia, Louisiana, Mississippi, and South Carolina. A Maternal and Child Health (MCH) Services grant paid the tuition of nurse-midwifery students who agreed to practice for at least one year after graduation in any of the six specified states. Federal funds were also used to help the new graduates find and establish clinical practice sites in one of those states, including a "seed team" agreement under which salaries for a team of nurse-midwives were paid for one year if a hospital or private medical practice promised to continue support after that time.

• Federal funds were used to establish a nurse-midwifery service to serve low- to moderate-income women who had no private physicians and lived in four specified southeastern Georgia counties. The program was started in 1972 in response to the high proportion of women from those counties who arrived at the Glynn-Brunswick Memorial Hospital for delivery having had little or no prenatal care. Working under the direction of the chairman of the obstetrics and gynecology department of the hospital, the nurse-midwives provided prenatal care, including referral of high-risk cases to physicians; delivered women with normal pregnancies; and coordinated postpartum follow-up, well-baby care, and family planning services with the county health departments (Reid & Morris, 1979).

An evaluation compared birth outcomes and estimated expenditures for perinatal care provided to women from the four-county service area during twelve-month periods before and after the program began. The infant mortality rate for the four counties decreased and the target population experienced decreases in preterm births, low birth weight, and neonatal mortality. The low birth weight rate went from 24 percent before to 14 percent after implementation of the nurse-midwifery service. Estimated expenditures for perinatal care in the four counties also decreased, even though costs of neonatal care were not included in the estimate. The birth rate dropped in the four-country project area but not in seven other nearby counties. The researchers hypothesized that the family planning services provided by the nurse-midwives may have accounted for this difference and a related decline in expenditures. However, there was also a reduction in expenditures per pregnant woman between the two time periods, including reductions in costs for personnel and for hospitalization following delivery (Reid & Morris, 1979).

• Other Children's Bureau MCH grants were used to help the Indian Health Service (IHS) develop its nurse-midwifery program. The IHS hired its first nurse-midwife in 1969. She was sent to Bethel, Alaska, a remote community that had the nation's highest infant mortality rate and was accessible only by airplane or boat. In 1971 the Bureau of Maternal and Child Health gave grants to the University of Utah and Johns Hopkins University to develop nurse-midwifery services in the Shiprock, Fort Defiance, and Chinle Service Units of the Navajo Reservation in Arizona and New Mexico. Nurse-midwives were also sent to Pine Ridge, South Dakota, and the Apache Reservation in Arizona (Milligan, 1995). A study of the outcomes of nurse-midwifery services provided to Navajo women at Fort Defiance, Arizona, between 1969 and 1974 reported a decline in the low birth weight rate—

from 10.7 percent during a period before the service was started to 5.5 percent during the first five years of the nurse-midwifery service (Ross, 1981). In 1977 the University of Arizona opened a nurse-midwifery education program and assumed responsibility for the Johns Hopkins Navajo Reservation services.

- In 1978 National Health Service Corps scholarships that paid a stipend for living expenses as well as all educational expenses became available to nurse-midwifery students who agreed to work in needy areas of the country.

Special Nurse-Midwifery Services for Care of Pregnant Adolescents

Special nurse-midwifery services were also developed to provide supportive care to pregnant teenagers and assist them in adapting to motherhood and avoiding additional unplanned pregnancies. Although the fertility rate for teenagers declined during the 1960s and 1970s, fertility of older women declined more sharply and, because of the post–World War II baby boom, large numbers of Americans were entering their teens. As a result, the proportion of all births in which the mother was a teenager increased and teenage pregnancy was seen as an "epidemic" with serious effects on young unmarried girls, their babies, and society in general. Younger and younger teens were getting pregnant; the fertility rate for girls younger than 15 increased until 1973, while fertility of all other age groups was declining (Centers for Disease Control, 1978). By the mid-1970s, approximately one million fifteen- to nineteen-year-olds were becoming pregnant each year, as well as thirty thousand girls younger than fifteen. Although many had abortions, more than six hundred thousand babies were born to teenagers in 1974 (Alan Guttmacher Institute, 1976). In addition, the proportion of teenage mothers who were unmarried was increasing. More than half of all out-of-wedlock births in 1974

were to teenagers; the problem was greatest among blacks.

The incidence of complications and bad outcomes was—and remains—much higher among teens. The maternal mortality rate was higher for teenagers than for women in their twenties—60 percent higher for girls younger than fifteen—and their infants were twice as likely to have a low birth weight and three times as likely to die (Alan Guttmacher Institute, 1976). Poor outcomes were associated with high-risk social situations; yet those at the highest risk seemed to receive the least adequate medical care (Chase, 1973). Responsibility for providing care to unwed pregnant teens fell heavily to government-subsidized services.

Many special programs were developed to try to provide care that would attract and engage pregnant teenagers and improve their pregnancy outcomes. This was and remains a complex challenge, requiring the ability to deal successfully with the nutritional and other physical needs and potential problems related to pregnancy, as well as the social, emotional, sexual, educational, and developmental needs and problems of adolescent girls, the latter compounded by the massive physical and social role changes inherent in being pregnant and becoming a mother. In many, if not most cases, these needs are compounded again by problems such as economic insecurity, if not outright poverty, inadequate social support, domestic violence, low self-esteem, depression, and poorly developed problem-solving, communication, money management, and homemaking skills.

State and local health agencies and various departments within academic medical centers and universities designed and pilot tested special programs, most of which utilized a variety of support services and the contributions of many disciplines. Although relatively few were available, nurse-midwives were utilized as the primary care providers in special programs in New Haven, Connecticut (Klerman & Jekel, 1973); Rochester, New

York (McAnarney *et al.*, 1978); New York City (Doyle & Widhalm, 1979; Chanis *et al.*, 1979); and Charleston, South Carolina (Corbett & Burst, 1976).

An evening clinic program for Hispanic and black adolescents at Lincoln Hospital in the South Bronx emphasized education about nutrition, efforts to discourage smoking, self-care during the postpartum period, family planning, and physical care and mental stimulation of the newborn. During the first two years of the program, the average maternal weight gain increased from twenty-one pounds to twenty-eight pounds, average newborn weights increased by a full pound, and the incidence of low birth weight decreased from 18.1 to 6.3 percent (Doyle & Widhalm, 1979).

The adolescent clinic run by the nurse-midwifery service at the Medical University Hospital in Charleston, South Carolina, was evaluated through a study that randomly assigned 270 teenagers who met criteria for the nurse-midwifery service to either the nurse-midwifery clinic or clinics run by ob-gyn residents (physicians in specialty training). Because the nurse-midwives emphasized prenatal education and nutrition counseling, the evaluation examined outcomes that might be expected to improve with better nutrition. The nurse-midwifery patients were less likely to develop preeclampsia (21 versus 26 percent), but were somewhat more likely to develop anemia (18 versus 13 percent). However, among teenagers who were anemic at some time during their pregnancy, those who received care from nurse-midwives were much more likely to have normal hematocrits when they delivered (83 percent) as compared with the physicians' patients (53 percent). The incidence of low birth weight (<2,500 grams) was small and the same (3 percent) for both groups of teenagers. However, infants whose mothers attended the nurse-midwives' clinic were more likely to weigh at least 3,000 grams, whereas most of the babies of the obstetric residents' pa-

tients weighed between 2,500 and 2,999 grams (Corbett & Burst, 1976).

A prenatal clinic for girls younger than seventeen years of age at Kings County Hospital Center in New York City tried to create opportunities for peer interaction and exchange of information between pregnant teens and emphasized education about fetal development, nutrition, hygiene during pregnancy, preparation for labor and delivery, infant care, and family planning. Evaluation of this program compared the incidence of low birth weight and perinatal mortality for ninety-eight low-risk girls who attended the nurse-midwifery clinic with outcomes for eighty-five teens who attended the regular clinic and fifty-one girls who delivered at Kings County but had not come for prenatal care. Teenagers who met high-risk criteria were assigned to a special clinic and were excluded from the study. The incidence of low birth weight was lower for teens cared for by the nurse-midwives (9 percent) than for either of the other groups—15 percent for those in the regular teen clinic and 14 percent for those with no prenatal care (Chanis *et al.*, 1979).

Grouping Nurse-Midwives with Nurse Practitioners and Physician Assistants

The development of two new categories of health care providers—nurse practitioners (NPs) and physician assistants (PAs)—had important effects on nurse-midwifery. The first training programs for both were started in 1965 in response to a shortage of physicians to care for people living in rural and inner-city areas.

Obstetrics and gynecology was one of the first fields to develop nurse practitioners. Obstetric and gynecologic nurse practitioners, sometimes called "women's health care nurse practitioners," are prepared to provide the routine and time-consuming ambulatory services that are such a large part of obstetric and gynecologic care: ten to twelve prenatal visits by each woman during pregnancy, a routine visit four to six weeks after the birth, yearly visits for cervical and breast cancer screening, and office or clinic-based care for contraception and a range of common gynecologic problems, including sexually transmitted diseases.

During the 1970s, nurse-midwives became grouped with NPs, and sometimes also with PAs, in a variety of state and federal laws and other initiatives aimed at supporting both or all three categories of practitioners. The combined group was first referred to as "physician extenders," then as "new practitioners," and, most recently, as "midlevel health care providers." The regulations developed to allow for the practice of these "new" categories of health professionals (nurse-midwives were not new) was not intended to create independent practitioners. Most required significant degrees of physician involvement, ranging from direct supervision to written agreements (Myers, 1986; Cohn *et al.*, 1984). *Most nurse-midwives now practice under state laws that regulate nurse practitioners.*

The Impact of Major Federal Government Programs

During the 1960s and 1970s the federal government started several programs that had significant impacts on nurse-midwifery. Medicare and Medicaid were signed into law on July 30, 1965. The objective was to allow the poor to buy into the mainstream of medical care. However, unlike Medicare, Medicaid set limits on the amount it would pay for specified medical services and did not allow physicians to charge more. Neither the federal government nor the states were willing to pay enough to attract large numbers of obstetricians to participate in Medicaid (Starr, 1982). This situation stimulated the creation of special programs to provide maternity care to Medicaid-eligible women. Those programs created greatly increased employment opportunities and demand for nurse-midwives and a wider base of political

support for changing state laws to enable them to practice.

The federal government also began to support the development of family planning services for the poor, beginning with the Office of Economic Opportunity in 1965. Enactment of the Family Planning Services and Population Research Act of 1970 (Title X of the Public Health Services Act) greatly expanded the number of sites providing contraceptive care. From the beginning of the political debate on the bill that resulted in this law, family planning advocates argued that it would be important to use nurse practitioners and nurse-midwives to staff the new family planning services—because of a shortage of physicians and because nursing-based practitioners would take a broader, more effective approach to family planning. Some physician leaders of the family planning movement were also important supporters of nurse-midwifery, and, except for those with religious objections, there was wide support for family planning among nurse-midwives, who had seen the ill effects of unplanned, unwanted pregnancies. Consequently, nurse-midwives were among the first health care providers to learn how to prescribe oral contraceptives and insert intrauterine devices (IUDs). Family planning is now one of the essential "core competencies" of a certified nurse-midwife.

The Children's Bureau began to fund selected nurse-midwifery education programs in about 1960; the Division of Nursing began to fund them in 1976. When the Children's Bureau was dissolved in 1970, its support of nurse-midwifery education was continued by the Maternal and Child Health (MCH) Bureau of the Health Resources and Services Administration, an agency of the Public Health Service. Both the Division of Nursing and the MCH Bureau still support some nurse-midwifery programs. More than half of the nurse-midwives who graduated during the 1960s and nearly two-thirds of those who graduated during the 1970s received financial aid through one of these two programs (Rooks *et al.*, 1978; Adams, 1984).

Federal funding for the training of nurse practitioners, physician assistants, and nurse-midwives began to increase in response to President Nixon's annual health message of 1971, which emphasized the need to increase the availability of primary-care manpower. A series of federal acts passed between 1971 and 1977 authorized federal funds to support training programs and stipends for trainees and developed the principle of linking the use of these funds to federal priorities related to the geographic maldistribution of physicians and other indicators of unequal access to health care.* Passage of the Nurse Training Act in 1975 provided a relatively stable source of funding, with bureaucratic management of funds for nurse-midwifery education based in the Division of Nursing.

Childbirth Care During the 1960s and 1970s

By 1960, hospitalization for childbirth was almost universal in the United States. Women had left their homes and families to have their babies alone in hospitals in hope of greater safety and decreased pain. Of nearly 56,000 pregnancies included in the National Institute of Neurological Disease and Stroke (NINDS) Collaborative Perinatal Study (data collected at twelve major hospitals between 1959 and 1965), all but 8 percent of the white women and 26 percent of the black women were anesthetized during the delivery (National Institute of Neurological Disease and Stroke, 1972). With routine obstetrical anesthesia and analgesia, labor was no longer "normal" and parturient women found it necessary to assume the hospitalized "sick patient" role. Groggy and stupe-

fied during labor and asleep or sleepy at delivery, women as cognizant individuals were no longer involved in the process of giving birth. Physicians delivered their babies and were thanked by the grateful fathers, who had not been present at the births. When she woke up the mother had to ask whether her baby, now in a central nursery, was a boy or a girl.

Eventually it was recognized that systemic painkillers depress not only the mother's but also the baby's respirations and nervous system, and general anesthesia for obstetrics was gradually abandoned. However, the spinal anesthesia that replaced it often slows the pace of labor, encouraging early artificial rupture of the fetal membranes and use of oxytocin to hasten the delivery. In addition, women whose lower bodies had been paralyzed had limited mobility and tended to labor and deliver on their backs—a position in which the pelvic outlet is tilted *up*. For that reason and because sleeping or paralyzed women could not use their voluntary muscles, forceps were often needed to deliver their babies. In some hospitals, use of forceps became routine. Forceps were used during 57 percent of the vaginal deliveries of white women in the NINDS Collaborative Perinatal Study. Episiotomies[†] also became routine, in part because they were necessary to accommodate forceps, and because of concern that perineal muscles and tissues stretched by childbirth would not return to their normal structure and function. This concern addressed health problems that could be serious but which became uncommon as couples began to limit the size of their families. Despite the declining proportion of high parity births, it was estimated

<hr>

* The Nurse Training Act of 1971, the Emergency Health Personnel Act Amendments of 1972, the Nurse Training Act of 1975, The Health Professions Education Assistance Act of 1976, The Health Services Extension Act of 1977, and the Rural Health Clinics Service Act of 1977.

† An episiotomy is an incision made to enlarge the vaginal outlet. The incision is usually made from the most posterior aspect of the vaginal opening in a straight line towards the anus. When a large episiotomy is needed, or when there is danger that the episiotomy might extend into the anus and rectum, the episiotomy may be cut so that it angles away from the anus.

that episiotomies were performed during more than 70 percent of deliveries that occurred in the United States in 1977 (Cogan & Edmunds, 1977).

A machine to enable continuous monitoring of the fetal heart rate (electronic fetal monitoring, or EFM) was introduced in 1960 (Hon, 1960). The fetal heart rate can be monitored externally, using ultrasound, or internally, by attaching electrodes directly to the fetus while in utero. When first used, EFM was applied mainly during high-risk or complicated labors. However, the desire to keep constant surveillance of every fetus throughout labor was almost irresistible. By 1979 EFM was being used during more than half of all labors and had been implicated in a rapid and alarming rise in the rate of cesarean sections (Banta & Thacker, 1979). Like anesthesia, EFM has a pervasive effect on women's experiences during labor. The electrical lines necessary for its use tether women to their beds and bedside equipment; many become hesitant to move because it is sometimes hard to maintain a clear EFM signal and the signal may become disrupted when the mother changes her position.

The natural childbirth, childbirth education, and breast-feeding movements entered the 1960s with a full head of steam. The 1956 founding of La Leche League led to the creation of a network of support for women interested in pregnancy, childbirth, and breast-feeding. Publication of *Thank You Dr. Lamaze* in 1959 resulted in greatly increased public interest in natural childbirth. The International Childbirth Education Association (ICEA), founded in 1959, and the American Society for Psychoprophylaxis in Obstetrics (ASPO), founded in 1960, began to certify childbirth educators and provide curricula for classes to prepare both parents for active roles during labor and delivery. *Husband-Coached Childbirth* was published in 1965, followed by *Awake and Aware* in 1966. Information and techniques promulgated through these publications

and organizations had the potential to completely change the role of hospitalized women during labor and delivery. Instead of being passively delivered by obstetricians, prepared women could be active participants who contributed to their infant's health by avoiding medications, assuming the most advantageous positions during labor, and using controlled muscle contractions to enhance the involuntary processes. Women could make a conscious and personal contribution to the safe births of their babies and be proud of their strength, self-discipline, and will. By the early 1970s, childbirth educators and the women and men who took their classes were fighting for the right of husbands to stay with their wives throughout labor and to be present in the delivery room (Bing, 1974).

The barriers to implementing these concepts were extraordinary. Most hospitals did not allow husbands into delivery rooms, separated mothers from their newborns, used interventions developed for high-risk or complicated cases on an ever-increasing proportion of women, and routinized the use of uncomfortable, disruptive procedures. Although some hospitals responded to women's criticisms and demands, the changes they made were superficial (Weitz & Sullivan, 1993). During the early 1990s a childbirth educator in Seattle interviewed twenty women who had taken her classes in the 1970s, during their first pregnancies. Although they had wanted natural childbirth, their childbirth care was "typical of that time," often including use of oxytocin to start or increase labor; enemas; perineal shaving; restriction to bed; nothing to eat or drink; intravenous infusions; manual pressure on the uterus during delivery; episiotomies; use of surgical drapes, masks, caps, and gowns; and frequent use of forceps, systemic tranquilizers and narcotics, and regional anesthesia. Few of the women had private rooms during labor. Their husbands were rarely present; if present during labor, they were asked to leave during vaginal examinations and the birth itself. The baby was kept in the nursery except for day-time feedings. The women were hospitalized for four or five days postpartum, during which heat lamps were used to treat their episiotomy pain (Simkin, 1991). There was little encouragement or help for breast-feeding. In many hospitals, the administration of a large dose of estrogen—to inhibit lactation—was part of the routine "orders" for all postpartum women; breast-feeding was not routine (Rooks, 1978).

Deep dissatisfaction and anger about this situation resulted in a variety of responses:

- A highly publicized lay and professional critique of American obstetric practices took place at professional meetings and in professional journals, as well as in books,* general newspapers, and women's magazines. In 1978 and 1979 this criticism culminated in congressional hearings on the risks and benefits of four common obstetric interventions† and a series of federal government agency reports.‡

- Several new organizations were started to support and promote midwifery and home births.**
- Some childbirth educators and members of La Leche League began to attend home births (Ventre, 1992).

Consumer criticism of aggressive medical management of childbirth occurred within the context of other significant social and cultural forces of the 1960s and 1970s, including the civil rights movement, the women's movement, the consumer movement, the antiwar movement, and the back-to-nature/health food movement started by the hippies. The ideas, experiences, and values resulting from these dynamic social movements led to a diminution of trust in authority figures and bureaucratic institutions, concern that technology was running rampant and would denigrate important human values, and increasing recognition of the importance of emotional, social, and behavioral factors as causes of disease and of the importance of psychological, cultural, and spiritual factors as sources of strength and healing. "The pill" was introduced in 1960. The availability of this and other effective methods of contraception, as well as other influences on the "baby boom" generation, resulted in a one- or two-child family norm. Together these changes led to the development of a clientele of well-informed, assertive, middle-class women who planned to have few or perhaps only one baby; wanted birth to be a very special, rich, and emotionally satisfying experience; believed that medicines and invasive techniques were used too often during childbirth and were dangerous; were accustomed to exercising choice as consumers; and sought a nonauthoritarian maternity care provider with

---

*For example, *Witches, Midwives and Nurses*, by Barbara Ehrenreich and Deirdre English (1973), which described women's historic roles as healers and the self-serving role of physicians in the demise of midwifery in the United States, and *Immaculate Deception*, by Suzanne Arms (1975), which questioned the medical profession's view of childbirth and the scientific validity of many obstetric practices.

†Obstetrical Practices in the United States, a hearing before the Subcommittee on Health and Scientific Research of the Committee on Human Resources, United States Senate, Ninety-fifth Congress, April 17, 1978.

‡For example, "Evaluating Benefits and Risks of Obstetric Practices—More Coordinated Federal and Private Efforts Needed," Report to the Congress by the Comptroller General of the United States; "Costs and Benefits of Electronic Fetal Monitoring: A Review of the Literature," published by the National Center for Health Services Research; and "An Evaluation of Caesarean Section in the United States," a report commissioned by the Office of the Assistant Secretary of Health for Planning and Evaluation.

**For example, the National Association of Parents & Professionals for Safe Alternatives in Childbirth, the Association for Childbirth at Home International, the American College of Home Obstetrics, and Home Oriented Maternity Experience.

whom they could deal on the basis of mutual respect.

Some of these consumers wanted and were willing to search for a midwife to take care of them. Before the mid-1970s, nurse-midwives had essentially taken care of the poor. Social and cultural changes during and since the 1970s created a receptivity and demand for midwifery care among private patients. However, it was difficult for a woman to find a source of nurse-midwifery care, and some of the women who wanted midwives were not satisfied with nurse-midwifery or criticized nurse-midwives for being unwilling to leave or condemn the practices of the institutions in which they worked (Myers-Ciecko, 1988). *Immaculate Deception*, one of the most influential books of this era, charged that nurse-midwives were more comfortable working in medically oriented obstetric services than providing family-oriented maternity care and that they had sold out to the "establishment" (Arms, 1975).

Unanticipated Effects of the Risk Approach to Maternity Care

Concern about the country's high infant mortality rate stimulated two large foundations, four medical associations, and the U.S. government to support development of a system to refer high-risk pregnant women and newborns to hospitals capable of providing the most sophisticated obstetric and neonatal care. The system they designed, called *regionalized perinatal care*, is predicated on the assumption that it is possible to predict with some degree of accuracy which women will experience serious complications during labor and delivery or will give birth to newborns who will need life-saving care. A systematic approach to making such predictions is referred to as *maternal risk assessment*. Certain maternal characteristics are associated with an increased likelihood of serious complications during pregnancy and a bad outcome for the mother or baby or both. The characteristics associated with

poorer outcomes include common factors, such as poverty and relatively young or old maternal age, and factors that are much less common but much more strongly associated with bad outcomes, including complications such as multiple gestation (twins, triplets, etc.) and the presence of maternal disease. If we could predict which pregnant women and newborns will experience serious problems during or soon after birth, we could send those women to special hospitals for labor and delivery—hospitals with special equipment and teams of specially trained doctors and nurses. This was and is the objective of regionalized perinatal care.

In 1972, the Robert Wood Johnson Foundation began to plan a national program to test and evaluate the effectiveness of using risk assessment and referral to concentrate the care of high-risk mothers and newborns in hospitals that could provide the newest forms of intensive intrapartum and neonatal care. The plan called for classifying all hospitals as level I, level II, or level III (Committee on Perinatal Health, 1976). The largest and most sophisticated hospitals were to be designated as level III (tertiary). They were usually associated with medical schools, were staffed for around-the-clock emergency care, and had the staff and equipment to care for serious illnesses and childbirth complications. Level II hospitals were the intermediate-sized private and community hospitals that provide most of the care to most of the patients in most of the cities in America. All smaller hospitals were designated as level I. Each perinatal regional network was to be based around a single level III hospital. In the regionalized perinatal care system, level III hospitals were expected to take care of their own clientele (many are tax-supported institutions that are responsible for providing health care to the poor) and to provide intensive care to high-risk women and infants referred to them from level II and level I hospitals. Level II hospitals were supposed to conduct normal deliveries and take care of most obstetric complications and some neonatal illnesses. Level I hospitals were restricted to uncomplicated deliveries and the care of healthy babies.

All maternity care providers within the region were to be trained to use a uniform risk assessment scoring system. Women were to be assessed at their first prenatal visit and at thirty-two weeks of pregnancy. High-risk women were to be referred from level I to level II or III , and from level II to level III, based on numeric risk assessment scores. In 1975 the Robert Wood Johnson Foundation (1978) funded a five-year test of this system in eight areas. At the same time, the National March of Dimes Foundation convened a committee composed of representatives of the American Medical Association, the American Academy of Family Physicians, the American Academy of Pediatrics, and the American College of Obstetricians and Gynecologists to develop specific, workable guidelines to implement regional planning for maternal and newborn care. The committee's report, published in 1976, was a blueprint for expanding perinatal regionalization throughout the country (Committee on Perinatal Health, 1976). Its recommendations were similar to the Robert Wood Johnson Foundation plan but added a new element by specifying that level III hospitals should have at least 8,000 to 12,000 deliveries per year, that level II hospitals should have at least 2,000 deliveries per year, and that, except under special circumstances (geographic remoteness and transportation difficulties), hospitals with fewer than 2,000 deliveries per year (i.e., level I hospitals) should close their maternity services in order to "consolidate" them into larger services. "Consolidation" meant eliminating the practice of obstetrics in as many small hospitals as possible.

In 1977 the federal government moved the process forward by incorporating recommendations from the March of Dimes report into proposed national guidelines for health planning [Department of Health, Education and Welfare (DHEW), 1977]. These were to

be powerful guidelines, which could not be ignored. The final guidelines called for closing small maternity units and consolidating services in high-risk acute care settings.

As the guidelines began to be implemented in more parts of the country, what happened in obstetrics was different from what happened in neonatal care. Although "regionalized perinatal care" merged high-risk obstetrics with high-risk neonatal care, they are very different specialties.

In the first place, most of the benefit ascribed to intensive perinatal care was based on the effectiveness of neonatal intensive care. Since publication of the first papers on this subject it had been clear that this kind of care reduces low birth weight mortality (Carrier *et al.*, 1972; Merkatz & Fanaroff, 1978; Meyer *et al.*, 1971). The only real question was whether and to what extent surviving babies would be neurologically damaged. In addition, neither the lower level hospitals nor the pediatricians who used them opposed transferring distressed babies to tertiary hospitals. Neonatal intensive care requires expensive equipment, 24-hour-a-day coverage by specially trained nurses, and neonatologists who are on the full-time hospital staff. Most hospitals cannot afford these units, and, because most pediatricians work out of their offices, they did not want to be responsible for this care. Also, once a baby is born, it is either sick or well. One is no longer dealing with levels of risk and the possibility of pregnancies that have been labeled "high risk" resulting in normal births. If a baby weighs only three pounds or cannot breathe, it is in trouble; it is not just "high risk." There are no false positives (high-risk women who deliver healthy babies without complications), and only a few babies need to be transferred. Level I and level II hospitals were happy to transfer their sick and tiny newborns to more intensive care. When the babies were better, they were discharged to the care of general pediatricians.

None of this is true with regard to obstetrics. The new obstetric techniques mainly provided better information about the condition of the fetus during pregnancy and labor. Although they allowed obstetricians to detect problems earlier and monitor them better, the main treatment was still to hasten delivery, by cesarean section if necessary. The benefits are not nearly as clear as the results from providing intensive neonatal care to low birth weight babies. [A recent study shows no benefit from delivery in a tertiary hospital for newborns who are not low birth weight (Mayfield *et al.*, 1990).] In addition, obstetricians did not want to refer their patients; they wanted to learn the new techniques. Intensive obstetric care did not require a new hospital unit with lots of equipment and around-the-clock special nursing care. The gradient between what could be provided in a university hospital and what could be provided in a good community hospital did not resemble the gradient between a regular nursery and neonatal intensive care. Obstetricians expected to deliver their patients' babies, and their patients expected it too. Referring a "high-risk" woman to another hospital and doctor causes the local hospital and doctor to lose face; this is particularly unacceptable when many women who are labeled "high risk" based on screening criteria go on to have normal births. Thus, although there was little resistance to sending sick babies to tertiary hospitals, obstetricians were more likely to pressure their own hospitals to buy the necessary equipment and to begin to employ the new techniques themselves and were less likely to refer their patients elsewhere.

An evaluation conducted at the end of the five-year program compared perinatal care and outcomes in the eight demonstration areas with those in eight similar areas that did not receive special regionalization funds (McCormick *et al.*, 1985). During the 1970s the percent of low birth weight deliveries, especially very low birth weight (VLBW) deliveries (less than 1,500 grams) had become significantly more concentrated in tertiary centers. But this was part of a national trend and was not greater in the eight project areas. As often happens, the intervention (regionalized neonatal care) was presumed to be better and became widely diffused before the evaluation had been completed. In this case, it was justified; concentration of the births of low-weight babies in hospitals with neonatal intensive care units was associated with a decrease in long-term morbidity and disability among children who had been low weight at birth. Although the evaluation found good results, when the foundation reviewed its experience with perinatal regionalization, it found that many perinatologists believed that further improvement in high-technology medicine could not contribute much to continued reduction in the country's infant mortality rate. Instead they looked for progress at the "low-tech" end of the spectrum, through prevention of low birth weight by family planning* and higher quality prenatal care (Robert Wood Johnson Foundation, 1978).

The United States does better than any other country at saving the lives of low birth weight babies; regionalization of perinatal care contributed to this achievement. However, regionalization did little or nothing to reduce the causes and, therefore, the actual incidence of low birth weight. Because of a high proportion of low-weight births, the international ranking of the United States with regard to infant mortality worsened during the 1970s. The underlying causes of preterm labor and intrauterine growth retardation (which are the immediate causes of low birth weight) must be addressed before labor begins. Despite fifteen years of efforts to organize and improve care during and after labor and delivery, the United States had

---

*Family planning is recommended because the child of an unwanted conception is at greater risk of being born at low birth weight, of dying it its first year of life, and of being abused (Brown & Eisenberg, 1995).

done little to improve prenatal care. In addition, some aspects of the effort to regionalize birth care may have impaired the United States' ability to provide prenatal care (Rooks & Winikoff, 1992):

- The closure of some small obstetric units drove obstetricians out of many small towns and discouraged family physicians from practicing obstetrics. This contributed to a situation in which there was no one to deliver the babies in many communities, (in combination with the stress and high financial cost of frequent malpractice suits against doctors practicing obstetrics).

- Providing prenatal care in many dispersed clinics while centralizing deliveries in a single large hospital creates a schism between prenatal and childbirth care. Pregnant women see prenatal care as preparation for the birth and value it more when it is provided by the people who will be with them when they have their babies. Prenatal clinics which are dissociated from intrapartum care lose power in the eyes of their patients; pregnant women who do not value prenatal care may not bother to use it, even when it is convenient and affordable.

- Regionalization contributed to overmedicalization of childbirth and to the high financial costs associated with excessive use of high-technology obstetric care. Risk assessment is imperfect. Some false negatives (low-risk women who experience serious complications or bad outcomes) are inevitable. When these occur, there is a desire to make the risk assessment system more sensitive. However, an increase in sensitivity (the ability of the risk assessment to identify as high-risk those women who will actually experience serious complications or bad outcomes) can only be achieved by a loss of specificity (the ability to identify as low risk those women who will not go on to experience serious complications or

bad outcomes). Concern about misclassifying even a small number of women who will ultimately experience problems leads to decisions that increase the sensitivity of the risk assessment system. Eventually some obstetricians argued that no pregnancy should be considered low risk until it is over; all pregnant women should be treated as high-risk.

- When small obstetric services closed and the percentage of deliveries in tertiary hospitals increased, many communities no longer had a model for normal maternity care. Medical students and obstetric residents learned a highly medicalized way to take care of women during labor and took that model with them when they finished their training. Over time, obstetric techniques that had been developed for use in high-risk cases were applied more and more broadly; in some cases their use became routine. The United States experienced huge increases in the use of continuous electronic fetal monitoring and oxytocin to induce or augment labor. Some labors were induced to avoid a last-minute rush for women who lived far from the hospital, which was more common where small obstetric services had closed. By the end of the 1970s medical authorities had become alarmed by the rapid increase in the rate of cesarean sections.

The application of maternal risk assessment in the United States increased the cost of pregnancy-related care and yielded problems as well as benefits. Some of the problems might have been avoided:

- There was no real focus on nutrition, efforts to help women stop smoking,* or other truly preventive measures.

---

*Cigarette smoking is associated with reduced infant birth weight, preterm delivery, intrauterine growth retardation, and sudden infant death syndrome.

- There was no real effort to find high-risk women and bring them into prenatal care. In this country, some of the highest risk women do not seek prenatal care.
- There were no criteria for low-risk pregnancy, labor, and birth; no attention to developing appropriate care for low-risk women; and no mandate for tertiary hospitals to refer low-risk women to lower level care.
- The system was in the control of the tertiary centers and physicians who specialized in high-risk care. Almost all of the efforts went toward developing the high-risk centers; little effort was aimed at improving primary care.
- The emphasis on closing small obstetric services was not necessary for achieving the goals of regionalization and caused many of the problems. A growing body of evidence finds that small-volume obstetric care is safe and less expensive (Fleck, 1977; Gray & Steele, 1981; Rosenblatt *et al*, 1985).

Home Births and the Origins of a New Kind of Lay Midwife

The proportion of births that occurred in hospitals rose from 37 percent in 1935 to 97 percent in 1960, and continued to increase during the 1960s, reaching its all-time high of 99.4 percent in 1970. But during the 1970s the percentage of out-of-hospital births more than doubled—from 0.6 percent in 1970 to 1.5 percent in 1977 (Institute of Medicine, 1982). The change was due to a small increase in the number of planned home births. A new phenomenon, these home births were of great interest to the press and to obstetricians, since they were neither accidental nor due to rural isolation or poverty but resulted from the deliberate choices of middle-class American women, many of whom were articulate and well educated. Women were choosing home births for a cluster of related reasons: to be able to control the circumstances of their births; to labor and deliver in supportive environments; to avoid procedures and other interventions that had become common or even routine during deliveries in hospitals; to allow families to remain together during the birth process, and because they wanted to experience the beauty and spiritual potential of a simple, natural birth. Two additional reasons were the lower cost of a home delivery and membership in religions that prohibit or discourage hospitalization, male birth attendants, or the use of allopathic medical care. Some home birthers were young people involved in the counterculture movement that began during the late 1960s. Some were members of traditional communities with conservative views of home and family. Some were highly educated women who had become convinced of the advantages of avoiding intervention during childbirth (Raisler, 1978).

Some physicians and a few nurse-midwives were part of the home birth movement. In addition, the demand for home births gave rise to a new kind of experientially trained lay midwife. Some of the new lay midwives had been childbirth educators, some were La Leche League members; most were mothers, many of whom had been "radicalized" by their own bad hospital or good home birth experiences. Some were members of communes and other alternative communities, in which individuals and families lived apart from the mainstream society, often in rural areas, and tried to develop a less expensive and more natural, satisfying, and healthful way of life. They were optimistic and committed to social change. When women in these communities became pregnant, they sought a kind of childbirth care that was consistent with their values.

Some women became involved almost by accident, often because they were the only person available when a friend or neighbor needed assistance during birth. Some began by going to home births as helpers and learners and assumed more responsibility as they gained more experience. Some asked labor-and-delivery-room nurses to attend a small number of home births with them (Jolly, 1996), or sought apprenticeship relationships with those few doctors who were doing home births. Others just read books and began attending births (Davis, 1981; University of Washington, 1981; Schlinger, 1992). Although all began as amateurs, over time some women took midwifery as a personal responsibility and special role in their communities, gradually learning from their own experiences and seeking knowledge from books and guidance and support from physicians and, as things developed, from other midwives. Although some midwives worked alone, many formed study groups with other developing midwives and some worked in formal or informal groups. The following sections describe three important examples.

The Farm in Summertown, Tennessee

The Farm was started as a rural counter-culture community by Stephen Gaskin and his wife, Ina May, and followers in 1971. During the late 1960s Stephen Gaskin taught at San Francisco State College, held regular evening classes on Zen and other spiritual subjects, and developed a following among the young people who congregated in San Francisco. During 1970, the Gaskins and hundreds of "hippies" formed a caravan of vehicles to begin a long, circuitous trip. Eventually they settled in Tennessee, where they established a spiritual community that was to be sustained by farming. During the trip, three babies were born to women in this group. Ina May observed the first birth and was thrilled by the sudden beauty of the mother. She was called to act as midwife for the second birth and began to study a midwifery manual; the baby was born blue and needed artificial respiration to begin breathing. By the time the third baby was born, she had memorized the manual (Mitford, 1992).

Shortly after their arrival in Tennessee, Ina May Gaskin sought and received the as-

sistance of the general practitioner from a nearby town when a woman from the commune went into preterm labor. He was sympathetic and became involved in the growing midwifery practice of the Farm, sharing his obstetrical knowledge with Ina May and other members of the community who were chosen to become midwives, and helping them during emergencies. In 1975, Gaskin published a book entitled *Spiritual Midwifery* based on her and the other midwives' experiences with pregnancies and births to women at the Farm. In it, she emphasized the spiritual aspects of birth and the importance of involving the family. The first half of the book includes personal accounts by parents, midwives, and attendants of more than 60 individual "birth tales"; the second half includes 200 pages of advice for midwives (Gaskin, 1975). More than a half million copies of the book were sold during the next twenty years (Gaskin, 1994).

In addition to taking care of women in their own community, the Farm offered free care to other women who had unwanted pregnancies; the purpose was to provide an alternative to abortion. Women accepting this offer could either keep the baby or leave it to be raised by people on the Farm. Many single women went to the Farm in response to that offer, and, as the word got out that the Farm would provide care to other people, some married couples began to go there to live during the last six weeks of pregnancy. In 1978 Gaskin reported on 838 deliveries conducted by herself and the midwives she trained during their first seven years on the Farm. Fifty-three percent of the births were to members of the community; the others were to people who went to the Farm specifically for care related to pregnancy and birth. At that time about 1,200 people were living as part of the Farm community; 90 of them were involved in the provision of health care, including two physicians, midwives, nurses, and 40 to 50 emergency medical technicians. They had two ambulances, an outpatient clinic, a laboratory, a pharmacy, and a pharmacist. Although most of the births occurred in homes, the Farm had a birth center, which was homelike but had incubators, oxygen, and other equipment. Women having twins or a breech or preterm delivery were encouraged to deliver at the birth center (Gaskin, 1978).

The Birth Collective at Fremont Women's Clinic in Seattle

The Fremont Women's Clinic was organized by a women's collective in 1971. The Women's Clinic grew out of the desire of women in the Fremont area of Seattle to learn about and exercise more control over their own sexuality and bodies. The clinic provided health education, discussion groups, counseling, and a regular schedule of prenatal, pediatric, geriatric, and gynecologic clinics and was part of a larger "free clinic" movement in Seattle. All aspects of the clinic's work were done by women who had trained themselves as "lay paramedics." They intended the clinic to model nonalienating, nonhierarchial relationships with "patients" and among themselves as health care workers. The clinic staff worked in teams, consulted one another about patient care, taught one another, established their policies through group discussions, and shared responsibility for all aspects of running the clinic. In addition to minimally paid part- and full-time staff, some physicians donated their time to attend specific clinic sessions (Fremont Women's Clinic Birth Collective, 1977).

The birth collective developed out of this milieu in 1975, when two family physicians committed themselves to working with five women who wanted to become midwives. The first seven months of their training included weekly classes and use of a classic midwifery textbook and books and journals from the University of Washington Health Sciences Library. A midwife with extensive home birth experience joined the collective and was the primary teacher in the "home" aspects of childbirth. The two physi-

cians shared their knowledge, which was based on hospital births. After seven months the members of the collective began attending births, usually with two midwives and one doctor at each birth. After each experience, all members of the collective reviewed the labor and delivery in detail. Within six months they had attended 120 births. After the first 70 to 80, the doctors no longer attended all of the births, although they continued to participate in weekly meetings during which all of the week's births were reviewed and there was a class or discussion on some topic. The midwives continued to attend births in groups of two or three, never only one.

The Birth Center of Santa Cruz

The Birth Center of Santa Cruz, California, was started in 1971. It was operated for five years as the practice of a collective of lay midwives, who provided prenatal care at the birth center and attended births in the mothers' homes. The training was informal. For example, one of the midwives first came in contact with the birth center when she went there for the birth of her own child. When her child was about three years old, she started to attend study groups and prenatal sessions at the birth center and then began to attend births with one of the midwives. Eventually she was asked to attend a birth alone. After that she was more or less on her own, although she could ask the more experienced midwives for help as needed (Merz, 1977). In 1974 the birth center was investigated by the California Board of Consumer Affairs and three of the midwives were arrested and charged with practicing medicine without a license. This was part of a series of arrests in California during the early 1970s of nonphysician health care providers, including acupuncturists, herbalists, chiropractors, massage therapists, and midwives (Bowland, 1993).

A study published in 1975 reviewed 287 consecutive home births attended by the Santa Cruz Birth Center midwives. Although they practiced with minimal medical back-up, 81 percent of the births occurred at home without significant problems. Eighty percent of the fifty-six women who experienced complications were transported to a hospital before delivery. All of the outcomes were good (Mehl *et al.*, 1975).

By 1976 the birth center had become a major local institution that attracted an increasingly wide group of midwives and clients. The original members of the collective became concerned about quality and closed the center because they realized that it lacked the structure necessary for quality control. Although the birth center closed, it led to the development of the Santa Cruz School of Midwifery, which ran educational workshops for midwives until about 1980. Most of the original members of the collective went on to obtain the formal training required to prepare them as fully qualified health professionals; three became physicians, five became CNMs, two became chiropractors, and two became qualified in acupuncture (Bowland, 1993).

By the middle of the 1970s, little enclaves of women from coast to coast were doing home births—quietly and largely unknown to each other. Slowly, by word of mouth and news articles, they learned of each other's existence. Some lay midwives did not want to "get organized," fearing that a national organization and efforts to set standards and make pronouncements could create an elite group within what was an inherently grassroots movement (Koons, 1977). Nevertheless, midwives in local areas began to meet to share information and access to training. State associations began to form and develop. During the last few years of the 1970s, lay midwives began to get together at meetings of organizations such as NAPSAC (National Association of Parents & Professionals for Safe Alternatives in Childbirth). Shari Daniels, a midwife in Texas, organized the first conference for the new midwives, which was held in El Paso in 1977. After that meeting, Ina May Gaskin

started a newsletter called *The Practicing Mid-wife*, which became an important, con-tinuing publication (Schlinger, 1992). Lay midwives began to publish home birth midwifery text-books, starting with *The Birth Book*, published by Raven Lang in 1972, followed by Ina May Gaskin's first edition of *Spiritual Midwifery*, in 1975.

During the 1970s many states repealed permissive lay midwifery laws, most of which dated from the early 1900s. By the end of the decade, only eleven states had statutes or regulations explicitly sanctioning the practice of midwives other than CNMs (University of Washington, 1980). A few states reactivated old laws to facilitate the practice of lay or direct-entry midwives, and legal decisions gave lay midwives in some states explicit permission to practice, for example:

- In 1975 a Danish midwife living in Seattle discovered a 1917 law that required the state Department of Licensing to administer an examination to graduates of any legally recognized foreign or domestic midwifery school with a training program of at least fourteen months duration and to license those who passed the examination for midwifery practice in Washington. She was soon joined by midwives trained in Chili, Australia, and England as the first licensed midwives (LMs) recognized in Washington since the law had fallen into disuse in the 1930s (Myers-Ciecko, 1988; University of Washington, 1980).
- The attorney general of Oregon held that midwifery independent of nursing does not constitute the practice of medicine as long as it does not involve the performance of surgery (including episiotomies) or use of prescription medications. Thus it is not illegal (Oregon Department of Justice, 1977).

Arizona, New Mexico, and Rhode Island enacted new laws or strengthened old ones to involve the state health department in licensing and oversight of lay midwives and to require training, a qualifying examination, case reports by midwives, and oversight by a professional advisory committee (University of Washington, 1980). For example, in 1978 Arizona adopted new rules and regulations for a 1950s law that had fallen into disuse due to aging of the state's granny midwives and the development of new services to care for the Hispanic women who had been the midwives' clientele. An increase in requests for midwife licenses prompted the Health Department to write new regulations. Under the new rules the Arizona Department of Health Services was responsible for licensing and supervising lay midwives and persons applying for licenses had to show evidence of midwifery training. Without requiring a particular educational program, the regulations specified the content of the necessary training; applicants also had to have observed at least ten births and delivered at least fifteen babies under the supervision of a physician, CNM, or licensed midwife. The Department of Health Services examined qualified candidates by means of a written test, an oral assessment of clinical judgment, and observation of the applicant's clinical midwifery skills. Midwives licensed under the new rules could accept only low-risk women and their clients had to be examined by a physician or a practitioner supervised by a physician during the last trimester of pregnancy. Prearranged medical backup for the delivery was required. Midwives were not allowed to administer any drugs, including herbs, or to perform any operative procedure other than cutting the umbilical cord (Sullivan & Beeman, 1983).

During this period lay midwives in California and some other states were arrested for practicing medicine or midwifery without a license or were prosecuted for murder following the death of a newborn. Although murder charges were usually reduced to a guilty plea on the charge of practicing medicine or midwifery without a license, a few midwives served some jail time. Some lay midwives during that period wanted recog-

nition through state laws. Others criticized credentialing and licensing as means by which professions such as medicine "hoard knowledge" and monopolize essential services (Fremont Women's Clinic Birth Collective, 1977). For all health workers except physicians legislative sanction is a double-edged sword that not only allows but restricts. The midwives attended home births and did not need access to hospitals; most were content to remain outside the system.

Most traditional or granny midwives practicing during the 1960s and 1970s were black or Hispanic women who lived and worked primarily in Texas and certain other southeastern states (Lee & Glasser, 1974). Of 2,350 lay or granny midwives known to health authorities in 1975, 43 percent lived in Texas, 12 percent in Alabama, and 9 percent in Mississippi (National Center for Health Statistics, 1976–77). Serving mainly poor, minority group women, they were largely invisible to mainstream Americans. Most participants of the counterculture, in contrast, were relatively well-educated members of the younger generation of America's white middle and professional class. All manifestations of the counterculture were of intense interest to the public and the press. Newspapers and women's magazines published many stories about the beautiful, spiritual experience of natural births attended by lay midwives in the company of the woman's family, in the warm, supportive environment of her home.

Criticism of Medicine and the Reaction of Obstetricians to Lay Midwives

Medicine, like many other centers of authority, "suffered a stunning loss of confidence" during the 1970s (Starr, 1982). This stemmed primarily but not entirely from widespread concern about seemingly relentless increases in the cost of medical care. Concerns about cost led to other criticisms, such as the overuse of surgery and hospitalization and the lack of effective peer review. Despite the enormous expense of American health care, Americans did not seem to be as healthy as people in other wealthy countries. America's poor international standing in infant mortality featured prominently in this critique.

The growing perception and rhetoric of a "crisis" in the cost, accessibility, and quality of health care coincided with the civil rights and women's movements. Extension of civil rights concepts to health care resulted in the assertion of rights to informed consent, to refuse treatment, to see one's own medical records, and to participate in therapeutic decisions. In 1972, the trustees of the American Hospital Association adopted a Patient's Bill of Rights, including rights to informed consent and considerate, respectful care (Starr, 1982).

Folk, non-Western, and other nonallopathic therapies gained a clientele and surprising respectability during this period. Holistic medicine was presented as a humane alternative to impersonal, overly technical, disease-oriented medical care.

"Since the Progressive era . . . reformers had assumed that professionals, including physicians, would act in the interest of the dependent; consequently, they were willing to give them wide discretion in institutions such as prisons and hospitals. By the 1970s, reformers had become intensely skeptical of professionals and the benevolent institutions they supervised" (Starr, 1982). Many writers portrayed the medical profession as a "dominating, monopolizing, self-interested force" (Starr, 1982). Advocates of self-care called for democratization of medical knowledge and more equality in the relationships between patients and health care professionals. The extreme authority and power of physicians, they argued, can and does result in abuse. The Federal Trade Commission extended its regulatory authority into the health care field in 1975. The medical profession, which had enjoyed a long period of unquestioned high esteem as a result of reforms made in response to the 1910 Flexner

report, was not prepared for expressions of doubt about the value of medical care and a serious challenge to the authority of physicians (Starr, 1982).

Discussing this era in *The Social Transformation of American Medicine*, Paul Starr described the distrust of medical domination as most apparent in the women's movement. "Feminists claimed that as patients, as nurses, and in other roles in health care, they were denied the right to participate in medical decisions by paternalistic doctors who refused to share information or take their intelligence seriously. They objected that much of what passed for scientific knowledge was sexist prejudice and that male physicians had deliberately excluded women from competence by keeping them out of medical schools and suppressing alternative practitioners such as midwives" (1982, p. 391). Although earlier feminists had rejected midwifery as a traditional, downtrodden women's role, the new form of midwifery was embraced by the feminist movement of the 1960s and 1970s. Feminists argued that medical care should be demystified and that normal female functions, such as childbirth and menopause, should not be treated like diseases.

The first edition of *Our Bodies, Ourselves* grew out of a group discussion on "women and their bodies" that was part of a 1969 women's conference held in Boston. Among other subjects, the members of the group discussed experiences as patients that had left them feeling dependent, like children, and undignified, as well as angry. In addition, they realized how little accurate information they had about their bodies, diseases, and health. Before the conference ended, some of the women decided to continue meeting as a group and to fight their feelings of dependence with knowledge. The group, which became known as the Boston Women's Health Book Collective, planned to research and write easily comprehended papers about medical and health-related subjects that women need to understand. The book was intended to be an instrument for social change. By 1984, more than 2.5 million copies had been sold and *Our Bodies, Ourselves* had been translated into twelve languages, including Braille (Boston Women's Health Book Collective, 1984).

The idea of educated, middle-class American women preferring and choosing to have midwife-attended home births was a severe affront to obstetricians. By 1977 the proportion of out-of-hospital births had more than doubled nationwide and was 5 percent or higher in several trend-setting states, including California. The American College of Obstetricians and Gynecologists (ACOG) went on the offensive by issuing a press release that asked all physicians to report deaths associated with intentional home deliveries to ACOG and a statement by the executive director that referred to home births as "child abuse" and "maternal trauma" (Pearse, 1977). Doctors who collaborated with home birth practitioners were threatened with loss of hospital privileges and, in some cases, their medical licenses. Physicians urged local police and prosecutors to arrest midwives for practicing medicine without a license. Starr described the conflict over home birth as an especially bitter battle (Starr, 1982). Lay midwives and home births became anathema in many academic obstetric departments.

The Reactions of Nurse-Midwives

Although nurse-midwifery had become somewhat more secure during the 1960s, nurse-midwives knew that their services and educational programs were vulnerable exceptions to standard obstetric care; the core of the widely accepted standard was that all care of pregnant women, especially delivery of the infant, should be managed by physicians. Most nurse-midwifery services were dependent on the personal support of a key obstetrician, who had to defend it to colleagues who were, at best, ignorant, but more often prejudiced and misinformed

about nurse-midwives. Most physicians regarded any kind of midwife as a substandard, stopgap measure for care of the poor. The emergence of high-profile lay midwives, well-educated women choosing home births, and other developments of the late 1960s and the 1970s added hostility to the equation. Although nurse-midwives were heartened by the feminist critique of high-tech obstetrics, they had to live with the anger it provoked in their medical colleagues.

In addition, nurse-midwives had a variety of reactions to the lay-midwives themselves. Many were strongly attracted to the kind of care modeled by lay midwives—care that allowed midwives, as well as women and their families, to experience the intensity and power of birth freed from the drab, institutional environment of the hospital, with its paperwork, uniforms, hierarchical working relationships, restrictions, routines, and medical procedures. At the same time, most nurse-midwives were concerned that the lay midwives' lack of training and practice standards and their reliance on the normalcy of childbirth would result in bad outcomes, and that confusion between lay midwives and nurse-midwives would destroy the hard and slowly won record and growing reputation of nurse-midwifery.

Many nurse-midwifery leaders of that time had been trained in the home birth services of the Maternity Center Association, Frontier Nursing Service, or Catholic Maternity Institute, or had other home birth experience. But, as hospitals became the predominant place of birth in the United States, nurse-midwives had eventually conformed to the trend. In addition, most nurse-midwives were practicing in public hospitals where they provided care to a population of women who have a relatively high incidence of complications. Many of them viewed home births "with a skeptical eye and questions of safety" (Burst, 1990). In 1973 the American College of Nurse-Midwives (ACNM) adopted a "Statement on Home Birth" that described the hospital as "the preferred site for childbirth because of the distinct advantage to the physical welfare of mother and infant"(ACNM, 1973). The initial motivation for the statement was to deflect arguments against legislation needed to allow nurse-midwives to practice in California (Sharp, 1995). However, it was an accurate reflection of genuine concern. The Statement on Home Birth was reviewed and sustained in 1976 (ACNM, 1976). No nurse-midwifery educational program in operation during the 1960s and 1970s provided home birth experience for its students.

Speaking at a 1978 conference of the National Association of Parents & Professionals for Safe Alternatives in Childbirth, ACNM President Helen Burst pointed out that the international definition of a midwife is incompatible with the idea of a "lay midwife." While acknowledging that many lay midwives are well trained, she spoke of the need for standards to ensure safe care: "While there are some lay midwives serving the consumer well throughout the maternity cycle with physician back-up arranged for, there are other lay midwives or birth attendants who quite frankly scare me and make me fearful for the unsuspecting consumer. This is the unprepared, inexperienced, unsupervised person who has been involved in a home birth from which she got an emotional high and now attends other home births as the 'midwife' focusing largely on repeat emotional experiences with little concern or knowledge pertaining to safety" (Burst, 1990). Her words reflected the anxiety of many nurse-midwives at that time. She went on, however, to explain that the lay midwifery movement had been good for CNMs, "painful as this may be, because it has crystallized some of our own frustrations and pointed out some of our own inadequacies which must be dealt with . . . . We also may be jealous of the lay midwife because of her freedom from professional restraints which sometimes frustrate us" (Burst, 1990). Nurse-midwives, she said, were caught in the middle of a conflict between the women who

were seeking changes and more control over their maternity care and physicians who opposed the changes and had most of the power (Burst, 1978).

Development of the ACNM's System of Quality Assurance

The American College of Nurse-Midwives used the 1960s and 1970s to develop clear, exclusive definitions, to implement quality control systems, to deepen nurse-midwifery's toe-hold in the mainstreams of health care, and to negotiate an agreement with the American College of Obstetricians and Gynecologists. The ACNM laid down strong standards for nurse-midwives and instituted disciplinary procedures to punish infractions of its rules.

Core Competencies and Accreditation to Ensure Quality Education

During the early 1960s most nurse-midwives viewed their field as a specialty of nursing. The American Nurses' Association (ANA) educational policies then (as now) called for all professional nurses to be educated in programs that lead to a bachelor of science degree in nursing (BSN) and for educational programs that prepare specialist nurses to require a BSN for entrance and grant a master of science degree in nursing (MSN) at conclusion of the program. Nurse-midwifery educators agreed with this policy and adopted it as a long-term goal. However, because only a small proportion of nurses actually had BSNs, they deferred that goal to the future. Of the seven nurse-midwifery educational programs operating in 1960, three were masters programs based in the graduate nursing schools or departments of Yale University, Columbia University, and Catholic University; four were "certificate programs" (not degree granting) based at the Frontier Nursing Service, the Catholic Maternity Institute, Johns Hopkins Hospital, and the Maternity Center Association (in conjunction with the State University of New York Downstate Medical Center). Thus the nurse-midwifery profession needed educational standards that would be flexible enough to apply to programs in diverse settings.

The need for an accreditation program specifically designed for nurse-midwifery education was discussed during the first workshop on nurse-midwifery education.* Nurse-midwife educators were not satisfied with the National League for Nursing's system for accrediting graduate nursing education programs, because it did not evaluate specialty practice (Sharp, 1983), and in 1962 the National League for Nursing announced that it could not accredit nurse-midwifery educational programs because some of them were not in graduate schools of nursing. The ACNM realized that it would need to develop its own accreditation program and began by conducting a survey to describe existing nurse-midwifery education programs and analyzing the nurse-midwife's role in health care. The ACNM Committee on Curriculum and Accreditation used the findings from these processes as the basis for drafting criteria for evaluation of basic certificate (nondegree) and master's degree education programs in nurse-midwifery. In 1965 the committee invited all nurse-midwifery education programs to seek accreditation. The first site visits were conducted in 1968. National accreditation of nurse-midwifery educational programs was in place by 1970 (Conway-Welch, 1986).

Development of a standardized curriculum was deemed infeasible because of the diversity of nurse-midwifery educational programs (Sharp, 1983). In particular, the need to provide nurse-midwives for practice in predominantly rural states made continuation of certificate programs—which do not require a college degree for admission—a necessity. Instead the ACNM established an Education Committee and charged it with

defining the essential, or "core," competencies of a nurse-midwife. The core competencies are the fundamental knowledge, skills, and behaviors expected of a new graduate; thus they are the expected outcomes of nurse-midwifery education (ACNM Education Committee, 1979). They apply regardless of the academic level of the nurse-midwifery program and serve as a guide for not only nurse-midwifery schools and students, but also for the employers of nurse-midwives.

The original core competency statement was approved by the ACNM Board of Directors in 1978; it has been revised periodically since then. It identified seven concepts that underlie all aspects of nurse-midwifery practice: a family-centered approach to client care; constructive use of communication, group dynamics, guidance, and counseling skills; communication and collaboration with other members of the health team; client education; continuity of care; use of appropriate community resources; and promotion of the positive aspects of health, including pregnancy as a normal physiologic process. The statement went on to describe the nurse-midwifery management process, specified the knowledge and skills needed to meet the needs of clients during each phase of the maternity cycle (and to provide family planning and well-woman gynecologic care), enumerated the professional responsibilities of a nurse-midwife, and described the nurse-midwife's responsibilities for recognizing and consulting or referring when complications or other deviations from normal occur (ACNM Education Committee, 1979). To become accredited, a nurse-midwifery education program must demonstrate that its curriculum will lead to achievement of the core competencies (Conway-Welch, 1986).

Ensuring the Competence of Nurse-Midwives at Entrance into the Profession

During the late 1960s, the ACNM created and charged a committee to develop, validate, administer and evaluate a national certification

---

*This workshop was held in 1958; it is discussed in Chapter 3.

examination for nurse-midwives. In 1970 the committee employed a test construction consultant. By 1971 ACNM had begun to require graduation from an accredited nurse-midwifery education program and a passing score on the national examination as criteria for certification. Both written and clinical examinations were administered to all candidates who took the test between May 1971 and January 1974. The clinical examination was discontinued because its results mirrored those of the written text so closely that clinical testing was not considered necessary to determine the safety and effectiveness of the candidate's practice. The purpose of the examination is to identify and fail candidates who do not possess the knowledge and cognitive skills necessary for safe and effective beginning level nurse-midwifery practice (Foster, 1986).

A Working Relationship with Obstetricians
In 1971 the ACNM, ACOG, and the Nurses Association of the American College of Obstetricians and Gynecologists (NAACOG) approved a "Joint Statement on Maternity Care," which asserted that the need for quality maternity care can best be met by the cooperative efforts of physicians, nurse-midwives, obstetric nurses, and other health personnel working in teams directed by obstetrician-gynecologists. This was the first official recognition and acceptance of nurse-midwifery by ACOG. The statement was revised in 1975 to clarify the recommendation requiring obstetrician direction of the team. The revision recognized that an obstetrician does not always need to be physically present when care is rendered and called for representatives of each of the separate disciplines to work together to develop written agreements that clearly specify the consultation and referral policies and "standing orders."

Clear Definitions and Exclusive Criteria for a Certified Nurse-Midwife
The title and definition of "nurse-midwife" were developed and formally adopted by the

ACNM in 1962.* A study to describe nurse-midwifery practices was conducted by the Children's Bureau with encouragement and support from the ACNM in 1963 (Thomas, 1965). A document that delineated the "Functions, Standards, and Qualifications of the Nurse-Midwife" was completed in 1966. The definition of a nurse-midwife was replaced with a more precise definition of a certified nurse-midwife, once certification was in place (1971). In 1975 the ACNM instituted a grievance procedure whereby any CNM could be censured, suspended, expelled, or decertified for conduct contrary to the objectives of the College or inimical to the welfare of women and infants. In 1977 the ACNM changed the wording of the definition of a certified nurse-midwife to specify that *a CNM is educated in the two disciplines of nursing and midwifery*. This action was taken to make it clear that *nurse-midwifery is not a specialty of nursing.*

Although nurse-midwives, like all other health care professionals, practice under a wide variety of state laws, the clear definition and exclusive criteria of a certified nurse-midwife do not vary from state to state. The clarity of this definition and the quality assurance programs that stand behind it allowed the ACNM and its members to use the 1960s and 1970s to begin to develop the legal and institutional supports necessary for nurse-midwifery practice.

Progress in Nurse-Midwifery Education During the 1970s

Seven nurse-midwifery education programs were in operation at the beginning of 1960. Four programs opened and four closed during the 1960s. By the late 1960s the demand for nurse-midwives exceeded the supply and

---

*The ACNM had to resist the advice of their medical supporters who thought the word "midwife" was too inflammatory and suggested "nurse obstetrical assistants" as a more acceptable term (Sharp, 1983).

the productive capacity of the education programs. Presidents of the ACNM during the early 1970s urged their colleagues to put their energies into education (Tom, 1982). Fifteen programs opened and only two closed during the 1970s, leaving nineteen programs in operation at the end of 1979. The number of both certificate and master's degree programs increased. Growth in nurse-midwifery education during this period was encouraged through federal financial support. That support was based in part on a shortage of physicians to provide primary maternity and other reproductive health care to poor women and women living in rural areas.

The demand for nurse-midwives put pressure on nurse-midwifery educators to expand their programs and make them more efficient. Nurse-midwifery education emphasizes extensive use of time-consuming tutoring and individual instruction. In 1972 the faculty of the nurse-midwifery education program at the University of Mississippi developed a modular curriculum based on the concept of mastery learning to make it possible for students with extensive previous educational and professional experience to complete the program in less time. The federal government provided financial support to assist the university in sharing this flexible curriculum with other programs. The curriculum included a comprehensive list of specific learning objectives that represented the essence of entry-level nurse-midwifery practice, self-contained packages of instructional materials that students could use for self-paced independent learning, and self-assessment tools to help students determine when they were ready to be tested for mastery of each module. In 1973 and 1974 the University of Mississippi program convened meetings to help other nurse-midwifery faculty adapt the Mississippi modules to the needs of their own programs. Nineteen of twenty-five programs in operation in 1987 were using some combination of mastery learning or modular curriculum (Decker,

1990). Such sharing became an ethic among nurse-midwifery education program directors, who in 1977 began what has become a continuing tradition of annual or semiannual meetings (Sharp, 1983).

Early pilot projects in the use of "off-campus" clinical learning sites for students enrolled in university-based nurse-midwifery education programs was another outcome of cooperation between the larger community of nurse-midwifery faculty. Two such pilot projects were conducted during 1979 and 1980: The nurse-midwifery program at the College of Medicine and Dentistry of New Jersey arranged for some of its students to obtain most of their clinical experience at a large, well-established private nurse-midwifery service in Reading, Pennsylvania, and the Georgetown University program arranged for several of its students to complete their entire clinical and educational experience at a high-volume CNM-run birth center in Harlington, Texas (Farr & Funches, 1982; Lonsdale *et al.*, 1982). The feasibility of an off-campus nurse-midwifery program "without walls" had been studied by faculty of the University of Mississippi Nurse-Midwifery Program, and faculty of the program at the Medical University of South Carolina had developed guidelines for a pilot test of an off-campus program prior to the start of either pilot program (Farr & Funches, 1982).

Some nurse-midwifery "internship" programs were also started during the 1970s. For example, the Los Angeles County/University of Southern California Medical Center's nurse-midwifery service offered a three-month program designed to facilitate "the transition from a student nurse-midwife to a fully functioning staff member" and to provide "further exposure and experience for new graduates who seek positions in the community or private practice sector" (Platt *et al.*, 1985). Internships also provided a way for nurse-midwives who had been out of practice to update their knowledge and skills in order to reenter active practice. The development of private nurse-midwifery practices run by education program faculty allowed students to become involved in the care of private patients while generating income for the program.

Changes in Nurse-Midwifery Clientele and Practice

Studies of nurse-midwives were conducted at approximately five-year intervals throughout the 1960s and 1970s—by the Children's Bureau in 1963 and by the ACNM in 1968, 1971, and 1976–1977. Although 750 nurse-midwives had graduated from U.S. nurse-midwifery programs by 1963, an extensive search revealed only 34 who were in clinical practice in this country. The principal investigator believed that those 34 represented "approximately 100 percent" of nurse-midwives in practice at that time (Thomas, 1965). The 1968 study found 126 nurse-midwives in practice, the 1971 study found 302, and the 1976–1977 study found 659. Twenty-two percent of employed nurse-midwives who participated in the 1968 survey were working in a foreign country, in part because few opportunities were available in the United States (Runnerstrom *et al.*, 1971).

Clinical practice opportunities for nurse-midwives increased significantly during the 1970s. Close to two-thirds of employed nurse-midwives who participated in the 1976–1977 study were in practice; all but 6 percent of those in practice were practicing in the United States. The nurse-midwives who participated in the 1976–1977 ACNM study had delivered more than 33,000 babies during the previous twelve months—slightly more than 1 percent of all babies born in the country during 1976 (Rooks & Fischman, 1980). By early 1977, nurse-midwives were practicing in forty-one states and the District of Columbia. This increase was due in part to the same social changes that resulted in a demand for home births and lay midwives during the 1970s and in part to growing concern about the need to provide effective care to women, especially young teenagers,

who were at high risk of poor pregnancy outcomes because of social and behavioral problems.

Nurse-midwives began to serve a wider spectrum of society. The number of nurse midwives in the 1976–1977 ACNM study who were in private practice with physicians was virtually the same as the number employed by public health agencies. In addition, 8 percent were providing care to military personnel and dependents, 5 percent were working with young women in a university or college health service, 3.4 percent worked for a health maintenance organization, and 2.4 percent had private nurse-midwifery practices. In addition, nearly 8 percent worked for a CNM-run maternity service. This growth in the number and diversity of nurse-midwifery practices occurred despite increasing numbers of physicians and the bursting of the post–World War II baby boom. More than one million fewer babies were born in the United States in 1976 than in 1960.

During the same period, there was a dramatic increase in pregnancies among girls aged fourteen or younger, and the number of reported cases of gonorrhea per 100,000 population more than tripled. Ninety percent of practicing nurse-midwives in the 1976–1977 study were providing family planning services; more nurse-midwives were prescribing oral contraceptive than were attending births. More than 90 percent were diagnosing and treating sexually transmitted diseases; sexual counseling was a routine part of the practices of 70 percent (Rooks *et al.*, 1978).

Only 8 percent of nurse-midwives who were managing births in late 1976 and early 1977 did so in a nonhospital setting (Rooks *et al.*, 1978). As a result of moving into hospitals, nurse-midwives had incorporated many medical techniques into their practice. The 1976–1977 ACNM study found nurse-midwifery practice to be somewhere between the technology-oriented care of physicians and the home birth practices of lay midwives. Nearly all study participants reported that they cut and repaired episiotomies; 88 percent worked in settings where the equipment for electronic fetal heart rate monitoring (EFM) was available, and of those who worked where EFM was available, more than two-thirds were responsible for implementing it when it was needed. Nevertheless, the practice of nurse-midwives remained different from the obstetric practice of physicians. Only 3 percent of nurse-midwives reported any use of forceps; 60 percent taught organized series of classes for their patients; almost all stayed with women throughout labor and delivery, and one-fourth conducted home visits after the mothers had returned home with their infants.

Nurse-Midwives Move into the Private Sector

Nurse-midwifery was developed as a way to provide effective care to women who lacked access to physicians. Private practice was not part of the ethic and culture of the profession and was discouraged, if not forbidden. The example of the lay-midwives helped to break this taboo. However, even after the taboo was broken, several factors slowed nurse-midwives' entrance into the private sector:

- The continuing commitment of nurse-midwives to care for the poor and other special-needs groups. The numbers of poor pregnant women were increasing, and the small number of CNMs were busy with the job at hand.
- Resistance to nurse-midwives' involvement with private patients by medical leaders of the institutions in which many nurse-midwifery education programs and services were based. Despite good outcomes of nurse-midwifery care provided to poor women, most physicians considered any form of midwifery to be inappropriate for women who could afford a doctor. Nurse-midwife leaders understood the circumstances within which they were "allowed" to educate midwives and serve the poor.
- The need for supportive or, at least, permissive changes in state laws, third-party payment rules, professional liability insurance coverage, and the regulations and practices that control access to hospital privileges. The ACNM began to work on several of these issues during the 1970s. In 1977, Mississippi passed a law that required all third-party payers in the state to cover services provided by nurse-midwives working in nonprofit clinics, if the midwives worked under protocols agreed to by physicians. In 1979 Maryland passed a law that required every health insurer to offer the option of paying for care provided by a nurse-midwife. The Maryland law did not allow third-party payers to require the nurse-midwife to be under the supervision, orders, or employ of a physician as a condition for payment of her fees.
- Few nurse-midwives felt prepared to deal with the financial risks and business-related responsibilities involved in starting a private practice, such as hiring accountants, lawyers, and consulting physicians and negotiating with hospital administrators and insurance companies (Middleton, 1986).

Nurse-midwifery faculty and service directors had neither the freedom nor the resources to respond to the demand for private sector midwifery care. At Johns Hopkins Hospital, for instance, nurse-midwifery faculty and students provided prenatal, labor, delivery, postpartum, and family planning care to a caseload of public sector patients, mainly women from the black, inner-city communities that surround the hospital, and taught prenatal and childbirth preparation classes for groups of women from the broader Johns Hopkins University community. When a woman attending those classes wanted a midwife to attend her during labor and delivery at the Johns Hopkins Hospital, it was not possible; "private patients" (not enrolled in Medicaid or some other public payment program) had to be admitted to the hospital under the name and responsibility of a private physician with hospital admitting privileges.

Nevertheless, during the 1970s, a few nurse-midwives began to provide care to private patients in various settings. The concept was initiated by overworked obstetricians and fed by a growing demand for nontraditional childbirth care among some groups of women, the example set by lay midwives, and the support of childbirth educators, who had grown frustrated by the inability of women prepared for natural childbirth to avoid interventions once they were in labor in a hospital. In some cases, nurse-midwifery services that had been developed to provide care to Medicaid-eligible women also began to accept women with private insurance. In 1970 Dr. John Burnett recruited nurse-midwives to open a service to meet the needs of indigent pregnant women in Springfield, Ohio (Burnett, 1972). The Community Hospital provided a building that could be converted into a clinic and allowed the nurse-midwives to deliver their patients at the hospital. Although the service was designed to serve Medicaid-eligible women, it was advertised to the entire community. Soon the Community Hospital Nurse-Midwives Center was serving one-third of the women in Springfield, including but not limited to Medicaid-eligible women. In 1971, Booth Maternity Center, a Salvation Army maternity home and hospital serving unmarried pregnant women in Philadelphia, developed a nurse-midwifery service to offer a family-centered maternity care program to private patients.

Some of the nurse-midwives who had been "seeded" into six southeastern states through the federally funded program at the University of Mississippi became long-term partners of the physicians with whom they had been placed. The chief of the Department of Obstetrics and Gynecology at the University of Mississippi invited the director of the Nurse-Midwifery Program to join his private practice to demonstrate that nurse-midwives were not limited to care of the poor (Meglen, 1993). In the words of two obstetricians practicing with nurse-midwives in Americus, Georgia, "What began not long ago as an expedient plan to relieve overburdened obstetricians of routine uncomplicated maternity cases had quickly come into its own as a first class 'quality' medical style—often preferred outright by mothers-to-be" (Gatewood & Stewart, 1975).

Nurse-midwives were brought into health maintenance organizations (HMOs) in some western states during the early 1970s. In 1971, the Kaiser Health Plan of Oregon began to offer nurse-midwifery care to its subscribers in the Portland area; the new service was motivated by Kaiser's inability to recruit additional obstetrician-gynecologists to meet a rising demand for obstetric and gynecologic services (Record & Cohen, 1972). The idea was supported by the chief of the department, who had visited nurse-midwifery programs in Baltimore and at Yale. In 1978, a group of women members of the Group Health Cooperative of Puget Sound requested the cooperative's board of directors to establish a nurse-midwifery service at Group Health. Although the Medical Advisory Committee did not support this idea, the consumers eventually prevailed (Rooks, 1983).

A few private hospitals hired CNMs as a way to attract obstetric patients; some busy private obstetricians employed them in order to reduce their "on-call" time without sharing their practice with another physician (Middleton, 1986). Others did so in order to meet the needs of women seeking a more natural, less technological approach to childbirth (Stewart & Clark, 1982). In addition, a few CNMs struck out on their own, developing home birth services and birth centers—both of which avoided the need for hospital privileges. Although some CNMs developed private practices that utilized hospitals for deliveries hospitals' refusal to grant privileges to nurse-midwives planning to provide care to private patients was (and remains) a significant barrier.

Nurse-midwives working in private practices, and the physicians they worked with, reported that nurse-midwives were less well accepted by poor women, who may have assumed that they were being assigned to a less qualified health care provider. This perception was especially common among African-American women, many of whom remembered or had heard tales of untrained granny midwives. To break down the association between midwives and the idea of second-class care for the poor, obstetricians practicing with CNMs in Americus, Georgia, asked that the nurse-midwives not work in the health department clinics, even though physicians in the practice had always done so (Gatewood, 1986).

Development of Free-Standing Birth Centers

The country's first birth centers were started by nurse-midwives serving poor families in rural areas. The first, called "La Casita," was started by the Catholic Maternity Institute in Sante Fe, New Mexico, in 1945 to provide a place where women who lived too far away for a home birth could be "at home" nearer to the hospital (Shoemaker, 1953; Ernst, 1986). It continued to operate until the mid-1960s (Burst, 1990). Several "maternity shelters" were opened and operated by nurse-midwives employed by public health departments (state and county) in Georgia during the 1950s, for example, the Barnesville-Lamar Maternity Shelter, which opened in 1951. A single building housed the local public health department offices, a clinic staffed by three nurse-midwives, and ten maternity beds. Although the shelter was well accepted by the community and reduced lay midwife deliveries and infant and maternal deaths, the long hours required of the nurse-midwives made it

hard to sustain staffing of the shelters (Melber & Malone, 1987).

The first urban birth center was opened in a modified townhouse in downtown Manhattan in 1975 by the Maternity Center Association (MCA), which had become concerned about "do-it-yourself" home births and home births attended by untrained lay midwives, both of which were increasing due to dissatisfaction with hospital obstetric care (Ernst, 1986). Two years of planning for the birth center had included an extensive review of the literature on the safety of out-of-hospital births. CNM Ruth Lubic, MCA's director, sought to confirm or reject her assumption, based on the long home birth experience of not only MCA but also the Frontier Nursing Service and the Catholic Maternity Institute, "that out-of-hospital birth can be safely managed providing there is professional supervision of a carefully screened population." She could find no evidence that "carefully planned, professionally supervised, out-of-hospital birth, in and of itself, had ever been demonstrated to be unsafe" (Lubic, 1979).

MCA opened its Childbearing Center as an alternative to both the hospital and the home and sited it in the middle of America's most populous and urbane city. It was described as "a place where women give birth" (as opposed to "being delivered") and "a place for the practice of midwifery." Nurse-midwives provided most of the care, which centered on prevention and early detection of deviation from normal. Acceptance and retention in the birth center program was based on evidence that the pregnancy was progressing normally (Bennetts & Lubic, 1982). Unlike the home births of that time, every effort was made to integrate the Childbearing Center into the existing health care system. Thus, in addition to establishing the physical facility and a functioning nurse-midwifery service, MCA sought to address rather than to avoid the strong medical opposition to the concept and went to work to develop licensure and third-party reimbursement, as well as obstetric and pediatric consultation, triage, transport to hospitals, and home nursing follow-up care (Ernst, 1986).

MCA intended the Childbearing Center to serve as a prototype; its processes and results were carefully documented. During 1978, the New York State Health Department, the Health Systems Agency of New York City, Blue Cross/Blue Shield of Greater New York, and MCA's own expert advisory committees examined outcome data from the center's first three years of operation. All agreed that it operated safely (Lubic, 1979, 1981, 1983; Faison *et al.*, 1979). In addition, Blue Cross/Blue Shield reported that the cost for complete maternity care at the Childbearing Center was less than 40 percent of the cost of care in New York City hospitals (Canoodt, 1982). In 1978, MCA's Childbearing Center was accredited as a Community Nursing service by the accreditation program operated by the National League for Nursing and the American Public Health Association. MCA was also active in developing a quality assurance program for birth centers, making site visits to fourteen of the twenty births centers that were known to be in operation throughout the country in 1979. Birth centers gave nurse-midwives, to their great advantage, the opportunity to develop their practice in a setting under their control.

Nurse-Midwifery in the U.S.
Military Services

All three major U.S. military services began to train some of their own officers as nurse-midwives during the 1970s. The ending of the draft after the United States' withdrawal from Vietnam cut off the military's supply of young physicians. The armed services, however, retained the responsibility to provide health care to their enlisted personnel, officers, and dependents. A study conducted by the Air Force in the early 1970s showed that it would be extremely difficult for it to recruit and retain enough obstetricians and other medical specialists. The need for maternity care was especially great, since many postwar soldiers, sailors, airmen, and Marines found their tour of military service a good time to start their families. All three services were interested in using "physician extenders"—nurse-midwives, nurse practitioners, and physician assistants—to provide some of the necessary services, and looked first at nurse-midwives, which was the only category with a well-developed system of quality control.

The Air Force was most assertive in training midwives and developing nurse-midwifery services. When it discovered that all of the ACNM-accredited nurse-midwifery education programs had long waiting lists of potential students, the Air Force started its own school at Andrews Air Force Base in Maryland. They staffed it by sending some of their Nurse Corps officers to existing nurse-midwifery education programs and recruiting experienced CNMs to open a certificate nurse-midwifery education program at Andrews in 1973. The ACNM refused to accredit the program, which needed to strengthen its faculty and did not meet the requirement for affiliation with an institution of higher learning. To satisfy that criterion, the Air Force program became affiliated with the certificate program that opened at Georgetown University in Washington, D.C., in 1975. In addition, to get some nurse-midwives with master's degree (necessary for higher rank in the military services), the Air Force bartered a deal in which the University of Utah reserved two positions for Air Force students in each class of its master's degree nurse-midwifery program in exchange for access to the high-volume nurse-midwifery service at an Air Force hospital near Salt Lake City as a clinical learning site for all students of the University of Utah program. In 1987 the Air Force and Georgetown programs merged and converted into a single program; the Air Force continues to use the nurse-midwifery service at Andrews Air Force Base as its main clinical-learning site and contributes its own faculty (Borgellaga, 1993).

In 1972 the Army Nurse Corps sent an Army nurse who had been trained as a midwife in another country to an ACNM-accredited "refresher" training program at Grady Memorial Hospital in Atlanta. After completing the program and passing the ACNM examination, she began to practice at Fort Knox with the intention of developing a nurse-midwifery service to support an education program. In 1974 the University of Kentucky started a master's degree nurse-midwifery program in collaboration with the Army. All students took their basic science courses at the University of Kentucky and then moved to Fort Knox, where they lived and had both the clinical and didactic aspects of the midwifery component of the program. At first most of the students were officers in the Army Nurse Corps; over time this changed, and most of the students were civilians (Lavery, 1977).

The Navy wanted to develop a program to train Navy nurses as midwives based on its own analysis of the services needed by the Navy, without reference to the ACNM's accreditation criteria. To prepare faculty for its program, the Navy sent several of its nurses to an ACNM-approved program. After they graduated and were certified, the Navy CNMs did not approve of the Navy's plans, and the program was never started. The Navy went ahead with plans to provide nurse-midwifery services, getting its CNMs by sending Navy nurses to ACNM-accredited programs (Borsellaga, 1993).

Early Models of Direct-Entry Midwifery Training

By the end of the 1970s, at least ten direct-entry midwifery training programs were in operation in the United States. A health-policy study conducted at the University of Washington in 1980 described them as "loosely organized"; noted that they varied widely in their sponsorship, structure, and teaching methods; and implied that many were unstable. In addition, none was "ac-credited or otherwise endorsed by a public or private body that could speak authoritatively on the quality of instruction provided" (University of Washington, 1980). The examples discussed on the following subsections are representative of the wide range of organized midwifery training programs in existence by 1979.

The Seattle Midwifery School

While lay midwives in most parts of the country were practicing illegally or outside the law, midwives in Washington had discovered a 1917 law that required the state to license midwives who were graduates of formal midwifery schools that met certain criteria. The law, which had lain dormant for decades, was reactivated in 1975 (University of Washington, 1980). Its existence made it possible for midwives from the Fremont Birth Collective in Seattle to conceive of developing a school to educate expert direct-entry midwives. They recognized "the absolute necessity of training" and were critical of "someone who has seen a few babies born and delivered some goats" and then calls herself a midwife. However, they were looking for means to develop "expertise outside of professionalism" (Fremont Women's Clinic Birth Collective, 1977). They used the general curricular design of direct-entry midwifery schools in the Netherlands as a starting point for designing a school in Seattle. The Seattle Midwifery School (SMS) was opened in 1978. The program included 350 hours of classroom instruction and clinical experience based on the school's home birth service and relationships with several of Seattle's publicly funded community clinics. The training took two to three years to complete, depending on the time needed to complete the clinical requirement (University of Washington, 1980). By 1980, five SMS graduates were practicing as licensed midwives in Washington State.

The Arizona School of Midwifery

This school was started by an experienced lay midwife from California. It was a free-standing school located in Tucson and supported by tuitions paid by students. An obstetrician-gynecologist in Tucson and several professors from the University of Arizona School of Nursing helped teach the courses. Clinical experience was based on home births in Tucson and the surrounding area. Six to ten students were enrolled at a time. The school operated between 1977 and 1981. Its curriculum met the requirements of the midwifery licensing rules adopted by the Arizona Department of Health Services in 1978 (Beeman, 1994).

After the Arizona School of Midwifery closed, its curricular materials were strengthened by a CNM on the staff of the state Department of Health Services and then were used as the basis for a midwifery program that was being developed at a community college. Special funding was used to develop the program, which was in an area with many Mormon families that needed midwives for home births. The midwifery program closed during the early 1980s, after the special funding ended. Few if any new students were applying by then, perhaps because enough midwives to meet the needs of that community had already been trained and licensed (Beeman, 1994).

Precepted Experience at a High-Volume Birth Center

Shari Daniels, a well-known lay midwife, organized a birth center to provide care to the many Hispanic women—citizens of both the United States and Mexico—who had been going to a particular area in Texas, near the Mexican border, to give birth with the assistance of indigenous *parteras*. She offered other lay midwives the opportunity to work at her birth center under her supervision for periods of from three to six months, giving them experience with a large number of births, including many involving complications.

Correspondence Courses

Apprentice Academics offered a correspondence course intended to provide the theoretical basis needed to complement an apprenticeship. It was operated by midwives based in Texas. This course is still ongoing, but is now based in Oklahoma.

Short Workshops

Informed Home Birth, based in Colorado, offered short workshops on childbirth to prospective parents, birth assistants, and childbirth educators at several locations around the country. Although the courses were not advertised as training for midwives, they were attended by many lay midwives, who were hungry for more knowledge. Informed Home Birth has moved but is still in operation.

Few lay midwives had access to any kind of organized midwifery course. Most read periodicals and books and/or arranged apprenticeships with physicians, CNMs, or more experienced lay midwives. Midwives in many places organized local midwifery study groups. Local and state midwifery organizations, which were beginning to form and meet on a regular basis, often incorporated educational sessions into their meetings.

Increasing Physician Resistance to Nurse-Midwives

The federal government responded to the physician shortage in the 1960s with generous financial support for medical education. The number of medical schools increased from 88 in 1965 to 126 in 1980, and the annual number of new medical graduates more than doubled—from 7,409 in 1965 to 16,327 in 1984 (Starr, 1982; Pearse, 1993). In addition, the Immigration Act of 1965 increased the flow of foreign-trained physicians into the United States. The increase in the number of physicians coincided with a slowing of population growth, raising concerns about the economic consequences of a surplus. In 1978 the secretary of the Department of Health, Education and Welfare told the Association of American Medical Colleges that the United States had enough physicians (*Nation's Health,*

November 1978). However, federal funds to encourage larger medical school classes continued until 1980 (Pearse, 1993),

A 1979 federal government report identified resistance from physicians and the inability of CNMs to find obstetricians to work with them as major obstacles to wider utilization of nurse-midwives (General Accounting Office, 1979). Physicians have many effective ways to "resist" midwives, including denial of CNM applications for hospital privileges, demands for unreasonable levels of professional liability insurance, refusal of hospital-based anesthesiologists and pediatricians to provide routine care to midwives' clients, misrepresentation of midwifery practice to the public, refusal of physician-controlled malpractice insurance companies to write policies for physicians who work with midwives, and professional ostracism of doctors who work with midwives (Tom, 1982). Physician opposition to nurse-midwives grew in proportion to the increasing numbers of physicians and heightening public awareness of midwifery as a viable option for middle-class women.

Chapter 5
Maternal and Infant Health and the Health Care System, 1980–1995

This chapter provides information about persistent problems affecting maternal and infant health and health care in the United States between 1980 and 1995. It sets the stage for Chapters 6, 7, 8, and 9, which focus on the development of midwifery within this complex milieu.

By 1980 the primary concern about medical and other health care had shifted from access and quality to an overriding concern about costs. Health care had become so expensive that few Americans felt secure about their ability to finance care for a serious medical problem without insurance, and many Americans were not insured.

Health care costs have risen at three times the general inflation rate for most of the past twenty years. By 1980 health care was consuming nine cents of every dollar spent in the United States, a higher percentage than in any other country [National Center for Health Statistics (NCHS, 1995)]. The rate of increase in health-care expendi-

tures accelerated each year between 1986 and 1989, peaked in 1990, and has fallen since then. Although the 5.4 percent increase during 1993 was the lowest in twenty years, it was twice as high as the overall inflation rate for that year. Fourteen cents of every dollar spent in the United States in 1993 was spent on health care (Zaldivar 1993; NCHS, 1995). The amount of money Americans spend on health care is equal to three-quarters of the amount spent for both food *and* housing (Center for Health Economics Research, 1993).

The proportion of Americans without any kind of health care insurance increased steadily throughout the 1980s; it was highest for people of reproductive age and their young children. Fourteen percent of fifteen- to-forty-four-year old Americans were uninsured in 1980; nearly 22 percent were uninsured in 1993 (NCHS, 1995). The rapidly increasing cost of health care insurance became a major concern of both business, which provides health insurance to most employed people and their dependents, and government, which pays for health care provided to the poor. A large part of the increase in uninsured people resulted from employers who decreased or entirely stopped coverage for their employees, throwing even more people into dependence on government programs (Bradsher, 1995). Health care accounted for almost 19 percent of the federal government's total expenditures in 1993, up from 12 percent in 1980 and 4 percent in 1965 (NCHS, 1995).

Another important influence during this period was a growing concern that the nation was producing too many physicians. This created intensified competition for private patients, intensifying medical organizations' determination to limit midlevel health care providers, including nurse-midwives, to the care of poor or rurally isolated people. Although the American Academy of Family Physicians took a strong position in favor of limiting the role of certified nurse-midwives (CNMs), the American College of Obstetricians and Gynecologists (ACOG) took a more positive path, updating its agreement with the American College of Nurse-Midwives (ACNM) regarding the appropriate role of nurse-midwives on the health care team and the necessary relationship between CNMs and obstetricians. Despite the agreement between ACOG and ACNM, many individual obstetrician-gynecologists were opposed to nurse-midwife involvement in the care of private patients. At the same time, nurse-midwives identified good working relationships with physicians, especially obstetrician-gynecologists , as key factors in their failure or success.

As the number and cost of medical malpractice suits soared during the early 1980s, physicians and, eventually, nurse-midwives were strongly affected. Many obstetrician-gynecologists and family physicians reduced or completely stopped the obstetric component of their practice, creating significant gaps in access to maternity care, especially for poor women and those without health care insurance. Interest in a variety of nonallopathic therapies and approaches to health enhancement increased societal understanding of the importance and potential benefits of the midwifery approach to pregnancy and childbirth.

Despite a growing body of research that has found no benefit to frequent or routine use of disruptive and invasive procedures during labor and delivery, application of obstetric interventions such as electronic fetal monitoring and epidural anesthesia continued to increase, and concern intensified about the high and growing rate of cesarean sections. Although the cesarean section rate finally stabilized and has begun to decrease, it remains much higher than in most other countries, and a high incidence of unnecessary cesareans has been widely acknowledged. Efforts to reduce the cesarean rate have encouraged still greater use of other labor and delivery interventions, and a strong focus on enhancing the forces and speed of labor.

America continued to have a high infant mortality rate relative to other industrialized countries. Our international ranking worsened regularly, falling virtually every year between 1980 and 1992. The reason for our country's relatively high infant mortality rate is a high incidence of low and very low birth weight. Low birth weight is caused by conditions that impair fetal growth and conditions that result in preterm labor; both occur more frequently among women who live with poverty and social distress. Scientists and health care policy makers studying the problem recommended that the country make a commitment to providing high-quality prenatal care to all women, and make it more accessible and attractive to women whose social and economic problems place them at particularly high risk. The Institute of Medicine and several other prestigious groups noted studies that had found a lower incidence of low birth weight among socioeconomically high-risk women who received their care from nurse-midwives and called for greater use of nurse-midwives as one of many actions needed to improve outcomes for babies born to these women. They also recommended changes to increase obstetricians' willingness to provide care to women on Medicaid—the federal program that pays for care provided to medically indigent pregnant women and young children. Despite implementation of many of these recommendations and much attention to these problems, the proportion of low birth weight infants increased during this time period.

High costs and lack of universal access made health care reform a major issue in the 1992 presidential election. Although Congress did not support President Clinton's proposed health care reform package and has not enacted any kind of national health care legislation, the widespread attention to health care cost and access problems during the election campaign and early years of the Clinton administration promoted and accelerated massive structural changes in the health care system and stimulated health care reform laws in some states. "Health care reform" is moving ahead on the momentum caused by the long-standing problems.

Managed care is the reform that the health care industry endorsed as the solution to these problems. Some form of "managed" health care is quickly becoming the norm throughout the nation. In most states, the move to managed care came first and fastest to health care that is paid for by Medicaid. Although costs declined slightly in response to the changes, no one knows how significant or lasting the savings may be. In the meantime, many health care providers and consumers are concerned about diminished quality of care, and access to care has declined. The persistence of these problems suggests that the country faces a long period of movement toward some kind of health care reform, including closer examination of the effects of managed care on access, quality, and costs; more government over-

sight of managed health care plans; and further experimentation within states and local areas (Lewin, 1995).

The move to managed health care has meant increased access to mainstream physicians and hospitals for medically indigent women who previously had to rely exclusively on public hospitals and other facilities and services designed especially for them. This has resulted in a critical reduction in the number of women using the obstetric units of large public hospitals and termination of some programs that had been developed for the specific purpose of providing care to poor pregnant women. The move to managed care has also spelled the end of small, unaffiliated private practices in many areas and resulted in a general tightening of the health care system's belt—downsizing resulting in closure of some facilities, reduced salaries and incomes, unemployment, and widespread feelings of insecurity among health care providers. Some physicians who had previously supported nurse-midwifery services that provided care to indigent women now see the midwives as financial competitors and have withdrawn their support.

High Cost of Hospital Care for Uninsured Pregnant Women and Newborns

The cost of providing health care to pregnant women and their babies is of particular concern. "Female with delivery" is the most common reason for hospitalization. There are approximately four million births per year; they account for 13 percent of all hospital admissions and more than 5 percent of all hospital days (Keeler & Brodie, 1993). Inability to pay for health care is more common among childbearing women, who tend to be young and either employed in or dependents of men employed in low-paying, entry-level jobs with few benefits or part-time jobs that provide no benefits at all. Twenty-six percent of women who were of childbearing age in 1985 were totally uninsured or had insurance that did not cover maternity care. Although pregnancy made some of these women eligible for Medicaid, 15 percent of deliveries were to women who were not covered by *any* health care plan (Gold *et al.*, 1987).

Hospitals discouraged uninsured women from using their facilities but could not turn away women who arrived in active labor. Although hospitals sent bills to uninsured women, much of the cost of their care had to be absorbed by the hospital. The actual cost of providing perinatal care to women and newborns in the United States in 1989 was estimated to be nearly $28 billion, averaging $6,850 for every mother and her baby. Payments made by patients or third parties came to slightly more than $25 billion, leaving a shortfall of about $2.4 billion (Long *et al.*, 1994). The cost of providing "uncompensated care" is ultimately passed on in the form of higher charges for services provided to patients whose bills *are* paid—by themselves or by insurance. Those costs, in turn, are passed on to individuals and employers in the form of higher health insurance premiums. The very expensive intensive care required by low birth weight newborns has been of particular concern, as are uninsured women, many of whom have no access to prenatal care and are more likely to give birth to low-weight infants.

Although the cost of all kinds of medical care increased rapidly between 1980 and 1995, a report by the U.S. Agency for Health Care Policy and Research identified pregnancy and newborn care as "areas in which expenditures have grown extremely rapidly" (Lewit & Monheit, 1992). Estimated costs for care of pregnant women increased by 88 percent between 1982 and 1987, and costs for care of infants increased by 95 percent. The increases were due to higher physician fees for obstetric care and the high cost of providing very sophisticated, intensive care to newborns with complications.

Medical Efforts to Constrain Midlevel Health Care Providers

A 1981 Harris poll of a representative sample of more than 1,800 physicians found them anticipating unwelcome change and concerned about the future. Most believed that the country was developing a surplus of physicians. Half had enough doubts about the future that they would not recommend medicine as highly then as they would have ten years earlier (Taylor & Yohalem, 1981). Although average medical fees increased by 12 percent between 1981 and 1982, most doctors saw fewer patients and average MD income increased less than inflation (Owens, 1982). Fear of a doctor surplus and increasing competition for patients heightened physicians' concerns about "midlevel" health care providers. In 1995 a commission established by the Pew Charitable Trusts published recommendations that 20 percent of medical schools be closed and that immigration of foreign medical graduates be restricted. These recommendations were based on the commission members' belief that up to half of the nation's hospitals will close while ambulatory and community health care settings will expand during the last half of the 1990s (Pew Health Professions Commission, 1995).

In 1985 the American Medical Association (AMA) resolved "to combat legislation authorizing medical acts by unlicensed individuals" and undertook a nine-point program of activities to assist state medical associations and medical specialty societies to oppose legislation that would allow health care providers who are not physicians to practice independently. In 1993 the AMA appealed to physicians for funds to help it respond to the "flocks of non-physician practitioner groups" who are "using the call for health care reform as a decoy to lower licensing requirements and broaden their scopes of practice." In 1995 the AMA House of Delegates added a statement that "The physician is responsible for the supervision of nurse practitioners and other advanced practice nurses in all settings" to its "Guidelines for Physicians/Nurse Practitioners Practice."

The American Academy of Family Physicians' Position on Nurse-Midwives

In 1980 the American Academy of Family Physicians (AAFP) issued a formal statement opposing nurse-midwifery licensure and asserting that "the use of nurse-midwives is not in the best interests of quality patient care . . .. The AAFP does not believe that the midwife can adequately substitute for the physician in obstetrics" and "has recommended abolishment of midwifery for many years while recommending production of sufficient competently trained family physicians to provide quality obstetrical services. Any trend from competently trained licensed physicians performing quality obstetrics back to midwifery must be considered a regressive step in the delivery of obstetrical service." In 1990 AAFP stated "strong opposition" to the "independent practice of obstetrics and gynecology by nonphysicians." CNMs "should be employed only as a means of providing limited care, always under the direction and responsible supervision of a practicing, licensed physician," with all payments going through the physician. In 1993 AAFP revised its stance slightly, noting that many family physicians work with nurse-midwives. However, the AAFP continues to oppose independent practice by nurse-midwives and upholds the principles that all nonphysician health care providers should be supervised by physicians and all payments for services should go through the supervising physician (AAFP, 1993).

The American College of Obstetricians and Gynecologists' Position

In a 1980 speech the executive director of ACOG urged family practitioners to cooperate with obstetrician-gynecologists to avert the "worrisome possibility" that CNMs would gain authority to practice independently. To ensure a large role for family physicians in deliveries, he said, it "is important for all of us in medicine to remember that the Indians are all outside the stockade and avoid taking shots at each other" (Pearse, 1980). His statement was not consistent with ACOG's formal position on nurse-midwifery in 1980, which was based on the Joint Statement on Maternity Care that had been worked out and agreed to by ACOG, the Nurses' Association of ACOG, and the ACNM in 1975.[*] In 1982 the ACNM and ACOG replaced this statement with a "Joint Statement of Practice Relationships Between Obstetrician/Gynecologists and Certified Nurse-Midwives." The new statement reiterated the two organizations' prior agreement that the maternity care team should be directed by an obstetrician-gynecologist, that appropriate CNM practice requires involvement of an obstetrician-gynecologist, and that the obstetrician's involvement should be specified in mutually agreed on written medical guidelines and protocols. In addition, the new document urged obstetric-gynecologic specialists to respond to nurse-midwives' requests for collaboration, encouraged hospitals to extend privileges to nurse-midwives, and asserted that quality of care is enhanced by the *interdependent* practice of obstetrician-gynecologists and CNMs (ACOG & ACNM, 1982).

In 1986 a distinguished obstetrician-gynecologist and public health leader addressed the relationship between nurse-midwives and obstetricians during a National Colloquium on Nurse-Midwifery in America. He spoke of a developing surplus of obstetricians and the reality that CNMs, family practice physicians, and obstetrician-gynecologists are all competing to be the primary-care providers for low-risk pregnant women

---

*See Chapter 4 for information on the Joint Statement on Maternity Care approved by ACOG, the ACNM, and NAACOG in 1971, and the supplementary statement approved in 1975.

(Cushner, 1986a, 1986b). Although he said that the leadership of ACOG stood behind every word of the ACOG/ACNM joint statement, he noted that those leaders were only about 50 people in an organization with approximately 25,000 members. "We cannot assume that all of the members of ACOG agree with the joint statement. Many, if not most of them, may disagree with it" (Cushner, 1986a). Approximately 8 percent of obstetrician-gynecologists surveyed by ACOG in 1987 employed nurse-midwives in full- or part-time staff positions (ACOG, 1988).

Importance of Nurse-Midwives' Relationships with Physicians

In 1985 the ACNM Foundation conducted a study to identify factors associated with success or failure of a nurse-midwifery practice. The nurse-midwives who participated in the study identified suitable physician collaboration and a good relationship between CNMs and physicians as the most important factors for success, and opposition from physicians as one of the most important obstacles. Practices without direct physician involvement were least able to attract an adequate number of clients (Haas & Rooks, 1986). In 1992 the Office of the Inspector General of the Department of Health and Human Services conducted a survey to determine what certified nurse-midwives perceived to be the most significant problems impeding a successful practice. CNMs who participated in that study considered attitudes and perceptions of the medical community to be the most significant barrier. The government investigators concluded that physicians probably also have an impact on most of the other barriers reported by nurse-midwives, especially inability to prescribe medications and obtain hospital privileges.

Medical Opposition to Lay Midwives

ACOG advocates active opposition to lay midwives. The California Medical Association conducted an anti-midwifery campaign throughout the 1970s and 1980s that re-sulted in prosecution of many lay midwives by the California Board of Medical Quality Assurance (Becker *et al.*, 1990).

The Medical (and Midwifery) Malpractice Liability Insurance Crisis

Both the number of medical malpractice claims and the amount of money awarded in malpractice suits increased dramatically during the 1970s. A crisis was declared during the early 1980s. Obstetrics was especially vulnerable because of the extremely high costs associated with permanent neurologic damage to an infant and the emotional shock when the awaited birth of a healthy baby turns into a frightening experience that ends with a dead or damaged newborn. In addition, the possibility that prenatal or birth-related injuries may not be fully appreciated until the child reaches the age at which most children begin to talk leaves those responsible for the care of pregnant women susceptible to liability suits that can be filed years after the pregnancy and birth. In 1983, ACOG surveyed a stratified random sample of its members regarding their experience with malpractice claims. Only 31 percent of obstetrician-gynecologists in California had never been sued; 27 percent had been sued three times or more. Nationally, 15 percent of obstetrician-gynecologists were being sued each year (Porter, Novelli, & Associates, 1983). Professional liability became a frightening part of obstetrics. It takes four and a half years to resolve a suit against an obstetrician, on average; even a single suit is a prolonged, stressful ordeal. Most doctors describe their feelings on first being caught up in a legal action as fear, followed by anger and bitterness (Enkin, 1994). There were many consequences:

- Some obstetricians and many family physicians dropped obstetrics from their practice; this created geographic gaps in the availability of maternity care.
- There were large and rapid increases in the cost of professional liability insur-

ance for physicians; these costs were passed to consumers in the form of increased fees.

- Most obstetricians increased their use of diagnostic procedures such as ultrasound examinations and continuous electronic fetal monitoring.
- Because poor women are more likely to experience complications and poor outcomes of pregnancy, many obstetricians believed that taking care of poor women would expose them to a higher risk of malpractice suits. In addition, Medicaid payments for maternity care were far below most physicians' usual fees. In combination, these factors caused many obstetricians to refuse to accept Medicaid-eligible women as patients.

Impact on Nurse-Midwifery

At first nurse-midwives believed they were immune to the problem. Since 1974 members of the ACNM had been able to purchase professional liability insurance policies that would pay up to one million dollars per claim for only $38 per year. Because the policy was available to all registered nurses, CNMs were part of a huge group of low-risk policyholders. In addition, until 1980 the company that issued these policies had paid a total of only $28,000 in insurance claims on behalf of CNMs. By 1982—only two years later—it had paid more than a million dollars for claims against policies held by nurse-midwives. As soon as the company could do so legally, it terminated its contract with the ACNM and offered a new contract within which it would write policies only for CNMs who did no out-of-hospital deliveries and were salaried (rather than self-employed); it projected an annual premium of $600 to $800 for the new policy. The ACNM Board of Directors wanted a policy that would be available to all nurse-midwives, and was able to obtain it— for one year—at the bargain price of $225 for one million dollars per incident coverage. One scant year later this policy was also canceled, even though there had been only one

suit against a CNM. Based on its experience with physicians, the insurance company had decided to get entirely out of the professional liability insurance business.

Only 5.2 percent of practicing nurse-midwives surveyed by the ACNM in 1982 had ever been named in a malpractice suit (Adams, 1984). Nevertheless, nurse-midwives became part of a national problem that was far beyond their control. Insurance companies were leery of insuring the risks of pregnancy and childbirth managed by physicians and were ignorant of midwifery. In 1982 the executive manager of the Association of California Insurance Companies wrote that, although the company carrying the ACNM-sponsored policy "tells us that the claim experience on this policy has been very good, . . . {w}hat this indicates is that someone else is paying for malpractice claims arising out of the CNM's function." The actuarial record of ACNM members was so good that the insurance company thought it was not true.

By 1985 the ACNM had worked with three different insurance carriers. The first quit because its $38 per year premium was too low; the second withdrew from the medical malpractice market; the third could not obtain reinsurance. As a result, in July 1985, insurance coverage was suddenly withdrawn from more than half of the ACNM's members. Most CNMs who continued to have insurance obtained it from local companies or through their employers and paid $1,000 annual premiums on average.

As a result of the unavailability and cost of professional liability insurance, some CNMs were forced to close their practices; some quit private practice and took jobs in institutions that provided insurance. Some who did only a few births a year stopped delivering babies; some dared to practice without insurance (Kraus, 1990; Gordon, 1990). In addition, liability concerns discouraged many physicians from working with nurse-midwives. Because ACNM standards require CNMs to demonstrate "a safe mechanism for obtaining medical consultation, collaboration and referral," anything that makes physicians reluctant to work with nurse-midwives may make it impossible for CNMs to practice in some areas.

The ACNM made constant efforts to negotiate a contract for the best possible insurance coverage of the largest possible number of CNMs for the lowest possible price and pursued a variety of activities to ensure the quality of care provided by nurse-midwives and to help them respond in the event of a poor outcome and lawsuit. After approximately one year without an ACNM-sponsored professional liability insurance policy, in July 1986 a consortium of insurance companies offered ACNM members a policy that would pay one million dollars per claim and $1 million for all claims in a year. Even this was not adequate, however, because many hospitals required nonemployee professionals on their staffs to have insurance that would pay at least one million dollars per claim and three million dollars per year ($1 million/$3 million policies). Inability to obtain that level of insurance prevented some CNMs from obtaining hospital privileges (Cohn, 1989).

Twenty-two percent of nurse-midwives practicing in 1987 had no liability insurance, and 10 percent had been sued. Although only 3 percent had been the primary defendant in a malpractice suit, the proportion who had ever been sued had doubled since 1982 (Adams, 1989). A study conducted in 1987 described the effects of the liability insurance crisis on ACNM members. Most respondents indicated that the increased cost and decreased availability and coverage of liability insurance was having a direct, negative impact on the financial viability of their practice and had resulted in increased use of defensive procedures, increased cost of care, decreased availability of care, restricted practice privileges, and stressed employer/employee relationships (Patch & Holaday, 1989).

Since 1993 the ACNM has had a stable, long-term professional liability program that offers $1 million/$3 million policies to CNMs in every state. Nevertheless, nurse-midwives and the ACNM have continued to struggle with the liability insurance issue. The following have been persistent problems:

- *Constantly increasing costs of insurance.* The cost of an ACNM-sponsored policy increases during each of the first five years of coverage and varies by the amount of coverage (four levels are available) and geographic region of the country. Nurse-midwives who do not attend deliveries receive a 50 percent discount. The least expensive policy (the first year of a policy with $250,000/ $500,000 limits of liability for a nurse-midwife who attends births in the region with the fewest claims) cost $2,132 in 1995. The most expensive policy (the fifth or later years of a policy with $1 million/$3 million liability limits for a nurse-midwife attending births in the region with the most claims) cost $13,500.

- *Restrictions related to the place of birth.* In 1991, the insurance company notified the ACNM that it would not renew or issue new policies for nurse-midwives who attend home births. Although the ACNM found another company to cover home deliveries, the cost is high and the policy provides only one-tenth of the maximum coverage available to nurse-midwives who attend births in hospitals or accredited free-standing birth centers. As a result, few CNMs attend home births, and many who do are not insured.

- *Insurance company practices that make it impossible or impractical for physicians to collaborate with nurse-midwives.* Some insurance companies refuse to write policies for physicians who work with midwives; charge higher premiums (a "surcharge")* to physicians who work with

---

*A 1987 ACOG survey found that 47 percent of the obstetrician-gynecologists who employed nurse-midwives had to pay a "surcharge" on their insurance (ACOG, 1988). This was less frequently required if the CNM was not employed by the physician; 10 percent of all physicians associated with nurse-midwifery practices in 1988 paid annual surcharges ranging from $94 to $23,000 (Cohn, 1989).

midwives; impose restrictions and requirements that limit and burden the practice of either the midwife or the physician to an extreme and unreasonable extent, for example, requiring the midwife to be employed by the physician; require the midwife to purchase her insurance from the same company (at a much higher cost than she would pay for similar coverage under the ACNM-sponsored program); do not allow the midwife to attend home births or births in a free-standing birth center, even if she collaborates with a different physician for those births; do not allow the midwife to serve as clinical preceptor for midwifery students; and require the physician to be in the hospital whenever the midwife is there to attend a woman during labor and delivery.

- *Misunderstanding of the legal concept of vicarious liability.* Malpractice insurance surcharges, denial or restrictive limitation of clinical privileges, and physician "supervision" requirements are often based on the mistaken belief that physicians who work with midwives and hospitals that grant privileges to midwives are legally liable for bad outcomes resulting from a midwife's care. If a nurse-midwife is employed by a physician or hospital, the doctor or hospital will probably be subject to vicarious liability. However, as of 1994, there had been no reported cases in which a hospital or physician had been held liable for the acts or omissions of a nurse-midwife who was not a bona fide employee (Jenkins, 1994).
- *Medical management of pregnancy and childbirth as the accepted "standard."* Midwifery care that differs from usual medical management has been considered to deviate from that standard. Failure to provide "standard care" is the *sine qua non* of malpractice. Care by a midwife is, *in and of itself,* nonstandard in the United States. Childbirth in any environment other than a hospital is non-

standard in the United States. The decision not to screen women for abnormalities through use of ultrasonograms and continuous electronic fetal monitoring is nonstandard in the United States, *even though these procedures and others that are used so commonly that they are "standard" have never been found to be associated with improved pregnancy outcomes when applied on a routine basis to all women* (Haverkamp *et al.,* 1979; Neutra *et al.,* 1978; Leveno *et al.,* 1986; Ewigman *et al,* 1993).

Despite these problems, nurse-midwives won some victories against unfair or unreasonable liability insurance company practices:

- In 1983 the Federal Trade Commission (FTC) intervened in a case involving two CNMs who attempted to set up a practice in Nashville, Tennessee, in collaboration with a physician. The practice was forced to close and the doctor to leave the state because the company that provided his medical malpractice insurance—which was owned and controlled by physicians and wrote 80 percent of the malpractice insurance policies in the state—canceled his insurance. The FTC entered the situation in response to a complaint that the insurance company's action constituted an unreasonable restraint of trade, hindered competition in the provision of health care in Tennessee, and deprived consumers of the benefits of competition—all violations of the Federal Trade Commission Act. Ultimately the FTC negotiated an agreement that prohibits the insurance company from any form of discrimination against doctors who collaborate with CNMs (Bailey, 1986).
- In 1992 the insurance superintendent for the District of Columbia ordered a malpractice insurance company to drop its $13,000 surcharge on policies for obstetricians who work with nurse-midwives (Washington Post, 1992).

Nurse-midwives continued to have a favorable liability record. Studies conducted in 1987 found that 71 percent of obstetrician-gynecologists but only 10 percent of CNMs had ever been named in a professional liability claim (ACOG, 1988; Adams, 1989). However, findings from these studies should not be directly compared. Liability arises from bad outcomes, most of which arise from complications; midwives are supposed to take care of normal cases and refer or transfer women with complications to physicians. In addition, nearly half of the claims against obstetrician-gynecologists came from their gynecologic practice (ACOG, 1988).

Impact on Direct-Entry Midwives

Most direct-entry midwives practice outside of the established health care system; to some extent, lack of malpractice insurance is just another aspect of that pattern. Most of them take care of well-educated, low-risk women who have sought their care and understand and accept any risk associated with birthing their babies away from a hospital and immediate access to medical intervention in case of an emergency. The pregnant woman is seen as the person with the greatest degree of responsibility for her own and her baby's well-being, an approach and attitude which surely helps to reduce, but cannot entirely eliminate the possibility of malpractice claims. Lack of insurance is not a serious barrier except for direct-entry midwives who seek access to the practice supports that are controlled by the guardians of the established health care system—payment by third-party health care financing plans, the ability to obtain and administer or prescribe controlled medications, and hospital admitting and practice privileges.

Where licensed midwives (LMs) have begun to acquire greater access to the system, lack of liability insurance can be a formidable problem. In anticipation of the implementation of Washington's health care reform law, the Midwives' Association of Washington State (MAWS), which includes direct-entry LMs and CNMs, supported legislation that authorizes a Joint Underwriting Association (JUA) for midwives and birth centers. When the state could not find an insurance company willing to write policies for midwives who attend home births in Washington, the insurance commissioner required all insurance companies authorized to write medical malpractice and general casualty insurance in the state to form a JUA to offer policies to birth centers and midwives who attend home births. The policy became available in 1995. As of October 1996, it provided insurance to several birth centers and approximately thirty midwives who attend home births—mainly LMs, but also some CNMs. The policy provides $1 million to $3 million worth of coverage and costs $2,400 per year for up to twenty-four births, and $100 more per additional birth. Insured midwives must participate in a quality review process that includes site visits and self-evaluation. Licensed midwives in Florida also have access to a state JUA, although most are insured through a local company. The Florida company is considering offering policies to licensed direct-entry midwives who are practicing in other states (Myers-Ciecko, 1996).

Increased Use of Alternative Health Care

In 1992 the *New York Times Magazine* published a chronology of events and research that had led to the gradual "mainstreaming" of alternative therapies during the 1970s and 1980s (Barasch, 1992). It included these items:

- The opening of China exposed many people to positive information about acupuncture, acupressure, and other aspects of Chinese healing.
- A book published in 1974 suggested that personality traits can increase the risk of heart disease.
- A 1975 book showed that meditation can lower blood pressure.

- In 1979 the editor of the *Saturday Review* described his recovery from an "incurable" disease by taking vitamin C and watching comedies.
- The first hospital program for therapeutic use of meditation and yoga was started in 1979.
- In 1981 a University of Rochester professor published a textbook on interactions between the immune system and the mind.
- In 1988 a Boston hospital established a Mind/Body Institute that uses relaxation techniques to help treat conditions such as cancer and chronic severe pain.
- In 1989 *The Lancet* reported a study of women who had metastatic breast cancer and were receiving regular medical care. Those who participated in therapies such as support group meetings and self-hypnosis lived twice as long as those with no psychosocial treatments.
- In 1990 *The Lancet* published research which demonstrated that a low-fat diet combined with techniques such as yoga and meditation can reverse the pathologic course of coronary heart disease for some people.

Growing distrust and disaffection between medicine and the general population, fed on the doctors' side by fear of malpractice suits and on the patients' side by cold and transient encounters with physicians in the increasingly bureaucratized health care system, increased interest in alternative sources of healing (Konner, 1993). These events, research results, and other changes increased both the demand and supply of unconventional forms of health care during the 1980s and early 1990s. A 1993 article in the *New England Journal of Medicine* estimated that one-third of all Americans had used some kind of alternative medical treatment during 1990 and had paid nearly fourteen billion dollars for the treatments (Eisenberg *et al*, 1993).

Although many European physicians combine the use of such treatments with allopathic medical therapies, most American doctors have disdained these methods, few of which have been subjected to rigorous, objective scrutiny. In 1993 Congress ordered the National Institutes of Health* to establish an Office of Alternative Medicine in order to begin to obtain data to evaluate the efficacy of these kinds of methods.

Increased understanding of the interrelatedness of the emotional, social, and spiritual aspects of wellness, illness, and healing have led to greater understanding of the importance of a woman's frame of mind and environment on pregnancy and childbirth. And increased public awareness and acceptance of "alternative" health care has weakened the assumption that the medical profession is the only source of valid information and effective methods to improve health and prevent and treat disease. These conceptual changes make it easier for people to understand and value midwifery.

By the end of 1995, forty-one states had passed laws that require all third-party health care financing plans that operate in the state to cover services provided by chiropractors, six states required coverage for services provided by acupuncturists, two states required coverage for naturopaths, and one required coverage for massage therapists and one for "providers of Oriental medicine." On January 1, 1996 Washington State implemented an unprecedented law that requires all health insurers and health maintenance organizations (HMOs) to provide access to all categories of health care providers who are licensed or certified by the state. Licensed direct-entry midwives are considered as a separate category from certified nurse-midwives in Washington; as a result, all health insurers and HMOs (which

---

*The National Institutes of Health (NIH) is the Public Health Service agency responsible for funding and guiding the nation's health research agenda.

have a large share of the health-care market in Washington) have to include some licensed midwives in the panels of health care professionals from whom their subscribers can seek care and expect to have it paid for by their health-insurance plan (Collins, 1996). One California-based insurance company offers a "wellness and preventive health care plan" which reimburses subscribers for alternative therapies such as homeopathy, herbal medicine, Shiatsu massage, acupuncture, hypnosis, and biofeedback (Barasch, 1992).

Development of a System of Supports to Ensure Quality Care in Birth Centers

During the early 1980s the leaders of the birth center movement created an organization for people who work in birth centers or want to start one, and used that organization to build a system to promote the quality of birth center care. They were emphatic in demanding that birth centers should not be isolated but should be part of the health care system—with the supporting structure necessary to provide stability to the centers and safety to their clients. In 1981 the Maternity Center Association (MCA) started a Cooperative Birth Center Network (CBCN) to promote guidelines, standards, licensure, and third-party reimbursement for birth centers; to inform the public about birth centers; and to provide direct assistance to existing birth centers and to persons interested in opening new ones. The CBCN knew of ninety-one birth centers that were in operation by the end of 1982.

In 1983 MCA obtained financial support from a foundation to assist the CBCN to establish the National Association of Childbearing Centers (NACC) as a not-for-profit membership organization. In addition to the activities started by its predecessor, NACC gathers, analyzes, and disseminates information about birth centers and conducts workshops for people who are interested in starting a birth center. The NACC Board of

Directors includes consumer representatives and some of the nation's leading health professionals. One of its first successes was to convince the Yellow Pages Heading Committee of the Bell Telephone Company to include "birth centers" as a heading in the nation's Yellow Pages.

NACC asked the American College of Obstetricians and Gynecologists to participate in a group to establish standards for birth centers. ACOG was unable to do so because of its official position against out-of-hospital birth. Instead, NACC worked with a multidisciplinary committee established by the Maternal and Child Health Section of the American Public Health Association (APHA), which included obstetricians. In 1982 the American Public Health Association issued its "Guidelines for Licensing and Regulating Birth Centers."

In 1983 ACOG and the American Academy of Pediatrics (AAP) published the first edition of the *AAP/ACOG Guidelines for Perinatal Care*, a manual outlining the two organizations' joint recommendations for the care of pregnant women and newborns. The guidelines asserted the following as the two organizations' official position regarding free-standing birth centers (i.e., those not located in a hospital): "The hospital setting provides the safest atmosphere for the mother, fetus, and neonate during labor, delivery, and the postpartum period. . . . Until scientific studies are available to evaluate safety and outcomes in free-standing birth centers, the use of such centers cannot be encouraged" except, perhaps, in geographically isolated situations "where special programs are necessary"* (AAP/ACOG). The guidelines approve of in-hospital birth centers that "function under the protocols of

---

*In 1982 the Institute of Medicine (part of the National Academy of Sciences) examined the same information available to AAP and ACOG and concluded that there was insufficient data to determine the relative safety and efficacy of *all* birth settings, *including* hospitals (Institute of Medicine, 1982).

the department of obstetrics and gynecology."

Although NACC supports the concept of in-hospital birth centers (units that have homey furnishings and follow some birth center practices), it asserted that a true birth center must have autonomy within whatever structure it is placed. If it is part of a larger acute-care facility, the organizational structure must give the birth center authority to establish its own policies, program, practices, and prices in keeping with the philosophy and purpose of the birth center. Few in-hospital birth centers meet this standard of autonomy. "Birth centers are an adaptation of the home rather than a modification of the hospital. It is not enough to hang plants and wall paper. Institutions may create a home-like environment within the obstetrical service unit but, although this is a first step and certainly to be encouraged, it is a far cry from the establishment of a birth center" (Lubic & Ernst, 1978). In 1995 New Jersey prohibited hospitals in that state from advertising in-hospital maternity units as "birth centers" unless the unit meets the state's standards and is licensed as a birth center. The director of Licensure, Certification and Standards took this action because "Such advertising is misleading to consumers" (Quickening, 1995).

Beginning in 1984, NACC has surveyed its members annually to obtain data to compare charges for birth center care with charges for a normal delivery with routine care in the referral hospitals used by the birth centers.* Although charges for all care have increased since 1984, total charges for care in birth centers are consistently 30 to 45 percent less than charges for care in hospitals in the same communities (Ernst, 1995).

The malpractice insurance crisis was a powerful impediment to the momentum created by the cost advantages of birth centers and the quality assurance system being

created by NACC. By 1985 NACC knew of 140 birth centers that had opened during the previous ten years. Twelve percent of them had closed—in some cases because they were undercapitalized, third-party payers refused to reimburse subscribers for the cost of birth center care, or local physicians and/or hospitals were unwilling to establish a referral relationship with the birth center. However, most birth center failures were due to inability to obtain liability insurance. Some centers closed because the obstetricians who had been working with them withdrew when their insurers threatened to cancel or not renew their malpractice insurance policies. Some physicians had to pay insurance policy surcharges because they provided consultation and accepted patients referred or transferred from birth centers. In 1984 NACC negotiated a master liability insurance policy that birth centers could buy into; because of unavailability of reinsurance, the company was unable to renew the policy in 1985 (Ernst, 1985).

Despite the malpractice insurance problem, by the mid-1980s hospital administrators, obstetricians, and for-profit health care organizations were showing significant interest in birth centers, as demonstrated by their participation in NACC workshops on how to open and run a birth center. By the end of 1985, two hundred birth centers had been opened, significant progress had been made in third-party reimbursement for birth center care, regulations for licensing birth centers had been drafted or adopted by more than half of the states, national standards for birth center care had been promulgated, and NACC had held the first of its now annual conventions and had begun a large prospective study of the safety of birth center care. A commission had been established to evaluate birth centers and accredit those that meet the standards.

The National Birth Center Study
Data collection for the National Birth Center Study started in June 1985. The research

---

*See Chapter 12 for additional information.

team's goals were (1) to have every birth center in the nation participate in the study; (2) to have the centers enroll every one of their clients into the study until twenty thousand women had been enrolled; (3) to collect detailed information on the women, their care, and the course and outcome of their pregnancies, including women who were referred or transferred to hospital care because of complications; and (4) to follow the condition of the mother and baby until at least four weeks after the birth. Many birth centers had closed because of the malpractice insurance crisis, and enrollment of study subjects was slower than expected. Enrollment was closed on the last day of 1987, by which time 17,856 clients of eighty-four birth centers throughout the United States had been enrolled.

The study was conducted in collaboration with investigators at the Columbia University School of Public Health. The first paper was published in the *New England Journal of Medicine* in 1989 (Rooks *et al.*, 1989). It reported outcomes for 11,814 women who had remained in birth center care throughout their pregnancies and were admitted to the birth centers for labor and delivery. Sixteen percent of the women or their newborns were transferred to hospitals during or soon after labor and delivery; however, only 2.4 percent of the women or infants had transfers that were considered to be emergencies. The intrapartum and neonatal mortality rate was 1.3 per 1000 births, no higher than rates from studies of low-risk births in hospitals. The cesarean section rate was only about half as high as rates reported by the studies of low-risk hospital births. The research team concluded that "birth centers offer a safe and acceptable alternative to hospital confinement for selected pregnant women."

How to Start a Birth Center Workshops

More than 2,400 people attended fifty-nine two-day "How to Start a Birth Center" workshops conducted by NACC between 1982 and 1995. In addition to 135 birth centers that were known to be in operation in 1995, the membership of NACC included nearly ninety individuals or groups who had joined the organization in order to develop new birth centers.

Trends in Hospital Care During Labor and Delivery

The 1980s saw a crescendo in interhospital competition for obstetric patients with insurance or other means to pay for their care. Although part of an overall increase in the marketing of hospitals, the competition for obstetric patients was especially acute. Health care marketing research found that childbirth is the first hospital experience for 38 percent of maternity patients and that women make 67 percent of all health care decisions, including where, how, and when health care is sought for family and friends, as well as for themselves. Market consultants advised that "catering to the maternity market segment is critical to patient acquisition, not only for the maternity department, but for other health services as well" (Dearing *et al.*, 1987).

Hospitals competed for the allegiance of obstetricians and advertised themselves as desirable places to give birth. In-hospital "birth centers" were developed to provide some of the changes women had been requesting, sometimes with the ambiance of a nice hotel. Institutional hospital decor gave way to wallpaper, curtains, framed pictures, double beds, rockers, and quilts. Routine enemas and perineal shaves were finally dropped in most, but not all, hospitals, and some hospitals developed "labor, delivery, recovery, postpartum" (LDRP) rooms, where some mothers can remain during their entire time in the hospital. Annual Inforum telephone surveys of one hundred thousand households throughout the country found that the proportion of women who were moved from a labor room to a special delivery room declined from about two-thirds in

1988 to about 40 percent in 1991. However, an even larger proportion—86 percent—said that they would prefer to use the same room for labor and delivery (DeWitt, 1993). In-hospital birthing rooms have a homey appearance and facilities to accommodate members of the woman's family—space for a television set (as well as an electronic fetal monitor). Fathers were welcomed during labor *and the birth,* and there was a new movement to allow fathers to watch their babies being delivered by cesarean section—a change made necessary by the increasing and then stable but high rate of births by major abdominal surgery.

Most physicians and their patients continued to believe that the use of ultrasounds and electronic fetal monitoring (EFM) reduces the chance of a poor pregnancy outcome, despite an unbroken sequence of studies that have found no advantage to routine use of either method.* In 1988 the chairman of the Department of Obstetrics, Gynecology and Reproductive Biology at Harvard Medical School described EFM as a "failed technology" but predicted that it would be difficult for obstetricians to stop using it in the absence of a substitute, in part because of the fear of being sued (Ryan, 1988). EFM was applied during 68 percent of all U.S. births in 1989 and 80 percent of births in 1994[†], with regular increases in use during each year in between, based on birth certificate data (NCHS, 1992; Ventura *et al.,* 1996). The actual percentage is probably higher, because it has been shown that obstetric procedures that were used are not always recorded on the certificate (Piper *et al,* 1993). The use of obstetric ultrasonography also increased steadily until it is now used during nearly 85 percent of all pregnancies. The Food and Drug Administration (FDA)

has expressed concern about the misuse of ultrasonic imaging of fetuses for making "keepsake" videos. Although ultrasound fetal scanning is considered safe for most usages, the FDA warns that "ultrasound energy delivered to the fetus cannot be regarded as innocuous" and that "exposing the fetus to ultrasound with no anticipation of medical benefits is not justified." There are strong incentives to adopt new obstetric technologies rapidly and apply them widely. Researchers, manufacturers, practicing physicians, and hospitals gain in prestige as well as financial rewards from the rapid adoption of these highly promoted procedures (Roy, 1993).

"Nothing by mouth" during labor remained the rule, necessitating routine intravenous infusions, and demand for "pain-free" birth increased. Obstetric nurses began to wear buttons with the word "pain" crossed out and encouraged patients to have epidurals during labor. A 1988 *New York Times* article entitled "Women Gain as Technology Becomes Part of Natural Birth" described epidurals (as well as EFM) as part of the new and improved modern approach to childbirth in this country (Brozan, 1988). However, epidural anesthesia may make the mother unable to assume an upright or semi-upright position during labor or to use voluntary effort to help push her baby out. Its use is associated with significantly longer labors, greater use of oxytocin, more frequent use of forceps, and more frequent need for cesarean sections (Kaminski *et al.,* 1993; Thorp *et al.,* 1993).

Efforts to Reduce the Rate of Cesarean Sections

Concerned because the cesarean section rate had tripled between 1968 and 1977, the National Institute of Child Health and Human Development (NICHD), a component of NIH, began the 1980s with a conference to develop scientific and professional consensus about the use of cesarean sections. The conference highlighted the rising cesarean

---

*These studies are described in Chapter 10.

†1989 is the first year for which national data are available on the use of obstetric procedures; 1994 is the year with the most recent data.

birth rate and produced consensus that the trend might be stopped, if not reversed, with no ill effects on pregnancy outcomes, through steps such as permitting women with a previous cesarean delivery to try to achieve a vaginal birth (NICHD, 1981). The conference also focused on dystocia (difficult and abnormally slow labor), which is the most common reason for primary cesarean sections. In 1982 the American College of Obstetricians and Gynecologists responded to the first recommendation with guidelines to encourage vaginal deliveries for women with prior cesarean sections (ACOG, 1982).

The cesarean section rate increased each year between 1980 (when it was 16.5 percent) and 1988, by which time nearly one of every four births (24.7 percent) was by cesarean section. Cesarean section became the most commonly performed surgical procedure in the United States in 1984, a position that it maintains (Keeler & Brodie, 1993).

In 1988 an American pediatrician working for the World Health Organization in Europe published an article in the *Journal of Public Health Policy* which argued that a national cesarean section rate in excess of 15 percent is probably not justifiable, based on data from other Western countries, all of which combine cesarean section rates that are lower than the U.S. rate with neonatal mortality rates that are also lower (Wagner, 1988). The U.S. rate in 1990 was approximately double the rate in three European countries; excess cesareans performed because of dystocia or a previous cesarean accounted for most of the disparity (Notzon, 1990). In 1990 the U.S. Public Health Service established an objective to reduce the cesarean section rate to 15 percent or less by the year 2000 (DHHS, 1991). On the basis of his review of the literature, one highly respected obstetrician suggested that the national cesarean section rate could be reduced to 8 percent without harming women or their babies (Quilligan, 1995).

The cesarean delivery rate declined slightly in 1989, but then remained at about 23 percent until 1992, when it dropped to about 22 percent. It remained at 22 percent during 1992 and 1993 and fell to 21 percent in 1994. All of the reduction between 1988 and 1991 was due to reduced repeat cesarean sections—those performed on women whose uteruses have been scarred by one or more prior cesarean operations. The proportion of women with previous cesareans who gave birth vaginally increased from 18.9 percent in 1989 to 26.3 percent in 1994 (Ventura *et al.*, 1996). Although the trend is in the right direction, the percentage of "VBACs" (vaginal birth after cesarean) is lower in the United States than in many European countries (Notzon, 1990). Data from two recent American studies indicate that as many as 75 percent of women with prior sections could deliver vaginally (Flamm *et al.*, 1994; Cowan *et al.*, 1994).

Despite some success in reducing repeat cesareans, the percent of primary cesarean deliveries* increased from 16.1 percent in 1989 to 17.8 percent in 1991 (NCHS, 1991). In 1992 the rate of primary cesareans began to decline for the first time—to 15.6 percent of all births in 1992. It declined to 14.9 percent in 1994 (Ventura *et al.*, 1996).

Average total charges (physician and hospital) for a cesarean section were more than three thousand dollars higher than for a vaginal delivery in 1991. Assuming that half of those cesareans were not necessary, a study conducted by the Public Citizen's Health Research Group concluded that unnecessary sections are costing society more than $1.3 billion per year (Wolf & Gabay, 1994). Unnecessary cesarean sections also have serious implications for the health of both mothers and babies. Maternal mortality rates are two to four times greater for women who have cesareans than for women who have vaginal births; about half of the deaths are due to the operation itself, rather than to an underlying

---

*The primary cesarean delivery rate is the percent of cesarean births among women who have not had a cesarean delivery in the past.

health problem (Miller, 1988; Lehmann *et al.*, 1987; Petitti *et al.*, 1982). There is also a substantial incidence of maternal morbidity. Four large studies have found that 1.1 to 3.8 percent of women who have cesarean sections experience major complications; 11.5 to 40.3 percent have minor complications (Sachs *et al.*, 1987). Cesarean sections may also result in problems during the mother's future pregnancies, including increased rates of placenta previa and placenta acreta, serious complications that require emergency intervention and may threaten the life of both the mother and the fetus (Clark *et al.*, 1985; Brenner *et al.*, 1978).

Cesarean birth may also have an adverse affect on the newborn, as shown in studies of infants delivered by elective repeat cesarean sections—in which the cesarean is not performed because of any pathology or complication during the current pregnancy. Such infants may be delivered prematurely if the surgeon miscalculates the length of gestation, a complication that should be avoidable through use of prenatal ultrasonography to document the size and gestational age of the fetus. However, it appears that newborns delivered by elective repeat cesarean sections at term are also at increased risk of compromised respiratory function. A study of infants with low five-minute Apgar scores* found that those delivered by repeat cesarean sections were 30 percent more likely to have low scores compared with babies delivered vaginally—a finding that could not be explained by differences in birth weight, gestational age, maternal health, complications during pregnancy or labor, or any other factors (Burt *et al.*, 1988). This study, based on births in Washington State from 1980 to 1983, echoed findings from the large Collaborative Study of Cerebral Palsy, Mental Retardation and Sensory Disorders, conducted between 1959 and 1966, which found fetal compromise and a higher incidence of low Apgar scores among infants delivered by elective repeat cesareans (Benson *et al.*, 1969), and similar studies conducted in Sweden (Hemminki, 1987) and England (Butler & Alberman, 1969). These findings suggest that vaginal delivery may help prepare the fetal lungs and endocrine system for breathing and the other rapid adaptations required at birth.

Factors Associated with Higher or Lower Cesarean Delivery Rates

Cesarean section rates vary with characteristics of the women, the health care system, the people who provide care and support to women during labor, and use of certain obstetric procedures. Maternal characteristics that influence cesarean section rates include maternal age (older mothers have higher rates, regardless of other factors), parity (the rate is highest for women having their first birth, regardless of age), education (women with more years of schooling have higher rates), and socioeconomic status (women with higher family income have higher rates). Hispanic women have a particularly low incidence of cesarean sections (Gould *et al.*, 1989; Stafford *et al.*, 1993). Women who are private patients and women with private health-care insurance have higher cesarean section rates, regardless of their risk status. Women who have no health-care insurance and women who attend publicly supported clinics have lower rates, regardless of risk status. Women who obtain their health care through a health maintenance organization (HMO) tend to have intermediate rates (Kizer & Ellis, 1988; Gould *et al.*, 1989; Haynes de Regt *et al.*, 1986; Wilner *et al.*, 1981; Stafford, 1990; Placek & Taffel, 1988; Zahniser *et al.*, 1991). Women who deliver in a "teaching hospital" are less likely to have cesareans than women who deliver in hospitals without an obstetric residency training program† (Sanchez-Ramos *et al.*, 1994).

---

*The Apgar score provides a rapid assessment of the newborn's condition based on heart rate, respiratory effort, muscle tone, responsive to stimulation, and color.

---

†See discussion in section on "Educational Approaches, Clinical Guidelines and Peer Review."

Studies in Britain and the United States have found significant variation in the tendency of individual obstetricians to use cesarean sections to resolve dystocia, even among physicians working in the same hospital, leading to the conclusion that "the individual clinician is a major determinant of the method of delivery" (Gullemette & Fraser, 1992; Goyert et al., 1989). Another study found a strong influence associated with qualitative differences in the care provided by labor and delivery suite nurses; care by certain nurses was associated with a much lower cesarean section rate (5 percent versus 19 percent), independent of the influence of physicians (Radin et al., 1993). Studies, in Guatemala and the United States have found that the continuous presence of a trained supportive companion shortens labor and reduces the cesarean section rate* (Kennell et al., 1991; Sosa et al., 1980; Klaus et al., 1986).

The increase in the national cesarean section rate paralleled increasing use of continuous electronic fetal monitoring (EFM) and epidural analgesia during labor in the 1970s and 1980s. Use of each of these procedures is associated with increased cesarean section rates among women who had no known complications at the onset of labor (Haverkamp et al., 1979; MacDonald et al., 1985; Leveno et al., 1986; Thorp et al., 1993). A prospective comparison of selective versus universal EFM of 34,995 labors at a major academic medical center in Dallas found a doubling of the primary cesarean section rate associated with continuous EFM (Leveno et al., 1986). A randomized, controlled, prospective clinical trial of the effect of intrapartum epidural analgesia on normal women having their first births at term found a tenfold increase in cesarean deliveries among women given epidural analgesia, compared with women given systemic anal-

gesics—2.2 versus 25 percent, $p < 0.05$ (Thorp et al., 1993). Use of epidurals prolonged both the first and the second stages of labor,[†] increased the need to use oxytocin to increase the strength of uterine contractions, and resulted in more cases of malposition (4.4 versus 18.8 percent, $p < 0.05$). The main cause of the increased cesarean section rate was a higher incidence of cesareans for dystocia.

Low Cesarean Rates Associated with Birth Centers and Care by Midwives

Women who are admitted to free-standing birth centers for labor and delivery and women attended by midwives have particularly low rates of cesarean section. This is to be expected, because both categories should include only women who anticipate uncomplicated births. However, the cesarean section rates associated with both birth centers and nurse-midwives are still lower when compared with rates for most groups of women from which all individuals with risk factors and complications that would preclude a birth center or CNM delivery have been excluded.

Only 4.4 percent of 11,814 women admitted for labor and delivery to eighty-four free-standing birth centers throughout the country between mid-1985 and the end of 1987 had cesarean sections (Rooks et al., 1989). Findings on the birth center clients were compared with data from five previ-

---

*See section on "Effect of a Constant Supportive Companion Throughout Labor."

†The first stage of labor includes the period that begins with the onset of true labor (frequent, intense contractions that are effective in thinning and dilating the cervix) and ends with complete dilation of the cervix. This stage may last for six to eighteen hours in a woman having her first baby and from two to ten hours in a woman having her second or higher-order baby. During the second stage, the woman feels the urge to push and senses the baby moving down and through the birth canal; this stage includes actual birth. The second stage is much shorter than the first stage, usually from thirty minutes to three hours in a woman having her first child, perhaps only five to thirty minutes in a woman who has given birth before.

ously published studies of outcomes of "low-risk" or "uncomplicated" hospital deliveries. In all five studies of hospital births, the low-risk or uncomplicated group was created by retrospective exclusion of women with certain characteristics (risk factors, complications, or outcomes) from data on a large group of women having deliveries in one or more hospitals. Some of the comparison studies even excluded women who had been considered low-risk at the onset of labor but developed complications such as meconium* or fetal distress during labor. Only two of the comparison studies reported cesarean section rates. The birth center rate of 4.4 percent was half or less than half of the rates found in those studies, even though the other studies were conducted between 1980 and 1985, when the cesarean section rate for the country as a whole was lower than it was when the birth center data were collected. Smaller studies comparing birth center outcomes with those of low-risk women in hospitals have also reported a lower incidence of cesarean sections associated with birth center care (Scupholme *et al.*, 1986; Feldman & Hurst, 1987).

Several studies have compared cesarean section rates resulting from care by physicians and CNMs. With few exceptions, they have reported lower rates associated with nurse-midwifery care. However, it has been difficult to rule out the possibility that the lower rates for CNMs are due to differences in the pregnant women themselves, especially differences in the incidence of complications that are indications for a cesarean section. This issue is discussed in detail in Chapter 10.

---

*Meconium is a dark greenish-black material that accumulates in the fetal gut during gestation. Lack of oxygen may cause the fetus to evacuate its bowels, resulting in the presence of meconium in the amniotic fluid. Meconium-stained amniotic fluid is a sign that the fetus experienced inadequate oxygenation at some point during the pregnancy or labor. Thick meconium may be a sign of fetal distress.

"Active Management of Labor" as a Way to Reduce the Cesarean Rate

The 1980 NIH Consensus Development Conference on Cesarean Childbirth's emphasis on dystocia drew attention to the work of Dr. Kieran O'Driscoll and his colleagues at the National Maternity Hospital (NMH) in Dublin, Ireland, who recommend "active management of labor" as an alternative to cesarean section for dystocia (O'Driscoll *et al.*, 1984). In contrast to the large and consistent increases in cesarean sections in the United States between the mid-1960s and the early 1980s, the cesarean section rate at NMH had remained at about 6 percent. Active management of labor as practiced at NMH includes the use of clear criteria for admitting women to the labor ward, early artificial rupture of the membranes, encouraging ambulation, continuous support by a nurse-midwife, early administration of oxytocin if there is not a steady and relatively rapid rate of cervical dilation, avoiding use of EFM, and selective (i.e., not routine) use of epidural analgesia (Boylan, 1989; Fraser, 1993). Two randomized clinical trials have been conducted in efforts to replicate the NMH results in the United States. The first study had positive results—a 26 percent decline in the cesarean section rate associated with use of active management of labor in a study conducted in Chicago (Lopez-Zeno *et al.*, 1992). The second study found no reduction in the cesarean section rate (Frigoletto *et al.*, 1995). The use of oxytocin to hasten delivery is increasing, probably in response to interest in active management of labor. Oxytocin was used to increase the force and speed of labor during 10.9 percent of births in 1989 and 15.1 percent in 1994 (NCHS, 1991; Ventura *et al.*, 1996).

Effect of a Constant Supportive Companion Throughout Labor

The reduction in the cesarean section rate found during the Chicago study of active management of labor was less than the reduction found in a randomized clinical trial of the effect of the presence of a supportive companion (doula) for the mother throughout labor. Two studies in Guatemala and one at an academic medical center in Houston found shorter labors and less need for many obstetric interventions, including cesarean sections, associated with the presence of a doula throughout labor and delivery (Sosa *et al.*,1980; Klaus *et al.*, 1986; Kennel *et al.*, 1991). A randomized controlled trial done in Houston found an 8 percent cesarean section rate among nulliparous women* with uncomplicated pregnancies who had a trained doula at their bedside, soothing and touching and encouraging them throughout labor and delivery. The cesarean section rates for similar women who had a noninteractive observer in their room during labor and for a control group of women who were usually unaccompanied and did not receive continuous support from the professional staff were 13 and 18 percent, respectively (Kennel *et al.*, 1991). The reduction in cesarean sections associated with constant support is both greater and more consistent than the reduction associated with active management of labor.

Educational Approaches, Clinical Guidelines, and Peer Review

Obstetric leaders in several kinds of settings have tried to reduce the cesarean section rate by influencing the behavior of physicians. Such efforts are most effective in hospitals where the obstetrician who wants to lower the cesarean section rate has clear and wide authority. Educational efforts are also more effective when backed up by clinical guidelines that require changes in practice, mandatory second opinions prior to performing cesarean sections, and/or retrospective peer review of all labors that end with a cesarean delivery. This approach has been used most frequently in university hospitals

in which the obstetric leader has authority over all clinicians and there are no private patients, although it has also been used to reduce the cesarean rate among patients admitted to the private service of a university hospital. In this case, the use of clinical guidelines to encourage a trial of labor for women with prior cesareans was reinforced by compiling each individual obstetrician's cesarean section record (total cesarean section rate, as well as primary cesareans, repeat cesareans, and the number of women with cesarean scars who had a trial of labor) and circulating this information to each member of the obstetrical staff. Educational approaches without the authority to implement clinical guidelines and/or mandated second opinions or peer review have not been effective (Porreco, 1985, 1990; Myers & Gleicher, 1988; Sanchez-Ramos *et al.*, 1990; Socal *et al.*, 1993).

No study has found worsening of infant outcomes as cesarean rates were reduced; several studies have reported improvements. Even though the U.S. cesarean section rate is declining, the current rate is too high.

Eliminating Financial Incentives

In 1995 Blue Cross/Blue Shield of New Jersey began paying physicians the same amount for a vaginal birth as for a cesarean section and $100 more for a vaginal birth after cesarean section (or VBAC). The vice president of the company noted that some other insurance plans have adopted similar policies. Although we do not know if these changes will reduce cesarean sections, in the words of one obstetrician, "It doesn't make sense to pay more for a 45-minute operation than to stay up all night with a patient in labor" (Flamm, 1996).

America's High Rates of Low Birth Weight and Infant Mortality

The infant mortality rate for the United States has been higher than rates in most European countries since the Children's Bu-

---

*A nulliparous woman is one who has not given birth before, including one who is in labor for the first time.

reau first examined the issue during the early 1900s. Despite much higher expenditures for health care, our ranking in relation to other countries has worsened over time. In 1973, the infant mortality rates of at least eleven other countries were lower than the U.S. rate. By 1980, at least eighteen countries were doing better. Twenty-one countries had lower rates by 1985, including Hong Kong and Singapore, both of which once had rates much higher than that of the United States. By 1990 the number of countries with lower rates had grown to 23 (NCHS, 1995). Part of the problem is higher infant mortality among certain groups of disadvantaged Americans. Black American babies are nearly 2.5 times more likely than white American babies to die before reaching one year of age. But even our white infant mortality rate is higher than the rates of many other countries (Office of Technology Assessment, 1988).

The primary reason is a persistently high incidence of low birth weight (less than 2,500 grams = 5.5 pounds) and very low birth weight (less than 1,500 grams = 3.3 pounds) among infants born in the United States. Low birth weight (LBW) babies account for two-thirds of U.S. infant deaths and a large share of infant morbidity. Serious, lifelong impairments such as cerebral palsy, blindness, seizure disorders, and mental retardation are three times more frequent among children who were low weight at birth. Even among survivors without obvious physical problems, LBW may be associated with developmental problems and is a significant predictor of learning disabilities and school failure. In addition, the economic costs of LBW are staggering. Special intensive hospital care for low birth weight babies can cost thousands of dollars a day, and most of the babies are hospitalized for weeks; some are in intensive care units for several months (IOM, 1985). Our infant mortality rate is as low as it is only because of the phenomenal ability of our neonatal intensive care units to salvage the lives, if not always the full, inherent potential, of tinier

and tinier babies. If we were not the best in the world at that, our infant mortality rate would be much higher.

The low birth weight rate for the United States declined slightly during the 1970s—from 7.6 percent of births in 1971 to 6.8 percent in 1980, was stable during the first half of the 1980s, and then began to increase—to 7.1 percent in 1991 and 1992, 7.2 percent in 1993, and 7.3 percent in 1994 (Office of Disease Prevention and Health Promotion, 1986; Ventura *et al.*, 1994, 1995, 1996). In 1983 the Institute of Medicine convened a multidisciplinary committee to study the causes and prevention of low birth weight. The two immediate causes are preterm births (when the baby is born too early) and conditions that deprive the developing fetus of an adequate blood supply or nutrition. Some things that cause these conditions are known, but the causes of many, if not most, cases are poorly understood. Some of the recognized causes of one or both conditions include smoking, maternal use of cocaine and other drugs, vaginal infections, subclinical genital tract infections, certain chronic medical diseases, inadequate diet, stress, physical labor, and especially long periods of standing, and unknown pathways that cause low birth weight to be much more frequent among women who are poor or black or unmarried or carrying babies they did not plan and may not really want, or a combination of these. Extreme prematurity is the most serious problem.

Focus on Prenatal Care

Most of the possible means to prevent low birth weight require the active participation of pregnant women. The ways to protect and maximize the health of an unborn baby lie mainly within its mother's power. She will ultimately decide whether to smoke, drink, or use drugs. What she eats; whether and how she works, exercises and rests; her hygiene; her exposure to sexually transmitted infections and violence; and how she copes with psychosocial stress all may affect the well-being of her baby and are beyond the direct control of her health care providers. In addition, to have any chance to stop the process once started, it is critical that pregnant women learn to recognize and report the earliest premonitory signs and symptoms of the beginnings of preterm labor. Effective means to prevent low birth weight must be implemented before the woman is in active labor. For these reasons, and because women who have little or no prenatal care are more likely to have LBW infants, the Institute of Medicine committee focused on the importance of prenatal care. Their main, overriding recommendation was for the nation to make a commitment to ensuring that all pregnant women, especially those at socioeconomic or medical risk, receive high-quality prenatal care (Institute of Medicine, 1985).

In 1989 an expert panel convened by the Public Health Service concluded that counseling about diet, smoking cessation, and the avoidance of use of illegal drugs is an important component of prenatal care and may be most effective if the counseling is received early. A more recent critical review of studies of the relationship between prenatal care and low birth weight cast some doubt on the strength of the beneficial effect of prenatal care. Other recent studies suggest that maternal infections may play a role in initiating some cases of preterm labor and that antibiotic treatment of high-risk women may reduce the incidence of preterm births. All of these conclusions and research suggest that we still have much to learn about how to use prenatal care to have an impact on low birth weight. These issues are discussed in greater depth in Chapter 10.

Access to Effective Reproductive Health Care for Socioeconomically High-Risk Women

During the 1980s there was a widening and deepening sense of crisis regarding the country's ability to provide adequate and effective maternity and other reproductive health care to all of its women. Racial and ethnic minority women, rural women, and women living with poverty and social distress were particularly likely to have limited access to effective care.

Although care during labor and delivery is important, childbirth is a dramatic, one-time per pregnancy event. Most American women are highly motivated to seek professional assistance during labor, and hospitals cannot turn away women who are in labor when they arrive. The greater challenge has been to provide access to prenatal care and family planning services that women are willing and able to use and return to over a period of time. Of women who gave birth in 1980, all but 0.35 percent did so in a hospital or had a physician or midwife to attend their out-of-hospital birth. Nearly four times as many women (1.3 percent) did not have a single prenatal visit before they delivered, 3.8 percent did not start prenatal care until they were seven or more months pregnant, and 18.4 percent of the births were to unmarried women, including 131,000 births to unmarried girls younger than eighteen (NCHS, 1982).

One-fourth of women who delivered babies in the United States during the 1980s did not start prenatal care until they were four or more months pregnant. The efforts to improve access to prenatal care began to show results during the early 1990s. By 1994, four of every five women started prenatal care by the end of the third month of pregnancy, and the proportion who did not begin until they were at least seven months pregnant or received no care at all had declined from 6 to 4 percent.

Health Objectives for the Nation
In 1980 the U.S. Public Health Service (PHS) assessed the nation's status with regard to fifteen measures of effort and success in promoting health and preventing disease, and established the first set of "Health Objectives for the Nation (DHHS, 1980). The objectives

included measurable goals to be achieved by 1990 for five preventive health services, five objectives related to the environment, and five related to personal health behaviors. The family planning objectives included reducing births to girls younger than fifteen to near zero by 1990 and reducing the birth rate for fifteen-to-seventeen-year-old girls and for single women of all ages. The pregnancy and infant health objectives included reducing the low birth weight rate to no more than 5 percent and increasing early use of prenatal care so that by 1990 there would be no county or racial or ethnic group in which fewer than 90 percent of women began prenatal care during the first three months of pregnancy.

In 1986 PHS made a mid-decade review of the country's progress toward the 1990 objectives. The nation was found to be well on its way to achieving most of the objectives that had been established for the fifteen areas of health promotion and disease prevention; the trend was worsening with regard to only eight objectives. Much of the bad news was concentrated in the areas of family planning and maternal and infant health care. There was no reduction in the birth rate for girls younger than fifteen, negligible declines in the rates for sixteen- and seventeen-year-old girls, and the birth rate for unmarried women was increasing. The low birth weight rate had declined slightly, but all of the decrease was in the moderate low birth weight group (1,500 to 2,499 grams at birth). The rate of very low weight births (less than 1,500 grams) remained unchanged, and it seemed unlikely that the country could reduce the overall low birth weight rate to 5 percent by 1990. In addition, we were far from the objective of having 90 percent of pregnant women in all racial and ethnic groups and counties begin prenatal care in the first three months of pregnancy. Of women who gave birth in 1984, 80 percent of white mothers and only 60 to 62 percent of black, American Indian, and Hispanic mothers started care in the first trimester (Office of Disease Prevention and Health Promo-

tion, 1986). A county-by-county study of maternity care found that, as of the mid-1980s, only 1 percent of all U.S. counties had met the 1990 goal (Singh *et al.*, 1994).

Comparing data from National Center for Health Statistics reports for 1980 and 1990 reveals no progress on any of the major family planning, pregnancy, and infant health objectives. In 1990 there were 11,657 births to girls younger than fifteen, and the birth rate for fifteen- to seventeen-year-olds was at its highest point since 1973, having increased by 23 percent between 1986 and 1990. That rate increase translated into 34,000 more births to girls fifteen- to seventeen in 1990 than would have occurred if the rate had remained at its 1986 level. A factor in this increase was the growing proportion of births to Hispanic women, who tend to have high fertility, especially during their teens. More than one million babies were born to unmarried women in 1990. The birth rate for unmarried women increased by 49 percent between 1980 and 1990, and the actual number of births to unmarried women increased by 75 percent (665,747 births to unmarried women in 1980 and 1,165,384 in 1990). The proportion of women beginning prenatal care during the first trimester of pregnancy remained unchanged at 76 percent. The percent who delayed care until the third trimester or had no prenatal care remained unchanged at 6 percent. Substantial racial differences in both percentages persisted throughout the decade; late or no prenatal care continued to be most common for women who were black, unmarried, or less than twenty years of age. The low birth weight rate increased during the 1980s, from 6.8 percent in 1980 to 7.0 percent in 1990. The very low birth weight rate increased by about 10 percent between the late 1970s and 1990, reflecting a steady rise in the proportion of preterm births (NCHS, 1982, 1993a).

In 1990 the Public Health Service developed a new set of national health promotion and disease prevention objectives—targeted for the year 2000 (DHHS, 1991). Many of the family planning and maternal and infant health objectives are the same as those originally set for 1990. We were further from some of the goals in 1990 than we had been in 1980. Two of the broad goals of the many specific objectives for the year 2000 are to reduce disparities in health between different groups of Americans and for everyone in the country to have access to preventive services. Although a thorough review of progress toward the specific objectives and general goals awaits compilation of data that were not available when this book was written, a review of selected objectives was published in 1995 (McGinnis & Lee, 1995). Of three maternal/infant and family planning objectives included in the early assessment, one showed improvement: The proportion of pregnant women beginning prenatal care during the first trimester of pregnancy increased from 76.0 to 77.7 percent between 1987 and 1992. However, the low birth weight rate also increased during the same period. A 5 percent increase in the rate of childbearing by adolescent girls was identified as one of the most alarming findings.

Reasons for Poor Access to Effective Care

The Institute of Medicine's 1985 *Preventing Low Birthweight* report identified several reasons why many women receive little or no prenatal care. The principal barriers were categorized as financial constraints, lack of maternity care providers, insufficient prenatal care services in sites routinely used by high-risk populations, factors that make women disinclined to seek prenatal care, inadequate transportation and child care services, and lack of systems to recruit hard-to-reach women into care.

In 1986 the Institute of Medicine convened another committee, this time to study how to draw women into early and continuous prenatal care. The committee report described an increase in the proportion of births to women with late or no prenatal care among women of all races, although

the trend was most pronounced among black women. By 1986, 11 percent of black pregnant women were entering care very late or delivered without having had even one prenatal visit (Brown, 1989).

Inadequate or no insurance and flaws in the Medicaid program were important but well-known financial barriers to care. Less well recognized obstacles included an inadequate supply of maternity care that is accessible to low-income women. Some communities did not have enough health department clinics, community health centers, or similar facilities to provide services to women who could not afford private care. This resulted in long waiting lists for initial appointments at some facilities, forcing women to delay their entrance into care. In addition, the supply of maternity care providers was limited by maldistribution of physicians, the unwillingness of some physicians to care for low-income women, including those enrolled in Medicaid, and disincentives to practicing obstetrics caused by the increasing expense of malpractice insurance. Reports from selected counties in California exemplified the problem: Between June and August of 1986, 1,245 women seeking prenatal care were turned away from publicly financed clinics in San Diego County, California (Brown, 1989). A 1988 study of problems experienced by women who had difficulty obtaining early prenatal care found that lack of system capacity was a problem for nearly one-third of the women (Center for Health Economics Research, 1993).

Reproductive Health Care Providers

Reproductive health care for women is provided by obstetrician–gynecologists (ob-gyns), family physicians (FPs), general practitioners (GPs), CNMs, nurse practitioners (NPs), physician assistants (PAs), lay and direct-entry midwives, and some naturopaths (NDs). The scope of practice of each group is different. Ob-gyns should play the most important role in the reproductive health care of women who have serious illnesses or complications and should provide consultation and accept referrals from all other care providers. In addition, many ob-gyns devote a large part of their private practices to the care of low-risk women. FPs, GPs, and CNMs can provide a full range of reproductive health care to low-risk pregnant and nonpregnant women, except for surgical services, such as sterilization. FPs and GPs also provide care to newborns, infants and children, and general medical care to all members of the family. CNMs provide care to newborns.

Several kinds of NPs, including family NPs, obstetric and gynecologic NPs, family planning NPs, and women's health care NPs, provide part or the entire scope of ambulatory reproductive health care to essentially well women—family planning, prenatal and postpartum care, breast and cervical cancer screening, health education and counseling, and management of genital tract infections and other common gynecologic problems. The scope of practice for PAs depends on each individual PA and his or her supervising physician; a small proportion of PAs provide obstetric as well as other kinds of reproductive health care. With additional training, some naturopaths and chiropractors also provide obstetric care. Most direct-entry midwives focus primarily on the care of pregnant women, although some provide advice and some therapies to nonpregnant women. They may provide family planning advice, but most cannot provide contraceptive methods that require prescriptions.

Prenatal Care

A county-by-county inventory of prenatal care conducted by the Alan Guttmacher Institute (AGI) during the mid-1980s estimated that approximately 24,000 ob-gyns and 18,000 GPs and FPs were providing obstetric services (Singh *et al.*, 1994). The geographic distribution of the physicians was very uneven; less than half of all counties had a least one ob-gyn with an office-based practice. Although 93 percent of the counties had at least one GP or FP, most of the GPs and FPs did not offer maternity care.

Nevertheless, 76 percent of all prenatal visits occurred in offices maintained by private physicians. Other important sources of prenatal care were clinics associated with hospitals (14 percent of visits) and other clinics (10 percent), including those operated by community action groups, family planning organizations, visiting nurse associations, and community and migrant health centers (Singh *et al.*, 1994).

Although women on Medicaid were less likely to utilize private physicians, 40 percent of their prenatal visits were to private doctors' offices. Women on Medicaid obtained 29 percent of their prenatal care at hospital clinics and 23 percent at health department facilities. Health departments were the largest source of prenatal visits (49 percent) for women with no health care insurance (Singh *et al.*, 1994). Health department clinics in the District of Columbia and eleven southern states constituted half or more of the sites at which women in those jurisdictions could obtain prenatal care. Community and migrant health centers accounted for half or more of the prenatal care sites in Idaho, Nevada, South Dakota, Vermont, Washington, and West Virginia. Six percent of births were to women who lived in 799 counties in which there was no apparent source of prenatal care (Singh *et al.*, 1994).

The AGI study focused on the sites at which prenatal care was provided, rather than the person providing the care. Because many ob-gyns employ nurse-midwives or nurse practitioners, it is not possible to determine who provided the care to women who made their prenatal visits to the offices of private doctors. CNMs and NPs were and continue to be very important providers of prenatal, postpartum, and family planning care at clinics operated by hospitals, health departments, Planned Parenthood affiliates, high schools and colleges, and community and migrant health centers. Reliance on these kinds of services increased during the 1980s (IOM, 1987).

Care During Labor and Delivery

Ninety-nine percent of births occur in hospitals. Obstetric nurses employed by hospitals provide most of the care during labor to most women who give birth in hospitals; they do so with and under the orders of physicians, who may or may not be present until shortly before the delivery. Physicians conduct most deliveries in hospitals, with nurse-midwives attending nearly all others. When all births are considered, physicians attended 93.9 percent of the births in 1994. CNMs attended 5.2 percent; other midwives attended 0.3 percent. The remainder (about half of 1 percent) were unattended or were attended by nurses, emergency medical technicians, naturopaths, chiropractors, physician assistants, family, friends or bystanders. The proportion of births attended by physicians is declining and the proportion attended by nurse-midwives is increasing. (See Table 2 in Chapter 7.)

Obstetrician-Gynecologists

Although ob-gyns deliver the majority of babies born in the United States, there are geographic gaps in their availability and they are least available to women who are poor. Many ob-gyns stopped practicing obstetrics as a result of the medical malpractice insurance crisis, choosing to focus on gynecology instead. As of 1988, only 72 percent of ob-gyns were practicing obstetrics. As of 1990, only one of four ob-gyns over the age of sixty was delivering babies, and they had begun to retire from practice entirely at younger ages (Pearse, 1993). A 1992 survey of two thousand members of ACOG found that one-eighth had dropped obstetrics during the previous year (ACOG, 1993).

Another problem was the refusal of many—eventually most—ob-gyns to take care of women on Medicaid. Reasons included unrealistically low Medicaid payments for obstetric care, denial of some claims, long delays in receiving payments, complex paperwork, the increased risk of a poor pregnancy outcome among socioeco-

nomically high-risk women, and obstetricians' belief that Medicaid clients are more likely to sue. Many indigent women are poorly educated, of a different race than their doctors, do not speak English, or are withdrawn and hard to talk to. Some obstetricians find it difficult to accept pregnant women who are not married, the immature behavior of pregnant teens, and women who have poor health habits that they seem unable or unwilling to change. Some poor women are illiterate, unable to read instructions, and lead stressful, disorganized lives, causing them to miss appointments or not follow the doctor's orders. They are sometimes referred to as patients who are "hard to serve." They have more problems than middle-class patients. They need more attention, more tests, more education, and more time. Instead of paying more to take care of them, because they need more care, Medicaid paid less, in some states as little as 60 percent or less of the doctor's usual fee. As of 1982, only 64 percent of obstetricians were willing to accept any Medicaid patients (IOM, 1985). Ob-gyn participation in the Medicaid program declined steadily from there. By 1987 fewer than half of practicing ob-gyns were accepting Medicaid payment for their care, by 1990 only 44 percent were willing to take Medicaid (Center for Health Economics Research, 1993).

In 1991 the Josiah Macy, Jr. Foundation convened a conference to examine the role of obstetrician–gynecologists in the twenty-first century. It was chaired by Dr. Edward Wallach from Johns Hopkins University School of Medicine. His introductory remarks recognized the need for dramatic improvement in the quality, cost, equity, efficacy, and access to health care for American women and the reflection of lack of access to care "in our country's unacceptably high infant mortality rate" (Wallach, 1993). Persons attending the conference discussed the need to motivate ob-gyns to care for women who are poor and to teach them how to provide effective care to poor women and women of color. There was agreement that "access to care depends on a team approach that includes nurse-midwives and nurse practitioners . . ." (Milliken, 1993).

In 1994, for the first time in the forty-three-year history of the American College of Obstetricians and Gynecologists, more women than men completed residencies in obstetrics and gynecology. Nearly as many women entered the specialty in that single year (N = 4,404) as the total number of female ACOG members who were already in established practices (N = 4,572). The proportion of women entering obstetrics has been increasing for more than a decade (O'Neill, 1995). In 1975, only 5 percent of all practicing obstetrician–gynecologists were women. By 1989, nearly one-fourth were women. ACOG has estimated that women will account for more than one of every three ob-gyns by the end of the first decade of the twenty-first century. Considering the increase in female ob-gyns, in 1991 the executive director of ACOG suggested that "to the extent that the choice of a nurse-midwife is a choice for a female provider rather than a choice for an approach to care, the woman ob-gyn may be a substitute for the midwife" (Pearse, 1993).

Family Practice Physicians

FPs provide "comprehensive medical care with particular emphasis on the family unit, in which the physician's continuing responsibility for health care is not limited by the patient's age or sex or by a particular organ system or disease entity (AAFP, 1994). FPs have provided a significant proportion of obstetric care in the United States, especially in rural areas. ACOG and the AAFP both acknowledge the need for the participation of family physicians (Stern, 1977). However, the proportion of physicians entering family practice residencies has been low and the participation of FPs in obstetrics declined drastically during the 1980s (Kruse *et al.*, 1989; Rosenblatt *et al.*, 1982; Smucker, 1988). ACOG estimated that FPs delivered

between 15 and 20 percent of the babies born in 1989 (Pearse, 1993).

Due to the high status and incomes of surgeons and specialists it has, until recent years, been difficult to attract enough American medical school graduates into family practice. The recent rapid reorganization of American health care resources into managed care organizations that give priority and the key "gatekeeper" role to primary care physicians has resulted in a dramatic reversal in that situation during just the past few years.* The number of first-year FP residents increased by less than 1 percent between 1980 and 1990 (2,365 in 1980, compared with 2,388 in 1990), but shot up to 3,494 in 1996—an increase of more than 46 percent in a period of six years. Nearly 15 percent of physicians graduating from American medical schools between July 1994 and June 1995 had entered FP residencies by October 1995. This proportion is the highest ever recorded (although the records only go back to 1980–1981), and it has been increasing each year since 1993. Approximately 12 percent of new American medical graduates entered FP residencies in 1993, and 13 percent in 1994. Nevertheless, graduates of foreign medical schools continue to fill many FP residency positions. The proportion of first-year positions filled by foreign graduates increased from 11 percent in 1980, to 18 percent in 1990, to 20 percent in 1996 (based on only the matches made by the National Resident Matching Program during March, which is the major matching period). A significant proportion of the foreign medical graduates who fill these posi-

---

*The "primary-care physician" category includes medical doctors (MDs) and doctors of osteopathy (DOs) who are general practitioners (physicians with no specialty training) and those who have completed residencies in family medicine, internal medicine, or pediatrics, except for pediatricians and internists who are qualified in subspecialties. See discussion of this subject in section on "Obstetricians as Primary Care Providers," in Chapter 14.

tions are U.S. citizens, for example, 30 percent in 1993 and 59 percent in 1992 (AAPF, 1994; Kahn *et al.*, 1996).

Individual FPs' decisions to include or not include obstetrics in their practice is a major factor affecting FP's contribution to the care of pregnant women. Although all family medicine residents receive some training in obstetrics, most do not deliver babies after they finish their training and go into practice (Rosenblatt *et al.*, 1997). A study from the late 1970s found 46 percent of FPs practicing obstetrics and great regional variation, from 61 percent in the North Central region of the country to 6 percent of those in the Northeast. FPs practicing by themselves or working in affluent counties or areas with many obstetricians were least likely to practice obstetrics (Rosenblatt *et al.*, 1988). In 1986 the AAFP reported that 23 percent of its members had stopped practicing obstetrics due to liability concerns (AAFP, 1986). Although a study conducted in 1987 found that 45 percent of FPs were delivering babies (virtually the same as during the late 1970s), 65 percent had practiced obstetrics at some time in their careers, 12 percent had stopped during the prior twelve months, and nearly half of those who were still doing obstetrics were thinking of dropping that part of their practice. The cost of malpractice insurance, fear of litigation, and the effects of delivering babies on the FP's lifestyle and office practice were the most important factors influencing their decisions (Kruse, *et al.*, 1989). Only 24 percent of FPs were delivering babies by 1992. Strong support for the role of maternity care in family practice by advocacy groups within the AAFP and the Society of Teachers of Family Medicine (STFM) was given credit for a reversal in the trend; the proportion practicing obstetrics increased to 29 percent in 1994. The proportion is higher among family physicians who practice in rural areas; 39 percent of rural FPs were practicing obstetrics in 1993 (Leeman, 1995).

Although declining FP participation in obstetrics was attributed primarily to concerns about malpractice, a 1988 editorial in the *Journal of Family Practice* identified the increasingly technological style of American obstetrics as a root cause of the problem. To decrease costs and make obstetric practice more rewarding, Dr. Roger Rosenblatt (from the Department of Family Medicine at the University of Washington) recommended that family physicians stop emulating the practices of high-risk perinatologists, "develop a style of obstetrical practice that recognizes that most pregnancies require no specific 'medical' intervention," and forge "closer ties with the growing number of well-trained midwives" (Rosenblatt, 1988). Although several studies have found that family physicians use somewhat fewer interventions than obstetricians (MacDonald *et al.*, 1993; Hueston *et al.*, 1995; Rosenblatt *et al.*, 1997), a 1988–1989 study of care provided to low-risk women in urban hospitals in Washington State found major differences between the care provided by CNMs and either kind of physician, but only small differences between labor and delivery care provided by FPs and ob-gyns, including similar rates of cesarean sections and operative vaginal deliveries—that is, use of forceps or vacuum to extract the baby (Rosenblatt *et al.*, 1997). The researchers were not surprised by these findings, because most family physicians in Washington State receive much of their obstetric training from obstetricians, often in tertiary medical centers, and all of the FPs in their study practiced in hospitals where most babies are delivered by obstetricians and use obstetricians for both consultation and referral. The family physicians were simply following the norms established by their specialist colleagues (Rosenblatt *et al.*, 1997).

Physician Assistants

PAs are licensed to practice medicine under the direction and supervision of a physician. Within the MD–PA relationship, physician assistants exercise autonomy in medical decision making and provide a broad range of diagnostic and therapeutic services. Their scope of practice depends on the agreement between each individual PA and his or her supervising physician. Although many PAs work directly with individual MDs, some operate primary health care clinics or work directly for hospitals. Many fill roles that would otherwise be filled by interns or foreign medical graduates, or they run clinics, in some cases far away from the hospital itself. Approximately 29,000 PAs were in practice as of 1995. Because early PA classes were recruited from the ranks of discharged military medical corpsmen, during the first fifteen years, most PAs were men. However, more than 60 percent of students admitted to PA training programs between 1983 and 1995 were women (Oliver, 1995). As of May 1995, Mississippi was the only state that did not provide legal recognition to physician assistants (ACOG, 1995).

Most PA education programs are associated with medical schools. Although most require students to have two years of college education and some prior health care experience before they enter the PA program, some nondegree programs accept high school graduates without additional formal education. The PA program itself usually consists of at least two years of classroom instruction and clinical rotations, usually including a six-week experience in obstetrics and gynecology. Five to ten percent of new graduates elect to enter six- to eighteen-month specialty training programs.

Approximately 4 percent of PAs specialize in obstetrics and gynecology. In addition, about one-third of those in family practice provide care to pregnant women (AAPA, 1993). Some PAs conduct vaginal deliveries for women who are expected to have uncomplicated births; however, there are no reliable data on how many PAs deliver babies. Fifteen percent of PAs practice in rural communities. Nine percent of ob-gyns who responded to a survey conducted by the Montana Department of Social and Rehabilitation Services in May 1991 indicated that they employed one or more PAs. It is common for PAs to assist physicians with complicated pregnancies and cesarean section deliveries.

There is growing interest in obstetric internships and residencies for PAs. Albert Einstein University offers a PA residency in obstetrics and gynecology at Montefiore Hospital in New York City, and the Department of Obstetrics and Gynecology at the New York Hospital–Cornell Medical Center plans to start one.

Access to Care for Rural Women
Nearly one-fourth of the population of the United States lives in rural areas—22.5 percent were living in nonmetropolitan counties in 1990. Poor roads and distance, often compounded by bad weather, make it difficult for women who live in rural areas to drive to cities to obtain maternity care. The people living in many rural areas are relatively poor, including a high proportion who have no health care insurance, making it difficult for physicians to make a living in those areas (Nesbitt, 1996). The number of physicians providing maternity care to poor women in rural parts of the country declined by 20 percent between 1984 and 1989 (Institute of Medicine, 1989). The number of rural hospitals that have labor and delivery units has decreased (Nesbitt, 1996).

Although obstetricians provide most of the maternity care in the country as a whole, family and general practice physicians have been the main source of obstetric care in rural areas. Less than 10 percent of obstetricians were located in rural areas as of 1989. In 1988, there was no obstetrician–gynecologist in 60 percent of rural counties. However, large numbers of FPs gave up obstetrics in response to the malpractice insurance crisis. Smucker documented a decrease in obstetrical practice by FPs in Ohio from 54 percent in 1975 to 16 percent in 1989 (Smucker, 1988). Similar declines were reported in

Alabama, Arizona, Missouri, Mississippi, Oklahoma, and Oregon (Allen & Kamradt, 1991). As a result, access to any kind of maternity care became a problem for women in many rural areas. A congressionally mandated 1989 review of health personnel shortages found that more than half of the states were experiencing shortages of maternity care providers in rural and disadvantaged areas. Thirty-one percent of the states reported that a shortage of nurse-midwives exacerbated the problem of providing adequate prenatal care. Predominantly rural states were especially likely to report the need for additional CNMs (Kolimaga *et al.*, 1992).

Women who have to travel a long time to visit a maternity care provider are less likely to receive adequate prenatal care (McDonald & Coburn, 1988). Several studies have found a correlation between lack of access to care for pregnant rural women and a higher incidence of complicated deliveries, low birth weight, and infant mortality (Nesbitt *et al.*, 1990; Allen & Kamradt, 1991; Larimore & Davis, 1995). Difficulty finding transportation has its greatest impact on rural indigent women, who may lack the means or funds to travel significant distances for prenatal care (Foster *et al.*, 1992).

Recommendations to Increase Use of CNMs to Increase Access to Care

In 1976 the Department of Health and Human Services convened a committee to determine how many physicians would be required to bring supply and need for each specialty into balance, to recommend ways to improve the geographic distribution of physicians, and to suggest mechanisms to finance graduate medical education. The Graduate Medical Education National Advisory Committee (GMENAC) completed and published its report in 1980. It predicted an overall surplus of physicians by 1990, but a shortage of primary-care physicians, and recommended expansion of residency training positions in family practice, general pediatrics, and general internal medicine. GMENAC also recommended that the country plan for CNMs to be handling 5 percent of all "normal, uncomplicated deliveries" by 1990. Midwives of all kinds delivered only 1.7 percent of all babies born in the United States in 1980, the year when that recommendation was made; the recommendation was considered to be quite visionary.

The Institute of Medicine's 1985 *Preventing Low Birthweight* report cited studies that had found a reduced incidence of low birth weight associated with nurse-midwifery care of socioeconomically high-risk pregnant women. The researchers suggested that these outcomes may result from CNMs' emphasis on education, support and patient satisfaction, and their nonauthoritarian approach to patients. A 1981 study had found that CNMs spent an average of twenty-four minutes with the woman during each prenatal visit and always devoted some of that time to patient teaching (Lehrman, 1981). In contrast, the 1975 National Ambulatory Medical Care Survey had found physicians spending an average of only ten minutes with each prenatal patient; 32 percent of their prenatal visits took five minutes or less, and they did little counseling (NCHS, 1980). Other studies had shown that CNMs' clients returned for a higher proportion of their prenatal appointments and were more likely than physicians' patients to carry out their care providers' instructions for self-care. The committee recommended that the nation rely more heavily on nurse-midwives and obstetric nurse practitioners to provide care to "hard-to-reach" high-risk women and that state laws be amended to support nurse-midwifery practice (IOM, 1985).

The Institute of Medicine's 1987 report on utilization of prenatal care noted that CNMs serve "disproportionate numbers of women who are poor, adolescent, members of minority groups, and residents of inner cities or rural areas" and that legal restrictions and "obstetrical customs" limit their numbers and scope of practice. The report characterized the country's maternity care system as "fundamentally flawed, fragmented, and overly complex. Unlike many European nations, the United States has no direct, straightforward system for making maternity services easily accessible." It urged the development of a new system, which should "rely on a wide array of providers, including both physicians and certified nurse-midwives, each of whom may practice in a variety of settings." It recommended increased use of CNMs and called for state laws and physicians to support hospital privileges and improved collaboration between physicians and nurse-midwives (IOM, 1987).

In 1988 the National Commission to Prevent Infant Mortality called on state universities to expand their nurse-midwifery training programs. The National Perinatal Information Center's 1992 report, *Perinatal Health: Strategies for the 21st Century,* states that nurse-midwives can and should play a major role in improving access to perinatal health care and should be represented at all levels of policy and decision making in the perinatal health care system. In 1993 the March of Dimes Birth Defects Foundation published a report entitled *Toward Improving the Outcome of Pregnancy: The 90s and Beyond.* Based in part on input obtained from nearly one thousand clinicians, policy makers, and community leaders during meetings in Atlanta, Denver, Los Angeles, New York, and St. Louis, it includes a blunt discussion of problems caused by the denial and delay of hospital privileges for certified nurse-midwives (March of Dimes Birth Defects Foundation, 1993).

In 1996 Dr. Thomas Nesbitt, a professor in the Department of Family Practice at the University of California, Davis, recommended collaborative practice between CNMs and family physicians as a means to extend access to high-quality maternity care in rural communities (Nesbitt, 1996). He cited a finding from a 1994 survey of the thirty northern-most rural hospitals in California to show that his idea was already be-

ing implemented to some degree: There was at least one nurse-midwife on the staff of one-third of the hospitals. Family physicians have been dropping out of obstetrics in part because of the negative effects on their families and practice from being constantly on call for labor and delivery. As more rural FPs dropped obstetrics from their practice, these problems have intensified for the declining number of FPs that continue to practice obstetrics. Dr. Nesbitt identified many clear benefits of associating with a CNM from the standpoint of a rural family physician, who may need a partner for obstetric coverage, but does not have a large enough general practice to bring in an additional FP (Nesbitt, 1996).

Implementation of the Recommendations About Midwives

The many recommendations to increase and facilitate the role of nurse-midwives in the care of socioeconomically high-risk women was heard and heeded by a variety of agencies and organizations. Philanthropic foundations weighed in with financial support to assist the start-up of nurse-midwifery services designed to meet the needs of specific groups of women. As a result, new CNM services were started in communities throughout the country during the last years of the 1980s. Foundations and governmental entities also developed special programs to encourage and support the recruitment and education of more midwives. The following are examples:

- *West Virginia.* In 1988 West Virginia obtained a Robert Wood Johnson Foundation grant to recruit and educate local nurses as nurse-midwives. The money was used for nurse-midwifery education scholarships for nurses who agreed to return to work in West Virginia after becoming qualified as a CNM. The number of CNMs practicing in West Virginia increased from four in 1989 to more than twenty in 1992.

- *North Carolina.* A study conducted in 1991 found no professional caregiver to deliver babies in 24 of North Carolina's 100 counties; all but three of the 24 counties were rural. To encourage the development of nurse-midwifery practices in underserved areas, North Carolina developed an incentive program that provides participating CNMs with malpractice insurance subsidies of up to three thousand dollars per year. CNMs in the program are authorized to receive payment from any type of third-party health care financing program for which her clients are eligible (Taylor & Ricketts, 1993).

- *Massachusetts.* Between 1991 and 1993 Massachusetts provided financial support to help more than thirty Massachusetts nurses undertake nurse-midwifery education in exchange for a commitment to work in underserved communities within the state for at least two years.

- *Florida.* Between 1985 and 1991 there was a 50 percent decrease in the number of obstetricians practicing in Florida and a 20 percent increase in the number of births. The Advisory Committee for the Florida Healthy Start Program recommended that the state establish an objective of having midwives provide care to half of all low-risk pregnant women in the state by the year 2000. In 1992 the Robert Wood Johnson Foundation provided funds to assist the University of Florida College of Medicine to determine how to best recruit, train, and retain state licensed midwives, as well as CNMs. In 1993, the Florida Midwifery Resource Center issued a "Call to Action" which established three goals: to educate six hundred additional CNMs in the State of Florida by the year 2000, to establish midwifery care as the standard of practice for the healthy pregnant woman, and to promote the development of family-centered birth centers. Strategies recommended to reach those goals include reducing barriers to nurse-midwifery education and increasing the capacity of nurse-midwifery education programs that are accessible to nurses who live in Florida, obtaining 100 percent Medicaid reimbursement for nurse practitioners and midwives, incorporating midwifery care into all aspects of state health care plans, identifying and eliminating barriers to the participation of midwives and birth centers in managed health care, providing incentives for the development of community-based birth centers, and integrating birth center experience into midwifery education.

- *Oregon.* During 1989 and 1990 a foundation in Oregon, made four grants for the purpose of establishing nurse-midwifery services to address unmet needs for quality maternity care for low-income women in three parts of Oregon and one community in southwestern Washington State. One of the programs served a large number of Hispanic migrant farm workers; one served low-income women in a sparsely populated rural area in central Oregon; one provided special care for pregnant women with drug and alcohol abuse problems and women involved in domestic violence. Follow-up in these programs demonstrated profound benefits to the women and their babies and communities. One program was credited with 50 percent reductions in both the low birth weight rate and the number of newborns admitted to the neonatal intensive care unit over a period of three years. Another was credited with a more than 80 percent reduction in the number of women who went to local hospitals in labor without having had any prior contact with the health care system (Meyer Memorial Trust, 1997).

Expansion of Medicaid Eligibility

Medicaid is the major means by which government finances health care for low-income pregnant women. It is a means-tested entitlement program financed by both the federal and state governments and administered by the states. Federal guidelines require states to provide specified benefits to specified groups of people. Although states must adhere to the federal eligibility and benefit guidelines to qualify for federal matching payments, individual states can be more generous than the federal guidelines, both in eligibility criteria and benefits. As a result, state-to-state variation in the program is significant. The federal share ranges from slightly less than 50 percent to 80 percent of the total Medicaid expenditures in various states (Kaiser Commission on the Future of Medicaid, 1995).

During the last half of the 1980s Congress enacted legislation to expand the number of women who are eligible for Medicaid and required states to make Medicaid-eligible women's access to obstetric care equal to that of other women. In addition to expanding eligibility for Medicaid, most states increased the amount they would pay for maternity care. The proportion of obstetrician–gynecologists who accept Medicaid-eligible women as patients increased along with the Medicaid payments (Piper *et al.*, 1994). The number of deliveries paid for by Medicaid more than doubled between 1985 and 1991, by which time Medicaid was financing almost one-third of all births in the United States (Singh *et al.*, 1995).

The expansion in eligibility resulted from changes that allow states to enroll low-income women and children who are not poor enough to meet the earlier criteria and "presumptive eligibility," which permits pregnant women to obtain prenatal care and other services immediately after they apply for Medicaid. This avoids a long waiting period while their papers are processed, which previously contributed to delayed entrance into care. A study to measure the impact of presumptive eligibility on Medicaid-eligible women in Tennessee found that women were enrolling in care earlier and were three times

more likely to fill a prescription for prenatal vitamins in the first three months of pregnancy. These changes were not associated with improvements in the outcomes of their pregnancies (Piper *et al.*, 1994).

The expanded access to health care for pregnant women achieved by these changes may be nullified, if not reversed, by cuts in federal funding for Medicaid that have been proposed by both the President and Congress in an effort to balance the budget.

Trends in the Numbers of Births and the Characteristics of Childbearing Women

The major determinants of birth outcomes are maternal race, ethnicity, social class, income level, marital status, and educational attainment. Disadvantaged women and their infants are most likely to have problems. Poor women may be at increased risk of poor pregnancy outcomes because of a complex, interactive mix of environmental, social, behavioral, medical, and health care correlates of poverty, including poor hygiene and nutrition, smoking and use of alcohol and drugs, physical and psychosocial stress, inadequate social support, violence, early and/or closely spaced pregnancies, high parity, and a higher disease burden due to less adequate diagnosis and treatment of some diseases, biological responses to stress, and a higher incidence of infections, including those resulting in sexually transmitted disease. The impact of these influences is compounded by lack of accurate information and obstacles to effective utilization of health care, including racial, cultural, gender, and language differences that impede the development of mutual trust and effective communication between care providers and women in need of care. Planning for the provision of effective maternity care should take into account the numbers, characteristics, and problems of childbearing women. These, in turn, are affected by the social, demographic and fertility characteristics of the population of the nation. This section provides a brief review of the current status and trends for some relevant characteristics.*

The "baby boomlet" that began in the late 1970s peaked in 1990, when there were 4.2 million births in the United States; it was the largest number in any year since 1962. The "baby boom" generation (Americans born between 1946 and 1964) is moving past the prime childbearing ages and is being replaced by a smaller group of women born during the "baby bust." There was a 1 percent decrease in births between 1990 and 1991, and the number has declined every year since then, falling below 4 million for the first time in many years in 1994. The number of births is expected to decline gradually for another decade. However, the decline should be small, with the number of births expected to remain at about 3.9 million per year until the year 2005, when it should rise back above 4 million. The current decline in fertility would be greater except for relatively high fertility among recent immigrants, most of whom are young (Savage, 1995). As a result of the rise of immigration into the United States from Latin America, Asia, and other regions, as of 1990, one of every seven U.S. residents (14 percent) spoke a language other than English in their homes. Seventeen percent of U.S. births in 1992 were to women who had not been born in this country. It is anticipated that racial and ethnic minorities will comprise 40 percent of America's youth by 2020.

The percent of births to women with some characteristics associated with increased rates of pregnancy complications is growing, especially the proportion of births to unmarried women and women at the upper end of the childbearing age span. The proportion of multiple births is also increasing, probably due to the use of fertility-enhancing drugs and a shift toward childbearing by older women (Ventura *et al.*, 1996). The percentage of births to women with other high-risk characteristics seems to be very stable, as shown in Table 1. The unmarried birth rate (births per 1,000 unmarried women) rose by 77 percent between 1980 and 1994. Thirty-three percent of 1994 births were to women who were not married, including the majority of births to black women (70 percent). Unmarried women are less likely than other mothers to get adequate prenatal care or gain sufficient weight during their pregnancy and are more likely to smoke.

Table 1
Percent of Births with Specific High-Risk Characteristics, United States, 1980–1994*

High-Risk Characteristic	1980	1990	1994
Mother's race:			
Black	15.7	16.5	16.1
Native American	0.8	0.9	1.0
Mother's age:			
<15	0.3	0.3	0.3
15–17	5.5	4.4	4.9
35–39	3.9	7.6	9.4
≥40	0.7	1.2	1.7
Mother with <12 years education	23.7	23.8	22.6
Unmarried mother	18.4	28.0	32.6
Mother's first birth	43.2	40.9	41.2
Fourth or higher order birth	9.9	10.5	10.5
Twins, triplets, etc./1,000 births	1.9	2.3	2.6
Less than 18 months since mother's last birth	13.2	13.6	NA

*Data are from the National Center for Health Statistics advance reports of final natality statistics for 1980, 1990, 1994, and 1995.

NA = data not available.

---

*Unless another source is given, all data are from reports of the U.S. Bureau of the Census and the National Center for Health Statistics.

Only 57 percent of births in 1988 resulted from intended pregnancies. Seven percent of the births were unwanted—births to women who, at the time they conceived, did not want to ever have another (or any) child. Thirty-six percent were births that were mistimed—the mother wanted to have a child some day, but not then. There is a strong association between poverty and whether or not a birth is planned, unwanted, or mistimed. The poorer a woman is, the more likely she is to have an unintended birth. The investigators who reported these data suggested that women whose pregnancies were not intended may need additional attention to help ensure their well-being during pregnancy and the birth of a healthy baby (Kost & Forrest, 1995).

A more recent study (data collected during 1990 and 1991) based on data from only four states (Alaska, Maine, Oklahoma, and West Virginia) also found that only 57 percent of births were intended, although the proportion that were unwanted (as compared to mistimed) was higher. Twelve percent of the mothers in the 1990–1991 study had not wanted to ever have another (or any) child (Gazmararian *et al.*, 1995).

The same study (data from stratified systematic samples of all births in Alaska, Maine, Oklahoma, and West Virginia in 1990 and 1991) found that 4 to 7 percent of the women reported that they had been physically hurt by their husband or sexual partner during the year preceding the birth. There was considerable variation by location; 7 percent of new mothers in Oklahoma had experienced physical violence during their pregnancies, compared with 4 percent in Maine. The incidence of physical abuse during pregnancy is higher for women who are young, single, of lower socioeconomic status, of higher parity (i.e., mothers with many other children), and did not want to be pregnant. Women carrying unwanted pregnancies were four times more likely to be physically hurt by their sexual partner, as compared with women with intended pregnancies—12 percent versus 3 percent (Gazmararian *et al.*, 1995). Studies that focus on women who use publicly supported inner-city clinics have found quite extraordinary rates of physical abuse during pregnancy. In a study of low-income women who obtained prenatal care at urban clinics in Virginia, Texas, and Maryland between February 1990 and January 1993, one-fifth of the teenagers and one-sixth of the adult women experienced physical or sexual abuse while pregnant. The abused women tended to start care later in the pregnancy, compared with women who were not abused, and their babies were 1.5 times as likely to be low birth weight (Parker *et al.*, 1994).

The proportion of pregnant women who smoke declined between 1989 and 1994. Fifteen percent of women who gave birth in 1994 smoked during their pregnancies (NCH, 1996). Cigarette smoking is associated with reduced infant birth weight, preterm delivery, intrauterine growth retardation, and sudden infant death syndrome. According to a survey conducted by the National Institute of Drug Abuse, 5 percent of American women who gave birth in 1992 used illegal drugs at some time during their pregnancy.

The number of HIV-infected women is increasing, as AIDS spreads into the heterosexual population of childbearing age. One recent study found that nearly 5 percent of adolescents attending an inner-city clinic were HIV-positive (Avery, 1995).

After many years of decline, breast-feeding increased during the early 1980s, when it became the dominant method of feeding infants during the first months of their lives. There was a sharp downward trend during the last half of the 1980s, especially among economically disadvantaged women and women of color. Breastfeeding is making a comeback: The proportion of all mothers who breast-fed their infants during the early postpartum period increased from 54 percent in 1988 to 60 percent in 1994; the proportion of mothers breast-feeding their infants at five or six months postpartum increased from 21 percent in 1988 to 23 percent in 1994 (NCHS, 1996). Young women with the least education, lowest income, and racial or ethnic minority status are least likely to breastfeed (Martinez & Nalezienski, 1981; Ryan and Martinez, 1989). Thirty-two percent of low income women breast-fed their babies during the early postpartum period during 1994; only 12 percent continued until their infants were at least five or six months old (NCHS, 1996). It is impressive that breast-feeding is increasing, even though most American women of reproductive age are in the workforce. Breast-feeding is an important factor for infant health and survival, even in industrialized countries such as the United States.

What Kind of Maternity Care Do Women Want?

The strident complaints of the home birth/natural childbirth movement of the 1960s and 1970s abated during the 1980s, as physicians and hospitals adopted some of the methods introduced by midwives and birth activists and as the politically active women who were having babies in the 1970s completed their families. Childbearing fell to a new generation of young women who are accustomed to using sophisticated equipment in many aspects of their lives and are more likely to trust the technical interventions that are now widely used during pregnancy and birth. Few American women have experienced or seen another woman give birth without substantial intervention. Most women expect prenatal ultrasounds (wanting to "see," know the sex of, and obtain a keepsake "picture" of their fetus), believe constant electronic fetal heart rate monitoring during labor is essential, and want epidural anesthesia and as little pain as possible. Most American couples plan to have only one or two children and believe that obstetric technology helps to ensure a perfect baby. Despite a cesarean section rate so high it is ridiculed by observers from other countries, it is rare for a woman to believe her own cesarean section was not a life-saving necessity.

Pregnant American women are hungry for advice and information. Books on pregnancy and childbirth sold well during the 1980s and early 1990s. Almost 2.7 million copies of *What to Expect When You're Expecting,* only one of many books and manuals on the subject, were sold between 1984 and 1993. In addition, there seems to be an ever-expanding market for childbirth education. The American Society of Psychoprophylaxis in Obstetrics (ASPO Lamaze) estimated that approximately forty thousand childbirth educators were working in the United States in 1993 and that half of all expectant parents were taking some kind of preparatory class. Many childbirth educators are diversifying their offerings, with special classes for adoptive parents, pregnant adolescents, siblings, and grandparents, and weekend retreats that offer busy professionals a relatively expensive but enjoyable alternative to a series of weekly evening classes (DeWitt, 1993).

In 1986 Penny Armstrong, a nurse-midwife with a long-term home birth practice in a rural Amish community in Pennsylvania, and coauthor Sheryl Feldman published a book about Penny's experiences and observations (Armstrong & Feldman, 1986). Trying to understand why one-fourth of all American women were having cesareans while the rate for Penny's Amish clients was only 6 percent, they "ruled out the possibility that it was all the physicians' doing. If one in four women had cesareans," they reasoned, "women must, somehow, be in agreement with them. . . . Society in general, including birthing mothers" must have "legitimate, if not particularly healthy, reasons for participating in and perpetuating the highly medicalized birth" (Armstrong & Feldman, 1990). They decided to interview well-educated white women who were intentionally pregnant or had recently given birth to planned babies— members of the trend-setting class of childbearing women—to try to understand their expectations and experiences regarding pregnancy and birth. Interviewing approximately sixty such women between 1986 and 1989 convinced them that many women do not want to give birth without technical interventions and drugs. Yet these were responsible women who had chosen to become pregnant and wanted to do the best they could for themselves and for their children. Somehow natural childbirth did not serve these women well. Women's natural power to give birth, which seemed to "flood" the rural Amish bedrooms, often "dried up" for women in hospitals (Armstrong & Feldman, 1990).

Epidural anesthesia bears part of the blame. Most of the women they interviewed wanted epidurals. One said that the "idea of avoiding anesthetics for the sake of 'some ideal' didn't wash with her. Sometimes you hear people obsessed with prepared childbirth say, 'The pain is good to feel.' If men said that, we'd say it was incredibly sexist." The authors agreed. To understand the situation better, they invited six midwives with a total of forty-six years of experience to talk about why even women who want normal births so often end up with medicalized deliveries or cesarean sections. They came to the disappointing conclusion that most American women have little confidence in their inherent capacity to give birth. As a result, only a few very strong, unusual, highly motivated women deviate from the usual hospital, medicated birth (Armstrong & Feldman, 1990).

Other studies that have asked women what they want during labor and delivery find that most expect and want the predominant pattern of care: delivery by a physician in a hospital. Midwifery is not well known or understood. Many women continue to associate midwives exclusively with home births and have no knowledge of the scope of practice or education of nurse-midwives. However, as more and more women have experience with midwives, the proportion who prefer them is growing. All surveys find a larger proportion of women who express an interest in using midwives, birth centers, or home births than the percent who actually use them:

- A 1984 survey asked 210 women who were planning to have children about their preferences for care during labor and delivery. Although most wanted to give birth in a hospital (79 percent) and be attended by a physician (85 percent), the proportions that had no preference or wanted to be attended by a midwife or deliver in a birth center were significant and higher than the percent of women for whom those options were available in 1984 (Jackson & Jenson, 1984).

- In *Birth As An American Rite of Passage* (1992), anthropologist Robbie Davis-Floyd reports results of interviews conducted between 1983 and 1989 with one hundred white middle-class women concerning their experience of pregnancy and birth in two cities in the South and Southwest. She found most of the women through obstetricians, childbirth educators, and La Leche League leaders. Although the majority said they wanted natural births, most thought it would be safer in a hospital and accepted interventions without complaint. If they were disappointed, they blamed it on themselves. Many of the women saw pregnancy as something to be managed in a way that would limit interference with their busy lives or expressed distaste at the idea of having to "drop down into biology." She found it understandable "that women with this attitude would welcome, even demand, the freedom from the body granted by the epidural" and sometimes even prefer "the orderliness and controllability of the cesarean section over the uncontrollable and chaotic biological process of birth" (Davis-Floyd, 1994). Twenty-four women actively strove to have natural births in a hospital; fifteen of them succeeded and felt personally empowered by their birth experiences. Nine ended up with cesareans and reported feelings of helplessness and victimization that lasted for years. Six women gave birth at home attended by midwives and were overjoyed with their experiences.

- During the early 1990s investigators interviewed 103 predominantly unmarried, young (average age of nineteen), white female first-year undergraduates at an upstate New York university about their expectations, feelings, and preferences regarding care during pregnancy and childbirth. Eighty-three percent wanted to be cared for by an obstetrician and 89 percent wanted to deliver in a hospital (Wallach & Matlin, 1992). Relatively small proportions wanted to have a midwife with them during labor and delivery (9 percent), or wanted to give birth in an out-of-hospital birth center (4 percent) or at home (3 percent). Asked to anticipate their feelings about labor and birth, they expected it to be closer to "awful" than to "wonderful." Using a scale in which 1 represented "awful, won't enjoy at all" and 5 represented "wonderful, couldn't be better," the mean response was 2.1. They anticipated the pain of labor (1 = no pain at all, to 5 = intolerable pain) as being almost intolerable; the mean response was 4.4.

Although there has been no overall increase in out-of-hospital births, free-standing birth centers have developed a niche in the increasingly competitive childbirth market. Their clientele are primarily well-informed members of the middle and upper-middle professional classes. The desire for epidural anesthesia and the belief that birth is safer in a hospital have created demand for hospitals to provide some of the amenities associated with birth centers.

Managed Health Care and the Changing Health Care System

Because of cost concerns, the federal, state, and local governments, which pay for government-subsidized care, and the business community, which pays the health insurance premiums for most employed people and their families, began to reject the fee-for-service health care system in which individuals select their doctors and individual physicians make all decisions regarding their patients' use of health care. The alternative is some form of "managed" health care. The prototype is a health maintenance organization that provides comprehensive preventive and treatment services to enrolled persons for a fixed monthly fee. The monthly premiums must cover the cost of providing all necessary services. HMOs that do not live within their incomes face financial failure; thus they are highly motivated to provide cost-effective care. In contrast, paying physicians on a fee-for-service basis encourages maximal use of health care resources. HMOs reverse the incentives, creating pressure to minimize unnecessary use of services. Passage of the federal HMO Act of 1973 stimulated growth of this kind of organization. In 1980, nine million Americans were enrolled in 235 HMOs. By 1994, there were more than forty-two million enrollees and 540 HMOs. There are significant geographic differences. More than 26 percent of the population of the western states were enrolled in HMOs as of 1994. Participation is lowest in the southern states—9 percent in 1994, although it is increasing in every region every year (NCHS, 1994).

"Managed health care" is based on the same principles as HMOs. The difference is that the functions of health care provider and health care insurer are combined within a single organization in an HMO, whereas managed health-care organizations unite separate health care facilities and providers under the umbrella of a health care insurance organization. Managed care was a central theme of most state and federal plans to reform health care during the early years of the Clinton administration. Although national-level health care reform was not feasible politically, the threat of health care reform combined with continuously escalating costs and declining access to health care—the problems that had stimulated interest in health care reform—led to dramatic and rapid changes in the organization and financing of health care during the first half of the 1990s, with more to come.

Aggressive Growth of Private For-Profit Managed Care Organizations

To position themselves for changes that seemed inevitable and to comply with new laws in some states, during the early 1990s hospitals, physicians, and other components of the fee-for-service health care system began to reorganize themselves into local managed health care organizations. A 1993 study found that 58 percent of the employees of companies that provide a health care plan were enrolled in some form of managed care (KPMG Peat Marwick, 1993). In the western third of the country, managed care accounted for 86 percent of people covered by employee health plans; in all regions, the managed care share of the market was growing. In 1995 a national commission studying challenges faced by the health professions predicted that 80 to 90 percent of all Americans who have any kind of health care insurance will be enrolled in a managed care system within a decade (Pew Health Professions Commission, 1995).

The transition into managed care is also a transition into the dominance of for-profit health care businesses. Most of the new managed care organizations are organized on a for-profit basis. During 1993 and 1994 for-profit organizations overtook nonprofit organizations as the major players in health care (Andrulis *et al.*, 1996).

The new organizations often result from fast-paced mergers and acquisitions and are run by managers who stress efficiency and make decisions that affect patient care and the working conditions of physicians. A March 30, 1995 article in the *Wall Street Journal* reported that mergers and acquisitions had affected twenty billion dollars worth of health

industry assets in 1994. On September 1, 1995, the *Wall Street Journal* reported that the big HMOs are "pulling in money faster than they can spend it" or figure out where to invest it. As a result, they are buying out their competitors; four large HMOs held cash reserves of more than one billion dollars. The article ran under the headline "Money Machines." The industry was described as moving toward a future in which "a few jumbo health plans" will dominate the market in most local areas. The bottom line is making money, with emphasis on reducing costs. This has had an impact on maternity care, including the highly publicized decision of many managed care organizations to require women to take their babies and leave the hospital within twelve hours after giving birth.

Effects on Medicaid

Medicaid has been the leading edge of this revolution in many states. By March 1995, all but eight states had Medicaid managed care programs; altogether they covered 7.6 million people, nearly one-fourth of those using Medicaid to pay their health care bills (*Nation's Health*, March 1995). By May 1996, one-third of Medicaid-eligible Americans were enrolled in managed care plans, mostly traditional HMOs that were not designed for the poor (*Nation's Health*, May/June 1996). Most states initially targeted AFDC recipients—pregnant women and children in the Aid for Families with Dependent Children program—as the first, if not the only, segment of the Medicaid-eligible population to be enrolled in managed care (*Nation's Health*, January 1995).

States hoping to shift their Medicaid programs to managed care ask the Health Care Financing Administration (which administers Medicaid at the federal level) to give them permission ("waivers") to make substantial changes in the eligibility or service standards that are part of the federal Medicaid law. The government grants the waivers to facilitate research and demonstration projects that promote the basic objectives of the Medicaid program, which are to broaden access to care for low-income people by reducing health care costs. By August 1996, thirteen states had received such waivers, and other applications were in the works (*Nation's Health*, August 1996). California now requires all Medicaid recipients to enroll in a managed care program and is encouraging private providers (physicians, hospitals, laboratories, etc.) to bid on contracts to provide the care (Andrulis *et al.*, 1996).

Effects on Public Hospitals

Public hospitals, usually in partnership with a medical school, have traditionally provided most of the health care to most of the poor people in most large American cities. The transition to managed care has had a devastating effect on many public hospitals, which are also under attack as part of government, which everyone wants to make smaller. Public hospitals that are not included in a managed care network are losing many of their Medicaid-eligible patients. This deprives them of the only large group of patients whose bills are actually paid, while leaving them as the only source of health care for low-income people who are not eligible for Medicaid or Medicare but have no other health-care insurance—the homeless and mentally ill, as well as people whose low-paid jobs do not provide benefits and people who have preexisting health problems that make them ineligible for health insurance (Andrulis *et al.*, 1996). Approximately one-third of public hospital patients are "self-pay" patients, which means that they are not covered by any source of payment for their health care; in this case, "self-pay" almost always means that the hospital will receive no payment. Revenue to support their care has come from "disproportionate share funds", the medical-education allowance, and the local government entity that owns and is responsible for the hospital (Kassirer, 1995). Since public teaching hospitals often run the most completely staffed and experienced emergency rooms,

they also get a high proportion of accident and violence victims, who may require extensive care and are often uninsured. In addition to losing a large proportion of their Medicaid patients, many public hospitals face reduced funding from state and local governments and elected officials calling for privatization (Andrulis *et al.*, 1996)

Public hospitals that lose their Medicaid-eligible patients also lose additional fees that Medicaid pays to hospitals that serve a "disproportionate share" of uninsured and Medicaid-eligible people. In 1992 the Medicaid "disproportionate share adjustment" paid to ninety-five public urban hospitals amounted to 12 percent of the hospitals' total revenues. States that have received Medicaid waivers in order to implement managed care for Medicaid-eligible people have negotiated to have the disproportionate share adjustment shifted from the public hospitals that had been taking care of most of the Medicaid population to the new managed care organizations (Andrulis *et al.*, 1996). During 1995 authorities in several major cities announced their intention to sell, close, or drastically cut the services provided in their large public hospitals (Kassirer, 1995).

Reduced Government Health Care Budgets

The desire to reduce the federal government's constantly increasing debt and limit taxes and changes in the political leadership of Congress ushered in by the 1994 elections have led to expectations of significant reductions in federal appropriations for Medicaid and other health and social welfare programs for medically indigent Americans, including pregnant and potentially pregnant low-income women and their children. State and local government budget problems have also become increasingly critical, resulting in grand-scale reductions of health services in some rural areas and in cities with many indigent people. In August 1995 the Los Angeles County Board of Supervisors voted to cut the county's six ambulatory care centers and close twenty-eight of thirty-nine health centers. Ten of the remaining centers will be scaled back. The cut required layoffs of 6,700 health department personnel and resulted in a 75 percent reduction in hospital ambulatory care and outpatient capacity (*Nation's Health*, September 1995).

Moving Medicaid-eligible people into managed care plans that make use of private hospitals and physicians has greatly increased the financial problems of public health agencies. Like public hospitals, public health departments have relied on Medicaid as a major source of funds. When Medicaid-eligible people go elsewhere, public health agencies lose their only paying patients, while retaining their responsibility to provide services to people who are indigent but not on Medicaid.

Primary Care Providers as Gatekeepers
A long-standing criticism of American medical care has been its overproduction and emphasis on specialists, with too little production and emphasis on primary-care physicians. Physicians in the primary care specialties (family medicine, internal medicine, and pediatrics) tend to have a relatively stable caseload of individual patients or families for whom they provide most of the necessary medical care over an extended period of time—the modern equivalent of the old-time general practitioner. This allows the physician to get to know his or her patients as individual human beings, and to take their medical histories, other medical problems, life circumstances, and personalities into consideration when diagnosing and prescribing treatment for health problems. Specialists, in contrast, tend to see individual patients for a specific medical problem and do not have a continuing relationship with most patients. As of 1993, only one-third of physicians practicing in the United States were generalists; the other two-thirds were specialists (NCHS, 1995). This situation often results in inappropriate health care that is considerably more expensive. HMOs and managed care organizations are trying to correct this by assigning every enrolled person to a primary-care physician. The primary-care physicians are expected to manage most of the health problems of the patients in their caseload and refer them for specialist care as necessary. Persons enrolled in this kind of health care organization cannot access the care of a specialist except through referral from their primary physicians. Some managed care organizations provide financial incentives to motivate gatekeepers to minimize use of specialist care.

Less than 15 percent of 1992 medical school graduates entered a postgraduate residency training program in one of the primary-care fields of medicine; this is not surprising because medical specialists typically earn 50 to 60 percent more than physicians in primary care (*Nation's Health*, August 1993). During the 1980s several medical schools began attempts to encourage more students to enter primary care. However, even if half of all medical students graduating during or after 1995 entered residencies in primary-care fields, the medical workforce would not achieve a 50/50 split between primary-care physicians and specialists until 2040 (Curran, 1994). This situation may lead to additional demand for nurse practitioners, nurse-midwives, and physician assistants as providers of primary health care, which is defined as "the first contact, whole-person medical and health services delivered by broadly trained, generalist physicians, nurses and other professionals" (*Nation's Health*, August 1993).

Small, Perhaps Transient Cost Reductions and Concerns About Choice, Access, and Quality of Care
Health insurance costs paid by private employers fell by 1.1 percent between 1993 and 1994. This was the first decline in a decade during which these costs had sometimes increased by as much as 18 percent in a year (Freudenheim, 1995). However, no one knows whether greater use of managed care retards the growth of medical costs permanently or produces a one-time reduction as

consumers shift into programs that cost less and deliver less care. In addition, some of the cost savings may have come from small businesses that dropped health insurance coverage for their employees. The number of working-age people without insurance increased by 10.1 million between 1988 and 1995, when there were more than 43 million uninsured people below sixty-five years of age. At least one million individuals lost their health insurance in 1994—after the collapse of President Clinton's plans for universal health care coverage (Bradsher, 1995).

A government study estimated that shifting the entire population into HMOs could produce a 5.5 percent reduction in medical costs, but questioned whether costs might then begin to grow at the same rate as before (Hage & Black, 1995). By April 1997 there were indications that the respite in health care inflation may be over; if so, it was very brief. A report prepared for the National Coalition on Health Care by a Tulane University health economist reported that "health care cost inflation is back" and projected that medical costs will rise more than twice as fast as general inflation during the next five years (Thorpe, 1997).

While managed care organizations emphasize cost containment, there are significant concerns about limiting consumers' ability to choose their own doctor and compromised quality of care. HMOs are a well tested and studied phenomenon; large-scale use of for-profit managed care organizations is not. At this point it is not known what effects the changes will have. Cost-conscious policies encouraging—often requiring—discharge of mothers and newborns within twelve or twenty-four hours of delivery were denounced by the American Medical Association, which insisted that such decisions "ought not to be relegated to the bean counters," and the American College of Obstetricians and Gynecologists, which warned that such policies imperil women and their infants. The U.S. Congress responded by passing federal legislation that requires hospitals to allow women and newborns to remain in the hospital for at least forty-eight hours after a delivery. Both the federal government and state governments are working on ways to either curb the growth of managed care or institute various kinds of safeguards. The insurance regulatory agencies of forty-three states have some authority over managed care organizations that operate in their state. But things have been happening too fast for the regulatory agencies to keep abreast of the changes. By July 1996, thirty-three states were considering or had already passed legislation to increase consumer protections related to managed health care (*Nation's Health,* August 1996). The association of state insurance regulatory agencies is designing a model state law. Some form of state control is coming.

Effects on Health Care Providers

The turmoil and uncertainty caused by large-scale cuts in government health care budgets, the rapid and massive move toward prepaid managed health care, and expected but uncharted future changes in the system have created a sense of insecurity among a wide range of health care providers. The components of the health care system are reshuffling themselves, trying to make new alliances, to be part of the action in newly developing managed care plans. It is like a continuing game of musical chairs in which every person and part of the system is trying to find a secure place, knowing that not everyone will end up with a seat. The whole system is tightening its belt.

Among physicians the insecurity caused by these changes is accentuated by a sense of lost control, reduced incomes, and calls for a reduction in the physician workforce. Most doctors used to be the owner-managers of their own small businesses. They are rapidly becoming employees of corporations. As such they are finding their working conditions under the control of corporate managers who use quantitative standards to monitor the performance of physicians.

Doctors' incomes fell by 4 percent between 1993 and 1994, the first drop in average physician income in more than a decade. The earnings of specialists dropped the most, 5.3 percent, compared with a drop of 1.7 percent for primary-care physicians. A spokesman for the American Association of Health Plans said that specialists' salaries are dropping because there are too many specialists "in the market," not because of managed health care. However, the overall reduction was widely ascribed to the country's transition to managed care (Meckler, 1996).

In December 1995 a commission that had been created and charged by the Pew Charitable Trusts released its report on challenges facing the health professions as the United States moves into the twenty-first century. Most of the anticipated challenges result from circumstances created by the shift to managed care. The commission predicted that changes in the health care system "will create difficult realities for many health professionals and great opportunities for others." It identified some of the conditions that will affect doctors and nurses; it ignored midwives. The following are among the changes predicted by the Pew Health Professions Commission (1995):

- As many as half of the nation's hospitals may close, with a loss of as much as 60 percent of the nation's current hospital-bed capacity.
- There will be big surpluses in the supply of many kinds of health professions, including a surplus of 100,000 to 150,000 physicians, as the demand for specialty care shrinks, and a surplus of 200,000 to 300,000 nurses, as hospitals close.

The commission recommended reducing medical school classes by 20 to 25 percent by 2005 (Pew Health Professions Commission, 1995).

Effects of For-Profit Managed Care on Indigent Pregnant Women

The move to managed care is having serious effects on the care provided to low-income pregnant women, including women whose care is paid for by Medicaid and women who have no way to pay for health care. Medicaid pays the medical bills for at least one-third of all women who give birth in the United States. Public hospitals, public health agencies, and private voluntary organizations try to meet the needs of pregnant women who cannot pay for care but are not on Medicaid for various reasons. This category includes many illegal immigrants, migrant agricultural workers, women who are addicted to alcohol or drugs, runaway teenagers, homeless women, and others who fall through the cracks of our pasted-together health care "system." Moving Medicaid-eligible women into managed-care plans that make use of private hospitals and physicians removes them from programs that were especially designed to meet their needs. There are significant concerns that the routine prenatal care provided in private physicians' offices is not adequate to meet the needs of many Medicaid-eligible women. Medicaid payment for services provided to Medicaid-eligible women has been a major source of funding for many agencies and programs that also take care of pregnant women who are not on Medicaid. As these programs lose their Medicaid patients, they lose their ability to provide care to the other women too. This dynamic is forcing closure of services that were the only source of care for some of the nation's highest risk pregnant women.

As a result of the rapid move to Medicaid managed care plans, many low-income women have left programs that were especially designed to meet their needs in favor of private practices and clinics designed for the general population. Some women who have always used publicly supported hospitals and services now have access to private hospitals and physicians. Women enrolling in a Medicaid managed care plan are typically offered a choice between several sources of care. Many start by choosing a hospital and say they will go to any doctor who uses that hospital (Curry, 1996). This is the first time that many of these women have been offered any choice in health care. Few want to return to the public facilities they have always had to use, many of which are old, crowded, and stigmatized as places that take care of the poor. However, it is not at all clear that for-profit managed care can serve these women as effectively as the programs and services they used before this change. Findings from two published studies, as well as unpublished data from several states, suggest that they do not.

The first study was based on births to Medicaid-eligible women in Kentucky during 1985 and 1986 and births to Medicaid-eligible women in North Carolina during 1986 through 1988 (Buescher & Ward, 1992). After controlling for other factors, the low birth weight rate was much lower for women who received prenatal care through public health department facilities than for those who received their care through other providers, mainly private physicians. The association between private care and low birth weight was especially strong for very low birth weight births (less than 1,500 grams, which is less than 3.5 pounds). These, of course, are the most serious cases—the most important to prevent.

The second study was based on births to low-income women who delivered babies at either of two large hospitals in Chicago during 1988 and the first half of 1989. The likelihood of giving birth to a preterm, low birth weight infant was more than three times greater for women who received their care from private physicians as compared with women who received their care from the Chicago Department of Health. This relationship remained after the data were adjusted for race, age, parity, history of adverse pregnancy outcomes, smoking, and use of drugs during pregnancy. When the data were adjusted to account for women who had been transferred to the care of a private physician because of complications, the relationship between source of care and preterm low birth weight was reduced somewhat, but was still more than twofold and the

difference was still significant (Handler & Rosenberg, 1992). Poor outcomes associated with private care in Chicago may reflect poor-quality care provided in certain high-volume medical practices that take care of large numbers of Medicaid-eligible people in some low-income areas of that city (Fossett *et al.*, 1990).

Public health agencies and other non-profit organizations that provide prenatal care to medically indigent women emphasize nutrition counseling and make special efforts to enroll low-income pregnant women in the Special Supplemental Food Program for Women, Infants, and Children (WIC). Women enrolled in WIC receive nutrition education and counseling and a regular supply of vouchers that enable them to purchase certain kinds of particularly nutritious foods. Several studies have found large decreases in low birth weight associated with participation in WIC (Kotelchuck *et al.*, 1984; Institute of Medicine, 1985). In the study from Kentucky and North Carolina, 79 percent of the women who received care through the health department were enrolled in WIC and thus received highly nutritious foods on a regular basis to supplement their diets. Only slightly more than half of the women who received their care from private physicians were enrolled in WIC.

Public sector prenatal care programs also emphasize other aspects of patient education ask women about habits and circumstances that can cause pregnancy complications (e.g., smoking, alcohol and drug abuse, domestic violence, other sources of stress; and provide access to special services (such as programs to help people quit smoking) and social work assistance as ways to help women deal with these problems. In discussing their findings, the authors of the Kentucky/North Carolina study concluded that, while the obstetrical medical care available through private physicians is adequate for most women with higher education and income, women with fewer resources need the additional services and multidisciplinary approach provided in health department clinics: health education, nutritional counseling and supple-mentation, social work, outreach, and other nonmedical ancillary services (Buescher & Ward, 1992).

Unpublished studies conducted in Florida, Oregon, and South Carolina have also found better pregnancy outcomes for low-income women who receive the comprehensive care provided by the health department, as compared with care provided by private physicians (Richter, 1996; Curry, 1996; Miller, 1996). Most long-term students of the problem of poor pregnancy outcomes among low-income women agree that brief prenatal visits that focus primarily on the physical aspects of pregnancy are not adequate to meet the needs of most low-income women.

A team of nurses and social workers involved in the maternity-care program at a health care plan organized around a hospital in Portland, Oregon, developed a questionnaire to help private obstetricians and the nurses who work in their offices identify pregnant women who need special attention. Because of changes in the way Oregon pays for the care of medically indigent people, large numbers of indigent pregnant women are now obtaining their care from private physicians who use that hospital. As a result, the proportion of deliveries paid for by Medicaid increased from 5 percent to nearly 30 percent. The questionnaire required the physician or nurse to ask questions related to risk factors that play a role in the etiology of low birth weight and other important pregnancy complications—questions about smoking, drinking, use of drugs, and exposure to sexually transmitted diseases and domestic violence. The physicians had a range of responses to this idea. A few said that the questionnaire is a good screening tool, which they should be using with all of their patients. Some said they could not afford to take the time themselves or even to pay for the time it would take their nurse to ask these questions. Some responded that "It's not my business to ask these things; and if I do, what do I do about the answers?" (*Nursing Progress*, 1996).

Many of the physicians who are now taking care of Medicaid-eligible women under managed care plans refused to accept them into their practices only a few years ago. Medicaid fees for obstetric care were increased during the last few years, making care of Medicaid-eligible women less unattractive to physicians, and women whose care is paid for by Medicaid are a huge part of the maternity care market. However, managed care has added other considerations. Managed care plans contract to take care of large groups of patients; individual physicians can no longer discriminate between who they are or are not willing to take care of. Obstetricians who refuse to treat Medicaid-eligible women could end up without a seat at the end of the game of musical chairs. But effective maternity care requires the development of a working relationship between a pregnant woman and her care provider. A disinclination to provide care to women who have many nonmedical problems is not a recipe for success.

Chapter 6
Midwifery in America: Philosophy, Objectives, and Body of Knowledge

Chapters 6 through 9 describe the development of midwifery in the United States from 1980 through 1995. Chapter 7 provides information on the growing role of midwives in childbirth in this country, and information about the women whose births are attended by midwives. Chapter 8 describes the development of nurse-midwifery, and Chapter 9 describes the development of lay and direct-entry midwifery [all midwives other than certified nurse-midwives (CNMs)]. This chapter—Chapter 6—presents information that is relevant to all midwives in this country during this period of time: the purposes and beliefs that underlie midwifery and how they lead to a practice that is distinct from the physician's practice of obstetrics, and the development and status of the body of knowledge that supports midwifery.

How Does Midwifery Differ from the Care Provided by Physicians?

There is much common ground in the knowledge base of midwives and physicians, some common ground in their practices, less in the philosophies that underlie their care. Midwives study books and read articles written by obstetricians, who, in turn, are influenced by midwifery. Both are influenced by their clients, some of whom are influenced by childbirth educators, who observe the work and study the writings of both midwives and physicians.

Many nurse-midwifery educational programs are operated as part of academic medical centers. Within those centers nurse-midwifery students, medical students, ob-gyn residents and nurse-midwife and ob-gyn faculty study, practice, and teach in the same clinics and delivery suites, attend some of the same lectures, and take care of women from the same general population. Physicians focus on the care of women with complications, and nurse-midwives take care of women with normal pregnancies, with collaboration provided by the obstetrician–gynecologists. In many teaching institutions, the obstetricians teach the nurse-midwifery students about complications, and the nurse-midwives teach the medical students and residents how to manage normal births.

There is a mixing of the knowledge and experience of midwives and physicians; no clear line can be drawn between the care provided by CNMs, other midwives, family physicians, and obstetricians. There is variation within each group—individual physicians who practice more like midwives and individual midwives who seem to practice more like doctors. Nevertheless, there are important general differences. This section attempts to describe those differences. The beliefs and values of midwives described here apply to all categories of midwives.

A Focus on What Is Normal Versus a Focus on Pathology

The main focus of medical education, training, knowledge, skills, and role is pathology—the diagnosis and treatment of disease and trauma. Physicians are expected to help us avoid sickness and to monitor our health, to reassure us when we are well and diagnose disease during its earliest, most treatable phases. Health education, health status monitoring, and disease screening are roles physicians share with health educators, nurses, and others. Health education and disease screening are not, however, the source of the authority, power, and wealth of physicians. The physician's unique and awesome role lies in his or her ability to diagnose and treat disease, especially the use of medications and surgery. The current edition of *Williams Obstetrics*, the quintessential textbook named for one of the "titans" of

twentieth-century American obstetrics described in Chapter 2, has 1,359 pages. Less than one-third of them are used to describe normal conception, pregnancy, labor and delivery, and appropriate care of normal pregnant women. Most of the book is devoted to abnormalities, disorders, and complications and methods to diagnose and treat those conditions (Cunningham *et al*, 1993). This emphasis is appropriate to prepare physicians for their unique, life-saving role. Closer examination of the content of *Williams Obstetrics* shows that its chapters on normal pregnancy focus primarily on the anatomy and physiology of the female reproductive system and development of the embryo and fetus *at the level of the body's organs and the cells*. This is the level from which the miracles of modern medicine arise.

In contrast to medicine, the midwife's education, training, knowledge, skills, and role focus on protecting, supporting, and enhancing *normal* childbearing and family formation. Midwives are expected to detect abnormal conditions and work with physicians in such a way that medical expertise is brought into situations involving a medical problem. Midwives are also expected to provide emergency management of complications that threaten the life of the fetus, mother, or newborn until a physician is available to provide definitive diagnosis and treatment. But midwives are not the experts in diagnosis and treatment of pathologic conditions. They are the experts in protecting, supporting and enhancing normal pregnancy and childbirth. As with the physician's focus on pathology, the midwife's focus on normal childbearing is grounded in knowledge of the anatomy and physiology of reproduction. However, a large part of the midwife's attention and concern focus on the woman as a person, a unique individual, in the context of her family and her life. The midwife is interested in the woman's expectations and experience of her pregnancy—her perceptions and beliefs; her knowledge, opinions, questions, and worries; her feelings, satisfactions and dissatisfactions, comforts and discomforts; her desires, decisions, and actions, and the effect of all of these on her pregnancy; the development of her fetus; her labor, delivery, breast-feeding, and postpartum recovery; and how she mothers her infant. In these realms, as well as in understanding the process of normal birth, midwives have made unique contributions to the body of knowledge about human reproduction.

Focusing on the normal aspects of pregnancy and childbearing does not mean that midwives cannot or should not play a role in the care of women who have complications and diseases. Having a problem such as diabetes greatly complicates pregnancy, increasing the risk of serious problems for both the mother and the baby. A pregnant woman with diabetes, or any other serious complication, needs a physician to control her disease and limit its impact on her pregnancy. But she is not just a diabetic; she is a pregnant woman who is preparing for childbirth and motherhood. Many aspects of her experience and needs during pregnancy are the same as they would be without the complication. She still needs a midwife to focus on the normal aspects of the process of bearing a child and becoming a mother.

Overlapping but Unique Fields of Knowledge

Physicians and midwives each gather a unique field of knowledge and skills appropriate to their particular role. Although their fields of knowledge overlap, with an area common to both, there are significant differences. Each profession uses the other's knowledge to varying degrees, and builds its unique expertise on knowledge from the clinical experience and research of its members and on knowledge from the basic and applied sciences. Physicians have more extensive knowledge of anatomy, physiology, pathology, biochemistry, pharmacology, anesthesiology, diagnosis, and therapy. Midwives have more extensive knowledge of nor-

mal labor and birth, the psychology and lives of women, family dynamics, lactation, methods of communication and teaching, and nonmedical methods to comfort women during labor. In addition, midwives are more aware of the limitations of the biological and physical sciences as a means to measure and understand the phenomenon of pregnancy and childbirth. Science cannot deal directly with subjective experience. Many of the things we experience and value in life are subjective and, therefore, beyond science. That does not mean that they are invalid or irrelevant; it only means that observations about them are dependent on the observer and cannot be measured objectively. The scientific method is not the only valid method of inquiry into the nature of things (Stewart, 1978).

Differences in Beliefs About the Nature of Pregnancy and Birth

Physicians and midwives differ most in their beliefs about the nature of pregnancy and childbirth, which physicians tend to view in terms of their potential for pathology. Focusing on pathology leads to certain perceptions: Women's bodies are very imperfect at giving birth; medicine can and should improve on nature. Although some women are at especially high risk of experiencing complications, every woman and her baby are at risk; you cannot assume that any birth is normal until it is over. Assumptions that underlie medical practice flow from this perspective: The main purpose of prenatal visits is screening for abnormalities. Childbirth must be closely monitored and controlled; it should start on or near the predetermined day, and each phase of labor should take no more than a specified amount of time. Some of the intensive methods developed for use in "high-risk" cases should be applied routinely. Consequences of these assumptions include lost opportunity to use prenatal care for purposes other than screening for pathology; frequent use of methods to induce labor and make women labor harder and faster; withholding food and drink from women who are working hard (i.e., in "labor") in case they might need cesarean sections; rupturing the bag of fluid surrounding the baby in order to "speed things up" and to make it possible to attach electrodes to the baby's head; and cutting women's vaginas and perineums on a routine basis.

Midwives have a different view. To understand this, it is important to understand the role that self-selection plays in determining who becomes a midwife. American women do not enter midwifery because it is a secure and highly esteemed position of power and authority that is likely to make them wealthy. Nor is it a role their mothers and fathers suggested when they were growing up. Midwifery is not a job young women go into when they could not decide what else to do. Most women who become midwives do so because they are fascinated and awed by pregnancy and birth. They come to the field predisposed to respect the natural birth-giving ability of women's bodies. Once committed to study midwifery, they inherit the wisdom and learn the methods of the field. Even though the vast majority of births attended by midwives in the United States occur in hospitals (89 percent of births attended by midwives during 1989–1994), the accumulated knowledge passed from midwife to midwife and teacher to student is based in part on midwives' extensive historic experience with home births. This experience has taught midwives that when essentially healthy women labor in a secure environment; receive physical and emotional support; eat, drink, rest, move, and position themselves as they want; and when little is done to add to their discomfort and they are respected and encouraged and *expected to give birth successfully,* most of them do.

Midwives believe that pregnancy and birth are fundamentally healthy processes, which have many normal variations (Steiger, 1987). They understand that there are risks and constantly observe for signs of abnormality, but treat childbearing as a normal physiological process that has profound meaning to many people. Treating it as a medical procedure has a detrimental impact on both the biological and social processes of reproduction.

Midwives believe that women's bodies are designed to give birth and know how to labor better than we understand, and that many of our attempts to control or improve the process end up disrupting it in ways that have unintended, often harmful consequences. Thus midwives endeavor to support and protect the normal process, because, as they have also learned, fear, discouragement, and seemingly harmless hospital routines and medical interventions can rob labor of its power. "There is power that comes to women when they give birth. They don't ask for it, it simply invades them. . . . But for all its mythic force, the power is vulnerable. It can be undercut" (Armstrong & Feldman, 1990). Although midwives have collected and published data to substantiate and support this understanding, such information has been better accepted when it came from doctors. The observations and conclusions of Dr. Michel Odent, a French surgeon who discovered these truths for himself during twenty years in charge of the maternity unit at the public hospital in Pithiviers, a small town south of Paris, have been particularly influential.

Dr. Michel Odent and "The Undisturbed Birth"

Dr. Odent went to Pithiviers in 1962 to take charge of general surgery and oversee a small maternity clinic in the hospital. Although he was not particularly interested in obstetrics, he wanted to reduce the number of women who needed cesarean sections because, as there was no obstetrician, he had to do the sections. For the most part, he relied on the midwives, who handled most of the births. Eventually his acute observations of their work led him to a deep and insightful involvement in obstetrics and led to development of his concept of "the undisturbed birth." Odent noted the good outcomes of the midwives and the contrast between the births at Pithiviers and those he had seen on the obstetrics ward of a large hospital in Paris. He was particularly interested in the approach of an older midwife, who was very patient with women during labor, and how it differed from the approach of a young midwife who was very enthusiastic about "prepared" childbirth. The more experienced midwife told women not to hold back, to relax and let themselves go, and then waited for the baby to come. The younger midwife coached her patients, but they had more problems, and needed more cesarean sections (Odent, 1994).

Dr. Odent and the midwives began to examine every labor and delivery intervention systematically, from breaking the membranous bag that contains the fluid surrounding the baby, to cutting the cord, in each case asking: "Why are you doing this? What do we gain, if anything, by altering the natural process? What happens if we let labor run its own course?" One by one, they let go of interventions. "They gave up epidurals, which depress the pushing reflex. They didn't break the bag of waters, which protected the baby's head and helped expand the opening of the uterus. They didn't cut the cord right after its birth. Its last pulses brought added rich stores to the baby and, at the same time helped to shrink the placenta so it could peel more easily from the uterine wall" (Armstrong & Feldman, 1990). They built a small, quiet, earth-toned room for women to labor and give birth in, gave up trying to teach women how to behave during labor, instead merely trying to make them feel at home in the hospital. They replaced weekly childbirth education classes with weekly gatherings at which Dr. Odent, the midwives, nurses, pregnant women, expectant fathers, and new mothers, fathers and grandparents met one another, exchanged information, sang, danced, and became friends. When women asked for advice about what to do during labor and delivery,

Dr. Odent told them that there is no one way to give birth: "The woman's body leads her and she need only follow it." The midwives and doctors would do whatever worrying was needed. Thus each woman labored in her own way. Many gave birth in a semisquatting position, supported by their husband's arms.

Observing these births, Dr. Odent concluded that the process works best in a small, dimmed, quiet, well-protected room where the woman is not intruded on by strange people and events and feels safe and free enough to abandon herself to the process, to surrender; birth goes best when it is "undisturbed." Odent referred to the "fetus ejection reflex" as "a spontaneous, natural process, like breathing, blinking your eyes, or having a bowel movement. As such, it is best managed not by our thinking mind, the neocortex, but by the hypothalamus," the part of the brain that controls the automatic functions of the body, and the pituitary gland, which releases oxytocin, the hormone that causes the uterus to contract. The body functions controlled by the hypothalamus work most efficiently when they are left alone. "The easiest birth comes . . . when the spontaneous process is not under the laboring woman's scrutiny; that is, when a woman can leave off neocortical consciousness— thinking, analyzing, monitoring her behavior for social purposes, or making decisions. If her birth environment is free from intellectual demands and control requirements, her labor will tend to be more powerful and effective" (Armstrong & Feldman, 1990). The hypothalamus makes oxytocin, which makes the uterus contract; it also produces endorphins—hormones that diminish pain and make us feel good. Warmth, quiet, darkness, and a feeling of security encourage the flow of endorphins; fear and stress inhibit their release.

Dr. Odent's work confirmed, amplified, and validated the body of knowledge about labor and birth which midwifery has gained from centuries of home births. Although most midwife-attended births occur in hospitals in the United States, and although even the most comfortable and homey birthing room bears little resemblance to the Pithiviers birthing room, American midwives try to reduce intrusive stimuli and to create a quiet, safe, sheltered environment for labor and birth.

Emphasis on Emotional, Social, and Environmental Factors

Biologic and social science research has shown that noxious environmental factors can affect a woman's pregnancy and the development of her baby. Thus society, employers, midwives, and physicians address the need for pregnant women to get enough rest, eat well, and avoid exposure to infectious diseases, radiation, occupational hazards, violence, strenuous work, and use of cigarettes, alcohol, illegal drugs, and many kinds of medications. We also recognize that the woman herself controls these positive and negative influences. Thus public health agencies try to educate pregnant women to take care of their babies by taking care of themselves. Midwives give particular emphasis and attention to educating and supporting women to make changes in their living habits that are conducive to a healthy pregnancy, baby, and family. In addition, they have been far ahead of medical skeptics in understanding that the hard-to-measure stresses and worries, satisfactions and pleasures of a woman's life can affect her pregnancy, labor, delivery, baby, self-esteem, and parenting skills. In 1993 a large prospective study documented an association between psychological distress and preterm births (Hedegaard *et al.*, 1993). Despite this and similar studies, most physicians pay inadequate attention to the emotional and social concerns of pregnant women.

Beliefs about the Role of the Client Versus That of the Health Professional

Midwives and physicians tend to differ in their view of the appropriate relationship between a pregnant woman and her care provider. Physicians are more likely to want to take charge of the interaction and are more likely to see themselves as the key decision makers, especially during labor and delivery. Midwives are more likely to see their role as educating the pregnant woman, giving her the information and support she needs to make her own decisions. The birth experience belongs to the mother, not the midwife or the doctor; she has the right and responsibility to be an active partner in her own care. The pregnant woman is not only a partner, she is the key member of the partnership, because it is she who has the most at stake (Barnes, 1994). Midwives' philosophy about their role is reflected in their use of words; many say that they "attend births" and "catch babies," while it is the mother who bears and, through her labor, delivers her baby into the world.

The midwife's role requires more than intellectual and manual skills; it requires personal involvement. Midwives endeavor to relate to each pregnant woman as a unique individual, not as a pregnancy, to develop personal relationships with their clients, to "be present" for them as a person, and to reduce the barriers that make it hard for people with less authority to open themselves to people in positions of greater authority. Midwives try to avoid using professional or institutional authority and roles to limit their involvement with women or to control them. Midwives use their own physical, emotional and spiritual energy to support and comfort women during childbirth. "Midwife" means "*with* woman."

Midwives put great importance on respect for human dignity; try to break through the barriers of race, ethnicity, and social class in order to achieve genuine communication; and try to see each situation from the woman's perspective, understanding that her subjective experience and beliefs are real and influence what she does. Midwives understand that women experience their pregnancies in the context of their relationships and roles in their families, work situations, and communities, and encourage members of the woman's family to be present during prenatal visits and be involved in all aspects of her pregnancy and care. The cultural and spiritual aspects of childbearing are respected. Midwives recognize that birth has different meanings in different cultures and believe that each woman has the right to experience this event in her own way (Fries, 1994).

Midwives strive to manifest respect for every woman and regard all women as having the right to complete and accurate information about their own condition and to make choices and decisions about their care. The desires of the woman and her family are valid concerns and objectives; safety comes first, but unnecessary hospital routines and schedules are not more important than the desires of an individual woman.

A large part of the midwife's role is teaching women to help them take better care of themselves during pregnancy and to know what to expect during labor and delivery, including understanding the pros and cons of alternative methods for achieving various objectives. Only the pregnant woman can affect the environment in which her baby is growing and developing; what she knows and believes will affect her behavior. Many midwives teach women how to assist in monitoring their own condition by weighing themselves, testing their own urine, and recording the information in their charts. The midwife and her client work on problems together, coming to mutual decisions on the woman's goals for her pregnancy and birth, and making plans to achieve her goals.

Less Narrow Definitions of Normal

Research has described common patterns for the progress of labor and delivery—relationships between progressive dilation of the cervix and the fetus's progress through the birth canal and how long it usually takes to achieve certain aspects of the process. Many facets of labor can be measured by time, or by the degree of progress per unit of time. If these measures are graphed for a large population of women, they will, like most biologic phenomenon, portray a "normal curve." The individuals whose measurements fall at either extreme of the curve are more likely to experience complications and poor pregnancy outcomes. For instance, labors that are either extremely short or long are more likely to have complications. However, there is a great deal of *normal* variation. For example, the fact that women with exceptionally long labors have a higher rate of complications does not mean that an individual woman who labors longer than usual will experience serious problems. Even if the *rate* of complications is two or three times higher than average, being at higher *risk* does not mean that a particular woman will experience the predicted complication. The medical model often calls for applying treatments as a preventive measure in the face of elevated risk. The midwifery model says to wait and apply treatments only as treatments, that is, only for actual complications.

Physicians tend to base their management of labor on relatively narrow criteria for what is normal, and to intervene when a particular woman's labor falls outside of those criteria. Midwives are more likely to accept greater variation as still within the "range of normal" as long as the woman and fetus are tolerating labor well. Individual labors that are further from the middle of the curve are cause for increased vigilance for early signs of actual complications, but not for automatic recourse to interventions. Treating more labors as normal may help them to remain normal; some of the interventions applied because a woman is high risk can actually cause complications. Treating normal labors as though they were complicated can make them complicated; being designated as high risk can become a self-fulfilling prophecy.

Midwives also accept a wide range of behaviors during labor as normal. Labor is an extraordinary time in a woman's life; she is not expected to behave according to usual social standards. She does not have to stay in bed, refrain from moaning or crying out, keep herself covered, or inhibit her self-expression.

Objectives of the Care

Midwives value childbearing, and birth itself, as an emotionally, socially, culturally, and often spiritually meaningful life experience—something to be experienced positively, with potential for making women feel stronger, and *be* stronger, and for strengthening bonds between the mother and the father, as well as other siblings, and the newborn. A healthy mother and baby are the highest priority, but not the only goals. Qualitative dimensions of the mother's subjective experience of giving birth are important. Pregnancy and childbirth cannot be separated from the rest of the woman's life; they may play an important role in her self-expression, sexuality, and psychological and spiritual development. The process, as well as the outcome, is important (Steiger, 1987). In assessing their work, midwives want to know if their clients were satisfied with their pregnancy and birth experience; satisfaction is viewed as an outcome, along with objective measures of the mother's and infant's health.

And giving birth is not the end of the process. Pregnancy is a time to prepare for the baby, as well as the birth, and the necessary but exciting changes that will be required in the woman's life, and in the lives of the baby's father and all members of her family. The time during which a woman carries and gives birth to her first child is a period of remarkable change. She changes from being merely a daughter to a mother; for many women that means changing from a child to an adult. This process demands a restructuring of her self-concept and of her relationships with her own parents, the father of her child, probably her siblings, and the external world of friends, school, and work. The kinds of adjustments women and their family members make during pregnancy, birth, and early parenthood may have long-term effects on

the quality of their family life and on the health of individual family members. Many women are particularly open to making positive changes in their lives while they are pregnant. Thus the goals of midwifery care are not only to protect and promote the physical health of the mother and baby, but also to assist pregnant women and their families to make emotionally healthy adjustments to the pregnancy and birth and to ensure that new mothers have the information, skills, and support necessary for them to successfully assume the roles and responsibilities of motherhood. Breast-feeding and mothercraft, in the widest sense, are part of the focus of the care.

Development of the Body of Knowledge

All professional practice rests on a body of knowledge. Every profession has a responsibility to refine and expand knowledge of the phenomena that are the *raison d'être* of its practice and to improve the efficacy of its methods. The core subjects of midwifery are normal pregnancy and birth, including breast-feeding and the complex processes by which women and families welcome, nurture, and protect their infants, and the mother's return to a healthy nonpregnant condition. Midwifery's body of knowledge encompasses these phenomena and methods to protect and enhance them. Modern midwives inherit a body of knowledge and methods that have been formally and informally developed and passed from midwife to midwife, as well as knowledge and methods developed by many fields of basic and applied biological and behavioral science, especially medicine.

Medicine's development within universities that were available only to educated upper-class males resulted in an enduring cleavage between medicine and midwifery based on gender, social class, and differences in how each field prepares new practitioners and expands its body of knowledge.

Midwifery began to lose social authority when medicine developed the institutional capacity to develop its body of knowledge and midwifery did not. Although midwives were known as a reservoir of powerful, uniquely female knowledge (the reason for the medieval church's fear and suspicion of midwives), medicine and its basic sciences became the main source of midwives' "scientific" knowledge. Women largely shifted their trust from midwives to physicians because of their belief that scientifically based medical practice was safer and better, and that whatever improvements would come would come from medicine. Despite problems associated with overuse of obstetric interventions and the many values that were sacrificed in this transition, the women were largely right. The high maternal and infant mortality rates of the past were felled by the discoveries and inventions of basic scientists, physicians, and public health professionals. The knowledge and methods that have made maternal mortality rare are now widely disseminated. New improvements in the care of pregnant women rest on that base. Acknowledging this history, it is fair to say that many of the methods that are improving childbirth today have come from midwives and others focusing on the purposes and subject matter of midwifery—normal pregnancy and birth, breast-feeding, and development of the bond between mothers and their newborns.

Data on the Effectiveness of Care During Pregnancy and Childbirth

Despite the great victories of modern medicine over maternal and infant mortality, many of the technical procedures and other elements of the care provided to most pregnant women by and under the authority of physicians in this country have been found not to be beneficial when applied to women whose pregnancies are normal. In 1979, Archie Cochrane, the former director of a prestigious epidemiology research unit in England, gave the "wooden spoon award" to obstetrics as the specialty that had demonstrated the least use of randomized, controlled trials to evaluate the effectiveness of patient care and treatment (Chalmers *et al.*, 1989).

In response to that challenge, three obstetrician epidemiologists—Iain Chalmers from England, Murray Enkin from Canada, and Marc Keirse from the Netherlands—undertook a systematic review of seventy journals in an attempt to identify all randomized clinical trials having to do with pregnancy and childbirth care that had been published since 1950. Their purpose was to evaluate and synthesize all valid evidence about the safety and effectiveness of each aspect of the care of pregnant women and newborns. In 1989 they published the results—a two-volume, 1,516-page book entitled *Effective Care in Pregnancy and Childbirth* and an electronic database covering the same material (Chalmers *et al.*, 1989). The second edition was published in 1995 (Enkin *et al.*, 1995). The electronic Cochrane Pregnancy and Childbirth Database, named after the epidemiologist who inspired their work, is updated regularly. Each chapter describes a particular procedure or practice, reviews and synthesizes the evidence about it, and presents conclusions and implications for practice and research. It includes information on how to evaluate research in order to determine which studies are most likely to provide valid information; the authors gave findings from randomized, controlled clinical trials the greatest weight in reaching their conclusions. The last chapter includes tables that list specific aspects of care under one of six categories, based on the evidence: (1) forms of care that have been demonstrated to be beneficial, (2) forms of care that are likely to be beneficial, (3) forms of care with a trade-off between beneficial and adverse effects, (4) forms of care with unknown effectiveness, (5) forms of care that are unlikely to be beneficial, and (6) forms of care that are likely to be ineffective or harmful (Enkin, *et al.*, 1995).

The purpose of this monumental continuing work is to "encourage the adoption of useful measures and the abandonment of those that are useless or harmful" (Chalmers *et al.*, 1989). Unfortunately, some of its most important lessons have not yet been applied to maternity care in this and some other countries. In a 1991 article on perinatal research, Iain Chalmers cited unsupported assertions by the author of a recently published standard obstetrics textbook and noted that it "is important to recognize the extent to which authoritarian and unsupported opinions are still offered as a basis for guiding both practice and research" (Chalmers, 1991). In 1993, Marc Keirse humorously pointed out that the pregnant uterus is treated differently in different countries: While 40 percent of pregnant women in France are given tocolytic drugs to stop labor and delay delivery, tocolytic agents are not even marketed in Ireland, where two-thirds of pregnant women receive drugs to increase the forces of labor and hasten the delivery (Keirse, 1993). It is difficult to believe that the underlying incidence of obstetric pathology is so high and yet so different in these two European countries. Many people also find it difficult to believe that one of every four or five American women really needs a cesarean section. Such extreme international differences remind us that the presence of actual pathology is only one of many factors that result in use of obstetric interventions.

Gaps in the Base of Essential Information
In addition to large-scale failure to implement the knowledge that has now been made explicit, there are significant gaps in the basic knowledge of normal pregnancy and birth. The gaps exist at every level, including physiology, as well as knowledge of whether many of the methods applied by physicians and midwives are effective and how some that are known to be effective work. Although much research has been conducted, we still do not really understand what triggers the initiation of labor (Cunningham *et al.*, 1993). We know that labor usually proceeds more slowly in first as compared with later births, but we do not really know why (Keirse, 1993). Although we know that social and psychological support during labor reduces the incidence of cesarean sections, we do not understand how support works to that effect. Nor do we understand the causes of postpartum depression or of many other biological and psychological phenomena.

Chalmers described several factors that dictate the research agenda. Although the safety and efficacy of drugs must be demonstrated before they are approved for use, this standard is not applied to any other aspect of medical care (Chalmers, 1991). He especially noted commercial influence on what research is done; treatments that use commercially produced products are the subject of much of the research. The Oxford research group's review of the worldwide literature found that, as of 1991, only 22 clinical trials had been conducted to find ways to *prevent* perineal pain during the postpartum period. In contrast, at least 112 studies had been conducted to test different methods to *treat* perineal pain. The story was the same for research on induction of labor. There had been only 30 controlled trials to identify the circumstances in which induction of labor might produce better outcomes than a more conservative approach. In contrast, there had been several hundred clinical trials to compare alternative methods for inducing labor. Epidural block for relief of labor pain has been provided by physicians, promoted by the media, and actively sought by pregnant women. Yet there had been only one systematic attempt to determine some of its potential long-term effects. Findings from that one study, which was not a randomized clinical trial, suggest that epidurals may nearly double the risk of chronic backache. Given wide use of epidurals, Chalmers asks if we can afford "to remain uncertain about whether epidural block is causing chronic backache on the sort of scale suggested by the only available evidence?"

Midwives have accused obstetricians of widespread implementation of unproved methods that interfere with normal birth. As time and science have progressed, many of the methods midwives questioned have been found to be unnecessary, and often harmful, when applied to women having normal pregnancies and births. Examples include advising pregnant women to restrict their weight gain and use of salt; restricting their position during labor and delivery; perineal shaving; routine enemas during labor; routine episiotomies; routine use of continuous electronic fetal monitoring; separating mothers from their newborns; giving sweetened water to breast-fed babies; and forcing breast-feeding mothers and babies to adhere to a schedule. Although midwives have introduced fewer procedures and thus are not nearly as guilty as obstetricians of using methods that have not been evaluated adequately, midwives use some methods that have not been objectively assessed, for example, perineal massage during the last months of pregnancy as a way to prevent tears during delivery. Although their methods are less likely to interfere with normal processes, midwives too need to examine the efficacy of their methods. The National Association of Childbearing Centers should be congratulated for insisting on a large prospective study to examine the outcomes of the care provided in free-standing birth centers. Although studies from individual birth centers had found that they were safe, a large prospective study was necessary to evaluate outcomes in this low-risk population.

Research on Normal Pregnancy

There seems to be new energy and interest in research about normal pregnancy, midwifery methods, breast-feeding, and the best ways to care for newly delivered mothers and their newborns. Although midwives are doing some of this research, much of it is done by others, including obstetricians, obstetric nurses, childbirth educators, pediatricians, public health nurses and physicians, nutri-tionists, psychiatrists, anthropologists, epidemiologists, and family practice physicians.

Research on Midwifery Practice

Midwives have probably been the subjects of more studies than they have conducted. Public health leaders were the first to suggest using nurses trained as midwives to help improve maternal and infant health. Mary Breckinridge collaborated with public health officials in Kentucky and inculcated careful record keeping and periodic analysis of service outcomes as a nurse-midwifery service norm. After publication of the excellent outcomes of the Frontier Nursing Service, public health officials came to view midwifery services as important examples of the application of key public health principles: emphasis on educating women to improve their own health and that of their children and families; emphasis on prevention and early detection of health problems; giving priority to those with the most problems and the least access to other health care; locating primary care in the communities where the people who need the services live; using administrative and referral relationships to link community-based services with other kinds and levels of care; recognizing the value of visiting pregnant women and new mothers and babies in their homes; focusing on individuals in the context of their families; recognizing the impact of social, economic, environmental, and cultural factors on maternal and child health; and relying on interdisciplinary collaboration to meet the complex needs of socioeconomically high-risk women and their babies. Public health authorities have conducted or supported many studies of the outcomes of midwifery care. The obstetricians who brought nurse-midwives into hospitals and supported them despite opposition from their colleagues have conducted or collaborated in many others.

Other physicians, such as Michel Odent, were stimulated to conduct studies and develop new approaches to maternity care based on their observations of the care provided by midwives. However, most of the research in which physicians have collaborated with nurse-midwives in the United States has been done to determine the safety and other outcomes of midwifery care—in order to defend it as adequate, that is, as being as safe as the care provided to similar women by physicians. Until recently the need to do this, and to do it over and over and in every kind of setting, has consumed most of the research energy of midwives. In 1986, Joyce Thompson, director of the nurse-midwifery education program at the University of Pennsylvania, published a review of studies about nurse-midwifery that had been published between 1925 and 1984 (Thompson, 1986). She found evidence that nurse-midwifery care is both safe and satisfying. Then she challenged the profession "to investigate the components of the care process and contribute to theory building and testing in nurse-midwifery. How does the way CNMs provide care during pregnancy differ from that of other providers? More important, do those differences contribute to better outcomes of care in terms of health and well-being of women and infants? If so, what is the relationship and which components can be replicated by other health professionals?" She and several colleagues then took a step in that direction by gathering information that allowed them to identify and define concepts that characterize nurse-midwifery care (Thompson *et al.*, 1989).

Much research is needed to identify and describe the methods used by midwives, how they differ from methods used by doctors and nurses in the absence of midwives, and the efficacy of particular methods. Beyond that, we ultimately need to know why and how these methods work. Although too little research has been done, some is being done. At least 65 percent of American nurse-midwives have master's degrees, at least 3 percent have doctorates, and most nurse-midwifery educational programs are based in universities, including some of the nation's leading institutions of health sciences research. However,

the high proportion of CNMs with advanced degrees is due to universities' demands that their faculty have advanced degrees. Many nurse-midwifery educators are exhausting themselves trying to earn doctorates while teaching and participating in practice. Although the doctorate is considered preparation for research, many CNMs with doctorates have done little research, and much of the research that has been done does not address clinical practice. Nevertheless, a few institutions (more accurately, a few individual CNMs) have substantial research experience and expertise and are making important contributions. As time goes on, more nurse-midwives are adding to the body of knowledge. The *Journal of Nurse-Midwifery* published sixty-nine research reports between 1987 and 1992, mostly reports of descriptive studies of clinical topics that used convenience or other nonprobability samples (Lydon-Rochelle & Albers, 1993). The proportion of studies with external funding increased from 11 percent in 1988 to 87 percent in 1992.

The following paragraphs provide examples of three kinds of clinical research being conducted by nurse-midwives in the United States and by professional midwives in other countries.

(1) Research that describes and analyzes a particular aspect of normal pregnancy, childbirth, or breast-feeding, for example:

- Studies of the relationships between fatigue and nausea and vomiting in women with no known medical problems (Reeves *et al.*, 1991; van Lier *et al.*, 1993), studies that describe healthy pregnant women's experience of nausea and vomiting (O'Brien & Zhou, 1995; O'Brien & Nabor, 1992), a study that described sleep disturbances and the impact of fatigue on women having their first pregnancies as compared with women having a second or higher order baby (Waters & Lee, 1996).
- A study of relationships between aerobic exercise, self-esteem, and physical dis-

comforts during pregnancy (Wallace *et al.*, 1986).

- Studies that describe the involuntary bearing-down efforts women make during the second stage of labor. Most women experience a desire to "bear down" or "push" during this phase. Childbirth educators, doctors, nurses, and midwives have a long history of giving women directions and encouragement to push in certain ways during the second stage (after the cervix is completely dilated, including the actual expulsion of the baby). During the late 1970s and early 1980s researchers began to report evidence that the bearing-down efforts women make spontaneously differ from those of women who have been coached to push while holding their breath, and that natural bearing-down is physiologically more advantageous to both the mother and the baby. CNMs at the University of Illinois conducted a series of studies to describe the second stage of labor for thirty-one healthy women who were having their first babies and had not been instructed or encouraged to bear down with contractions. Data were collected to describe (1) the women's respirations, bearing-down efforts, vocalization, and behavior, (2) the obstetric conditions and intrauterine pressure associated with the bearing-down reflex, and (3) the duration of the second stage of labor, the fetal heart rates, and the neonatal outcomes. Allowing the women to push spontaneously had no negative effect on the progress of their labors. Uninstructed women seemed to use their voluntary muscles to push in a way that complemented the involuntary bearing-down reflex (Roberts *et al.*, 1987).
- A study to describe the feelings, concerns, conflicts, and other aspects of the experience of twelve women who breastfed their infants for more than a year (Wrigley & Hutchinson, 1990).

(2) Research to assess the accuracy and side effects of methods used by both midwives and physicians to determine if pregnancies are progressing normally. Several of these studies compared the accuracy of clinical assessments with the results of ultrasounds. Although most women who give birth in this country have at least one ultrasound, routine ultrasonography is not recommended in *Effective Care in Pregnancy and Childbirth:* "The place, if any, for routine ultrasound has not been established as yet. In view of the fact that its safety has not been convincingly established, such routine use should be considered experimental for the present, and should not be implemented outside the context of randomized controlled trials" (Enkin *et al.*, 1995). The following are examples of this kind of reseach:

- A study to determine if asking low-risk women to count and record the frequency of fetal movements increases their anxiety about the well-being of their babies (Gibby, 1988).
- A study to describe the accuracy of Leopold's maneuvers in screening for malpresentations. (Leopold's maneuvers are a precise set of manual examinations to determine the position of the fetus within the uterus. Anything but the usual head-down position is a malpresentation.) Four experienced CNMs examined 150 women during the third trimester of pregnancy to determine the fetal presentation. The same women then had ultrasound examinations, which provide the most accurate determination of fetal presentation. The CNMs identified twenty-three of the twenty-six actual malpresentations (Lydon-Rochelle *et al.*, 1993).
- A study to describe clinicians' ability to identify the uterine fundus. (The fundus is the top of the uterus. It is necessary to identify the fundus in order to measure the fundal height. The fundal height is measured at every prenatal

visit. The pattern of uterine growth observed in this way is used to monitor the growth of the fetus. Abnormal findings may mean that the fetus is not growing as expected, that the pregnancy is more or less advanced than previously estimated, that there is more than one fetus, that there is too much or too little fluid surrounding the fetus, or other problems.) In this study, one obstetric resident, three CNMs, and two nurse-midwifery students examined 126 pregnant women (Engstrom *et al.*, 1993). The examiners made a small mark on the skin at the top of the uterine fundus. The researchers then used ultrasonograms to measure the actual level of the fundus and determined the extent of clinician error and factors associated with excessive error. The amount of error they found—1.25 centimeter, on average, with one error of almost nine centimeters—surprised the researchers, who conducted a follow-up study to determine whether clinicians' expectations about a particular patient's fundal height influence the accuracy of their measurements. Based on findings from that study, the research team concluded that seeing the numbers on the measuring tape and knowing the presumed length of gestation biases clinicians in a way that contributes to error (Engstrom *et al*, 1994).

- Studies to determine the accuracy of assessing fetal well being by listening to the fetal heart rate with a fetoscope (similar to a stethoscope) as compared with use of an electronic fetal monitor (Paine *et al.*, 1986).
- A study to determine how well Dutch midwives' assessments of meconium-stained amniotic fluid agree with a standard assessment, with each other's assessments, and with their own assessments when presented with the same sample more than once. (See footnote about meconium on page 97). Some

studies suggest that perinatal risk is increased when the amniotic fluid is heavily rather than lightly stained with meconium. In addition, meconium inhaled during the newborns first gasps after birth may cause very serious pneumonia. Both physicians and midwives describe meconium-stained fluid as "thick" or "thin" meconium and respond differently depending on that distinction. The study found that grading the severity of meconium staining by visual assessment is so inaccurate and imprecise that it does not provide a valid basis for assigning different care to different degrees of meconium staining (van Heijst *et al.*, 1995).

(3) Research to determine the effects of methods that are used more commonly by midwives than by physicians:

- A study to assess the ability of a particular exercise to relieve a common source of abdominal pain during pregnancy (Andrews & O'Neill, 1994).
- Studies to determine the safety and effects of immersing women in warm water during labor. In the book he published in 1984, Dr. Odent claimed that warm water immersion induces physical and mental relaxation, which promotes more efficient first-stage labor. Water immersion is being utilized in various places around the world; consumer advocates are recommending it, and hospitals are installing tubs in renovated or newly constructed obstetric units. However, immersion in water is not mentioned in leading obstetric textbooks, and scientific data on the practice are limited. A nonrandomized controlled study found faster cervical dilation among women who sat in warm water for one-half to two hours during early labor, although there was no effect on the total duration of labor. In 1993 two CNMs and a physician published results of a randomized study. Although most women in the experimental group

enjoyed relaxing in the tub, there were no significant differences between the groups in cervical dilation, contraction pattern, time from admission to delivery, or infection (Schorn *et al.*, 1993).

- Nurse-midwives have conducted several studies of the effects of instructing women to hold their breath while pushing during the second stage of labor. One study compared the length of the second stage, the newborn's condition as measured by Apgar scores (based on breathing, heart rate, color, muscle tone, and responsiveness), and the mother's perception of second stage labor for five women taught the breath-holding method of pushing and five women who were encouraged to push spontaneously. Outcomes for both groups were similar except that all of the women instructed to hold their breath while pushing required episiotomies, compared with only one woman in the spontaneous pushing group.

  Women taught to hold their breath while pushing described pain, backache, cramps, and a sense of not accomplishing anything. Women who pushed spontaneously described relief that came with pushing; it was hard work and hurt, but also felt good in a way, and there was a sense of satisfaction, accomplishing something, making progress (Yeates & Roberts, 1984). A later study compared the effects of these two ways of instructing women on the level of oxygen in the fetal blood and the length of second stage labor; the pushing method had no effect on either outcome (Paine & Tinker, 1992). Another study followed women who had taken childbirth education classes. Most women taught to hold their breath while pushing did not do it if they delivered in an environment that encouraged them to respond to their own instincts during labor (Lindell & Rossi, 1986).

- Two Swedish midwives conducted a randomized trial to compare the effect of encouraging women to use a birthing stool with encouraging use of the conventional semirecumbent position. A birthing stool allows the woman to sit upright or squat and makes it possible for her husband to sit close behind her and support her back. Although the midwives provided different advice and encouragement to the women in one group as compared to the other, they did not try to persuade a woman to use a position that she found to be uncomfortable. In fact, slightly less than half of the women who were encouraged to use the birth stool actually did so, and 9 percent of the women in the control group used the birth stool although they were encouraged to use the conventional position. The women who were encouraged to use the birthing stool reported less pain than women in the control group, and they and their husbands tended to be more satisfied with the mother's position during the birth. Ninety percent of those who actually used the birth stool said that they would like to use it during any future birth. However, they had a tendency to bleed more and there was no difference in the length of labor or the use of oxytocin (Waldenström & Gottvall, 1991).

- Results of the Swedish study just described differed from those of a nonrandomized retrospective study conducted by two American CNMs and an American obstetrician: two hundred women who squatted during second-stage pushing were compared with one hundred women who delivered in other positions. The women who squatted had shorter second-stage labors, significantly fewer and less severe perineal lacerations, and no increase in the incidence of postpartum hemorrhage. However, the women who delivered in the semirecumbent position were more likely to have received oxytocin either to induce labor or to strengthen it during the first stage. The differential use of oxytocin could have contributed to the observed difference in the length of the second-stage (Golay *et al.*, 1993).

These studies exemplify the wide range of subjects investigated by midwives, the variety of research methods, and the incremental growth of the body of knowledge

Contributions of American Direct-Entry Midwives

Direct-entry midwives have contributed by retaining and teaching some safe and effective alternatives to more invasive obstetric interventions, thereby saving methods that might otherwise have been lost in the transition to high-technology childbirth. In addition, because of their separation and independence from medicine, they have the opportunity to develop a body of knowledge and practice "that reflects women's subjective experiences, in contrast to externally imposed obstetrical models," including "largely unrecognized but often time-honored solutions to the tasks and problems of childbearing" (Sakala, 1993). Carol Sakala, a sociologist at Boston University, has described methods that direct-entry midwives in Utah use to prevent and treat dystocia (and therefore reduce the need for cesarean sections) and to reduce and help women cope with pain (see Chapter 9) (Sakala, 1988). Another sociologist, Barbara Katz Rothman, stresses the impact of context on our knowledge about birth. Birth at home is different than birth in a hospital. The setting affects the "knowledge" that emerges because "the birth process itself is shaped by the settings in which it occurs" (Rothman, 1984). To support her point, she cited several obstetrical "facts" that may be largely or in part artifacts caused by medical management of childbirth in hospitals. Anthropologist Robbie Davis-Floyd (1995) similarly believes that out-of-hospital practice is necessary for women to "rediscover" their own ways of birthing, and for midwives to rediscover how best to support them. The few studies of care provided by direct-entry midwives describe a practice that *is* different from that of most nurse-midwives.

These are the observations of social scientists. Direct-entry midwives in the United States have done little research themselves. This is beginning to change and will change with their circumstances. Anne Frye, a midwife who is writing a three-volume textbook for independent midwives, has asked other midwives to share their "valid techniques" and "tricks," as well as cultural customs, "blessingways, ceremonies, rituals and rites of passage" with which they are familiar. The first volume of her trilogy—on midwifery care during the prenatal period—was published in 1995. The second will focus on care during labor and delivery, the third on postpartum care. Other midwives are sending her information, especially for the book on midwifery care during childbirth (Frye, 1996). Descriptive studies being conducted by the Midwives Alliance of North America (MANA) will also make a contribution. However, much more research is needed even to describe direct-entry midwifery practices and the concepts and theories that underlie the practice. Another level of research will be needed to assess the effectiveness of methods that are unique to direct-entry midwives.

The studies being conducted by MANA will describe the practices and outcomes of care provided by MANA members—CNMs as well as direct-entry midwives. In 1992 MANA adopted a data-collection form developed by their Research and Statistics Committee in conjunction with a Canadian epidemiologist. The form is used to record more than four hundred details about an individual woman's pregnancy, labor, and birth and both the mother's and the baby's condition during the first six weeks after the birth. The same form is being used for three purposes. All members of MANA who were in active practice when the study was started were invited to participate in all three studies. Data collection began in May 1993 (Johnson & Daviss, 1996).

- *A retrospective study.* Midwives who agree to participate in this aspect of the study are asked to complete data-collection forms for each of their five most recent births. As of May 1996, ninety-five midwives had contributed data. Most sent data on only their five most recent births, but several midwives completed forms for a more extended retrospective series of consecutive clients.
- *A prospective study.* Midwives participating in this aspect of the study are asked to list all births they expect to attend during the next three months on a study registration form. This process is repeated every three months; an individual midwife may participate in the study for as long as she wants but is only committed to three months at a time. They are expected to complete data-collection forms on every pregnant woman in their practice. The completed form is sent to the study coordinator after each woman's six-week postpartum visit. The midwives must account for every client whose name has been entered on the study registration form. Between 30 and 60 midwives have participated in the prospective aspect of the study during each three-month period since the study started (May 1993). As of May 1996, a total of 312 midwives had contributed prospectively collected data on more than 2,300 births.
- *Retrospective studies using data collected by state and provincial midwifery associations.* Midwifery associations in more than a dozen states and provinces are using the MANA form to collect retrospective data to document all births attended by their members during a defined time period. Using the MANA form allows data collected by local midwifery associations to be analyzed readily and compared with findings from the larger MANA data set. Local midwifery associations had submitted data on more than 1,500 births as of May 1996.

Including all three studies, data on more than six thousand midwife-attended births had been collected as of May 1996. Eighty-eight percent of the women were planning to have home births; 6 percent were planning to give birth in a free-standing birth center. Eight percent were planning to have hospital births. Because some MANA members are nurse-midwives, the data set includes some births attended by CNMs (Johnson & Daviss, 1996)

In addition to describing direct-entry midwifery practices and outcomes, these studies should yield new information about labor when women are in familiar and supportive environments and are attended by midwives who are patient and are comfortable with variation outside of medically defined norms. The number of births anticipated is large enough that the investigators expect to be able to describe direct-entry midwifery care and response to complications that occur relatively rarely, such as shoulder dystocia, a long second stage of labor, and retained placenta, and to describe practices that are not required often, such as attempts to turn a fetus from the breech to the head-down position. The number of births should also be large enough to provide a reliable picture of situations requiring emergency transport to a hospital and the incidence of perinatal mortality. It may also be possible to compare practices and outcomes of births attended by direct-entry midwives in different parts of North America and in different kinds of settings (Johnson & Daviss, 1996).

Preliminary analyses have been initiated to examine associations between the length of second-stage labor and perinatal outcomes; the effect of massaging and stretching the perineal tissues during the third trimester of pregnancy on the incidence and severity of perineal tears; the success of attempted vaginal birth after cesarean section (VBAC) at home as compared with VBACs attempted in hospitals; the success of various techniques for resolving shoulder dystocia;

and the effect of restricted use of episiotomy on the incidence of third- and fourth-degree perineal tears. In each analysis, the data from the prospective and retrospective components of the study are analyzed separately; where the results are similar, the data are combined. In the preliminary VBAC analysis, more than 90 percent of the women who attempted a VBAC at home were able to deliver vaginally. Examination of the data on perineal massage or stretching during the third trimester suggests that this practice does not reduce the incidence of third- and fourth-degree perineal tears and may even increase the risk (Johnson & Daviss, 1996).

The most well-known and important example of midwives preserving low-intervention skills is Ina May Gaskin's development of a videocassette on assisting a vaginal breech birth. First produced in 1981, it became available at a time when cesarean sections for breech presentation had become a standard for obstetricians. As the occurrence of vaginal breech deliveries declined, the knowledge and skill required to assist in such a birth became in danger of extinction. Physicians who knew how to manage a vaginal breech delivery retired or lost confidence in skills they no longer practiced; young physicians not only were not taught these techniques, but had never even seen them being used. As the cesarean section rate continued to increase, the presumed advantages of delivering breech babies abdominally was scrutinized more carefully. Three studies designed to identify the best way to deliver babies in breech presentation at term (i.e., excluding preterm babies, who have additional problems) were published during the 1980s. All found no advantage of cesarean sections for the babies and much higher rates of significant complications among the mothers delivered by cesarean section (Cunningham *et al.*, 1993). Despite this new knowledge, lack of skills to assist a

vaginal breech birth made it hard to reverse the trend. As stated in the 1993 edition of the *Williams Obstetrics* textbook, "one important criterion for safe vaginal delivery is becoming more and more difficult to fulfill; that is, most resident training programs within the near future will not provide sufficient opportunity for acquisition of skills essential for successful vaginal breech delivery" (Cunningham *et al.*, 1993).

Breech presentation is a serious complication. An episiotomy, anesthesia, and possibly intensive resuscitation of the newborn may be needed, and there is an increased rate of perinatal mortality—whether the delivery is vaginal or by cesarean section (Cunningham *et al.*, 1993). Thus most home birth midwives refer women with persistent breech presentation to a hospital for labor and birth. However, it is not always possible to identify a breech presentation during early labor. Physicians, as well as midwives, are sometimes surprised by the sudden appearance of fetal buttocks, when they had anticipated a fetal head (Cunningham et al., 1993). Some obstetrical authorities buttress their objection to home births with the possibility and danger of an unanticipated breech, while some direct-entry midwives believe that breech deliveries can be as safe at home as in a hospital. This issue is discussed further in Chapter 9. Whether to be prepared for unexpected breech deliveries or to attend breech deliveries at home intentionally, there is need for an effective way to teach midwives how to manage a breech delivery. The fifty-five minute video, produced at the Farm Midwifery Center in Tennessee demonstrates external version (a method to turn the fetus into the head-down position by manipulating it through the abdominal wall) and shows and explains the management of six breech births that occurred at the Farm. The video was and remains a unique teaching tool, appreciated by physicians and CNMs as well as direct-entry midwives. It has done much to keep these methods alive.

Direct-entry midwives value "Grand Midwives" (often referred to as granny midwives) for the experience-based knowledge they have developed and passed from one to another. Grand Midwives are often invited to speak at direct-entry midwifery conferences. They are old; there is a desire to learn from them before their special knowledge "slips away" with the passage of time (Tully, 1993).

Chapter 7
Midwifery in America, 1980–1994: Percent of Births, Place of Birth, and Clientele

This chapter provides information on where babies are born, who (physician, midwife, or "other" person) attends births in the United States, and how and to what extent these things changed during the fifteen-year period between 1980 and 1994. It also describes women whose births are attended by midwives demographically and by some characteristics and factors that are associated with perinatal risk. The data that provide both kinds of information come primarily from birth certificates.

Birth Certificates—Source of National Natality Data

The individual birth certificates of infants born in the United States yield the most reliable available information about the mother, the birth attendant, and the place of birth. Birth certificate data are compiled in each state and then aggregated by the National Center for Health Statistics (NCHS),

which publishes annual reports of natality data at the national level. These data have several limitations with respect to births attended by midwives:

- Most states did not distinguish between CNMs and other midwives or between various out-of-hospital birth sites until the U.S. Standard Certificate of Live Birth was revised in 1989. Thus 1989 is the first year for which there are national data on the number and percent of births attended by CNMs and other midwives and on the number and percent of home births and births in freestanding birth centers.
- Some births attended by CNMs in the State of Illinois and by nurse-midwifery students in many states have been categorized as births attended by "other midwives." All data presented in this book have been adjusted to attribute those births to CNMs.

- Some midwives do not sign the birth certificates of the babies they deliver. In studies conducted between 1982 and 1994, between 7 and 13 percent of CNMs who were attending births reported that they did not sign birth certificates.* Underreporting of births attended by direct-entry midwives is assumed to be higher, especially in states where their practice is illegal. In this situation no birth certificate may be filed until one is actually needed, when the child is older, or a birth certificate may be filed and someone other than the midwife may be identified as the attendant. Some states suggest many possible categories of birth attendants on the birth certificate form. Oregon, for instance, provides space to indicate whether the primary attendant at an out-of-hospital birth was a medical doctor (MD), doctor of osteopathy (DO), naturopathic doctor (ND), doctor of chiropractic (DC), certified nurse-midwife (CNM), registered nurse (RN), midwife (any except a CNM), "other licensed medical" person, or "non-medical" person. The National Center for Health Statistics collapses the information collected by states into six categories: doctors of medicine, doctors of osteopathy, CNMs, "other" midwives, other birth attendants, and unspecified. Some out-of-hospital births attended by direct-entry midwives are probably included within the numbers of births that fall into the "other birth attendant" and "unspecified birth attendant" categories.
- Birth certificate data cannot distinguish between births that occur at home by intention and births that occur at home by accident. The lack of distinction between intended and unintended home births undermines attempts to use national natality data to determine the

safety of home births. The hospital is listed as the place of birth for births that occur in a car or ambulance en route to a hospital (Johnson, E., 1996).
- It takes NCHS about two years to aggregate, analyze, and report the national data. The *Advance Report of Final Natality Statistics, 1994,* was published in June 1996 (Ventura *et al.,* 1996). It provides data on place of birth and birth attendant. In addition, *Births and Deaths: United States, 1995,* was published in October 1996 (Rosenberg *et al.,* 1996). It is a preliminary report that provides some information on births but does not include data on place of birth and birth attendant. These publications are the sources of the most recent birth data reported in this chapter and elsewhere in this book.

Underreporting of Births Attended by Midwives

As already noted, the number of births attended by both kinds of midwives is underreported. However, the proportion of CNMs who do not sign the birth certificates of infants whose births they attend is relatively low and is decreasing—from 13 percent in 1982 to 7 percent in 1994.

Underreporting of births attended by direct-entry midwives is assumed to be more significant. Although most Americans eventually need a birth certificate, it is possible to obtain the certificate many years after the birth. Data from retrospective birth certificates are not folded back into the natality data provided by the National Center for Health Statistics. This causes some underreporting of home births in areas where direct-entry midwives have been harassed and try to be discreet about their practice. Only 25 percent of home births attended by direct-entry midwives in Santa Cruz County, California, between 1971 and 1973 were registered with the Bureau of Vital Statistics. Later studies

---

*See Table 7 in Chapter 8.

Later studies found that birth certificates had been filed for 20 to 100 percent of the home births attended by midwives and physicians in California, with reporting more likely for births attended by physicians and less likely for births attended by direct-entry midwives. These studies were conducted during the Vietnam War, and it was assumed that some parents did not file birth certificates because they wanted to protect their sons from ever being drafted into military service. A study of home births attended by physicians and lay midwives in and around Madison, Wisconsin, during the late 1970s found that, even with strong encouragement from the birth attendants, birth certificates had been filed within six months for only 60 percent of the babies (Mehl *et al.*, 1980). A social scientist who collected information on births attended by twelve direct-entry midwives in Massachusetts during 1986 and 1987 could identify birth certificates for only about one-fourth of the babies when she tried to find them three years later (Sakala, 1996).

A high degree of underreporting of direct-entry home births is not universal, however, and reporting probably became more complete after people adjusted to termination of the draft in 1973. Recent data from Vermont and Oregon suggest relatively complete reporting of births attended by direct-entry midwives in those states. Birth certificates had been filed for all but eight of 253 home births (4 percent) included in a prospective study of direct-entry midwifery practice in Vermont from 1981 to 1985 (Carney, 1990). Although Oregon has a long tradition of home births attended by lay and direct-entry midwives (approximately two thousand home births per year during the early 1980s, falling to about one thousand per year during the early 1990s), only about twenty-five people seek retrospective birth certificates in Oregon each year (Herman, 1996).

Table 2 provides information on the number and percent of out-of-hospital births attended by direct-entry midwives for each year from 1989 through 1994. The minimal number is the actual number of birth certificates on which "other midwife" (other than a CNM) was indicated as the birth attendant. This is a minimal number that does not acknowledge any underreporting. The "maximal estimate" is based on the assumption that midwives other than CNMs attended half of the out-of-hospital births for which birth certificates were filed but no birth attendant was specified or the birth attendant was someone other than a physician or a midwife. Applying this assumption increases the number and percent of births attended by direct-entry midwives by about fifty percent; it is the same as assuming that a correct birth certificate is filed for only two of every three births actually attended by a direct-entry midwife. The validity of the assumption on which the estimates are based is not known. It is unlikely that the actual degree of underreporting is greater than this. The proportion of all U.S. births attended by direct-entry midwives during each year between 1989 and 1994 probably varied between about 0.3 and 0.45 percent. Increasing the numbers based on the assumptions that produce the maximal estimate increases the estimated proportion of births attended by direct-entry midwives but has no effect on the stability of the proportion. There has been no increase or decrease, whether one considers the birth certificate data or estimates based on the assumption of significant underreporting.

All further discussion of the number of out-of-hospital births in this chapter, and elsewhere in the book, is based on data provided by the National Center for Health Statistics, that is, data derived from birth certificates. The true numbers and percentages of out-of-hospital births, especially home births attended by direct-entry midwives, may be somewhat higher but could not be less than the numbers and percentages presented.

Trends in Place of Birth and Birth Attendants

Table 3 provides information on all births in the United States by birth site and birth at-

Table 2
Minimal (Reported) and Estimated Maximal Numbers and Percents of Births Attended by Direct-Entry Midwives, 1989–1994*

| | Numbers and Percents of Births, by Attendant, Based on Birth Certificates | | | | | | Maximal Estimate for "Other Midwives"† | |
| | "Other Midwives" | | "Other" | "Unspecified" | "Other" and "Unspecified" | | | |
Year	Number	% of all U.S. Births	Attendant	Attendant	All	50%	Number	% of all U.S. Births
1989	12,400	0.31	11,707	771	12,478	6,239	18,639	0.46
1990	11,575	0.28	9,661	751	10,412	5,206	16,781	0.40
1991	12,085	0.29	11,547	804	12,351	6,176	18,261	0.44
1992	11,767	0.29	11,512	646	12,158	6,079	17,846	0.44
1993	12,281	0.31	11,341	617	11,958	5,979	18,260	0.46
1994	11,846	0.30	10,856	808	11,664	5,832	17,678	0.45

*Based on all out-of-hospital births for which birth certificates were filed for 1989–1994. All data are from the Monthly Vital Statistics Report series, *Advance Report of Final Natality Statistics*, for 1989, 1990, 1991, 1992, 1993, and 1994. These reports are published annually by the National Center for Health Statistics.

†These numbers and percents are maximal estimates derived by adding half of the births attributed to "other" and "unspecified" attendants to those actually attributed to "other midwives".

Table 3:
Live Births by Birth Site and Birth Attendant, United States, 1980 and 1989–1994*

Year and Site	All Births		Percent of Births by Specified Attendant				
	Number	Physicians	All Midwives	CNMs	Other Midwives†	Other or Unspecified
All Births						
1980	3,612,258	97.2	1.7	Unknown	Unknown	1.0
1989	4,040,958	95.4	3.6	(3.3)	(0.3)	0.9
1990	4,158,212	95.0	3.9	(3.6)	(0.3)	1.1
1991	4,110,907	94.7	4.4	(4.1)	(0.3)	0.9
1992	4,065,014	94.3	4.9	(4.6)	(0.3)	0.8
1993	4,000,240	94.0	5.3	(5.0)	(0.3)	0.8
1994	3,952,767	93.8	5.5	(5.2)	(0.3)	0.7
Hospital	*Percent of All*					
1980	99.0	97.0	1.4	Unknown	—	0.7
1989	98.8	96.3	3.1	(3.1)	—	0.6
1990	98.9	95.7	3.5	(3.5)	—	0.8
1991	98.9	95.5	4.0	(4.0)	—	0.6
1992	99.1	95.1	4.4	(4.4)	—	0.5
1993	99.0	94.7	4.8	(4.8)	—	0.5
1994	99.0	94.6	5.0	(5.0)	—	0.4
All Nonhospital	*Percent of All*					
1980	1.0	33.4	30.9	Unknown	Unknown	35.7
1989	1.2	27.5	46.1	(19.8)	(26.3)	26.4
1990	1.1	29.2	44.8	(20.1)	(24.7)	26.0
1991	1.1	25.7	47.4	(21.0)	(26.4)	26.9
1992	1.1	23.7	48.0	(20.6)	(27.4)	28.3
1993	1.0	19.9	50.2	(19.8)	(30.7)	29.9
1994	1.0	17.4	53.5	(24.0)	(29.5)	29.1

(*continued*)

Table 3:
Live Births by Birth Site and Birth Attendant, United States, 1980 and 1989–1994* (Continued)

Year and Site	All Births	Percent of Births by Specified Attendant				
	Percent of All	Physicians	All Midwives	CNMs	Other Midwives†	Other or Unspecified
Birth Centers						
1980	Unknown	Unknown	Unknown	Unknown	Unknown	Unknown
1989	0.35	35.1	63.0	(39.8)	(23.2)	1.9
1990	0.36	40.4	58.0	(38.7)	(19.3)	1.2
1991	0.35	33.6	64.7	(43.3)	(21.3)	1.7
1992	0.33	30.4	67.1	(43.1)	(24.0)	2.4
1993	0.28	20.0	76.9	(44.6)	(32.2)	3.2
1994	0.30	15.3	82.8	(56.7)	(26.1)	1.8
Home Births						
1980	Unknown	Unknown	Unknown	Unknown	Unknown	Unknown
1989	0.69	20.9	41.0	(12.3)	(28.7)	38.1
1990	0.67	21.0	41.3	(12.4)	(28.9)	37.6
1991	0.67	19.4	42.2	(11.8)	(30.4)	38.4
1992	0.64	17.7	42.5	(11.3)	(31.2)	39.7
1993	0.63	17.4	42.9	(10.1)	(32.8)	39.7
1994	0.62	15.9	44.7	(10.5)	(34.2)	39.4

*All data are from the national natality statistics compiled by the National Center for Health Statistics and published as issues of the Monthly Vital Statistics Report series, *Advance Report of Final Natality Statistics*, for 1980, 1989, 1990, 1991, 1992, 1993, and 1994.

†These percentages do not include any in-hospital births attributed to "other midwives": 2,559 for 1989; 2,724 for 1990; 2,663 for 1991; 2,420 for 1992; 1,543 for 1993; and 1,567 for 1994. Many of these births result from an error in the attribution of CNM births in the State of Illinois. National Center for Health Statistics officials believe that the others are births attended by nurse-midwifery students. No in-hospital births are known to have been attended by lay or direct-entry midwives between 1989 and 1994.

tendant for 1980 and every year between 1989 and 1994.* The number of births increased until 1990 and has fallen each year since then.

Birth Sites

The proportion of births in hospitals has remained stable at approximately 99 percent; likewise, the proportion of births in all out-of-hospital birth sites has remained stable at approximately 1 percent. The proportion of births in free-standing birth centers stayed at 0.35 to 0.36 percent during 1989 to 1991, declined between 1991 and 1993, and regained some of that loss during 1994. There are more than twice as many home births as births in free-standing birth centers. The proportion of home births declined very slightly but steadily between 1991 and 1994. Out-of-hospital birth sites not shown in Table 3 include clinics and doctor's offices, which accounted for 900 to 1,100 births during each year shown on this table.

Birth Attendants

The proportion of babies delivered by physicians fell slowly but steadily throughout this period, dropping by 3.4 percent between 1980 and 1994. The decline occurred in births in hospitals and births in nonhospital settings. Although most of the births affected by this change occur in hospitals, the role of physicians in nonhospital births fell much more sharply—by almost half. Physicians attended one-third of all out-of-hospital births in 1980, but only 17 percent in 1994.

Most of the decline in births in free-standing birth centers was due to declining participation by physicians. The number of birth center births attended by "other midwives" also declined between 1989 and 1994 (3,312 births in 1989; 3,079 in 1994), while

the number attended by CNMs increased (5,678 in 1989; 6,686 in 1994).

Midwives' overall role in childbirth increased more than threefold during this period, from 1.7 percent of all births in 1980 to 5.5 percent in 1994. Births attended by nurse-midwives in hospitals account for nearly all of the increase. By 1994, CNMs were attending 5 percent of all in-hospital births.

The number of out-of-hospital births attended by midwives increased from 17,456 in 1980 to 21,766 in 1989, and then fell a little each year until 1993 ($N = 20,114$), and rebounded in 1994 ($N = 21,476$). This fluctuation was due to changes in the number of out-of-hospital births attended by CNMs. Both the number and the percent of births attended by lay and direct-entry midwives were extremely stable throughout this period; the number varied between 11,575 and 12,400, while the proportion remained at 0.3 percent of all births in the nation. We know that the number of births attributed to direct-entry midwives is underreported. If we assume that birth certificates are filed for most of the births they attend, that most of their uncounted births are home births attributed to an "other" or "unspecified" birth attendant, and that half of the home births in those categories were attended by lay and direct-entry midwives, the number of births they attended would increase to about 17,500 per year—approximately 0.5 percent of all births in the country each year between 1989 and 1994.

Complete national data on cesarean sections have been available only since 1991. If only vaginal births are considered, the proportion of births attended by midwives is higher than the figures shown in Table 3. Midwives attended 5.9 percent of noncesarean births in 1991, 6.4 percent in 1992, 6.8 percent in 1993, and 7.1 percent in 1994.

What Kinds of Women Use Midwives?

Nurse-midwifery in the United States began with services designed for women who

---

*Unless other attribution is provided, all data in this section are from the national natality statistics compiled by the National Center for Health Statistics and published as issues of the Monthly Vital Statistics Report series, *Advance Report of Final Natality Statistics*, for 1980, 1989, 1990, 1991, 1992, 1993, and 1994.

lacked access to medical care because they lived in isolated rural areas or because they were poor. Nurse-midwives have always provided care to a disproportionate number of women who are members of racial and ethnic minority groups and have gained respect for the special effectiveness of the care they provide to these women and to pregnant adolescents. The nation's continuing need to provide attractive, cost-effective care to these groups of women motivated federal funding of nurse-midwifery education and contributed to the development of a high proportion of nurse-midwifery services. The development of demand for midwifery care among well-educated middle-class and professional women added another group to the picture. Nurse-midwives' growing role in health maintenance organizations brought in a wider spectrum of middle-class women, so that all groups are now represented. Nevertheless, nurse-midwives continue to take care of a relatively high proportion of women who are poor, unmarried, young, and black, and play a special role in the care of Native American women. CNMs delivered 15 percent of the babies born on Indian reservations in 1984 (Taffel, 1987). CNMs also fill a lot of local niches—small groups of women who are separated from the mainstream by geography, culture, or religion; recent immigrants; women from other countries who are in the United States temporarily; and women who are in prison or jail.

Lay midwifery's development at a different time, for different reasons, in a different context resulted in a different clientele. Direct-entry midwives attend home births and operate their own birth centers. They are the only experienced home birth attendants in many communities. With few exceptions, they practice outside of the established health care system, to which they provide a clear alternative. Women and families seek their care for many reasons: because they have strong faith that birth is a normal process that requires no intervention, because they want to control their birth environment and prevent intervention, because

they do not have access to mainstream health care, because giving birth at home is very important to them, because they reject and/or fear physicians and hospitals, because they need assurance that no men will be present during labor and delivery, because they want their family matters to be private and distrust and try to avoid involvement with "the system," or because they anticipate birth as a very significant experience, know what kind of experience they want, and are determined to achieve it. Most direct-entry midwifery clients are white, married, and have had several previous babies. Beyond these very general characteristics, they are a rich mixture: traditional, conservative, home-oriented women; college-educated, middle-class professionals and intellectuals; "New Agers;" members of certain religious groups; women who live in rural areas; women who need inexpensive care because they are not covered by any third-party health-care payment plan; "survivalists" and other people who are trying to live apart from the mainstream of American society; and Mexican women who want to give birth in the United States.

The following studies used national birth certificate data to describe the women who use midwives:

- An analysis of ethnic differences in the women whose births were attended by midwives between 1982 and 1989 (Parker, 1994)
- An analysis of births attended by midwives in hospitals and in out-of-hospital birth sites between 1975 and 1988 (Declercq, 1992)
- Demographic information on all women who had midwife-attended births in 1989, by category of midwife and place of birth (Declercq 1993)
- Information about women who had home births between 1989 and 1992 (Declercq *et al.*, 1995).
- Information on the number of births attended by CNMs and "other midwives" in 1994, by state (Clarke *et al.*, 1997).

The following sections summarize the information from these five studies and from an analysis of home births to black women from 1989 through 1994.

Women Whose Out-of-Hospital Births Were Attended by Midwives, 1975–1988

A high proportion of all out-of-hospital births attended by midwives occurred to white Hispanic women who were originally from Mexico. Texas alone accounted for one-third of all out-of-hospital births attended by midwives during this fourteen-year period. Out-of-hospital births attended by midwives accounted for at least 1 percent of all births during this period in nine states. Eight of the nine states are in the rural West: Alaska, Washington, Oregon, Idaho, Montana, Nevada, New Mexico, and Texas, plus New Hampshire (Declercq, 1992).

Ethnicity of Women Whose Births Were Attended by Midwives, 1982–1989

Native American women were most likely to have their babies delivered by a midwife. Black women and Hispanic women were the next most likely group; and non-Hispanic white women and Asian women were least likely (Parker, 1994).

Women Whose Births Were Attended by CNMs in Hospitals, 1988 and 1989

As a group, women whose babies are delivered by nurse-midwives in hospitals are very different from women whose births are attended by midwives in birth centers or homes, as shown in Table 4. Compared with all women who delivered babies in the United States in 1989, women whose births were attended by CNMs in hospitals tended to be younger (18 percent were teenagers), were more likely to be unmarried (38 percent), and a higher proportion were black (21 percent). One-third had not completed high school, and they were less likely to have been to college (Declercq, 1993). Births attended by CNMs in hospitals accounted for at least 7 to 10 percent of the births in three

states (Alaska, Florida, and New Mexico) in 1988 (Declercq, 1992).

Women Whose Births Were Attended by CNMs in Birth Centers, 1989

In contrast to the women they take care of in hospitals, nurse-midwives' birth center clients were highly educated (half had been to college and more than one-fourth were college graduates), predominantly white (95 percent), and less likely than all women who gave birth in 1989 to be teenagers or unmarried (Declercq, 1993). See Table 4.

Women Whose Births Were Attended by Other Midwives in Birth Centers, 1989

Five states accounted for 91 percent of births attended by direct-entry midwives in free-standing birth centers in 1989. Nearly three-fourths of the births occurred in centers located in Texas, close to the Mexican border; most of the clients were Mexican-American women and women who are citizens of Mexico. Another 19 percent occurred in birth centers located in Arizona, Pennsylvania, Florida, and Washington. The age distribution for women whose births were attended by direct-entry midwives in birth centers was similar to that of all women giving birth in the United States. However, they tended to have many children; they were more than twice as likely to being giving birth to their fourth or a higher order child. Almost all were white and married; most had not graduated from high school (Declercq, 1993).

Women Who Have Home Births

Women who gave birth at home in 1989 were similar to other women who had babies that year with regard to race (see Table 5). However, they were less than half as likely as all U.S. mothers to be having their first birth and were three times more likely to be having their fourth or a higher order child. Home birth mothers were much less likely to be teenagers and nearly twice as likely to be at least thirty-five years of age. They were somewhat less likely to be unmarried and

Table 4
**Demographic Information on Women Who Had Midwife-Attended Births in Hospitals
and Birth Centers, Compared with All Births in the United States, 1989***

Demographic Characteristic	CNM Births in Hospitals	CNM Births in Birth Centers	Other Midwife Births in Birth Ceners	All Births in the U.S.
Race:				
White	72.3	95.0	98.2	79.0
Black	21.0	2.9	0.5	16.7
Other	6.7	2.0	1.2	4.3
Age:				
<20	18.3	7.6	12.1	12.8
>34	7.2	10.9	8.4	8.4
No. of previous births:				
None	39.4	34.1	33.2	41.0
Three	12.6	13.6	21.7	10.3
Unmarried	38.3	11.7	8.5	27.1
Education:				
Less than high school	33.3	18.6	59.1	23.2
Some college	17.3	24.5	11.2	20.3
College graduate	14.1	26.3	7.4	17.3

*Data are adapted from Declercq ER. Where babies are born and who attends their births: Findings from the revised 1989 United States Standard Certificate of Live Birth. *Obstet Gynecol* 1993;81:997–1004.

somewhat more likely to have less than a high school education (Declercq, 1993).

Compared with all home birth mothers, women whose births were attended by CNMs were more likely to be white and to have had more education (34 percent college graduates), and only half as likely to be unmarried. Although they tended to be older, they were less likely to have given birth to many children (Declercq, 1993).

Very few nonwhite home births were attributed to "other midwives;" less than 2 percent of their clients were black, and relatively few were unmarried or less than twenty years old. In other ways they were quite similar to the total group of home birth mothers (Declercq, 1993).

Data from 1989 through 1992 regarding race, age, parity, marital status, and educa-tion were similar to those for 1989 alone. In addition, women who gave birth at home during 1989 to 1992 tended to have shorter intervals between pregnancies (compared with all women who gave birth in the United States during that period), were somewhat less likely to drink alcohol, and were much less likely to smoke. Fewer were Hispanic (12 versus 14 percent of all U.S. births during 1989–1992). Women who lived in the West and Southwest had the highest proportion of home births. Nevertheless, the percent of births occurring at home decreased in twelve of the fifteen western states between 1989 and 1992. The proportion of home births was higher than 1.5 percent in only seven states: Alaska, Montana, Vermont, Idaho, Oregon, Nevada, and Washington. All of these states have relatively low popula-

Table 5

Demographic Information on Women Having Midwife-Attended Home Births, United States, 1989*

Demographic Characteristic	Attended by CNMs	Attended by Other Midwives	All Home Birth Mothers	All Women Giving Birth in the United States
Race:				
White	93.2	96.0	80.9	79.0
Black	4.2	1.5	15.1	16.7
Other	2.5	1.9	4.0	4.3
Age:				
<20	2.1	4.7	7.8	12.8
>34	19.5	14.8	15.6	8.4
No. of previous births:				
None	19.3	20.9	19.9	41.0
Three	26.0	30.6	31.8	10.3
Unmarried	11.8	8.7	23.7	27.1
Education:				
Less than high school	17.6	28.9	28.6	23.2
Some college	25.7	24.3	21.0	20.3
College graduate	33.7	18.8	18.1	17.3

*Data are from Declercq ER. Where babies are born and who attends their births: Findings from the revised 1989 United States Standard Certificate of Live Birth. *Obstet Gynecol* 1993;81:997–1004.

tion densities. Only 30 percent of home births occurred in cities with populations of 100,000 or more (Declercq *et al.*, 1995).

The small proportion of black home births attributed to lay midwives is somewhat mysterious and may be an artifact. When all home births to black women from 1989 through 1994 are the unit under consideration (i.e., all home births by black women = 100 percent), the largest proportion—48 percent—were attended by physicians, with the next largest proportion (43 percent) being attributed to "other attendants." Some midwives believe that, especially in rural parts of some southeastern states, black women who are members of certain church congregations assist at the home births of other women from their church. They think of themselves as church women, rather than

as midwives, and check the box for "other attendant" on the baby's birth certificate (Davidson, 1995). The number of home births to black women declined by 23 percent between 1991 and 1994. Most of the reduction came from births attended by physicians. Physicians accounted for 52 percent of home births to black women in 1991, but only 42 percent in 1994.

Although there are no data to quantify it, religion is an important factor in determining which women have home births. As many as one-third to one-half of the women who have home births attended by lay and direct-entry midwives are members of religious groups that consider birth to be an important spiritual and family event and prefer to avoid medical intervention and control of the process. Some religious groups that favor home births include the Amish, Mennonites, Orthodox Jews, evangelical Christian denominations, Mormons, Moslems, Jehovah's Witnesses, and Christian Scientists. In some churches, the midwife has a role within the religious community, for which she is accountable to the church and to God.

States That Have a Relatively High Proportion of Midwife-Attended Births

Utilization of midwives varies greatly between states. Midwives attended at least 10 percent of all births in each of nine states in 1994. New Mexico had the highest proportion (19 percent), followed by Alaska (16 percent), New Hampshire (15 percent), Utah (12 percent), Delaware (11 percent), and Georgia, Massachussetts, Vermont, and Florida, each with 10 percent (Clarke, *et al.*, 1997).

The jurisdictions with the highest proportion of births attended by CNMs were: New Mexico (18 percent), Alaska and New Hampshire (14 percent each), Oregon (11 percent), and Massachusetts, Delaware, and Georgia (10 percent each). The relatively high proportion of births attended by nurse-midwives in New Mexico is due primarily to the large role of nurse-midwifery on certain American Indian reservations. Nurse-midwives attended births in every U.S. jurisdiction in 1994 (Clarke, *et al.*, 1997).

Direct-entry midwives accounted for at least 1 percent of the births in ten states in 1994: Alaska (2.2 percent), Idaho and Montana (1.6 percent each), Nevada and Vermont (1.5 percent each), Washington (1.4 percent), Utah (1.2 percent), Texas (1.1 percent), and Oregon (1.0 percent). Although direct-entry midwives attended only 1.1 percent of the births in Texas, Texas accounted for 27 percent of all births for which a birth certificate was filed with "other midwife" marked as the birth attendant ($N = 3,562$). The only other states with at least 1,000 births attributed to direct-entry midwives were Pennsylvania (1,301) and Washington (1,096). Direct-entry midwives accounted

for the majority of births attended by midwives in Kansas in 1994 (108 births attended by direct-entry midwives, 79 attended by CNMs), and for at least one-fourth, or more, of the births attended by midwives in Missouri, Arkansas, Texas, Idaho, and Nevada (Clarke *et al.*, 1997).

Risk Factors Among Women Served by Midwives

During the early 1990s the Robert Wood Johnson Foundation funded a study to provide information on demographic characteristics of the women who obtain maternity care from CNMs. Questionnaires were mailed to more than 4,000 nurse-midwives (all those known to the ACNM) in May 1991. More than 2,400 were completed and returned by CNMs who were eligible for the study (Scupholme *et al.*, 1992). The study focused on the extent to which nurse-midwives provide care to eight categories of women considered "vulnerable" based on poor access to care and poorer than average pregnancy outcomes: women who are adolescent, black, native American, Asian or from one of the Pacific Islands, Hispanic, poor, immigrant, or without health care insurance. Ninety-nine percent of the nurse-midwives provided care to at least some women with one or more of the "vulnerable" characteristics. Ninety-five percent took care of adolescents, 89 percent provided care to black women, 36 percent to Native American women, 57 percent to Asians or Pacific Islanders, 79 percent to Hispanics, 89 percent to indigent women, 51 percent to immigrants, and 79 percent to women without health insurance. Seven percent of the CNMs attended home births. Those attending home births were less likely than the others to provide care to adolescents, blacks, Asians, Hispanics, or immigrants, but they were much more likely to take care of women without insurance. Half of the payment for the care provided by the CNMs in this study came from Medicaid or other forms of government subsidy. Only 20 percent came from private health care insurance. Fifty-six percent of the nurse-midwives' clients lived in areas considered to be medically underserved; 34 percent lived in inner-city areas, 22 percent in rural areas (Scupholme *et al,* 1992).

There are many ways to be "vulnerable." A study based on middle-class women from a small university-centered city in the Midwest found that women with a history of sexual or physical abuse were more likely to want a female care provider during pregnancy. Given a choice between a private nurse-midwifery practice and a private obstetrician, most of the women who had been abused selected the CNM practice, even though six of the twenty-two obstetricians were women (Sampselle *et al.*, 1992; Oakley *et al.*, 1995).

A study based on all U.S. births in 1989 calculated the incidence of several risk factors for six groups of women: mothers whose births were attended by CNMs in hospitals, birth centers, and homes; mothers whose births were attended by direct-entry midwives in birth centers and homes; and all women giving birth in the United States in 1989 (Declercq, 1995). The risk factors analyzed in this way included timing of entry into prenatal care, smoking, consumption of alcohol, weight gain during pregnancy, and the occurrence of specific diseases and prenatal complications. All of this information is recorded on birth certificates. The findings reflect the risk status of women *whose births were attended by midwives;* women who began care with a midwife but were referred to physicians because of their risk status or complications are not included. The following generalizations summarize the findings from this study:

- Women whose births are attended by nurse-midwives in hospitals have a higher-than-average concentration of risk factors associated with poor pregnancy outcomes. Compared with all women giving birth in the United States, they are more likely to have had a previous low birth weight baby; they are also more likely to have had a very large

baby. They are less likely to start prenatal care during the first three months of pregnancy and are more likely to arrive at the hospital having had no prenatal care at all. Higher proportions smoke, are anemic, or have kidney disease or a hemoglobinopathy. They are as likely as other women to have a disease that affects their heart or lungs.

- Women whose births are attended by nurse-midwives at home or in a free-standing birth center are low risk in most respects. Although they are less likely to start prenatal care during the first three months of pregnancy compared with all U.S. mothers, they are more likely to start care early compared with women whose births are attended by direct-entry midwives. Virtually all women who use birth centers operated by CNMs and more than 98 percent of those who have home births attended by CNMs had at least some prenatal care (similar to all women who gave birth in 1989). Women having home births with CNMs are more likely than those in any other group to have had a large baby during a previous pregnancy, and they have the highest average weight gain. This combination puts them at high risk for having large babies during the current pregnancy.

- Only one-third of the women who delivered babies in birth centers run by direct-entry midwives started prenatal care during the first three months of pregnancy. Thirty percent did not start until they were at least seven months pregnant, although almost all of them had at least one prenatal visit before they went to the birth center in labor. Most of these birth centers are near the Texas–Mexico border, a factor that may be associated with the relative lack of prenatal care. Data recorded on the babies' birth certificates indicate low rates of most medical problems, including a very low rate of diabetes. Since diabetes is generally higher among Hispanic women, this finding may reflect inaccurate or incomplete recording of information on the babies' birth certificates, due either to lack of prenatal care or lack of access to the prenatal records of women who live in Mexico. Women in this group are least likely to smoke or drink. They report the lowest average weight gain.

- Women who had home births attended by direct-entry midwives are the second least likely to start care during the first trimester.* Almost 3 percent had no prenatal care prior to labor and delivery. Although most direct-entry midwives insist on prenatal care, some feel that they cannot refuse a woman who calls them for help during labor, even if they have not seen the woman before (Tritten, 1996). Very few women who have home births attended by direct-entry midwives smoke or drink alcohol. They are somewhat more likely to gain at least twenty pounds during pregnancy, compared with the general population of childbearing women. The proportion who have given birth to large babies prior to their current pregnancy and the proportion with genital herpes were higher than in the general population of childbearing women in 1989. They were less likely to have most of the other medical conditions listed on birth certificates.

These findings reflect the effects of (1) the significant role of in-hospital nurse-midwifery services in the care of socioeconomically high-risk women, (2) the demographic characteristics of women who choose to have midwife-attended home births (predominantly white, married women, who tend to

---

*In 1989, 33 percent of women who gave birth in birth centers operated by direct-entry midwives started care during the first three months of pregnancy, compared with 56 percent of women who had home births attended by direct-entry midwives and 75 percent of all women who gave birth in the United States.

be of relatively high age and parity), and (3) midwives' referral practices: Midwives refer most women who develop conditions that have serious ramifications for pregnancy to physicians but take care of women who have some medical-risk factors.

Two studies examined associations between perinatal risk factors and the care provider chosen by pregnant women in Washington during 1988 and 1989. Nineteen percent of pregnancies in the state during the study period were included in the analyses. One study focused on risk factors recorded in the prenatal records of clients of stratified random samples of urban and rural obstetricians (ob-gyns), urban and rural family physicians or general practitioners (FPs/GPs), and urban CNMs. The majority of the women (57 percent) had at least one risk factor. Most of the differences in risk status among the five groups of women were due to socioeconomic status. Women with private insurance and no risk factors were most likely to seek care from an urban ob-gyn. Rural women and those who were poor and young were most likely to seek care from an FP or GP. Overall, the clients of urban CNMs had an intermediate level of risk (Dobie *et al.*, 1994).

The other study from Washington examined risk factors for low birth weight (a slightly different set of factors) among Medicaid-eligible women who obtained prenatal care from ob-gyns, GPs, FPs, CNMs, licensed direct-entry midwives, or a clinic in both urban and rural areas (Cawthon *et al.*, 1992). The data were used to determine what proportion of the clients of each kind of care provider had no risk factors, social risk factors only, medical risk factors only, or both social and medical risk factors. Urban women who received prenatal care from CNMs had the highest incidence of social risk factors. Rural clients of obstetricians had the highest incidence of medical risk factors. However, the differences among the groups were relatively small. Only 13 percent of the total group had no risk factors at all.

Chapter 8
Nurse Midwifery in America, 1980–1995

This chapter focuses on the development of nurse-midwifery in the United States between 1980 and 1995. It describes the laws that regulate the practice of nurse-midwif-ery, nurse-midwifery education, the systems the American College of Nurse-Midwives (ACNM) uses to ensure the quality of nurse-midwifery education and practice, how and where nurse-midwives practice, expansions in their scope of practice during this period of time, the nature of their collaboration with physicians, and circumstances that either support or create barriers to their practice.

Concerns about the country's persistently high infant mortality rate coupled with inadequate care for many high-risk pregnant women and the high cost of maternal and newborn health care led to a more widely and urgently recognized need and demand for nurse-midwives during the 1980–1995 period. By 1990 a variety of new or revised state and federal laws strength-ened support for nurse-midwifery practice throughout the country. Nevertheless, the malpractice insurance crisis constrained growth of the profession during most of the 1980s.

With implementation of an adequate and stable liability insurance program and a growing national awareness of a "maternity care crisis," there was an upsurge in the number of new nurse-midwifery educational programs during the early 1990s, including a large, national distance learning program that made it possible for students to complete an accredited nurse-midwifery education program while continuing to live and work in their own communities. The Community-based Nurse-midwifery Education Program made nurse-midwifery education accessible to hundreds of experienced nurses for whom becoming a midwife had been a long but impossible dream. The ACNM and the Department of Health and

Human Services Division of Nursing (source of most federal funds for nurse-midwifery education) continued to support certificate programs as well as those that lead to a master's degree. At the same time, nurse-midwifery educators built increasing flexibility into many programs, enabling students with a variety of educational backgrounds (e.g., college graduates who are not nurses, nurses without a bachelor's degree, nurses who already have master's degrees, CNMs with no degree) to obtain needed educational experience and credentials without wasting time and money on redundant learning or degrees. The average number of new ACNM certificates awarded each year increased by 150 percent between the last half of the 1980s and 1995.

Increased demand for CNM services resulted in gradual expansion in the scope of nurse-midwifery practice: use of new procedures, more responsibility for care of women with complicated pregnancies, and some responsibility for managing common nonreproductive health problems. Providing care to relatively high-risk women in collaboration with obstetricians in some of the nation's busiest academic and other tertiary-hospital obstetric departments had effects on nurse-midwifery: CNMs became more heavily involved in the care of women with significant obstetric complications and were under pressure to increase the number of patients they could take care of in a given period of time. They were taught and expected to use the obstetric interventions practiced in all academic obstetric departments. Most obstetricians believed these interventions were necessary to assure the health of pregnant women and their newborns and thought it would be negligent and unethical for nurse-midwives not to use them. Although nurse-midwives' philosophy about the nature of pregnancy made them less eager to use these procedures, most of the data which has since shown that these procedures are inappropriate in the care of normal women was not available at the beginning of this period. Physicians are the dominant force in hospital obstetric departments,

with authority to establish protocols that apply to everyone who works there. As CNMs were drawn into the care of more and more women with complications, some became accustomed to using some of the medical methods.

Individual nurse-midwives and nurse-midwifery services used various means to cope with the dissonance evoked by these pressures. Some adapted their practice to fit into and complement the predominant medical model. Others avoided these circumstances by joining or establishing practices that do not require them to exceed the traditional definition of midwifery. The desire to avoid routine use of medical interventions played an important role in midwives' motivation to develop free-standing birth centers as places for the practice of midwifery. Some CNMs were able to develop midwifery birth centers as separate units within larger institutions, including academic tertiary hospitals—a feat that requires inspired leadership on the part of the medical, as well as midwifery, authorities within the institution.

Nurse-midwives developed a variety of distinct practice models—practice in free-standing birth centers; high-volume services within the obstetric departments of tertiary academic hospitals; in-hospital birth centers that are run by CNMs and are physically separated from (but still close to) a labor and delivery suite run by obstetricians; private group nurse-midwifery practices; small rural practices with consultation by a family physician; special services developed to meet the needs of specific populations of women; working in close collaboration with physicians in large health maintenance organizations (HMOs), and a small but persistent practice of home births. Nurse-midwives in these settings work in collaboration with medical doctors (MDs), primarily obstetrician–gynecologists, but also family physicians and pediatricians.

Two distinct kinds of MD/CNM working relationships evolved: (1) the nurse-midwifery service model, in which CNMs are responsible for the care of a caseload of women whom they have screened and determined to be eligible for midwifery care, and (2) the CNM/MD team model. Nurse-midwives made significant progress in putting the laws, rules, regulations, and policies needed to support their practice into place. Although opposition from physicians underlies most of the remaining barriers, most physician opposition arose from physicians outside of the collaborative relationship. As a result of increasing experience with CNMs during medical school and in various work settings, a growing proportion of physicians understand and respect midwifery.

The rapid transition to managed care began to threaten the stability of many long-standing nurse-midwifery services during the mid-1990s, and is constraining the rate of growth of the profession. Insecurity arising from these rapid, widespread uncharted changes and new incentives for physicians to provide care to medically indigent women created new challenges for nurse-midwifery.

Laws that Regulate the Practice of Nurse-Midwifery

Nurse-midwives practice legally in every U.S. jurisdiction. However, the laws that sanction, regulate, and restrict their practice in different states vary considerably. The laws of most states address the educational requirements, credentialing process, scope of practice, authority to dispense or prescribe medications, and the manner and degree of required collaboration with physicians. Some states also mandate continuing education or peer review, give nurse-midwives specific authority to sign birth certificates, or designate CNMs as primary-care providers (permitting managed care subscribers to engage the services of a nurse-midwife without referral by a primary-care "gatekeeper"). Many states require third-party health care payers to cover services provided by nurse-midwives, and five states and the District of Columbia prohibit hospitals from discriminating against nurse-midwives in decisions about the grant-

ing of hospital admitting privileges. A few states restrict CNMs to delivering babies in hospitals or licensed birth centers, that is, they prohibit them from attending home births.

CNMs in almost every state practice under different laws than those that affect other kinds of midwives. There are a few minor exceptions; for example, CNMs and direct-entry midwives practice under the same statute but different regulations in New Mexico, and the only lay midwife with a permit to practice in Washington, D.C., does so under the law that regulates nurse-midwives. In addition, there is one exception of considerable importance: In 1992 New York passed the first state law written with the intention of creating a legal umbrella to cover all formally educated professional midwives.

Prescription Privileges and Mandated Third-Party Payment

The ACNM published summaries of the laws affecting nurse-midwifery in every state in 1976, 1984, 1992, and 1995 (Forman & Cooper, 1976; Cohn *et al.*, 1984; Bidgood-Wilson *et al.*, 1992; Barickman *et al.*, 1992; Jenkins, 1995b). Changes have been in the direction of greater autonomy for nurse-midwives:

- The number of jurisdictions that grant prescriptive authority to CNMs increased from eighteen in 1984 to thirty-nine in 1995.
- The number of states that require private third-party health care payers to cover services provided by CNMs increased from fourteen in 1984 to thirty-one in 1995.
- Federal law requires all state Medicaid programs to pay for care provided by nurse-midwives.

New Legislative Issues

With prescription privileges and mandatory third-party payment in place for most nurse-midwives, the ACNM turned its attention to prohibiting discrimination against CNMs who apply for independent hospital privileges, obtaining legal authority to prescribe controlled substances (a category that includes the most effective pain-killing medications), and establishing the legal basis for independent practice by replacing "supervision" or "direction" with references to "consultation, collaboration, and referral" in legal descriptions of the required relationship between a CNM and a physician (Jenkins, 1995a; Bidgood-Wilson, 1992).

During 1994 and the first half of 1995 several jurisdictions changed their laws to recognize the independence of nurse-midwifery practice. Most of the new laws utilize concepts expressed in ACNM documents that define nurse-midwifery as "the independent management of women's health care, focusing particularly on pregnancy, childbirth, the postpartum period, care of the newborn, and the family planning and gynecological needs of women" and state that the nurse-midwife "practices within a health care system that provides for consultation, collaborative management or referral as indicated by the health status of the client" (ACNM, 1993). Some states adopted the exact wording of the ACNM standards or incorporated the standards by referencing them in the law. Independent practice laws make it clear that nurse-midwifery practice is authorized by the nurse-midwife's license and does not flow from the authority of a physician (Williams, 1994b).

As of June 1995, nine states had enacted "any willing provider" laws to require managed care organizations to include any licensed nurse-midwife who is willing to participate in a particular managed care plan in the list of health care providers available to people enrolled in the plan (Jenkins, 1995b). Washington State's new law requires managed care organizations to offer the services of at least some individuals from every category of qualified health providers. Although this approach is less inclusive, it should guarantee access to midwifery for women enrolled in managed care.

What Boards Regulate Nurse-Midwifery Practice?

As of June 1995, nurse-midwifery was regulated by the board of nursing in thirty-six states and the District of Columbia; nurse-midwives in most of those jurisdictions practice under the rules and regulations that apply to nurse practitioners. CNMs in the other states were regulated by the board of medicine (two states), the board of nursing *and* the board of medicine (five states), the department of public health (five states), a special "Registered Nurse Certified Nurse-Midwifery Board" (Utah), and a Board of Midwifery (New York) (Jenkins, 1995b).

Legal Requirements for ACNM Certification

Eighteen states and the District of Columbia require certification by the ACNM or ACC (ACNM Certification Council) for licensure to practice as a nurse-midwife. Six states recognize ACNM/ACC certification as meeting the state's requirements but do not exclude the possibility of another certifying entity; 21 states require certification but do not specify a particular certifying agency and accept ACNM/ACC certification. Five states do not require any kind of national certification for authorization to practice as a nurse-midwife (Jenkins, 1995b).

Mandated Master's or Bachelor's Degrees

Although most CNMs have master's degrees, usually in nursing, some ACNM-accredited education programs are based in institutions that do not grant degrees. In 1992 the American Nurses' Association, National Council of State Boards of Nursing, and American Association of Colleges of Nursing recommended that each state require CNMs, nurse-anesthetists, nurse practitioners, and clinical nurse-specialists to be licensed as "advanced practice registered nurses" (APRNs) and that APRN licenses require a master of science degree in nursing or a related field. Since then these organizations have lobbied to implement this concept in every state. The ACNM uses other, very effective means to ensure the competence of nurse-midwives and does not require any kind of academic degree.* The organization that represents nurse anesthetists also resisted the master's degree mandate at first, but then fell into line, leaving the ACNM and the Association of Nurse Practitioners in Reproductive Health the only opponents among the organizations that represent the targeted groups (Rooks & Carr, 1995). Oregon was the only state that required all nurse-midwives to have master's degrees in nursing in 1989. By June 1995 four other states had enacted laws that will require master's degrees at some time in the future—not until July 1, 2008, in the case of Colorado. In addition, three states require a bachelor's of science degree in nursing. Two states that do not require degrees for licensure require MSNs for prescriptive privileges (Jenkins, 1995b).

Defining Episiotomies as Surgery and Thus as the Practice of Medicine

Controversy about episiotomies arose in California and Washington during 1995. An opinion by the attorney general for California states that nurse-midwives may not perform episiotomies as a "standardized procedure" because the California Nursing Practice Act specifies that "a nurse-midwife is not authorized to practice medicine and surgery" and episiotomies are surgical procedures (Church, 1995). The California Board of Registered Nursing allows CNMs to perform episiotomies because the procedure is within the scope of practice of a nurse-midwife based on common practice and because the Nursing

---

*In 1996 the ACNM Division of Accreditation amended the criteria for accreditation of nurse-midwifery education programs. As of June 1999 all accredited programs must either require a baccalaureate degree for entrance or grant no less than a bachelor's degree on completion of the program (Burst, 1996). Information on the circumstances leading up to this decision is provided later in this chapter.

Practice Act requires nurse-midwives to have completed an education program that prepares them to cut episiotomies and repair both episiotomies and lacerations as needed. As of November 1995, the issue had not been resolved.

The same issue arose in Washington State subsequent to an effort by ophthalmologists to prevent optometrists from using laser surgery. Legislation to define incisions as the practice of medicine was proposed but was opposed by nurse practitioners and others and was not passed.

New York's New Midwifery Law

The governor of New York signed a new Professional Midwifery Practice Act into law in July 1992. The act defines midwifery as a profession with a specific scope of practice and calls for a Board of Midwifery to regulate the profession. The board must include two obstetrician–gynecologists, a family physician, a pediatrician, an at-large member, and at least seven midwives who represent a broad range of midwifery practice and education. The board functions as part of the New York State Education Department. Although passage of the law was seen as a victory for direct-entry midwifery, no direct-entry midwives were appointed to the board, in part because the law requires midwives appointed to the board to be licensed and CNMs were the only midwives licensed by the state of New York when the board was appointed. The board met for the first time in February 1994. The law and its implementing rules and regulations became effective in February 1995.

Licensure as a professional midwife in New York requires (1) completion of a midwifery education program that has been registered by the New York State Education Department (NYSED) or that has been determined to be equivalent to a program registered by the NYSED and (2) passing a professional licensing examination that is acceptable to the NYSED. Although *the law does not require an academic degree, the reg-*

ulations state that the midwifery education program must lead to a bachelor's or higher degree. Other standards written into the regulations are similar to those of the ACNM, and the state plans to use the ACNM Certification Council examination. CNMs with current permits to practice in New York were grandfathered into the new law.*

The new law gives licensed direct-entry midwives essentially the same scope of practice as a CNM: management of normal pregnancies and childbirth; primary, preventive reproductive health care of essentially healthy women; and evaluation, resuscitation, and referral of infants for other care as needed. Licensed midwives who have completed an appropriate pharmacology course may prescribe and administer certain drugs, immunizing agents, and diagnostic tests and devices and can order laboratory tests. Licensed midwives must work with a consultant physician who practices obstetrics or work in an institution that provides obstetric care and has a physician on its staff. The law places no limitations on the place of birth.†

Nurse-Midwifery Education

The Role of the ACNM Core Competencies

The ACNM's statement of *Core Competencies for Basic Nurse-Midwifery Practice* delineates the fundamental knowledge, skills, and behaviors expected of a nurse-midwife at entrance into practice. The core competencies statement guides the curricula of nurse-midwifery education programs, the process for assessing and accrediting nurse-midwifery education programs, and development of the national nurse-midwifery certification examination. In addition, the core competencies statement serves to inform all interested parties (e.g., clients, colleagues, employers) of the competencies that can be expected of every CNM. By focusing on the core competencies, nurse-midwifery education programs that are in diverse institutional settings and grant different degrees (or no degree at all) produce graduates with the same basic scope and level of clinical ability.

The 1979 article in which the ACNM Education Committee presented the original core competencies stated that "creativity, individuality, and experimentation in nurse-midwifery education are essential to the vitality of the profession" and encouraged educational programs to be innovative in developing the means to help students achieve the core competencies (ACNM Education Committee, 1979). Whether in response to changing circumstances or that encouragement, the 1980s and early 1990s were a period of introspection, concern, innovation, growth, and change in nurse-midwifery education.

Nurse-Midwifery Education During the Early 1980s

In 1980 there were twenty-one accredited basic nurse-midwifery educational programs, three programs seeking accreditation, and two precertification programs; the latter prepare and qualify nurse-midwives trained in other countries to take the ACNM national certification examination‡ and assist CNMs who have been inactive to update their knowledge and skills. Most of the basic programs were either certificate or master's degree programs. Certificate programs took nine to eighteen months to complete, accepted nurses without a college degree, and

---

*CNMs in New York previously practiced with registered nurse (RN) licenses and a "permit to practice" under a clause in the public health code.

†This law has had severe effects on direct-entry midwives who were already practicing in New York State. See Chapter 9 for further information.

‡Programs to prepare foreign-trained nurse-midwives to take the ACNM examination have been relatively important: 13 percent of nurse-midwives who were in clinical practice in 1976–1977 had received their original midwifery education in another country, as had 9 percent of those in practice in 1982 (Rooks *et al.*, 1978; Adams, 1984).

gave a certificate in nurse-midwifery. Master's degree programs usually took two academic or calendar years to complete, required a bachelor's of science in nursing (BSN) degree as a prerequisite to enrollment, and awarded a master's of science in nursing (MSN) or master's in nursing (MN) degree on completion of the program. There were only three significant exceptions:

- The Yale University School of Nursing offered a three-year program by which college graduates who were not nurses could become prepared and licensed as RNs, qualify to take the ACNM national certification examination, and earn a MSN degree.
- A two-year program at Johns Hopkins University School of Hygiene and Public Health combined a one-year master's of public health curriculum with education and clinical training that qualified the student to take the ACNM examination.
- Education Program Associates opened the nation's first distance learning nurse-midwifery education program in 1980. It was a demonstration project designed to provide midwifery education to family nurse practitioners (FNPs) and primary care physician assistants (PAs) employed in publicly funded clinics in medically underserved areas of California. A joint project of the Stanford University Medical Center and a nearby community college, it broke new ground by allowing students to study part time while continuing to live and work in their own communities, giving students experience in out-of-hospital births as well as hospital deliveries, basing midwifery education on the knowledge and skills of experienced FNPs and PAs, and allowing students to complete the program quickly by not having to take courses for which they could demonstrate previously acquired mastery of the objectives (Stark *et al.*, 1984).

The decade opened with publication of the first American nurse-midwifery textbook (Varney, 1980). This was an important step, because the book gathered, examined, and shared the profession's body of knowledge for the first time. The first revision was published in 1987, the third edition in 1996.

Identifying Problems and Setting Goals
In 1982 the Maternity Center Association (MCA) celebrated a half-century of nurse-midwifery education in the United States by convening a seminar to consider the current conditions and future of nurse-midwifery education. During the seminar, Kitty Ernst, a past-president of the ACNM who was then director of the National Association of Childbearing Centers, identified as two of the most important problems the limited availability of clinical experience for students and the siting of most nurse-midwifery educational programs in medical centers that specialize in the care of high-risk women and babies (Ernst, 1982).

Student recruiting and the inefficiencies of nurse-midwifery education were also important problems. Although the number of nurse-midwifery educational programs increased during the 1980s, the number of applicants declined dramatically between 1984 and 1986, when seventeen programs reported reductions of 6 to 70 percent. The reasons seemed to arise from the malpractice insurance crisis, increasing costs and reduced government support of nurse-midwifery education, and expanding opportunities for intelligent, well-qualified women to enter a wider variety of fields (Raisler, 1987). Nine percent of places in nurse-midwifery educational programs went unfilled in 1990 (Rooks *et al.*, 1991), when there were, on average, fewer than eight new graduates per nurse-midwifery program. The profession could not play a major role in solving the nation's maternity-care problems with such limited capacity to produce CNMs. In 1991 the ACNM established a task force to identify barriers to increasing the number of nurse-midwives. In 1992, the ACNM set a goal of educating enough nurse-midwives to have 10,000 in practice by 2001 and created a commission to design a strategy to achieve the goal.

Innovations in nurse-midwifery education during the 1980s aimed at solving the problems identified by Ernst and making nurse-midwifery education more efficient and more accessible to nurses who want to become nurse-midwives. Nurse-midwifery educators also focused on clinical education itself, especially the critical role of the clinical preceptor, and devoted increasing energy to research, recognizing the need to further develop the professional body of knowledge.

Expansion of Clinical Learning Sites

The development of quantitatively and qualitatively adequate clinical learning sites presents a major challenge and the greatest ongoing constraint to any effort to produce significant numbers of competent midwives. Given permission and cooperation, most nursing and medical schools could use patients receiving care in most of the nation's hospitals and clinics to provide useful student learning experiences. Arranging appropriate clinical practice for midwifery students is much more difficult in a country where midwifery is still an "alternative" to standard care. Midwifery students need a sufficient volume of patients, opportunity to provide care to some women throughout the maternity cycle, experienced midwifery role models, and a clinical learning environment where the role they are trying to learn is practiced and accepted (Beebe, 1980).

For almost fifty years, the first step in developing a nurse-midwifery education program was to develop a nurse-midwifery service; almost invariably, the service was based in a hospital or health care system dedicated to care of the poor. These settings had many advantages for students, including high numbers of patients and opportunities to see and have experience with serious obstetric complications. In addition, working with poor women challenged nurse-midwifery faculty and students—indeed, the profession as a whole—to find more effective ways to intervene in some of the nation's most constant and, in the long run, most serious maternal health care problems. But there are also disadvantages, if these are the only clinical opportunities available to students. Midwifery students benefit from experience with clients from a variety of social, economic, and educational backgrounds, and many students wanted to have at least some involvement in out-of-hospital births. In addition, there was simply a need for more clinical learning sites in order to produce more CNMs.

Solutions included further development of some of the innovations that had been started during the last half of the 1970s—developing private nurse-midwifery practices run by the faculty of a nurse-midwifery education program, placing students in private nurse-midwifery practices and services that are not otherwise associated with the education program, and experimenting with distance learning. In 1980 the director of nurse-midwifery at the University of Pennsylvania School of Nursing made an important contribution by publishing a thoughtful article on selection and maintenance of clinical experience sites for nurse-midwifery educational programs (Beebe, 1987). She discussed her expectations of all parties involved in the use of a clinical learning site that is distant from the home institution, that is, the on-site CNM who accepts responsibility as a member of the clinical faculty, the university-based program that uses an off-campus clinical site, and the student who is obtaining clinical learning experience at a distant location.

Focus on the Role and Skill of the Educator

Those who teach any clinical practice should be both proficient in practice and able to teach. From their inception, nurse-midwifery education programs have been affiliated with some of the nation's leading universities, giving nurse-midwifery educators access to theories and methods of teaching and learning. They have been influenced by Knowles' theories and work on how adults learn; Schön's work on how professionals can become increasingly competent, even "artistic" in their practice by observing and reflecting on their actions; Benner's work on how nurses learn from experience, evolving from novice to expert; and research on how women judge and assimilate knowledge (Knowles, 1980; Schön, 1987; Benner, 1984; Belenky *et al.*, 1986). The original work in the training of clinical perceptors was spurred by needs arising from the use of off-campus clinical learning sites by university-based programs, with the first work done at the University of Pennsylvania. Development of an entire nurse-midwifery educational program based on distance learning (by EPA in 1980) made the need to train clinical preceptors ever more clear.

The First Distance Learning
Program for Nurse-Midwives
Unlike programs that developed off-campus clinical sites as an extension of an on-campus program, the Education Program Associates (EPA) program was designed explicitly for distance learning. It began as a two-phase program, with the first phase focused on ambulatory care. Eighty hours of didactic training were packed into five intensive two-day sessions at Stanford University Medical Center. Students used modular curricular packages (learning objectives, required reading, and instructions for written assignments) to study at home between those sessions. Phase 1 ended with a sixteen-week preceptorship with a physician, during which a CNM from the EPA faculty provided at least twenty-four hours of direct clinical instruction and evaluation. Additional on-site teaching or an intensive clinical preceptorship with a CNM or another physician was organized for individual students as needed (Stark *et al.*, 1984). The second phase focused on childbirth and care of the newborn and followed a similar pattern of learning

activities: a series of intensive didactic sessions, modular written assignments to be completed at home, and a preceptorship under the supervision of a CNM. Students had intrapartum (i.e., labor and delivery) experience in out of hospital settings, as well as in hospitals, and took care of high- and low-risk pregnant women.

In 1987 EPA severed its affiliation with Stanford Medical Center and moved to San Jose, where it became affiliated with the San Jose State University School of Nursing. As a result, EPA students can earn upper division academic credit for their midwifery courses. The program consists of a three-phase sequence: Common Adult Health Problems, Ambulatory Women's Health Care, and Intrapartum, Postpartum and Newborn Management. Students who enter the midwifery program as a family nurse practitioner, obstetric–gynecologic nurse practitioner, physician assistant, or foreign-trained midwife can skip either or both of the first two modules by passing a written examination, demonstrating clinical proficiency, and completing selected written assignments. The faculty screen clinical preceptors and orient them to the program and their responsibilities for student learning.

The EPA program is accredited by the ACNM; its nurse practitioner graduates are qualified to take the ACNM's national certification examination. PAs who complete the program receive continuing education units from the American Academy of Physician Assistants and can apply for a license to practice midwifery in California under the supervision of a physician (Stark *et al.*, 1984).

Distance Learning for Nurses
Throughout the Nation
In 1989 the Frontier School of Midwifery and Family Nursing (associated with the Frontier Nursing Service in Hyden, Kentucky) expanded the distance learning concept into a national program. The Community-based Nurse-midwifery Program (CNEP) was developed in response to the need to prepare more

nurse-midwives, to prepare nurse-midwives for practice in birth centers, and to make it easier for nurses living in small towns and rural areas to become nurse-midwives. It tapped into a deep reservoir of experienced obstetric nurses who want to become midwives but could not because of where they live.

Students must be nurses who are college graduates (not necessarily in nursing) with average grades of B or higher and high scores on the Graduate Record Examination (GRE). Each applicant must have identified a CNM in active, full-scope practice who agrees to serve as her preceptor and provide her primary clinical learning site. A student can complete the course while living at home if her clinical site is close; many work part time during at least the first half of the program. Self-contained self-instructional course modules are used to deliver most of the didactic content of the curriculum. Faculty who live throughout the United States design and continually update the courses and read and grade students' worksheets, papers, and tests. The distance learning structure allows the program to use a wide spectrum of nurse-midwives as teachers—experienced clinicians practicing in a variety of settings, educators who are nationally recognized experts in particular areas, and leaders of the profession. In early 1996, CNEP had at least one student in every state in the nation.

The program starts with a three-day orientation during which members of the incoming class go to Kentucky where they meet each other, meet key members of the faculty, learn more about the program and how to succeed as self-directed learners who are physically separate from their teachers and classmates, and are introduced to the first set of courses by the faculty members who design and teach each course. Levels I and II are home-study courses. Level III is a two-week intensive workshop during which small groups of students and faculty come together for seminars and clinical skills training. Level IV is an extended practicum

with clinical teaching provided by each student's own preceptor(s). CNEP regional clinical coordinators (RCCs) provide each student and preceptor with oversight and support of the student's clinical learning experience. Each RCC is an experienced nurse-midwife who is in active clinical practice in her region.

CNEP uses many methods to overcome the barrier of distance, including two periods of intense, face-to-face interaction with students, telephone communication (faculty maintain telephone "office hours"), copious responsive notes on students' written products, and an electronic bulletin board by which students and faculty communicate with and transmit documents to all other members of the school community using personal computers located in their homes. Teaching methods include case studies, information searches, and journal writing; videos and recorded tapes augment other forms of communication. The program is developing interactive forms of computer-assisted learning. Students and their preceptors gather in regional groups for "case-presentation days" during which they discuss nurse-midwifery practice issues. Module post-tests and closed-book, proctored midterms and final examinations evaluate each student's mastery of the material.

The program intends to prepare students who will be safe, effective practitioners in any clinical setting, including out-of-hospital sites and rural areas; thus it demands very thorough clinical learning. Students are required to have twice as many clinical experiences as the minimum recommended by the ACNM, are encouraged to have clinical experience in more than one setting (e.g., a birth center and hospital), and must have experience with patients with complications as well as low-risk patients. Twenty part-time RCCs ensure that clinical sites and preceptors are appropriate for student learning and meet CNEP's criteria.

CNEP began formal training of students' clinical preceptors in 1992. Clinical preceptors attend a two-day workshop to develop or update skills for clinical instruction of adult learners, to become oriented to CNEP, and to learn a common approach and language (to make it easier for preceptors, students, and faculty to communicate clearly about the students' progress) and a common set of pathways for dealing with problems. The conceptual framework and language are shared with students, who are recognized as the most important members of the teaching/learning team. Students are expected to take responsibility for their own learning, while the school exercises oversight and is responsible for guiding students in identifying and solving learning problems. Preceptors are paid and assume significant responsibility. While students are in the clinical practicum, usually about six to nine months, the RCCs monitor their progress through written evaluations, observations, and frequent communication with each student and her preceptor; help to identify problems; and use student learning plans and performance contracts to resolve identified problems (Treistman *et al.*, 1993). Full-time faculty oversees the Clinical Department, including arranging for new or additional sites for particular students as needed. One full-time faculty member focuses exclusively on quality assurance. The program uses a nurse-midwifery faculty practice at Johns Hopkins Hospital in Baltimore for intensive assessment and intervention for students with serious clinical difficulties.

Because their students recruit and CNEP encourages, trains, and supports the development of new clinical preceptors, lack of clinical learning sites—a previously perennial constraint on the number of students accepted by any and all nurse-midwifery programs in the country—does not limit enrollment into CNEP. Forty-two students were admitted in 1989, 44 in 1990, 92 in 1991, 112 in 1992, and approximately 150 per year during 1993, 1994, and 1995. CNEP has had more than 300 current students at all times since 1993 and has had students in

more than 450 clinical sites. Many new sites developed by CNEP and its students have also become available for use by traditional (university-based) programs in their local areas. More than seven hundred CNEP preceptors, as well as faculty from many other programs have attended CNEP's Preceptor Training Workshop. Thus the profession's overall capacity to prepare nurse-midwives has been enhanced by breaking down institutional and geographic barriers to involve a much larger proportion of practitioners in nurse-midwifery education. Bringing this wide variety of practitioners into the educational process also makes the process richer and more closely attuned to the realities of the field. Since 1993 the federal Bureau of Primary Health Care has provided three rural health outreach grants to support CNEP's efforts to make rural practices available for clinical education of nurse-midwifery students and to develop technology to increase access to education for rural midwifery students and CNMs. As of 1995, 25 percent of CNEP students lived in and 35 percent of CNEP graduates worked in rural areas.

CNEP acquires its required academic affiliation through a relationship with the Frances Payne Bolton School of Nursing at Case Western Reserve University (CWRU) in Cleveland. All CNEP courses meet criteria for graduate-level credit applicable to either a master's or doctoral degree in nursing at Case Western. All CNEP students are eligible to enroll in a program that leads to a master of science degree in nursing. Additional work to earn the master's degree includes two intensive on-campus courses (one that requires one week on campus, one that requires ten days), assignments that can be completed at home, and participation in a nursing research project. All students who complete CNEP receive a certificate in nurse-midwifery from the Frontier School of Midwifery and Family Nursing. The master's degree is separate, optional, requires additional tuition, and is granted by Case Western Reserve University.

In 1995 CNEP and the Frances Payne Bolton School of Nursing initiated a distance learning program to enable nurses who are not college graduates to enroll in CNEP. Nurses who have associate degrees can earn a bachelor of science in nursing (BSN) in one calendar year by taking two intensive courses (two weeks each) at the CWRU campus in Cleveland and completing other courses at home using distance learning methods. Students seek provisional acceptance into CNEP when applying for the BSN completion program. CNEP received more than one hundred telephone inquiries about the new program during the first month after it was announced, most from experienced nurses who were working in women's health care and lived in small towns and rural areas. Two-year community college programs offering an associate degree constitute the largest educational route to practice as a registered nurse in the United States.

Increasing Numbers of Educational Programs, Students, and Graduates

Although the number of basic nurse-midwifery educational programs increased from twenty-one in 1980 to twenty-eight in 1984, the yearly output of newly certified nurse-midwives remained relatively stable from 1980 through 1984. In 1984 the number of applicants to nurse-midwifery programs began to decline. As a result, the number of new nurse-midwifery certificates* awarded each year dropped from an average of 243 per year during 1980–1984, to 201 per year during the last half of the 1980s. Alarm about inadequate access to maternity care during the late 1980s drew attention to the slow production of nurse-midwives and motivated rapid development of new programs. Thirty-five accredited or preaccredited[†] nurse-midwifery education programs (thirty-four basic and one precertification[‡] program) were in operation in 1993. Forty-seven programs (forty-four basic and three precertification) were in operation as of March, 1996 (Slattery & Burst, 1996). Fifty programs were in operation by the end of 1996 (Patamia, 1996). The average number of new ACNM certificates awarded each year increased from 201 per year during 1985–1989 to 258 per year during 1990–1992, and 417 per year in 1993–1994. The largest number of new certificates (506) were awarded in 1995. The ACC expected to certify somewhat fewer new CNMs in 1996, probably about 400.

Unlike the medical specialties, which control the number of approved residencies, the ACNM controls the quality but not the quantity of nurse-midwifery programs. Most CNM programs are developed in response to local needs for midwives or a specific institution's desire to expand into an increasingly popular field. Demand for nurses is declining, and many nursing schools are shifting their attention to training nurse practitioners, which is the growth industry of nursing; nurse-midwifery is the highest profile component of this trend. The number of positions in nurse-midwifery education programs results from the sum of local decisions rather than a centralized analysis of current and long-term national need. However, it seems clear that nurse-midwifery educators responded to the

---

*The term *certificate* is used in two very different ways, which can be confusing. Nurse-midwifery education programs that do not grant academic degrees have traditionally been referred to as "certificate" programs; students earn a certificate from the school, instead of a degree. Graduates of both degree and certificate nurse-midwifery education programs become "certified nurse-midwives' or CNMs based on meeting criteria that include passing the national nurse-midwifery "certification" examination.

†Preaccreditation status is the designation for an education program that intends to initiate a nurse-midwifery curriculum and has been found to meet the ACNM Division of Accreditation criteria based on an evaluation conducted before any students are admitted.

‡Precertification programs are primarily intended to prepare and qualify nurse-midwives who received their midwifery education in another country to take the ACNM Certification Council examination in order to become certified.

ACNM's goal of educating enough CNMs to have 10,000 in practice by 2001.

The Controversy Regarding Mandatory Degrees

The ACC has not required candidates for the national certifying examination to have a university degree. The ACNM Division of Accreditation criteria require all nurse-midwifery education programs to be affiliated with an institution of higher education; however, the programs are based in a wide variety of degree- and nondegree-granting institutions. Of forty-four basic programs in operation in March 1996, thirty-one programs (70 percent) were operated by a university-based school, college, division or department of nursing. Thirty percent were in other kinds of institutions: two were operated by a college or school of medicine, four by a hospital or medical center, three by a college of allied health sciences or health-related professions, two by a private nonprofit educational program or school, and one by a school of public health; one is a joint undertaking by the nursing school in one university in Texas and the medical school in another (Slattery & Burst, 1996; Routledge, 1997). The ACNM's openness to this variety contradicts the American Nurses' Association (ANA) long-standing position that all nurse practitioners should have master's degrees in nursing, and the 1992 recommendation by the ANA, the National Council of State Boards of Nursing (NCSBN), and the American Association of Colleges of Nursing that state laws should require master's degrees for licensure of all advanced practice registered nurses (APRNs), including CNMs.

Early nurse-midwifery leaders were highly educated women who believed that midwifery education should be based in universities. When that objective conflicted with the need to recruit students from areas with a particular need for midwives, they developed alternative means to ensure the quality of the education of nurse-midwives. But as the general level of education among Americans has increased, nurse-midwives have been under pressure to require master's degrees for entry into their profession. By the end of 1995, all but nine nurse-midwifery education programs led to a master's degree. Five of the nine required or planned to require a baccalaureate degree for admission, and one gave preference to applicants with bachelor's degrees (Burst, 1996).

During the mid-1990s, this issue was made more complex by the ACNM's decision to establish educational and certification standards for direct-entry midwives.* In 1994 the ACNM Division of Accreditation (DOA) published criteria for accreditation of basic *direct-entry* midwifery programs, *including a requirement that midwifery education be part of "a program of professional studies which culminates in no less than a baccalaureate degree."* This criteria brought criticism from within the profession because it put the ACNM in the position of requiring an academic degree for professional direct-entry midwives while not requiring a degree for certification of nurse-midwives (Rooks & Carr, 1995). The DOA did not perceive this to be an unfair discrepancy because it considered the nursing education and experience required for entrance into a nurse-midwifery education program equivalent to requiring a bachelor's degree for direct-entry midwives. Other reasons for the decision included the DOA's commitment to not devalue the three years of academic work required for preparation as a direct-entry midwife, recognition "that increased education yields increased professionalism which equals increased ability to compete, and survive, in today's health care system," and the common-sense conclusion "that the provision of primary health care to women requires more, not less, education" (Burst, 1995). In 1996 the DOA amended the criteria for accreditation of nurse-midwifery education programs to apply the same

---

*See Chapter 9 for information on the history leading up to this decision.

criteria to nurse-midwifery programs. As of June 1999, all accredited nurse-midwifery programs must either require a baccalaureate degree for entrance or grant no less than a bachelor's degree on completion of the program (Burst, 1996).

The ACNM's long support for nondegree ("certificate") programs was based on the need to keep the profession open to a wide range of nurses and to avoid unnecessary barriers and expense for qualified RN applicants. Although the proportion of nurses with BSNs is growing (from 23 percent of the RN workforce in 1980 to 30 percent in 1989, and 42 percent in 1996), the majority of nurses (58 percent in 1996) were prepared in diploma or two-year associate-degree programs (Division of Nursing, 1997). The proportion of newly registered nurses who obtained their basic nursing education through a four-year university or college program hovered at about 30 percent throughout the period between 1980 and 1994. Although the proportion graduating from nondegree hospital-based programs is declining (from 19.2 percent of 1980 graduates to 7.5 percent of 1994 graduates), the shift is to associate degree programs based in community colleges, which produced 48 percent of new graduates in 1980 and 62 percent of new graduates in 1994 (National League for Nursing, 1995). The characteristics needed to excel in midwifery are not exclusive to nurses with college degrees. There is a particular need to recruit into nurse-midwifery nurses who would like to live and practice in rural communities. Nurses with a rural background may be even less likely than others to obtain their basic nursing education in a four-year college.

The ACNM's core competencies and accreditation process undergird the quality of all nurse-midwifery educational programs, regardless of the degree. Although the research orientation of master's degree programs provides important benefits, there is no evidence that nurse-midwives with master's degrees provide safer, more effective, or more satisfying care to women. Nor are CNMs with master's degrees more likely than certificate program graduates to pass the national nurse-midwifery certification examination. A 1995 study of factors associated with higher scores on the national certification examination found that graduates of certificate nurse-midwifery education programs had a higher average score on the test than graduates of master's degree programs (Fullerton & Severino, 1995). In addition, a 1985 study of factors affecting the level of success experienced by individual CNMs found no association between type of nurse-midwifery education and the level of professional success (Haas & Rooks, 1986). Nevertheless, the percentage of nurse-midwives with master's degrees is high; 67 to 70 percent of nurse-midwives who responded to surveys conducted by the ACNM between 1990 and 1993 had graduate degrees, including 4 or 5 percent who had doctorates.

Flexible Programs That Accept Students with a Variety of Backgrounds

During the past 15 years, many nurse-midwifery education programs developed special tracks to accommodate the needs of students with different educational backgrounds and objectives. Three of the forty-seven nurse-midwifery education programs that were accredited or had received preaccreditation status from the ACNM Division of Accreditation as of March 1996 were precertification programs that prepare and qualify nurse-midwives who received their basic midwifery education in a foreign country to take the ACC examination in order to become CNMs.

Only four of the forty-four basic nurse-midwifery education programs in operation in early 1996 offered only one option or "track": Three accepted only nurses with bachelor's degrees and offered programs that combined nurse-midwifery education with work leading to a master's degree in nursing (two programs) or a master's degree in public health (one program). One accepted RNs without college degrees and offered a program that culminated in a nurse-midwifery certificate. All of the other programs offered at least two, and in some cases as many as five different tracks to meet the needs of students who enter with different educational backgrounds and want to earn different kinds and levels of degrees. The most common track provides nurse-midwifery education and a master's degree in nursing (MSN) to students who have BSNs when they enter the program; some accept nurses without BSNs, so long as they have a bachelor's degree in something. A common (and shorter and less expensive) track provides nurse-midwifery education to nurses who already have MSN degrees. A few programs make it possible for RNs with diplomas or associate degrees (ADs) to obtain nurse-midwifery education while earning a BSN. A few programs accept students who have college degrees but are not nurses; on completion of the program, they receive an MSN degree and are qualified to take the ACC examination. A few programs offer nurse-midwifery education to students who are already prepared as nurse-practitioners. Students completing these programs may earn a diploma in nurse-midwifery, a BSN, an MSN, an MA or MN (master in nursing) degree, a master in public health (MPH) degree, and, in a few cases, a nursing doctorate or a PhD in nursing (Slattery & Burst, 1996). In addition, a program that opened in 1996 hopes to eventually offer a master of science in midwifery (MSM) degree (Carr, 1996).

Financial Support of Nurse-Midwifery Education

The federal government has been an important source of financial support for nurse-midwifery education. Federal support comes from two components of the U. S. Public Health Service: the Maternal and Child Health Bureau,* which has funded

nurse-midwifery education programs since 1960, and the Division of Nursing,[†] which began to support nurse-midwifery education in 1972.

The Maternal and Child Health Bureau (MCHB) supports relatively few programs, targeting its resources at preparation of nurse-midwives who will teach, run programs, be advocates, and contribute to the development of public policy. The purpose is leadership, not increasing the number of practitioners; the funds go only to programs that give master's or higher degrees. MCHB has given grants to nurse-midwifery programs at Columbia University, Emory University, Georgetown University, the University of Illinois, Johns Hopkins University, the University of Pennsylvania, and Yale University. The number of programs supported by MCHB declined during the 1980s and early 1990s. Of $1.26 million awarded by the MCHB for nursing projects to be completed between July 1993 and June 1998, $500,000 (40 percent) has been allocated for grants to three nurse-midwifery programs. The amount allocated to nurse-midwifery education during 1988–1993 was approximately the same, although the total for all nursing education projects is down slightly (from $1.4 million for 1988-1993).

The Division of Nursing's support for nurse-midwifery education programs comes from an allocation dedicated to supporting programs that prepare either CNMs or nurse practitioners (NPs). The purposes are to increase and equalize access to health care and to nursing education and careers, especially for racial and ethnic minorities and other groups that have had limited access to health care. Programs that prepare nurse-midwives to serve populations in special need have been given high priority. The Division of Nursing (DN) provided more

---

*Maternal and Child Health Bureau, Health Resources and Services Administration, Public Health Service, U.S. Department of Health and Human Services.

†The Division of Nursing is part of the Bureau of Health Professions, Health Resources and Services Administration, Public Health Service, U.S. Department of Health and Human Services.

than $48 million to support nurse-midwifery education programs between 1976 and 1995. The number of nurse-midwifery programs receiving DN funds increased along with the total number of ACNM-accredited programs during the 1970s and 1980s. For example, two programs were funded in 1976, eight in 1980, thirteen in 1985, and twenty in 1990. The 30 percent increase in funds for nurse-midwife programs between 1990 and 1995 was no match for the rapid increase in the total number of programs. The proportion of funds going to nurse-midwifery programs has remained at about 25 to 30 percent for many years; 70 to 75 percent is used to support programs that train NPs.

The DN limits its funding of all other graduate nursing education to programs that lead to a master's degree in nursing. Although it has continued to support certificate programs in nurse-midwifery, there is a trend toward restricting DN support for nurse-midwifery education to "post-master's" certificate programs (for people who already have a master's or doctoral degree). The ANA and other nursing organizations want to write this limitation into the federal law that underlies the program.

In addition to program support, both the DN and the MCHB provide stipends to nurse-midwifery students. Some nurse-midwifery students also receive National Health Service Corps scholarships that require recipients on graduation to accept assignments to work in underserved areas, at the discretion of the Public Health Service. Sixty-six percent of 2,246 CNMs who participated in an ACNM survey conducted in 1987 reported that they had received federal financial assistance during their basic nurse-midwifery education (Adams, 1989).

The 1993 report of the National Commission on Nurse-Midwifery Education (established to develop a strategy for preparing 10,000 nurse-midwives by 2001) concluded that, although nurse-midwifery education was well positioned for growth, current levels of funding were inadequate to meet the needs at that time and in the future. The commission particularly identified needs for financial support to expand clinical teaching sites, increase faculty, collect data, and conduct research (National Commission on Nurse-Midwifery Education, 1993).

The combination of more nurse-midwifery programs and no increase in DN funds means that individual programs have less access to federal financial support. At the same time, many of the academic medical centers in which most nurse-midwifery programs are based are experiencing the loss of large numbers of their obstetric patients, who are being shifted into the new managed health care organizations. Either of these effects may undermine the viability of some nurse-midwifery educational programs. The combined effects of both circumstances may result in the closure, consolidation, or shrinkage of some programs.

Some states also support nurse-midwifery education, either providing funds for a program located in the state or giving scholarships that allow nurses from that state to enroll in other programs. State funds were instrumental in the initiation of new programs at Boston University, Marquette University, the University of Washington, and the State University of New York at Stony Brook during the first half of the 1990s (Patamia, 1996). State scholarship programs are usually designed to meet specific needs within the state. For instance, Texas provides scholarships that pay half of the tuition for nurses who live in rural parts of Texas and enroll in CNEP.

Quality Assurance

The ACNM has established an interwoven set of definitions and processes designed to ensure the quality of nurse-midwifery education and practice. The ACNM core competencies statement identifies the basic knowledge and skills required for safe and effective nurse-midwifery practice. The ACNM standards of practice specify the necessary behaviors. The ACNM Division of Accreditation evaluates and accredits nurse-midwifery education programs based on their ability to transmit the core competencies and meet other criteria. Eligibility to take the national certification examination requires licensure as an RN in at least one U.S. state or territory, graduation from an accredited nurse-midwifery education program, and a document signed by the program director which states that the individual has completed the nurse-midwifery component of the program satisfactorily and is capable of safe practice. The examination is designed to assess the knowledge required to provide safe care according to the ACNM core competencies and standards of practice. Other skills and abilities are assessed by the educational programs and must be documented before an individual is allowed to take the examination (Fullerton & Severino, 1995). ACNM certification requires eligibility to take the examination and passing the examination. A process has been developed by which nurse-midwives who received their midwifery education in other countries can demonstrate their competency and, if necessary, acquire additional didactic knowledge or clinical skills. Completion of this process makes them eligible to take the national certification examination (Fullerton *et al.*, 1996).

Nurse-midwives have many means to acquire continuing education, including articles published in the *Journal of Nurse-Midwifery*, workshops and educational sessions offered before and during the ACNM annual meeting, and regional workshops organized by the Continuing Education Committee. Participation in peer review has been incorporated into the *ACNM Standards for the Practice of Nurse-Midwifery*. The Peer Review Committee has developed sample documents to help structure peer review by CNMs and to provide consultation to ACNM members and chapters that are trying to develop peer review. The ACNM philosophy, code of ethics, and procedures for incorporating new elements into nurse-midwifery practice also contribute to

the organization's efforts to ensure quality in the practice of nurse-midwifery.

Until 1991 the ACNM had the capacity to suspend or revoke certification as a way to discipline a nurse-midwife who is unable or unwilling to practice according to its standards. The ACNM lost the authority to decertify nurse-midwives when it created the ACNM Certification Council and released its authority to certify nurse-midwives to the new entity. Antitrust considerations made it necessary to separate certification from the other functions of the College. The ACC does not have the authority to decertify. A nurse-midwife can be removed from practice by action of the licensing agency in her state.

Accreditation of Nurse-Midwifery Education Programs

The ACNM Division of Accreditation establishes the standards for nurse-midwifery education and accredits programs that meet those standards. The U.S. Department of Education recognizes the DOA as an accrediting agency for basic nurse-midwifery programs. The DOA also accredits programs that prepare and qualify individuals who have already completed a nurse-midwifery educational program in another country to take the national certification examination in order to practice as a CNM in the United States.

The accreditation process involves a periodic review conducted by the DOA and the faculty of the educational program. The DOA publishes documents that present its standards for assessing the quality of a nurse-midwifery education program, including criteria relevant to an educational program's philosophy, organization, faculty, students, curriculum, resources, and facilities. The criteria require programs to be located within or to be affiliated with an accredited institution of higher learning. The program must teach a curriculum that is designed to lead to development of the ACNM's *Core Competencies for Basic Nurse-Midwifery Practice*. An

Advisory Committee composed of members representing nursing, medicine, education, the public, and nurse-midwifery students provides input to the DOA Governing Board regarding the accreditation criteria, policies, and procedures. Following the DOA guidelines, faculty of the education program evaluate their own program in relation to the DOA criteria and their own stated objectives. They use their findings to improve the program and incorporate them into a self-evaluation report, which they submit to the DOA. Then members of the DOA Site Visitors Committee visit the program to validate, amplify, or clarify information in the faculty's self-evaluation report. The DOA Board of Review determines the accreditation status of the applicant program based on the faculty's self-evaluation and the site visitors' report (Conway-Welsh, 1986).

The DOA accredits nurse-midwifery education programs that it recognizes as carrying out the philosophy, purpose, and objectives set forth by its faculty and as having met the standards established by the profession for the preparation of competent nurse-midwives (Slattery & Burst, 1995). The assessment for accreditation cannot be conducted until the first class of students has graduated. Programs seeking DOA accreditation must submit their self-study report and application for accreditation within six months of graduating their first class. Although the accreditation process is voluntary, only graduates of ACNM-accredited programs are eligible to take the certification examination.

The DOA grants "preaccreditation" status to an educational program that intends to initiate a nurse-midwifery curriculum and has met the criteria intended to ensure the development of a high-quality program. A nurse-midwifery education programs must receive preaccreditation status before it is allowed to admit students. Preaccreditation status gives the first class of students confidence to enroll in a new program and guarantees successful students the right to take the ACC examination.

Examination and Certification of Nurse-Midwives at Entry into Practice

The early development of the national nurse-midwifery certification examination was described in Chapter 4. The ACNM first assigned responsibility for developing and administering a mechanism to measure entry-level competence to the ACNM Testing Committee. The Testing Committee became the Division of Examiners in 1974. The name was later changed to the Division of Competency Assessment. In 1991 the ACNM created the ACNM Certification Council as a separate organization that is responsible for developing and administering the examination and certifying successful candidates under agreement with the ACNM.

The first version of the national certification examination included an observation and assessment of clinical skills as well as a written test. The clinical examination was discontinued based on analysis of the results of tests conducted during 1971–1973; results from the clinical examinations mirrored those of the written tests. Consequently the Testing Committee determined that clinical tests were not necessary to determine the safety and effectiveness of the practice of a person who has passed the written test; the Testing Committee conducted no further clinical testing after 1974 (Foster, 1986). Since then the examination has been a paper-and-pencil test. The "pass/fail" break in the scores is determined for each new form of the examination based on the advice of experienced test readers (each a knowledgeable CNM) that tests with scores above the breakpoint reflect knowledge and judgments associated with safe and effective practice while tests with scores below the breakpoint reflect misinformation suggestive of hazardous or ineffective practices (Holley & Cameron, 1978).

From 1974 to 1995 a modified essay or short-answer format was used. The examination was constructed, read, and scored in accord with a highly structured answer key that had been assessed for congruity with the contemporary medical and nursing literature (Fullerton *et al.*, 1989). The ACC began using a multiple-choice and short-answer format in 1995.

The examination derives its validity from information about the clinical activities and problems involved in actual current nurse-midwifery practice. To identify the necessary knowledge and competencies, the ACC conducts periodic analyses of the critical tasks of nurse-midwifery practice. The ACC began the 1993 task analysis by developing a preliminary list of tasks based on information in ACNM documents, nurse-midwifery education program curricula, survey reports, state agency codes and regulations, textbooks, and the list of tasks used in the previous analysis. A list of tasks considered essential for direct-entry midwives was also considered. A panel of CNM educators, service directors, and clinical experts reviewed and revised the list; tasks related to advanced, rather than entry-level practice, were eliminated. The revised list specified 189 clinical tasks that are within the scope of American nurse-midwifery practice. Data collection forms were sent to a stratified random sample of all CNM members of the ACNM, each of whom was asked to indicate how frequently she performs each task on the list and how critical it is to safe, effective practice. The information was used to determine average frequency and "criticality" scores for each task, and its overall importance. The importance index was lowest for items with low frequency and low criticality and highest for items with high frequency and high criticality. Tasks that are performed infrequently but are critical to patient well-being received high importance scores. The ACC used information from this analysis to develop a blueprint of the examination. The blueprint guides the development of test items (Fullerton, 1994).

Since 1989 the examination has been criterion referenced. "The goal of a criterion-referenced test is to discriminate between those individuals who have acquired the desired level of knowledge and those who have not. How well a particular test-taker's performance compares to others who take the same test is considered irrelevant" (Fullerton *et al.*, 1989). The exam is designed to distinguish between candidates who do or do not possess the knowledge and cognitive skills necessary for safe and effective beginning-level nurse-midwifery practice (Foster, 1986). Of 4,885 candidates who took the test for the first time between 1971 and 1995, 487 failed—a failure rate of 10 percent. The rate was consistent throughout that period. Candidates who fail may retake the test twice. Those who retake it are given a different version of the test, with completely different questions. Some who fail it once do not chose to take it again. The failure rate for those who take it a second time may be higher than 10 percent, although some information on this is missing. Only nine individuals are known to have failed the examination three times (ACNM Certification Council, 1996).

Certification of Nurse-Midwives Educated in Other Countries

Nurse-midwives who received their midwifery education in other countries have played important roles in the profession in the United States—beginning with Mary Breckinridge, founder of the first nurse-midwifery service in America, who received her midwifery training in Great Britain. The ACNM has encouraged the development and maintenance of "precertification" education programs designed specifically to meet the needs of foreign-educated nurse-midwives, who constituted 17 percent of the U.S. nurse-midwifery workforce in 1976–77 (Rooks *et al.*, 1978). Although that proportion fell to 10 percent in 1982 and has declined with the growth in American nurse-midwifery education programs and graduates (Adams, 1984), there is a strong commitment to providing opportunities for foreign-educated nurse-midwives to become certified and able to work in this country. Precertification programs provide both didactic and clinical training based on the core competencies; most take about six months to complete. They have always been limited in size and number, and there have been periods when none was in operation. Some foreign-educated nurse-midwives have had to complete a basic nurse-midwifery education program in order to become qualified to take the certification examination (Fullerton *et al.*, 1996).

In 1990 the ACNM Board of Directors appointed an ad hoc committee to explore the development of an alternative path that could be made cost effective and widely available. The committee proposed a pilot study of a partial reciprocity process, which they called the "Assured Equivalency Option" (AEO). A pilot test of the proposed plan was approved for a maximum of thirty-six individuals—estimated to be enough to determine the applicability and success of the process (Fullerton *et al.*, 1996).

The AEO process was designed to assess the knowledge and clinical competency of an individual foreign-educated nurse-midwife and to provide the didactic and clinical education needed to bring her knowledge and skills into equivalency with graduates of ACNM-accredited basic nurse-midwifery education programs. The AEO process is available to foreign-trained nurse-midwives who have practiced nurse-midwifery for at least two years within the ten years prior to application and who have had at least one year's experience working as a registered nurse in the United States. Applicants must document their nursing and midwifery education and experience and their English-language competency, provide letters of reference, and be interviewed. Those accepted into the AEO program must complete courses in well-women gynecology and family planning, physical assessment, and pharmacology. They are also advised to take a course in professional issues affecting nurse-midwifery in this country. Several basic nurse-midwifery education programs make these courses available to AEO candidates. The

next step is to take the AEO qualifying examination; those who pass the examination may begin a clinical nurse-midwifery practicum. The purpose of the practicum is to demonstrate and validate the clinical competency of the candidate and familiarize her with the realitites of nurse-midwifery practice in the United States. When the CNM who serves as her primary clinical preceptor can document that the candidate performs as a safe beginning-level nurse-midwife and has signed a statement to that effect, the candidate is eligible to take the national certification examination (Fullerton *et al.*, 1996).

As of March 1996, seventeen individuals had completed the pilot program. Fifteen of them had been certified and were practicing as CNMs. It was anticipated that all individuals admitted to the program would complete it by the end of 1996. Continuation of the option will depend on the results of a program evaluation conducted by the ACNM Division of Research. As many as 10,000 foreign-educated nurse-midwives may be living in the United States (Fullerton *et al.*, 1996).

Incorporating New Procedures into Nurse-Midwifery Practice

In 1992 the ACNM issued a statement on expansion of nurse-midwifery practice and skills beyond the basic core competencies and published a six-step process to guide a nurse-midwife who is considering expanding her practice to include a new procedure. The 1992 document was actually an update of a procedure in effect since 1972. As early as 1970, the ACNM Clinical Practice Committee had begun to focus on the need for guidelines to aid in the assessment of possible extensions of nurse-midwifery practice. Realizing that practice would be constantly evolving, the committee rejected the "laundry list" of procedures approach in favor of a process that would allow nurse-midwives to use their own judgment, in their own settings, to determine what is safe and appropriate (Summers, 1992). The 1992 statement noted that advances in science and technology create changes in health care that require some nurse-midwives to possess knowledge and skills beyond the basic core competencies and that some CNMs need or want to specialize in particular areas of practice. "In order to assure that new technical skills remain within the scope and safety of nurse-midwifery practice, the ACNM requires that the incorporation of these skills be accomplished in accordance with the current *ACNM Standards for the Practice of Nurse-Midwifery* and *Guidelines for Incorporation of New Procedures into Nurse-Midwifery Practice,* including proper documentation of the process of incorporating new technical skills" (ACNM, 1992b).

The 1992 ACNM *Guidelines for Incorporation of New Procedures into Nurse-Midwifery Practice* call for the following steps: (1) Identify the need for the new procedure, taking consumer demand, safety, institutional requests, and the availability of other personnel to perform the procedure into consideration. (2) Gather and examine relevant laws and other documents (e.g., regulations, institutional bylaws, legal opinions) that would constrain or support performance of the procedure by a CNM. (3) Evaluate the procedure as a nurse-midwifery function by examining the relevant literature regarding risks and benefits, whether the procedure is being performed by other CNMs, and the need to manage any complications that might result from use of the procedure. (4) Develop a process to educate nurse-midwives to perform the procedure. (5) Plan a method to evaluate the effects of nurse-midwives' performance of the procedure. (6) Notify the ACNM Clinical Practice Committee after completion of the process (ACNM, 1992).

Peer Review

In 1985 the ACNM mandated all practicing CNMs to participate in peer review. An ACNM *Guide to Quality Assurance/Peer Review* was first produced in 1984; it was revised in 1994. Many ACNM chapters (state or local units of the organization) operate peer review programs. Several chapters have published reports of their approach to peer review (Thompson, 1986; Stein, 1996). The ACNM gives one continuing education unit (CEU) for participation as a peer reviewer. Participating in peer review is a learning experience for everyone involved but is time consuming. Receiving CEUs is helpful, because many health-care organizations restrict paid educational leave to activities for which CEUs are earned (Stein, 1996).

Data Describing Nurse-Midwives

The ACNM Division of Research conducts periodic surveys to describe CNMs and various aspects of nurse-midwifery practice. Table 6 summarizes data from surveys conducted in 1982 (Adams, 1984), 1987 (Adams, 1989), 1988 (Lehrman & Paine, 1990), 1990 (Lehrman, 1992), 1991 (Walsh & DeJoseph, 1993), and 1993 and 1994 (Walsh & Boggess, 1993). Much of the information in this section is taken from those studies, including information not shown on Table 6. An effort was made to include all certified nurse-midwives in the studies conducted in 1982 and 1987. Ninety percent of the CNMs who participated in the 1982 survey were members of the ACNM; 84 percent of those who participated in the 1984 survey were members of the ACNM. Surveys conducted since then have been limited to ACNM members. Data are also collected on student members. The numbers of nurse-midwives included in the surveys do not reflect the number of CNMs practicing in the United States during specific years. A small proportion of nurse-midwives are not members of the ACNM, and some members do not complete and return the survey forms. However, the response rate has been high in recent years. The 1994 survey is based on questionnaires completed by 4,399 ACNM members, of which 3,830 were CNMs, and 569 were nurse-midwifery students. The

Table 6

Personal Information About CNMs Based on National Surveys Conducted by the ACNM Between 1982 and 1994*

	1982	1987	1988	1990	1991	1993	1994
Data source reference number	1	2	3	4	5	6	6
Number of CNMs in survey	1,684	2,278	1,735	1,877	1,722	3,452	3,830
Mean number of years practicing as RN before CNM	7.7	8.5					
Mean age when certified as a nurse-midwife	30.1	31.4					
Mean age at time of survey (years)				41.8	42.3	43.0	42.9
Percent female	99.0	98.5	98.7	97.9	98.0	99.1	99.1
Highest educational degree (percent)							
Diploma only, no degree	14.7	10.3		8.3	7.3	7.9	
Associate degree	4.8	6.3	14.3	4.7	5.6	5.5	
Bachelor's degree	23.2	21.0	19.2	18.7	17.6	19.4	
(in nursing)	(17.8)				(13.6)	(15.0)	
(in another field)	(5.4)				(4.0)	(4.4)	
Master's degree	54.6	59.0	63.5	64.6	65.0	63.4	
(in nursing)	(44.9)				(54.4)	(53.6)	
(in another field)	(9.7)				(10.6)	(9.8)	
Doctorate	2.7	3.4	3.0	3.7	4.5	3.8	
(in nursing)	(0.8)				(1.8)	(1.5)	
(in another field)	(1.8)				(2.7)	(2.3)	
% completed midwifery internship and/or "refresher" program	28.0	22.2					
Race/ethnicity (percent)							
Caucasian	90.7	94.5	95.1	96.0	95.1	93.3	92.1
Black/African-American	3.2	2.8	2.2	1.8	2.1	3.6	3.9
Hispanic	1.2	0.9	1.0	1.1	0.8	1.7	1.6
Asian/Pacific Islander	0.8	0.6	0.8	0.6	1.1	1.0	1.1
Native American	0.2					0.2	0.2
Other	3.9	1.2	0.8	0.5	0.9	0.2	1.1

Data sources: 1, Adams, 1984; 2, Adams, 1989; 3, Lehrman & Paine, 1990; 4, Lehrman, 1992; 5, Walsh & DeJoseph, 1993; 6, Walsh & Boggess, 1996.

* Percentages were calculated based on numbers presented in each published paper; individuals with missing information were excluded from the denominator.

questionnaires had been sent to 5,060 ACNM members; 87 percent responded (Walsh & Boggess, 1996). The exact number of CNMs in practice each year is not known. It was estimated that about 4,000 nurse-midwives were practicing in 1995.

Most CNMs have extensive experience as registered nurses before they enter a nurse-midwifery educational program and are mature women when they graduate (see Table 6). As the 1980s progressed, new nurse-midwives entered the field with even more experience. Most CNMs are women; only one percent are men.

Most CNMs have college degrees; at least two-thirds have graduate degrees (Table 6). The proportion with less than a baccalaureate degree declined steadily during the 1980s, to about 13 percent during the first half of the 1990s. The proportion with a graduate degree increased from 57 percent in 1982 to 68 percent in 1990. There was relatively little change in those percentages during the first half of the 1990s. Most nurse-midwives whose highest degree is a bachelor's or master's degree earned the degree in nursing. Most CNMs with doctoral degrees earn them in fields other than nursing, for example, public health or education.

Although most nurse-midwives are non-Hispanic Caucasians, there is a great need for nurse-midwives who are members of racial and ethnic minority groups, and nurse-midwifery education programs and the ACNM have been trying to recruit ethnic-minority nurses. As shown in Table 6, they are having some success. Data on the race and ethnicity of nurse-midwifery students is also encouraging: Of 569 students included in the 1994 survey, 5 percent were black, 3.3 percent were Hispanic, and 1.2 percent were Asian (Walsh & Boggess, 1996). Approximately 10 percent of nurses holding RN licenses in the United States in 1996 came from racial or ethnic minority backgrounds (Division of Nursing, 1997).

Nurse-Midwifery Practice as Defined by the ACNM Core Competencies

Nurse-midwifery draws its knowledge, philosophy, and practices from midwifery, medicine (especially obstetrics), and nursing. Midwifery contributes its core belief in pregnancy as a special, but normal, usually healthy life process and experience with profound physiological, emotional, social, and, for some women, spiritual ramifications and meaning, and its belief in engaging women in their own care. Advances in the science and methods of obstetrics are continually being assessed and selectively incorporated into modern nurse-midwifery practice. Nursing contributes a strong emphasis on patient education, effective communication with clients, advocacy and empowerment of patients, and a focus on the family (Lops *et al.*, 1995). In addition, nurse-midwives have always been committed to developing midwifery as an integral part of the mainstream health care system of the United States. As each of these influences on their role continues to evolve, so does the practice of nurse-midwives.

The document that defines the core elements of nurse-midwifery practice is the ACNM statement on *Core Competencies for Basic Nurse-Midwifery Practice*. The Clinical Practice Division of the ACNM is responsible for periodic revision of the core competencies statement. The following description of the practice of a certified nurse-midwife comes from the statement adopted in 1992. Twelve basic concepts and skills from the social sciences and public health permeate all aspects of nurse-midwifery practice: (1) promoting family-centered care, (2) facilitating healthy family and interpersonal relationships, (3) constructive use of communication and guidance and counseling skills, (4) communicating and collaborating with other members of the health care team, (5) providing health education, (6) promoting continuity of care,

(7) using community resources, (8) promoting health and preventing disease, (9) recognizing pregnancy as a normal physiologic and developmental process, (10) advocacy for informed choice and decision making, (11) consideration of bioethical issues related to women's health, and (12) knowledge of and respect for cultural variations. The scope of practice of a CNM includes preconception care (of women planning and preparing to become pregnant), antepartum care (also called prenatal care), intrapartum care (during labor and delivery), neonatal and postpartum care of the mother and baby for several weeks after the birth, and meeting "the family planning and gynecologic needs of well women," including those who are peri- and postmenopausal. There are three important aspects to nurse-midwifery management of care:

1. *Primary management.* Independent management of the complete care of a woman or newborn by a nurse-midwife, including identification of the need for consultation or referral to a physician or other member of the health care team. Primary management includes initiating care during emergencies and managing some kinds of complications.

2. *Collaboration* (also called "comanagement"). Identifying problems that require the involvement of a physician or other member of the health-care team, obtaining consultation, planning and implementing care that involves inputs from both the nurse-midwife and a physician or other health care provider, continuing to manage the midwifery aspects of the care, and serving as a consultant or comanager for other health care providers.

3. *Referral.* Identifying the need for ongoing care that is outside of the nurse-midwife's scope of practice, selecting appropriate sources of that care in collaboration with the woman, and transferring responsibility for the client's care to another health professional.

ACNM standards require nurse-midwives to practice within a health care system that provides for consultation, collaborative management, or referral as indicated by the health status of the client.

An Expanding Scope of Practice

Changes in nurse-midwifery practice are both reflected and stimulated by changes in the official definitions and policies of the ACNM. The ACNM made small but important changes in the definition of nurse-midwifery practice during the fifteen years between 1980 and 1995, and adopted several other policies that permit or encourage expansion of the scope of practice. This section describes ACNM policies and activities during that period of time which permit or facilitate expansions in the scope of practice. Although it includes information on ACNM statements about home births and abortions, these policy changes addressed philosophical concerns and neither reflected nor resulted in significant changes in the actual practice of nurse-midwives. However, the other policy changes are consistent with a significant increase in the scope of practice during this period.

ACNM Support for Home Births

The ACNM had a relatively negative position on home births during the 1970s (see Chapter 4). In 1980 the College retracted its earlier position, asserted consumers' rights to freedom of choice and self-determination, issued a statement endorsing nurse-midwifery practice in all settings (hospitals, homes, and free-standing birth centers), and developed guidelines for establishing "alternative" birthing services. The proportion of CNMs attending home births and births in free-standing birth centers rose during most of the 1980s, but began to decline at the end of the decade, falling to 7 percent in 1991, when the ACNM's professional liability insurance company announced that it would no longer issue policies to nurse-midwives who planned to attend home births (see discussion in Chapter 5). In addition, some third-party health care financing plans either stopped paying for home birth services or reduced their payments; for example, CHAMPUS* pays for home births but set the reimbursement lower than the cost of providing the care. Some state Medicaid programs pay for home births; many others do not.

In 1991 the ACNM created an Ad Hoc Committee on Home Births. The committee presented an all-day workshop on how to organize a home birth practice during the ACNM's 1991 convention and has presented a workshop or session on home births during every subsequent annual convention. The committee used information from its first workshop to develop guidelines for home birth, including examples of the essential documents for a home birth practice, a list of conditions that make women ineligible for home births, a list of equipment needed during home births, and a discussion of the importance of distance (expressed as time) to the nearest hospital. The ad hoc committee was changed to a standing committee in 1994. The committee is scheduled to publish a handbook on home birth in 1997; in addition to updating the issues addressed in its earlier publication, the handbook will include a section on the business aspects of operating a home birth practice.

In 1992 the Home Birth Committee began to make plans for both retrospective and prospective studies of home births attended by CNMs. Findings from the retrospective study—10,176 home births attended by seventy-eight CNMs with solo home birth practices and twelve CNM group home birth practices between 1987 and 1991—were published in December 1995 (Anderson & Murphy, 1995).† Data from the smaller

prospective study is being analyzed by a CNM/epidemiologist at Columbia University in New York City.

The Home Birth Committee's greatest challenge has been the lack of adequate liability insurance for home births attended by nurse-midwives. The committee has made limited progress: In 1995 the insurance company that offers policies to other ACNM members found a company willing to write policies for CNMs who attend home births. However, the cost is much higher and the maximum payment for damages is only $250,000; this is less than one-tenth of the coverage available to nurse-midwives who attend births in hospitals or accredited birth centers, and it is much less than is needed. One insurance company is willing to issue adequate ($1 million/$3 million) policies to ACNM members who attend home births in several states in the middle section of the Eastern seaboard. Joint underwriting associations make insurance available to CNMs who attend home births in Pennsylvania, Florida, and Washington; a few companies issue policies to CNMs in Arizona and California.

The *Journal of Nurse-Midwifery* devoted one entire 1995 issue to home birth. In addition to a report of the Home Birth Committee's retrospective descriptive study, the special issue included articles on informed consent; quality assurance, documentation, and peer review; guidelines for selecting clients for a home birth practice; practical suggestions for preparing couples for home births; care of the infant born at home; CNM/physician collaboration in a home birth practice; and a home birth curriculum guide to assist nurse-midwifery educational programs in preparing students for home birth practice.

---

*CHAMPUS pays for the health care of the legal dependents of members of the U.S. military services.

†See discussion in the section on Home Births later in this chapter for additional information and a summary of findings from this study.

Extending Nurse-Midwifery Practice Beyond the Age of Reproduction

Taking care of private patients created a desire and demand for nurse-midwives to expand their practice into the care of peri- and postmenopausal women, many of whom want to retain their relationship with the CNM who took care of them during pregnancies and provided their family planning care. Many nurse-midwives feel the same, as do many obstetricians, who tend to deliver fewer babies and take care of more postmenopausal women as both they and their patients age. During the mid-1980s, the ACNM changed the definition of basic nurse-midwifery practice to accommodate the desire of many CNMs to extend their practice to include gynecologic care of women during and after menopause.

New Procedures and Approaches: Care of Women With Complications

Data from surveys conducted by the ACNM in 1976–1977, 1982, and 1987 documented nurse-midwives' increasing use of obstetric procedures and growing role in the care of women with complications (Rooks *et al.*, 1978; Adams, 1984, 1989). The studies also found that some nurse-midwives were incorporating certain holistic health care methods into their practice. Nurse-midwives were increasing the variety of practice styles. Some CNMs were working in close collaboration with physicians in high-technology, high-volume academic medical centers, where many of the women had high-risk factors or serious complications; others were developing free-standing birth centers or working to create a place for low-intervention care of low-risk women within various kinds of hospitals.

Nurse-midwives' commitment to the care of socioeconomically high-risk women and their role in the obstetrics and gynecology departments of many urban medical centers involved them in collaborative care (with physicians) of women who have serious medical and obstetric complications. Their role as the main maternity care provider in some rural areas also required involvement in the care of women with complications. The ACNM survey conducted in 1982 found that most CNMs who were pro-

viding care to women during childbirth were responsible for some women with complications: 14 percent of those who attended births sometimes managed breech deliveries; 41 percent repaired fourth-degree lacerations (tears involving the rectum), if necessary; and 63 percent performed manual removal of the placenta. In addition, most CNMs used some obstetric interventions when they thought the procedure was needed, for example, attaching fetal scalp electrodes, inserting pressure monitoring devices into the uterus, and cutting episiotomies (Adams, 1984).

A similar study conducted in 1987, five years later, found that nearly all CNMs who were providing prenatal care accepted women with some "high-risk" characteristics. For example, 91 percent took care of fifteen- to seventeen-year-old girls; 95 percent took care of women older than thirty-five; and 89 percent took care of women having their sixth or higher order baby (Adams, 1989). Most CNMs were providing prenatal and childbirth care to women with post-term pregnancies, anemia, diabetes, or hypertension, and were attending births of women with preterm labor or an increased risk of infection because the membranes surrounding the fetus and amniotic fluid had ruptured more than twenty-four hours before the onset of labor. Nearly one-fourth of the nurse-midwives attending births reported that they "first assist" during cesarean sections; 42 percent indicated that they would like to learn to do so.

Many nurse-midwives had learned some aspects of the care they were providing after they graduated from their basic nurse-midwifery education programs, presumably through on-the-job training and continuing education. The procedures and responsibilities they had adopted since graduating included some "high-tech" procedures, some "high-touch" procedures, and providing care to women with certain kinds of complications independently or through comanagement (Adams, 1989):

- Examples of "high-tech" obstetric procedures and skills more often learned after rather than during their basic nurse-midwifery education included performing and interpreting the results of real-time ultrasonography, conducting and interpreting the results of various tests of fetal well-being, obtaining blood samples from a vein in the scalp of an unborn fetus, serving as the first assistant during cesarean sections, performing circumcisions, performing cryosurgery (using an instrument to freeze the surface layers of the cervix as a treatment for abnormal, possibly precancerous, conditions), and performing artificial insemination.
- Examples of "low-tech" or "high-touch" methods more frequently learned after graduation included use of acupressure, acupuncture, biofeedback, hypnosis, therapeutic touch during labor, and attending underwater births.
- Several procedures used to avoid the need for cesarean sections were more frequently learned after graduation: external version (manual manipulation of the fetus through the woman's abdomen in an attempt to turn it from a breech presentation to the normal head-down position) and conducting a trial of labor for vaginal delivery of women with previous cesarean sections (i.e., vaginal birth after cesarean—a "VBAC").
- Most nurse-midwives who were managing the prenatal care of women with diabetes, managing preterm labor, managing labor for women whose membranes had ruptured more than twenty-four hours before the onset of labor, or delivering twins had not learned to do so during their basic nurse-midwifery education.

In 1993 the *Journal of Nurse-Midwifery* published an issue devoted to advanced nurse-midwifery practice. It discussed the ACNM statement on collaborative management of women with complications and the *Guide-lines for Incorporation of New Procedures into Nurse-Midwifery Practice* and presented articles on nurse-midwives' use of ten "advanced practice" procedures: amnioinfusions, colposcopy, endometrial biopsy, external cephalic version, circumcision, vacuum extraction, third-trimester ultrasonography, fetal scalp sampling, subdermal contraceptive implants, and use of prostaglandins during labor. An editorial shared the Editorial Board's concern that many CNMs may "feel that the Journal is betraying the art and soul of midwifery and venturing too far into the medical model. Yet, we feel confident that other CNMs will welcome this information as vital to their professional development and to the demands of their practice setting . . . . There are those of us who guard our position as experts in the care of low-risk clients in low-risk settings and others who, either by choice or necessity, are venturing further into the gray areas between low- and high-risk care. Although the most traditional of us may try to resist, we find that technology is creeping into our existence on many fronts and is, in fact, a reality that can often be used to advantage" (Sinquefield, 1993). The editorial cautioned that the information in the journal was not sufficient to equip CNMs to perform the new procedures.

All of the ACNM documents included in the special advanced nurse-midwifery practice issue had been adopted or revised during 1992. They included 1992 revisions of the official ACNM *Definition of Nurse-Midwifery Practice* and the *Core Competencies for Basic Nurse-Midwifery Practice,* and a statement on *Expansion of Nurse-Midwifery Practice and Skills Beyond Basic Core Competencies* (Avery & DelGuidice, 1993). "Essentially normal" was removed as a modifier of appropriate clients in the definition of nurse-midwifery practice. The old definition limited "the independent management" aspect of nurse-midwifery practice to the care of "essentially normal newborns and women." The new statement is less restrictive, defining nurse-midwifery practice as "the independent management of women's health care, focusing particularly on pregnancy, childbirth, the postpartum period, care of the newborn, and the family planning and gynecological needs of well women."

In 1994, the *Journal of Nurse-Midwifery* published a supplementary issue devoted to nurse-midwifery management of a selected group of obstetric complications. The introductory editorial noted that "prevention and identification of complicated pregnancies have always been a part of nurse-midwifery's repertoire," that CNM/MD teams are providing collaborative management of many obstetric complications, that "basic CNM education programs have traditionally included the recognition of deviations from the expected norm, as well as the initial management and follow-up of problems within their curricula," and that, whereas "CNMs who practice in remote rural areas often play primary roles in the management of specific complications because of the dearth of health care practitioners . . . CNMs who practice in large urban teaching institutions may be forced to transfer their patients to the physician as soon as an initial identification of a problem is made" (Zeidenstein, 1994). The entire supplementary issue and much of the regular issue that accompanied it were devoted to articles that presented up-to-date summaries of information on the etiology, pathophysiology, diagnosis, and nurse-midwifery management of specific complications.*

Nurse-Midwives as Primary Care Providers
A 1994 report by the Institute of Medicine defined "primary health care" as "the provi-

---

*Gestational diabetes, iron-deficiency anemia, pregnancy-induced hypertension, preeclampsia, premature rupture of membranes, preterm labor, postdate pregnancy, intrauterine growth retardation, shoulder dystocia, meconium-stained amniotic fluid, postpartum hemorrhage, and articles on methods for early detection of preterm labor and the risks and benefits of invasive prenatal diagnostic procedures.

sion of integrated, accessible health care services by clinicians who are accountable for addressing a large majority of personal health care needs, developing a sustained partnership with patients, and practicing in the context of family and community" (Institute of Medicine, 1994). Primary care includes health assessment, health promotion and disease prevention services, routine and "first contact" health care, and management and coordination of services provided by specialists. A continuing criticism of American health care is that it devotes too many resources to specialized disease care and not enough to primary care. Lack of sufficient numbers of primary care professionals and facilities contributes to high health care costs, inadequate access to care for millions of Americans, and poor quality of care (Alliance for Health Reform, 1992). A major objective of all efforts at health care reform, and a result of the move toward prepaid managed health care, is to encourage all Americans to initiate and maintain a continuing relationship with a "primary health care provider" who is capable of handling most common health problems and refers patients to specialists only as needed. In addition to providing most of the actual health care, primary care providers are the designated gatekeepers of the newly evolving health care system; many health care plans will not pay for specialist care unless the patient was referred to the specialist by his or her primary care provider.

Because of the low priority given to primary care in the United States, obstetrician–gynecologists and family planning clinics are the only health care providers with whom many women have had an ongoing relationship. They see an obstetrical care giver while pregnant and for vaginal infections or concerns about their sexual organs, obtain contraception from them, go to them for annual Pap smears and breast examinations, and see other specialists for other kinds of problems. This approach fails to meet some of the preventive health care needs of women, especially low-income women and members of racial and ethnic minorities (Commonwealth Fund, 1993). For example, women who use obstetrician–gynecologists as their primary care provider are more likely to be screened for breast and cervical cancer, but are less likely to get nonreproductive health services such as immunizations and screening for high blood cholesterol (Bartman & Weiss, 1993; Horton et al., 1993). As a result, many women have to visit several doctors or other health care providers in order to obtain basic care and some women do not receive important preventive health care services (Murphy, 1996).*

As increasing numbers of women are obtaining their reproductive health care from CNMs, some want and expect to use a nurse-midwife as their primary care provider. And, whether or not women intend to utilize nurse-midwives as primary care providers, CNMs working in ambulatory care settings encounter women with health problems that are not related to their reproductive system. Because a high proportion of the women they take care of are poor and poor women have more health problems and are even less likely than other women to have a continuing relationship with a physician, many CNMs see patients who have health problems that require care that is not included in the ACNM core competencies.

During 1992 the ACNM asked the chairs of each of its chapters, committees, and divisions, and the directors of all nurse-midwifery education programs and services to complete a questionnaire on the adequacy of the current Core Competencies for their own clinical practice. Most of the respondents stated that the core competencies should be expanded to include "primary care content" similar to the content of family nurse practitioner (FNP) programs. Investigation of this issue led to identification of

several problems, including the lack of universally acknowledged definitions of "primary health care" and a "primary care provider." While there is wide agreement that physicians specializing in general internal medicine, family medicine, or pediatrics are primary care providers, there is little agreement about other kinds of MDs and other kinds of health professionals. Also, most programs to prepare FNPs are about one year in length, making it impractical to simply add their content to a nurse-midwifery education program, and FNPs have not defined the core competencies of their practice.

In October 1992, the ACNM approved a formal statement which declares that CNMs provide primary health care for women and newborns. The statement points out that nurse-midwifery care includes assessment, treatment, and referral; emphasizes health promotion, education, and disease prevention; focuses on the woman as a whole; and provides continuity of care throughout the childbearing years and into the peri- and postmenopausal periods. "CNMs are often the initial contact for providing health care to women, and they provide such care on a continuous and comprehensive basis by establishing a plan of management with the woman for her ongoing health care. Such care by the CNM is inclusive and integrated with the woman's cultural, socioeconomic and psychological factors that may impinge on her health status" (ACNM, 1992a). The National Health Service Corps and the Federal Office of Rural Health Policy recognize CNMs as primary health care providers.

Two studies have been conducted on nurse-midwifery involvement in primary care. The first tried to determine the extent to which CNMs practicing in 1993 were involved in dealing with certain common nonreproductive health problems. More than three hundred CNMs attending the 1993 ACNM annual meeting were asked to indicate whether and how often they identify

---

*This issue is discussed in Chapter 14.

and manage each condition on a list of twenty-six common specific health problems (Scupholme & Carr, 1993). The majority of them indicated that they managed seven of the conditions (sinusitis; viral syndromes affecting the ears, nose, and throat; strep throat; chronic anemia; indigestion; obesity; and viral syndromes affecting the gastrointestinal tract) at least once for every fifty clients. They were less likely to manage the care of women with rashes, ringworm, warts, conjunctivitis, otitis, laryngitis, tonsillitis, bronchitis, chest infections, minor asthma attacks, chronic hypertension, acute or chronic abdominal pain, mild depression, domestic assault, and sexual abuse. Most of them never treated women with superficial burns, sties, muscular strains and sprains, or minor injuries.

The other study focused on the health assessment, health promotion, and disease prevention practices of CNMs. Almost 350 CNMs completed and returned questionnaires mailed to a stratified random sample of ACNM members in 1994 (Murphy, 1996). Ninety-seven percent of them were providing prenatal care; 87 percent were providing family planning and gynecologic services. Eighty-five percent thought of themselves as primary care providers. Like obstetrician–gynecologists, the nurse-midwives were most likely to provide health promotion and disease prevention services related to reproductive health and were less likely to focus on other aspects. For instance, 89 percent of the CNMs asked their prenatal clients to examine their breasts in order to determine if the women were doing it correctly; only 37 percent examined almost all of their prenatal clients for gingivitis and tooth decay. Most of the nurse-midwives screened almost all of their family planning/gynecology clients for hypertension and asked them about smoking and use of alcohol and drugs. When findings from this study were compared with data from a national survey conducted in 1991, it was evident that women who obtain their care from CNMs are more likely than most

American women to receive counseling about common health problems as part of their health care. The CNMs met or approached most of the Public Health Service objectives for provision of health promotion and disease prevention services by the year 2000.*

The ability of CNMs to provide a wide scope of care to women is making them attractive to the new managed health care organizations that are emerging from the rapid systemic, but nonsystematic transformation of health care that is occurring in the wake of the failure of national legislation for health care reform. For example, when the University of Southern California terminated its agreement to place ob-gyn residents in the California Hospital Medical Center's clinics (in Los Angeles), the hospital decided to replace the physicians with nurse-midwives. By employing twenty-four nurse-midwives, the hospital could staff each clinic with one physician and four or five CNMs; this change not only decreased the number of physicians needed by the hospital, it greatly increased the number of patients seen in the clinics every month. The CNMs' ability to handle a wide scope of practice was essential to making this change (*Inside Ambulatory Care*, 1995).

Nurse-midwives (and ob-gyns) need additional training to prepare themselves for a larger role in primary health care. Continuing education programs on "primary care

---

*The U.S. Public Health Service has established 523 quantified health promotion and disease prevention objectives and subobjectives for the nation to achieve by the year 2000. Some of the objectives call for achieving specified reductions in disease conditions (e.g., reducing the coronary heart disease death rate among blacks to a certain level) or reducing the percent of people who practice a risky behavior (e.g., smoking). Some of the objectives call for certain clinicians to provide certain health services as part of primary care, for example, increasing the proportion of primary care providers who ask their patients about smoking and counsel them for smoking cessation to 75 percent (National Center for Health Statistics, 1994).

for women's health care providers" began to be offered widely in about 1994. In 1995 the *Journal of Nurse-Midwifery* published the first of two issues comprising a home-study program on comprehensive assessment and management of common health problems in women. The first issue focused on elements of a comprehensive health assessment.* The editorial that introduced the special issue challenged CNMs to integrate the full scope of primary care services into nurse-midwifery practice (Williams, 1995). The subjects for the articles included in the second issue devoted to primary care (published in 1996) were selected based on information regarding the twenty most frequent reasons for women's visits to physicians during 1992 and the twenty most frequent diagnoses given to women during those visits.†

Rescinding a Policy That Prohibited Performing Abortions

The subject of abortion is as tortured and complex among nurse-midwives as among any other group of Americans. Nevertheless, a majority of the members present at the 1990 annual meeting of the American Col-

---

*The special issue on primary care published in 1995 included overview articles on tests and procedures to screen women for a variety of medical conditions (breast, colorectal, cervical, skin, ovarian, endometrial and other cancers, high blood cholesterol, renal problems, and seven specific diseases); environmental assessment of the home, community and workplace; the art of interviewing; comprehensive sexual health assessment; individual articles on assessment of hematologic disorders, common musculoskeletal disorders, and gastrointestinal disorders; individual articles on comprehensive assessment of the head and neck, and the respiratory, cardiovascular, and neurologic systems; and assessment and management of genitourinary tract disorders in women.

†Articles in the 1996 special issue on primary health focused on common problems of the head and neck, headaches, common mental health problems, common respiratory problems, gastrointestinal disorders, and musculoskeletal disorders.

lege of Nurse-Midwives voted to "recommend to the Board of Directors that the ACNM statement prohibiting CNMs from performing abortions be rescinded, thereby allowing individual CNMs to utilize the guidelines for the incorporation of new procedures into nurse-midwifery practice if she/he decides to provide that service."

In 1991 a sample that included half of all ACNM members was polled to determine their attitudes about performing abortions. More than 1,200 completed questionnaires were returned—a 71 percent response rate. A slight majority, 52 percent, indicated that they would or possibly would vote in a secret ballot to permit CNMs to perform abortions; 24 percent would, or possibly would, incorporate abortion procedures into their practice; and 19 percent would, or possibly would, perform abortions in an abortion clinic (McKee & Adams, 1994). Fifty-seven percent would be willing to prescribe RU 486, and 56 percent would perform dilation and curettage for spontaneous abortion. CNMs who supported the idea of nurse-midwives performing abortions were more likely to have practiced well-woman gynecology and to have provided services such as abortion referrals, pre- and postabortion examinations and consultation, and treatment of complications of legal or illegal abortions.

The ACNM's policy prohibiting certified nurse-midwives from performing abortions had been in effect since 1971. It was rescinded in 1992. Reasons for rescinding it included nurse-midwives' philosophical support for each woman's right to self-determination (a basic precept of the ACNM philosophy) and doubts that it is appropriate for a professional organization to impose this kind of restriction on its members. The latter reason is consistent with the ACNM's long policy of providing a procedure to assist individual nurse-midwives to make careful, fully informed decisions regarding the components of their own particular practice.

Nurse-Midwives' Practice Circumstances

Studies conducted by the ACNM Research Division provide data on the employment and practice arrangements of CNMs during the 1980s and early 1990s. Selected findings from those studies are summarized in Table 7. Several other studies conducted during this period but not shown on Table 7 also provided information on the practice circumstances of nurse-midwives during this time period.

The proportion of employed CNMs who were practicing or teaching nurse-midwifery increased from 74 percent in 1982 to between 85 and 90 percent during the early 1990s. More than five hundred CNMs who responded to the 1987 survey and were employed but not working as nurse-midwives were asked to give the reason. The most common reasons included the difficult hours required for nurse-midwifery practice, lack of nurse-midwifery positions in some communities, not being current in practice (therefore needing to take a refresher course in order to return to practice), and the high expense of malpractice insurance (Adams, 1989).

Less than two-thirds of the CNMs in the first two studies conducted during the 1980s were attending births. The proportion attending births has since increased to about three-fourths. Most CNMs who do not attend births work in ambulatory care settings (e.g., prenatal or family planning clinics), function primarily as administrators or researchers, or practice or teach nursing.

Where Do Nurse-Midwives Work?

Table 7 shows the employer or other primary practice arrangement for most of the CNMs who were working and participated in the seven ACNM studies.* The categories are arranged in order of descending importance based on findings from the most recent study. Hospitals were the largest employers of nurse-midwives throughout this period, employing from 26 to 36 percent of the CNMs in every study. The next largest number of CNMs were in practice with physicians, mainly as employees, but sometimes as partners. Approximately 10 percent worked for educational institutions, mainly in nurse-midwifery education, but also in medical and nursing education. The proportion of CNMs working for HMOs and other prepaid health care plans increased during this period, and the proportion of CNMs working in private nurse-midwifery practices declined. The proportion of CNMs working for one of the military services or another part of the federal government (such as the Indian Health Service), or for state and local health departments declined as the number of nurse-midwives in other positions increased. However, the actual number of nurse-midwives working in government health care systems increased during this time. The vast majority of CNMs are salaried employees whose income is not directly based on the fees they bring into a practice.

Sixty-four percent of the nurse-midwives who participated in the 1987 study worked in settings in which individual clients could choose to be cared for by either a physician

---

*Percentages are based on employed CNMs only. Some CNMs have part-time positions in addition to their primary position. The information in Table 7 refers to their primary employment. The wording of the questions changed a little over time, so that the categories are not entirely consistent. Categories that were included in only one study and categories that account for very small proportions of employed CNMs are not shown on Table 7, for example, employment in a university health service or mission. The employer categories shown in Table 7 account for 86 to 90 percent of employed CNMs in all seven studies.

Table 7
Nurse-Midwives' Employment and Practice Arrangements Based on National Surveys of CNMs in Clinical Practice, Surveys Conducted Between 1982 and 1994

	1982	1987	1988	1990	1991	1993	1994
Data source reference number	1	2	3	4	5	6	6
Number of CNMs in survey	1,684	2,278	1,735	1,877	1,722	3,452	3,830
Percent practicing or teaching nurse-midwifery*	74.4	80.3	77.9	87.6	90.5	86.6	84.9
Percent attending births†	65.6	65.6	64.8	77.2	83.4	76.8	74.8
Primary employer/practice arrangement (%):							
Hospital or medical center	35.9		25.6	25.7	25.6	29.1	29.5
Private practice with physician(s)	19.7		18.6	22.1	23.3	20.8	21.3
Educational institution			13.1	10.6	10.7	9.7	9.5
Prepaid health care plan	6.0		6.4	6.8	7.2	8.8	8.2
Private nurse-midwifery practice	14.1		9.6	10.1	9.4	7.5	7.2
Military and/or other federal agency	5.8		9.2	5.5	5.7	4.9	4.5
Public health department/agency	9.0			4.7	4.1	3.5	3.1
Free-standing birth center			3.1	3.7	4.3	2.9	2.8
In-hospital birth center						1.2	1.2
Basis of income from work as a CNM:							
Salary (per hour, monthly; may include bonus)				89.5	91.4		
Fees for services rendered				4.4	4.1		
Of those attending births, percent who:‡							
Sign birth certificates	87.4	89.4			94.5	89.4	93.1
Attend births in hospital			96.0	91.7	92.8	91.7	93.0
(in hospital delivery rooms)	(81.4)	(78.4)					
(in an in-hospital birth center)	(34.0)	(42.9)					
Attend births in free-standing birth centers	12.0	13.5	18.8	10.5	9.5	15.9	21.5
Attend home births	14.2	13.0	10.0	7.4	7.0	5.0	4.9
Must have a physician in room for delivery	5.9	5.3					
Mean annual number of births/CNM	75	75			81		

Data sources: 1, Adams, 1984; 2, Adams, 1987; 3, Lehrman & Paine, 1990; 4, Lehrman, 1992; 5, Walsh & DeJoseph, 1993; 6, Walsh & Boggess, 1996

*Percent of employed CNMs; i.e., retired and unemployed individuals were eliminated from the denominator

†Retired and unemployed individuals were excluded from the denominator in all studies. In addition, only CNMs in clinical nurse-midwifery practice were included in the percentages shown for the study conducted in 1982.

‡Percent of employed CNMs who attend births; includes CNMs attending births in part-time secondary jobs, as well as in their primary employment.

191

or a CNM. Women served by the other nurse-midwives in this survey were directed to the nurse-midwifery service by the institution providing their care and did not have the option of choosing a physician (Adams, 1989).

CNMs Who Attend Births

The bottom third of Table 7 provides additional information about nurse-midwives who deliver babies. As they grow older, many CNMs discontinue clinical practice or limit their practice to ambulatory care, that is, they withdraw from labor and delivery (Fullerton, 1994). The same trend is found among obstetricians.

The proportion of nurse-midwives who sign the baby's birth certificate increased from 87 percent in 1982 to 93 percent in 1994 (Table 7). Until this figure reaches 100 percent, the number of births attributed to nurse-midwives will be undercounted in data derived from birth certificates.

Nurse-midwives' role in out-of-hospital birth is declining. Nevertheless, some CNMs attend births in several settings; this allows them to offer a choice to women who remain low risk (Scupholme & Walsh, 1994). Although only 3 percent of births attended by CNMs in 1994 occurred in a free-standing birth center (Ventura *et al.*, 1996), more than 21 percent of CNMS who were attending births in 1994 attended at least some of them in a birth center. Inability to purchase adequate liability insurance has driven many CNMs away from attending home births; the proportion attending births in homes fell from more than 14 percent in 1982 to less than 5 percent in 1994.

The average (mean) number of births per CNM per year increased during the 1980s and early 1990s—from 75 per year in 1982 and 1987 to 81 per year in 1991 (Table 7). Another study (data collected from a random sample of 545 ACNM members) found an average of 119 births per CNM doing deliveries in 1993 (Franklin Communications, 1994). The increase may be associated with the growing proportion employed primarily

in a private CNM practice or free-standing birth center. The 1982 and 1987 studies showed higher average numbers of births for nurse-midwives working for a military service or public health agency and the lowest averages for those in private practice, whether with physicians or other CNMs (Adams, 1984, 1989).

In addition to collecting data from individual CNMs, the 1982 survey gathered information on 357 nurse-midwifery practices. Forty-one percent of the practices that provided care during labor and delivery had only one CNM—often working with one or more physicians (Adams, 1984).

Nurse-Midwives' Use of Time During Clinical Care

During the early 1990s, the Robert Wood Johnson Foundation funded a study to find out what kinds of women and infants were receiving care from CNMs and more about the services they were receiving. The first phase of the study described certain demographic characteristics of the clients of a large national sample of nurse-midwives in active clinical practice ($N = 1,879$). Findings from that phase of the study were discussed in Chapter 7 (Scupholme *et al.*, 1992). The second phase of the study described the clinical services provided by the CNMs and the amount of time they spent providing specific kinds of services. Data for phase II came from a subsample of the large phase I sample; 369 CNMs in the subsample recorded precise information about the services they provided during 16,729 contacts with clients during a two-week period in September 1991 and a two-week period in June 1992. The phase II data set describes 15,993 of the 16,729 CNM/client contacts reported by the respondents, including 828 births. A small number of contacts could not be classified and were omitted from the analysis (Scupholme *et al.*, 1994).

Eighty percent of the nearly sixteen thousand CNM/client contacts were for pregnancy-related care; 17.5 percent were for gynecologic care of nonpregnant women, and 2.5 percent were contacts with newborns. The nurse-midwives spent 83 percent of their work time in direct contact with clients. The mean amount of CNM/client face-to-face time during an initial visit (a new client or an old client with a new condition) was 41 minutes, with a median of 35 minutes.* Return visits averaged 22 minutes (median = 20 minutes). The mean time devoted to counseling and education during ambulatory visits was 5 minutes (median = 7.9 minutes). The mean time spent interviewing the patient to obtain information about her condition was 6 minutes (median = 8.8 minutes). The mean time spent attending a birth was 4 hours and 24 minutes (median = 3.5 hours) (Scupholme *et al.*, 1994).

Findings from the Public Citizen's Health Research Group 1994 Survey

In 1995 the Public Citizen's Health Research Group published a report based on its 1994 survey of 618 nurse-midwifery practices—419 practices that attend births in hospitals and 39 practices based in free-standing birth centers. The Health Research Group estimated that the nurse-midwifery practices included in its survey were responsible for 50 to 60 percent of the births attended by CNMs in 1994 (Gabay & Wolfe, 1995).

The Public Citizen's Health Research Group became interested in nurse-midwifery because of its earlier research about unnecessary cesarean sections (Wolfe & Gabay, 1994). During that research they had collected data on method of delivery for live births in 3,159 hospitals in forty-one states. Nurse-midwives were practicing in 175 of those hospitals. The cesarean section rate for the hospitals with CNMs was 19.3 percent, compared with 22.3 percent for all hospitals in the study, that is, the rate was 13

percent lower in the hospitals with CNMs. In addition, the VBAC rate in the hospitals with nurse-midwives was nearly one-third higher than the average for all 3,159 hospitals (Gabay & Wolfe, 1995).

Findings from the 618 CNM hospital birth practices included in the Health Research Group Study are summarized here. (Findings from the birth center practices are summarized in the section on nurse-midwifery practice in free-standing birth centers.) The average number of CNMs in the 618 practices was 3.4. About 35 percent of the practices had only one CNM; in half of those practices, the CNM was employed by a physician. Four percent of the practices had 10 or more CNMs; most of the large nurse-midwifery practices were operated by a hospital or university. Thirty-eight percent of the practices were private practices involving one or more CNM and one or more physicians. The next largest group was hospital-owned practices (22 percent of the total), followed by private CNM practices (11 percent), and practices based in HMOs (7 percent) and universities (6 percent).

All of the practices provided prenatal care and care during labor and delivery. Almost all of them provided postpartum care (98 percent) and family planning and well-woman gynecologic services (92 percent). Only 14 percent were responsible for care of the babies. Twenty percent offered additional services as well, such as the routine physical examinations women often need for entrance into schools or sports, breast-feeding instruction and support, infertility services, preconception counseling, and childbirth education (Gabay & Wolfe, 1995).

Most of these practices take care of some moderate- and high-risk women through co-management with physicians. Only 4 percent of the practices indicated that all of their clients are low risk.

Continuity of care means that the same care provider or a small group of care

---

*This means that half of the visits took 35 minutes or less and half took 35 minutes or more.

providers sees each woman throughout her pregnancy. Almost 90 percent of the practices included in the Health Research Group survey reported that the nurse-midwives established a prior relationship with most or all of the women they admit for labor and delivery. A little less than 10 percent worked in systems where the person who provides prenatal care is not part of the nurse-midwifery service that attends the woman during childbirth (Gabay & Wolfe, 1995).

Sixty percent of the practices usually provide care on a one-midwife-for-one-patient basis during labor and delivery. In 35 percent of the practices, one CNM is often responsible for the care of more than one woman during labor.

The practices were asked to provide information on options they offer clients during labor and delivery and the extent to which the same options are available to women who give birth at the same hospital under the care of physicians. All or almost all women in these hospitals could have a family member with them throughout labor and delivery, rooming-in, and open postpartum visitation regardless of whether their care provider was a nurse-midwife or a physician. However, the nurse-midwives' clients were significantly more likely to be offered each of the eleven other options: drinking fluids during labor, walking during labor, delivery in a birth room (usually the same room as the labor room) instead of in a delivery room, having friends (in addition to family) with them during labor and delivery, taking a shower or tub bath during labor, using alternative positions during delivery (e.g., squatting or lying on her side, rather than delivering with her feet up in stirrups), use of intermittent rather than continuous fetal monitoring, waiting to clamp and cut the cord (which ensures that the infant is not deprived of its natural allotment of blood), breast-feeding on demand (instead of scheduled feedings), and early and very early discharge (Gabay & Wolfe, 1995).

Nurse-Midwifery Practice Models

This section describes and provides examples of nurse-midwifery practice in a variety of settings: free-standing birth centers, practices based in academic tertiary-care hospitals, small CNM or CNM/MD practices in small towns and rural areas, special programs designed to meet the needs of particular groups of women, CNM services in health maintenance organizations, and home birth practices. These are not the only kinds of nurse-midwifery practices. Other models include CNM group practices in urban settings; CNMs who are partners or employees of a single physician or a group of physicians; CNMs in the Indian Health Service or one of the U.S. military services; CNMs who provide only ambulatory care and work for public health agencies, local Planned Parenthood affiliates, and so on. However, the models and examples featured here represent a wide range of practice styles, settings, and arrangements. In addition, because most of the descriptions come from published research findings, they provide very accurate, specific information.

Nurse-Midwifery Practice in Free-Standing Birth Centers

The National Birth Center Study described care provided to nearly eighteen thousand women in eighty-four birth centers nationwide during 1985–1987.* CNMs provided prenatal care to 81 percent of the women, and CNMs and obstetricians working in teams provided prenatal care to another 5 percent. CNMs or nurse-midwifery students provided care to 79 percent of the women who labored in the birth centers and attended the births of 81 percent of them (Rooks *et al.*, 1989).

Prenatal care provided to the birth center clients stressed education and the

---

*The methods and major findings of the National Birth Center Study are described in Chapter 5.

women's responsibility and ability to monitor and improve their own health; many birth centers taught women to test their own urine and record their own weight at each visit and to understand and use the information in their charts. The women were observed for early signs and symptoms of complications and had access to all necessary diagnostic and therapeutic measures (such as Rhogam for Rh-negative women, tests to diagnose genetic fetal abnormalities, and treatment for preterm labor). But the emphasis was on preventing problems and maximizing health; preparing women for labor, delivery, breast-feeding, and mothering; and dealing with each woman's particular discomforts and concerns. Nearly all of the women completed a childbirth education course. Most of the women gained an appropriate amount of weight. Noninvasive methods were often used as the first effort to solve problems: castor oil to stimulate labor in women whose membranes had been ruptured for many hours; exercises and positioning or external version to convert persistent breech presentations; fetal movement counting and simple monitoring of the fetal heart rate in preference to fetal adaptability tests that require stimulation of contractions. Prenatal sonograms were used selectively, not routinely; 8 percent of CNM clients had two ultrasonograms, compared with 24 percent of the obstetricians' birth center clients (even though women who used birth centers run by obstetricians were of higher socioeconomic status and had fewer complications than clients of birth centers run by CNMs).

Care provided by nurse-midwives to women during childbirth in a birth center differed significantly from usual hospital care. Birth center clients were relatively unlikely to receive central nervous system depressants, epidural anesthesia, continuous electronic fetal monitoring, oxytocin induction or augmentation of labor, intravenous infusions (IVs), amniotomies, or epi-

siotomies, and had relatively few vaginal examinations. The fetal heart rate was usually monitored by a small hand-held "doppler" that can be temporarily pressed against the woman's abdomen. All but 5 percent of the women drank or ate while in labor at the birth center; 43 percent took showers or baths and 35 percent had massages. Ninety-seven percent labored in the company of friends or family, often including children. One-fourth of the first-time mothers, and only 6 percent of those who had given birth before, required an analgesic, tranquilizer, or sedative during labor. Pain relief was considered inadequate for only 2 percent of the women, most of whom were transferred to hospitals so that they could have an epidural. Twelve percent of the women were transferred to hospitals before they gave birth for one reason or another, most often first-time mothers whose labors "failed to progress." Forty-three percent of the women who gave birth in the centers were in an upright or semi-upright position during the actual birth. Only 18 percent had episiotomies, and there were few significant lacerations (Rooks *et al.*, 1992).

The survey conducted by the Public Citizen's Health Research Group in 1994 provides additional and more recent information (Gabay & Wolfe, 1995). Survey questionnaires were completed by staff of forty-one "established" CNM birth centers that are members of the National Association of Childbearing Centers (1993). CNMs at about half of the birth centers also attend births in hospitals or, in a few instances, also attend home births. The number of CNMs working for these birth centers ranged from 1 to 14, with a mean of 3.5. Fifty-four percent of the birth center CNMs had hospital admitting privileges. All of the birth centers offered well-woman gynecologic care, as well as complete maternity care. Ninety-seven percent also provide family planning services; 69 percent give childbirth education classes, and 36 percent provide well-baby care. Data were collected for births at these centers during 1991, 1992, and 1993. They averaged 177 births per center in 1991, increased to 218 births per center in 1992, and declined to 198 per center in 1993. About 18 percent of the women who began labor care at the birth centers were transferred to hospitals during labor or shortly after giving birth. The cesarean section rate was 6.7 percent (Gabay & Wolfe, 1995).

Nurse-Midwifery Services in Tertiary Academic Hospitals

The largest numbers of CNM clients and deliveries during the 1980s were in large nurse-midwifery services based in academic and other publicly supported hospitals for care of medically indigent people in the nation's largest cities, for example, Cook County Hospital in Chicago, Jefferson Davis Hospital in Houston, the Los Angeles County/University of Southern California Woman's Hospital in Los Angeles, Jackson Memorial Hospital in Miami, the Downstate Medical Center and North Central Bronx hospitals in New York City, and Grady Memorial Hospital in Atlanta (Wente, 1986). In addition, most nurse-midwifery education programs are based in or affiliated with academic medical centers, which provided most of the clinical experience for nurse-midwifery students. These environments exerted an important influence on nurse-midwifery practice.

This section includes information from four important studies of nurse-midwifery practices within three of the country's leading academic departments of obstetrics and gynecology during the period from 1973 to 1993. The earliest study (data on 10,766 births attended by CNMs at the county hospital in Atlanta from 1973 to 1982) describes two distinct models for providing nurse-midwifery care to patients in this kind of setting and raises issues about the effect of the academic tertiary medical center environment on nurse-midwifery. Two studies from a large CNM service at the Los Angeles County/University of Southern California

Women's Hospital provide the physicians' perspective on the role of nurse-midwives in this kind of setting (data from 1979 to 1980) and describe the development and performance of a separate in-hospital nurse-midwifery birth center (1981–1992). The most recent study (1988–1993) compares care provided by CNMs to private patients at an academic medical center in the midwest with care provided by physicians to similarly low-risk private patients at the same university hospital.

Grady Memorial Hospital, Atlanta, Georgia, 1973-1982 A 1984 report on a decade of nurse-midwifery practice at Grady Memorial Hos-pital in Atlanta, Georgia, described two patterns for providing nurse-midwifery care to women in a high-volume tertiary-level university-affiliated county hospital for the indigent. It also documented changes in nurse-midwifery practice in response to both the general increase in use of obstetric interventions during this period, especially in academic medical centers, and nurse-midwives' growing criticism of routine use of some of those procedures (Sharp & Lewis, 1984).

The two models of care at Grady were called *comprehensive care* and *episodic care*. In the comprehensive care model, patients without serious complications or high-risk conditions were assigned to the CNM service during the prenatal period and received nurse-midwifery care throughout the rest of their pregnancies unless they developed a prenatal complication that required ongoing medical care, at which time they were transferred to the obstetric service. If women in this group developed complications during labor and delivery, the nurse-midwives usually retained them in their service and provided their care in collaboration with physicians. In the episodic care model, women who were low-risk at the onset of labor but had not been assigned to the CNM service for prenatal care were assigned to the midwifery service for labor and delivery.

Combining the two models allowed the nurse-midwives (and nurse-midwifery students) to provide continuity-of-care to a caseload of patients, increased the number of births for students, and made it possible for the nurse-midwives to provide relief when the obstetric service was overwhelmed with women in labor. As the number of deliveries at Grady climbed during the early 1980s, the obstetric residents became busier and asked the nurse-midwives to assume more and more responsibility for women not in their prenatal caseload (Sharp & Lewis, 1984).

Outcomes for both groups of patients were good, but they were better for women assigned to CNMs during labor (episodic care) than for women in the nurse-midwives prenatal caseload (comprehensive care); women with prenatal complications were retained in the comprehensive care group but were excluded from the episodic care group. The study was important in demonstrating that it is safe to screen women into nurse-midwifery care during labor and the practical advantages of combining both models in a single setting (Sharp & Lewis, 1984).

Ten years of data from this service suggest the complexity of practicing—and teaching and learning—midwifery in this kind of setting. Use of electronic fetal monitoring and epidural anesthesia increased steadily over the ten-year period. Use of oxytocin to induce labor increased in the episodic group and remained stable but relatively high in the comprehensive care group. The decision to induce ultimately rests with the collaborating physician; the nurse-midwives' care in these matters was clearly influenced by the beliefs and practices of their obstetric colleagues. However, the use of episiotomy decreased over time in both groups of patients, as the nurse-midwives grew more skeptical of "routine episiotomies," which were still a widely practiced obstetric standard. The publication of findings from this large data set (information on 10,766 nurse-midwifery deliveries) and earlier publication of data

from the large nurse-midwifery service at Jackson Memorial Hospital in Miami (Scupholme, 1982), contributed to an ongoing intraprofessional dialogue about the appropriate role of nurse-midwives in the complicated obstetrics practiced in the nation's leading teaching hospitals and the effect of collaborative management of high-risk women by ob-gyn CNM teams on the role of midwives as "the guardians of normal pregnancy" (Sharp & Lewis, 1984).

LA County/University of Southern California Medical Center Women's Hospital, Los Angeles, 1979–1980 Physicians working with nurse-midwives in these settings had their own perspective. In 1985, members of the faculty of the Department of Obstetrics and Gynecology at the University of Southern California School of Medicine described the nurse-midwifery ser-vice at the Los Angeles County/University of Southern California (LAC/USC) Medical Center Women's Hospital (Platt *et al.*, 1985). The physicians' report on this service (published in *Obstetrics and Gynecology*) reflects the concerns of leaders of an academic obstetric and gynecology department that is responsible for providing safe, effective care to a large population of low-income women while fulfilling its responsibilities for teaching and research.

Although the nurse-midwifery service was started in 1974, it did not become part of the "mainstream" of health care at the hospital until 1979. The department wanted the nurse-midwives to assist in providing care to the hospital's large volume of obstetric patients and to create "an identity as providers of alternative obstetric services for Hispanic women," (who are the main clientele of the hospital). It was essential that the nurse-midwives establish a reputation among the professional staff of being capable of "productivity on many levels." The paper reported the following accomplishments from a two-year period during which twelve CNMs held clinical or academic appointments in the School of Medicine (Platt *et al.*, 1985).

- The CNM/ob-gyn team operated two nurse-midwifery educational programs, a twelve-month basic program and a three-month internship to help recent nurse-midwifery graduates in "the transition from a student nurse-midwife to a fully functioning staff member" and to provide "further exposure and experience for new graduates who seek positions in the community or private practice sector." In addition, the nurse-midwives were active participants in departmental conferences and clinical rounds and assumed responsibility for some parts of the clinical teaching of medical students on the labor and delivery unit. The director of the nurse-midwifery service gave lectures on normal labor and birth to the medical students.
- Clinical services provided by nurse-midwives included participation in a breastfeeding clinic, family planning clinics, satellite clinics, a special clinic for pregnant adolescents (staffed entirely by CNMs), and labor and delivery.
- The nurse-midwifery service accepted women who had no known medical problem when they presented for labor and delivery even if they had not received any prenatal care. Women who were low risk at admission to the delivery suite and had been seen by a midwife during prenatal care were delivered by a nurse-midwife whenever possible. All teens who had attended the special clinic for pregnant adolescents were delivered by nurse-midwives. CNMs delivered 14 percent of all babies born at Women's Hospital during 1979–1980. Electronic fetal monitoring was used routinely.
- The perinatal mortality rate was low, only 1 percent of the infants demonstrated clinical signs of fetal distress, and the cesarean section rate was less than 2 percent.

The authors commented on the nurse-midwives' ability to provide safe, effective care "for slightly higher risk patients than traditionally accepted by the established standards for nurse-midwifery. Whereas the presumed role of the nurse-midwife is with the normal, low-risk patient, the perinatal mortality in the higher risk group of patients cared for by the service was favorably low at 1.8 per 1000." They attributed the nurse-midwives' good outcomes to the "extended nursing role," exposure to continued postgraduate education provided by teaching conferences, "integrated medical/midwifery care," and the effect of continuous peer review on the quality of care. The authors assumed that the low cesarean section rate was largely due to the process for selecting patients for nurse-midwifery care but noted that, "even taking these factors into account, the difference observed in the primary cesarean section rate is not fully explained" (Platt *et al.*, 1985).

The Normal Birth Center at the LAC/USC Medical Center Women's Hospital, Los Angeles, 1981–1992 The second study from the LAC/USC Women's Hospital described the policies and practices of the Normal Birth Center, which was opened in 1981 as an in-hospital unit staffed by nurse-midwives, nurses, and pediatric nurse practitioners. The hospital developed the new unit in response to an ever-increasing demand for obstetric services at Women's Hospital. The article reported outcomes of more than thirty thousand births at the Normal Birth Center between 1981 and 1992 (Greulich *et al.*, 1994). More than 90 percent of the women cared for at Women's Hospital were on Medicaid or some other form of government assistance; 95 percent were Hispanic.

The Normal Birth Center (NBC) is three floors above the high-risk labor and delivery unit. It has six birth rooms, each with a private bathroom, and three 4-bed postpartum rooms. Babies stay with their mothers; there is no separate nursery. All women who come to Women's Hospital for childbirth are examined by a nurse-midwife or an obstetric resident. Those who meet the NBC criteria are admitted if there is room; they can not choose to be admitted to the regular obstetric unit. Criteria for selecting women into the NBC results in a "mixed risk" caseload; although women with complications such as preterm labor, hypertension, or twins are excluded, women with some high-risk conditions (e.g., prior cesarean section, anemia) deliver at the NBC. Two CNMs and five or six registered nurses and support staff are on duty during every shift; no physicians work on the unit. Women admitted to the NBC are encouraged to have the support person(s) of their choice with them throughout labor and delivery; children may be present. Women are encouraged to be up and about, to walk. All women have twenty minutes of electronic fetal monitoring (EFM) immediately after admission to assess the condition of the fetus; however neither internal EFM nor intravenous fluids are used routinely. Women are encouraged to drink fluids throughout labor; food may be consumed. Analgesics and tranquilizers are available but are not used often. Walking, showering, changing positions, and emotional support are the main methods of pain relief. Women who want epidural anesthesia are transferred to the high-risk unit. Oxytocin is not used to strengthen contractions, although nipple stimulation may be used (Greulich *et al.*, 1994).

Mother and baby stay in the birth room for two hours after the birth and then go to a postpartum room for twelve to twenty-four hours. Women are told to return to the main Women's Hospital admitting room if they have problems after discharge, are asked to bring their babies to the NBC follow-up clinic to be examined by a pediatric nurse practitioner two to three days after discharge, and are given appointments for a four-week family planning visit at Women's Hospital or a health department clinic. Women whose social situation indicates the need for additional assistance are referred to visiting nurse or public health services (Greulich *et al.*, 1994).

More than 36,000 women were admitted to the NBC between June 1981 and the end of 1992. Seventeen percent were transferred to the high-risk obstetric unit; 83 percent gave birth in the NBC ($N = 30,311$). There were no intrapartum maternal or fetal deaths among all 36,410 admissions. The transfer rate was 13.1 percent for women admitted during 1985–1992 ($N = 25,890$). The primary cesarean section rate was 1.8 percent; the overall operative birth rate (cesareans, forceps, and vacuum extractions) was 4.1 percent (Greulich *et al.*, 1994). These results were similar to those from the National Birth Center Study, except that there were no intrapartum fetal deaths among women admitted to the LAC/USC Women's Hospital Normal Birth Center, and the cesarean section rate was lower. (The difference in cesareans is not surprising because the NBC population consisted almost entirely of low-income Hispanic women, who have a particularly low cesarean section rate.) This study shows that nurse-midwives can provide the low-intervention/good-outcome care associated with free-standing birth centers in an in-hospital birth center within a tertiary academic medical center—if the in-hospital unit meets the autonomy criteria for an authentic birth center (see Chapter 5).

The University of Michigan Hospital, Ann Arbor, May 1988–February 1993 A study from the University of Michigan differs from the others by describing care provided within an academic medical cen-ter to *private* nurse-midwifery patients, com-paring it with care provided to low-risk private patients of obstetricians in the same hospital and health care system, and analyzing the data to determine whether differences in care were due to factors other than the care provider (Oakley *et al.*, 1995).

The major differences in prenatal care involved use of ultrasounds and the proportion of women receiving education and counseling on a variety of subjects: The nurse-midwives' clients had only about half as many prenatal ultrasounds (0.9 per woman, on average) as the physicians' clients (1.7 per woman), but were more likely to receive education and counseling about sexuality during pregnancy (97 percent versus 69 percent), smoking (65 percent of smokers in the group cared for by CNMs versus 38 percent of smokers cared for by physicians, but no difference in the proportion who actually stopped smoking), nutrition (98 percent versus 81 percent), and specific suggestions about food choices (92 percent versus 71 percent). The nurse-midwives provided most of the nutrition counseling to their clients (97 percent), whereas nurses provided most of the nutrition counseling to the physician's clients (85 percent).

The physicians' clients had more frequent use of ten kinds of interventions during labor and delivery: intravenous fluids, continuous EFM, internal placement of intrauterine pressure gauges and electrodes, artificial rupture of the membranes, use of analgesics during labor, epidurals during labor, transfer to a delivery room (instead of giving birth in the labor room), episiotomies, use of forceps, and cesarean sections (13.0 percent versus 19.3 percent for the physicians' patients). The nurse-midwives' clients were much more likely to consume fluid and food by mouth during labor, to have the fetal heart rate monitored by noncontinuous methods (doppler or fetoscope), to use a variety of comfort measures during labor (frequent changes of position, relaxation techniques, massage, ambulation, taking showers, listening to music), and to give birth without anesthesia. The nurse-midwives' clients reported a greater sense of empathy with their main care provider (Oakley *et al.*, 1995).

The researchers used multivariate analysis to determine whether differences in the women's prenatal medical condition, personal characteristics, and preferences about

their care could account for the differences in the care provided to the nurse-midwives' clients as compared with the physician's clients. Taking all of the other factors into account helped to explain the differences between the care experienced by the two groups of women. The woman's own expectations about the use of comfort measures was the single most influential factor in determining how many measures were actually used (Oakley *et al.*, 1995). When a wide variety of socioeconomic factors, and the woman's evolving medical condition and preferences regarding her care were considered in the analysis, the difference in the cesarean section rate between the two groups of women declined to just below the level of statistical significance (Oakley, 1996). But whether the primary care provider was an obstetrician or a CNM remained a statistically significant factor for most of the differences, even when all of the other factors had been controlled. Whether the woman was taken care of by an obstetrician or a nurse-midwife was by far the single most important factor associated with her perception of empathy with her care provider (Oakley *et al.*, 1995).

These examples demonstrate the wide range of nurse-midwifery practice styles possible within tertiary/teaching hospitals. They also show (1) the evolution of nurse-midwifery practice during a twenty-year period of time, (2) the influence of the patients themselves on the care provided, and (3) the impact of establishing a midwifery unit that is physically separate from the high-risk obstetric unit.

Nurse-midwifery practice in these settings changed over time—over calendar time (as new research gave midwives a stronger basis for resisting the routine use of some procedures) and as nurse-midwifery services were in operation for longer periods of time within specific institutions. Nurse-midwives' use of episiotomy at Grady Hospital in Atlanta decreased steadily between

1973 and 1982; nurse-midwives used EFM routinely for births they attended at Women's Hospital in Los Angeles during 1979 and 1980 but did not use it routinely in the birth center they established at the same hospital in 1981. Nurse-midwifery services in each of these settings were small and tenuous when they started. They were in institutions led by academic obstetricians, most of whom believed that routine episiotomies and EFM are part of a high standard of modern, effective maternity care. Evidence to the contrary exists now, but did not exist then. Midwives who criticized routine use of those methods at that time could only cite their philosophical beliefs about pregnancy and their own experience, which were different from the philosophy and experience of tertiary hospital obstetricians. It took reports of large randomized, controlled clinical trials published in the most prestigious medical journals to convince academic obstetricians that these methods are not necessary. In fact, both of these methods are routinely used in most academic hospitals even now, despite the evidence.

In addition, over time nurse-midwifery services, such as those at Grady and at Women's Hospital, proved their worth and earned the respect needed to buttress the midwives' requests to practice somewhat differently from the obstetricians. Nurse-midwifery was still quite small and new at the beginning of this period—not well known or understood by obstetricians, many of whom were initially very skeptical. In both cases, the nurse-midwives earned respect as they made substantial contributions and met the standards and expectations of their particular environments: The nurse-midwives at Grady developed the episodic model of care to make it possible for them to fill in as the obstetric residents became busier and busier. In the words of the obstetric leaders at Women's Hospital in Los Angeles, it was essential that the nurse-midwives prove themselves capable of "productivity on many levels."

Practice in Small Towns and Rural Areas

Some CNMs have established small practices of their own or have been invited into physician's practices in small towns and rural communities. The following examples exemplify CNM practices in rural settings.

In 1986, all obstetricians at St. Claire Medical Center in Morehead, Kentucky, announced their intention to exclude Medicaid patients from their practice, threatened to do so, or threatened to leave the area. The hospital arranged for four family physicians (FPs) to establish a maternity clinic near the hospital, which they staffed on an alternating basis. After three years, the FPs felt overwhelmed with maternity patients, and two of them left. By this time it had become clear that the continuous presence of a single care provider was needed, and the hospital hired a CNM. Ten months later they hired another. The result was a three-tiered maternity care program. CNMs provided routine prenatal care and attended uncomplicated births. FPs assumed responsibility for complicated pregnancies, conducted instrument-assisted deliveries, tended to the nonobstetric problems of pregnant women, and took care of newborns and infants. The obstetricians performed cesareans and consulted on particularly high-risk cases, often during biweekly meetings at the maternity center (Hueston & Murry, 1992).

During the first five years, the number of deliveries at the hospital increased because the program attracted women from surrounding areas. In addition, there was a decrease in deliveries to women with no prenatal care and a trend toward women starting care earlier. The proportion of births attended by obstetricians declined from 83 percent in 1984 to 27 percent in 1989. During that year each of the two nurse-midwives attended an average of ninety deliveries; each of four FPs attended an average of fifty-eight deliveries, and two obstetricians attended forty-two, including all cesarean sections (Hueston & Murry, 1992).

Declining deliveries at Mary Imogene Bassett Hospital in Cooperstown, New York, resulted in closure of the hospital's obstetric residency program in 1986. The hospital, which serves ten rural counties in upstate New York, developed a CNM service to fill the gap left by the obstetric residents. The CNM service has functioned continuously at this hospital since 1986; by 1996, it employed nine CNMs. Although the nurse-midwifery service is part of the department of obstetrics and gynecology, the director of the service reports to both the vice president for nursing and the chief of obstetrics and gynecology (Stone *et al.*, 1996).

Ob-gyns provide care to women who request to have all of their care provided by a physician. Management of all other women is determined by their risk status. CNMs take care of low-risk women; CNMs and ob-gyns comanage the care of high-risk women. Ob-gyns consult with the CNMs as needed. CNMs provide prenatal care at four of the fourteen clinics that provide primary care to people in the area served by the hospital. A CNM and an ob-gyn are always on call for the hospital's birth center (Stone *et al.*, 1996).

The number of babies born at the hospital increased from 336 in 1986 to 793 in 1994. CNMs attended 98 percent of the nonsurgical births in 1994. Other outcomes included decreases in the incidence of episiotomies (accompanied by reductions in third- and fourth-degree lacerations) and cesarean sections; the latter was accompanied by increases in the proportion of vaginal deliveries for twins, babies in breech presentation, and women with prior cesareans (Stone *et al.*, 1996).

Judith Kurokara has practiced in Wolf Point, Montana, as a nurse since 1978, as a family nurse practitioner since 1982, and as an FNP and CNM since 1988. She obtained both her FNP and nurse-midwifery education through distance learning programs that allowed her to continue to live and raise her family in Wolf Point while preparing herself to become a major part of the local health care system. Wolf Point is part of the Fort Peck Indian Reservation; about three-fourths of Kurokora's patients are Native Americans. She provides prenatal care at the local Indian Health Service (IHS) clinic and at the local level I hospital (not run by the IHS), where she attends about one hundred births per year.

Although pregnant women account for about 70 percent of her work, Kurokara believes that the FNP/CNM combination is essential for practice in Wolf Point. The two elements weave together; she takes care of a woman during pregnancy and then takes care of the baby, other children in the family, and the father. The IHS sends an obstetrician to Wolf Point to provide consultation on high-risk IHS patients. Wolf Point's only physician, an FP in private practice, provides most of the other backup, including cesarean sections. It is also possible to fly a woman to the nearest tertiary hospital, which is hundreds of miles away. Kurokara now has a CNEP student and stays linked to other CNMs practicing in rural areas through CNEP's electronic bulletin board (Kurokawa, 1996).

Barbara Kaye has practiced nurse-midwifery in Cottage Grove, Oregon, since 1977. She went there to work in a free-standing birth center that closed a year after she arrived. Wanting to stay, she approached all physicians practicing obstetrics in Cottage Grove; all were FPs, and none had enough maternity patients to absorb a partner. The local level I hospital hired her, gave her an office in the hospital and privileges as a member of the "allied professional staff," and collected the fees for her services. All seven physicians who delivered babies at the hospital agreed to provide her with clinical collaboration and consultation. Each of her clients was asked to select a backup doctor and to meet him during the prenatal period. Eventually Kaye learned to help women choose a physician whose philosophy and practice would be most consistent with the woman's hopes for her own birth (Kaye, 1991).

This arrangement continued for six years, during which Kaye attended about one-third of the births in Cottage Grove. In 1984 she became an employee of a family medicine group practice; she stayed with them for another six years. In 1990 the family physicians moved their practice out of town, to a city. Kaye went back to her previous arrangement at the hospital, attending about half of the births in Cottage Grove and using whatever physicians were practicing obstetrics there for consultation. In 1995 a part-time CNM joined the practice, allowing Kaye to be "on call" for less than twenty-four hours per day, seven days per week, for the first time in eighteen years.

Nurse-Midwifery Services to Meet the Needs of Special Populations

Many nurse-midwifery services have been developed for the purpose of meeting the needs of a specific group of women. These services are often initiated by officials and staff of local public health departments, university medical centers, and not-for-profit private/voluntary organizations with responsibility or special concern about particular groups of socioeconomically distressed women (or girls) and their babies. In recent years, some nurse-midwifery services have specialized in the care of HIV-positive women. Evaluations of services devoted to the care of adolescents in settings as diverse as Chicago and rural North Carolina have found better outcomes, especially a lower incidence of low birth weight, for very young teenage mothers when their care is provided by nurse-midwives (Brucker & Muellner, 1985; Piechnik & Corbett, 1985). Special nurse-midwifery services have also been developed to care for particular populations of Hispanic women, especially migrant farm workers. Nurse-midwifery services within the Indian Health Service also fall within this category.

Nurse-Midwifery in Health Maintenance Organizations

HMOs have been leaders in developing innovative approaches to cost-effective health care. They were among the first components of the health care system to offer nurse-midwifery care to women who can exercise choice in their use of health care.* Unlike services that separate patients into "low-risk" and "high-risk" groups and assign low-risk women to a CNM service and high-risk women to an MD service, many HMOs use a multidisciplinary team to provide care to the entire group of women. Although obstetrician–gynecologists have primary responsibility for complicated pregnancies and high-risk deliveries and CNMs manage the care of most uncomplicated pregnancies, nurse-midwives may comanage the care of women with complications, patients are not classified as "nurse-midwifery clients" and "physician clients," and there may be no special "nurse-midwifery service" (Goings, 1986).

A 1989 report described the role of CNMs in the Kaiser Permanente Medical Center in Anaheim, California (Bell & Mills, 1989). Women see a CNM or ob–gyn nurse practitioner (NP) at their first prenatal visit and a physician at their second visit, after which they see whomever is available, although every woman sees a physician at least once during each trimester (third) of her pregnancy. Although physicians concentrate on the care of women with medically complicated pregnancies, CNMs and NPs provide education, guidance, and additional support to women with complications. At least one obstetrician and one CNM are on duty in the labor and delivery unit at all times. The physicians deliver all women with serious complications and women who want to be delivered by an MD, and assist the CNMs with unexpected complications. In 1982 the Kaiser Permanente Cost/Benefit Analysis Department conducted a cost analysis of the obstetrics and gynecology departments at each of the eight Kaiser medical centers in Southern California, includ-

---

*See Chapter 4 for a discussion of the development of the first HMO nurse-midwifery service.

ing the one in Anaheim, which was the only Kaiser hospital in Southern California using CNMs at that time. The study documented significantly lower costs at Anaheim than at the other hospitals, with no adverse effect on maternal and perinatal mortality. In addition, the majority of the clients at Anaheim (suburban, mainly affluent women) who expressed a preference indicated that they would prefer to be delivered by a nurse-midwife if they had another pregnancy. By 1992 a total of sixty-six nurse-midwives were working in all ten Kaiser hospitals in Southern California, where they were handling 70 percent of all normal births.

Home Births

Nurse-midwives attended 3,412 home births in 1989 and 3,429 in 1990. The number then declined each year until 1993, when it dropped to 2,539. It increased slightly—to 2,591—in 1994.

A retrospective descriptive study conducted by the ACNM Home Birth Committee provides information based on ninety CNM home birth practices between 1987 and 1991, including seventy-eight solo practices and twelve group practices (Anderson & Murphy, 1995). The data collected describe the care provided to 11,788 women who were planning to have home births between 1987 and 1991, including information on women who were transferred to hospitals during the course of a home birth. The study captured between 61 and 72 percent of all home births attended by CNMs during 1989–1991, including home births attended by CNMs in 29 states. The largest numbers occurred in California (28 percent of the total), Pennsylvania (10 percent), and New York (7 percent). More than half of the CNMs had been attending home births for at least five years. Eighty-seven percent of the practices had collaborative agreements with physicians; 86 percent had written protocols or practice guidelines. Most of the midwives (88 percent) always brought an assistant, most often a registered nurse, to help with the birth.

All but one of the practices (99 percent) would not attempt a home birth for women who go into labor at less than thirty-five completed weeks of gestation. Ninety-six percent would not attempt home births for women carrying twins or babies in breech presentation. Only a few practices would consider a home birth for women with these conditions; all of those practices were run by CNMs who had been attending home births for at least five years. Other conditions that were considered contraindications for home birth included hypertension (excluded by 93 percent of the practices), gestation exceeding forty-two weeks (excluded by 61 percent), and previous cesarean section (excluded by 59 percent). Ninety-one percent of the practices transported the woman to a hospital if there was thick meconium in the amniotic fluid (Anderson & Murphy, 1995).

Six percent of the women were referred to other care providers during the prenatal period or at the onset of preterm labor, which accounted for 17 percent of the referrals. Other frequent reasons for prenatal referrals were pregnancy continuing beyond forty-two weeks (11.5 percent of all referrals), breech or other malpresentation (9 percent), hypertension or preeclampsia (8 percent), twins or other multiple gestation (4 percent), gestational diabetes (4 percent), placenta previa or placental abruption (3.5 percent), and diagnosed congenital anomalies (3 percent). In addition, 18 percent of the women left the care of the home birth CNM during their pregnancies because they wanted a different care provider or changed their minds about having a home birth (8 percent), moved outside of the area (7 percent), or their third-party health care plan refused to pay for a home birth (3 percent). This left 11,081 women who began home births under the care of the ninety CNM practices that were included in this study (Anderson & Murphy, 1995).

Ten percent of the women, or their newborns, were transferred to hospitals during labor or shortly after the birth. There were no maternal deaths. The intrapartum and neonatal mortality rate was 1.6 per 1000 births; this is similar to the rate for women in the National Birth Center Study and no higher than rates from studies of low-risk births in hospitals. (See Table 13 in Chapter 11.)

Collaboration with Physicians

Ideal renditions of the role of a midwife and the role of a physician are complementary. Most women have uncomplicated pregnancies, but some do not, and even the healthiest are at risk of unexpected complications. Thus some women actually need—and all should have—access to medical care throughout their pregnancies. In addition, all women, even the sickest, need the education, respect, comfort, and personal support provided by a midwife. Healthy women involved in the labor of birth benefit greatly from avoiding unnecessary interventions, intrusions, and deprivations that can frighten or discourage them, sap their energy, diffuse their focus, and rob them of their rightful wonder at the experience of giving birth. Packaging the services of midwives and physicians in a way that facilitates appropriate use of the capabilities and expertise of both professions provides the best possible care to women. Midwives and physicians also benefit by being able to focus on providing the kinds of care that each is most interested in and is best prepared and suited to provide. Because midwives have a limited scope of practice, knowing their limits and when to involve a physician are important aspects of each midwife's practice.

One of Mary Breckinridge's first actions in developing the Frontier Nursing Service was recruiting physicians into that part of Kentucky and developing protocols that outlined a collaborative relationship between the midwives and the physicians. The assumption that nurse-midwifery practice serves clients best when it occurs within a system that guarantees access to medical care has been a central principle from the beginning (Tom, 1982). The philosophy, definitions, standards, and other key documents of the ACNM all address the concept of collaboration and cooperation between physicians and nurse-midwives. Although the ACNM defines nurse-midwifery practice as "the independent management of women's health care," it requires nurse-midwives to practice "within a health care system that provides for consultation, collaborative management or referral as indicated by the health status of the client." The *ACNM Standards for the Practice of Nurse-Midwifery* require CNMs to have "a safe mechanism for obtaining medical consultation, collaboration and referral" and written policies or practice guidelines that describe the limits of independent nurse-midwifery management and the conditions and circumstances that require medical consultation, collaboration, and referral. Nurse-midwives queried in 1985 identified "suitable MD collaboration" and "basic philosophical agreement among the CNMs and physicians in the practice" as the first and second most important ingredients for success, ranking ahead of the "absence of unreasonable constraints from state laws and regulations" and "access to practice settings," that is, the ability to get hospital privileges (Haas & Rooks, 1986).

In 1985 an ad hoc ACNM committee collected data on 361 of 664 CNM practices listed in the *1985 ACNM Nurse-Midwifery Service Directory*; 288 of the practices provided information on medical collaboration. Eighty-nine percent had backup from one or more obstetrician–gynecologists, 11 percent from a family practice physician. Five percent also had a formal collaborative arrangement with a pediatrician (Burst, 1987).

Although there are many possible administrative mechanisms for achieving collaboration, there are really only two basic models: (1) medical collaboration in a midwifery practice or service and (2) medical/midwifery joint practice. Each model has its own characteristics, advantages, and potential problems.

Medical Collaboration in a Nurse-Midwifery Practice or Service

In this model the primary ongoing responsibility for the woman's care rests with the nurse-midwife. The CNM's responsibilities include identifying the need for physician input in the care of a specific patient and obtaining the necessary input, whether by consultation, comanagement, or referral (sometimes called a "transfer"). The midwife retains primary responsibility for the patient unless and until an agreement is made to turn part or all of that responsibility over to a physician. It is her responsibility to seek information from a physician (i.e., consultation) when needed, and what she does as a result of the consultation is her responsibility. She could decide not to follow his* advice, fully or in part, or to seek the opinion of another physician. Once the midwife has involved a physician in the care of a particular woman, she and the physician may jointly decide to comanage the woman's care, that is, to work as a team and share responsibility. Or they may agree to a referral or transfer; in that case the midwife relinquishes primary responsibility to the physician, although she may continue to provide certain aspects of the patient's care, with the physician's agreement.

Although it is up to the nurse-midwife to initiate the physician's involvement in a patient's care, both parties work under an agreement that requires the CNM to seek physician consultation (at a minimum) in specific situations. It is important for the CNM to make clear whether she is asking for an opinion (i.e., consulting) or asking the MD to make a plan for the patient's care (comanagement or transfer of primary responsibility from the midwife to the physician). If she is consulting, the MD may not have the right to take over. If she is asking for a plan, the nurse-midwife may not have the right to refuse the plan he suggests (King, 1995).

This model of collaboration is used when there is clear assignment of responsibility for specific patients to a particular CNM or nurse-midwifery service, for instance, as the means to provide medical collaboration to a private practice composed entirely of CNMs. With this model, women who seek or are assigned to midwifery care during the prenatal period expect to see a particular midwife or a member of the midwifery practice or service at most prenatal visits and to be attended by a midwife during childbirth. This means that one or more midwives must be on duty or on call for labor and delivery at all times. A physician must also be available ("on call") at all times; however, it is not necessary for the physician to be constantly present at the hospital.

Arrangements for medical collaboration in a nurse-midwifery practice or service vary with the size, institutional setting, and other characteristics of the practice and the community. Midwifery practices or services that are part of large institutions usually obtain their medical backup from the obstetrics and gynecology department of the institution; in this situation, the midwifery service is often a unit within the ob-gyn department, for example, the Normal Birth Center at the LAC/USC Women's Hospital in Los Angeles. Private midwifery services arrange for medical collaboration in a variety of ways, including contracts with individual physicians or groups of physicians. Midwives in rural areas may need several layers of physician participation, for instance, a local family physician for medical problems, an obstetrician or surgeon close enough to perform a timely cesarean section, and a perinatologist with privileges at a level III hospital for telephone consultation and referral of women and newborns with complications that require more sophisticated care. For example, the CNM in Wolf Point, Montana, uses the services of an itinerant Indian Health Ser-

---

*For convenience, female pronouns are used in reference to midwives and male pronouns are used in reference to physicians, despite the fact that there are both male and female members of both professions.

vice obstetrician; a private, local FP who can perform cesareans; and a life/flight service to provide emergency transportation to the nearest tertiary hospital.

Several potential problems may arise in relation to medical collaboration for a nurse-midwifery practice or service:

- Obstetrical collaboration may not be available, either because no appropriate* physician is available (as in an isolated rural situation) or because no appropriate physician will agree to collaborate. A nurse-midwife cannot practice if she cannot find a physician who is willing to work out a satisfactory collaboration agreement. As a result nurse-midwives have been unable to practice in some communities.
- Dependence on physician participation makes nurse-midwives vulnerable to coercive restraints on their practice. For example, a CNM who provides care to poor women may not be allowed to take care of women who have insurance; the CNM may not be allowed to attend home births; the CNM may be required to use intravenous infusions and continuous EFM on every patient.
- Nurse-midwives may have to use backup from physicians whose practice style or standards are incompatible with nurse-midwifery practice. As a result, clients who experience complications may be confronted with an authoritative or interventionist style of care that is offensive to them and is what they went to the midwife to avoid.
- CNMs may have to provide emergency care to patients whose conditions are beyond their scope of practice if the physician fails to meet his obligations.

The *Joint Statement of Practice Relationships Between Obstetricians and Gynecologists and Cer-*

tified Nurse-Midwives[†] states that "quality of care is enhanced by the interdependent practice of the obstetrician/gynecologist and the certified nurse-midwife working in a relationship of mutual respect, trust and professional responsibility" and that "the appropriate practice of the certified nurse-midwife includes the participation and involvement of the obstetrician/gynecologist." It urges ob-gyns to respond when CNMs ask for their participation. However, the "interdependence" between CNMs and obstetricians (or other physicians) is lopsided, that is, not mutual, and thus not real interdependence. Physicians have support from nurses in their offices and in the hospital and can practice without collaborating with a midwife. A nurse-midwife, in contrast, cannot practice if no physician is willing to work with her. Many potential nurse-midwifery practices and birth centers have been stopped before they started and others have closed because no physician in the community was willing to collaborate.

Lack of physicians willing to back up a nurse-midwifery service can even be a problem when the midwifery service is part of an institution that includes a department of obstetrics and gynecology. If key leaders of the obstetric department are not in favor of midwifery, it is difficult to establish and sustain a nurse-midwifery service over a long period of time, even if the administration of the hospital or other organization is sincere in its desire to have one. In addition, if a nurse-midwife is determined to establish a practice in a particular community, she may have no choice but to work with a physician whose practice style is incompatible with hers.

Another kind of problem can result when the institution is eager for a midwifery service, usually to take care of large numbers

---

*A backup physician must practice obstetrics, have hospital privileges, and be capable of performing cesarean sections.

---

†The ACOG/ACNM joint statement was developed and approved by the American College of Obstetricians and Gynecologists (ACOG) and the American College of Nurse-Midwives (ACNM) in 1982. See Chapter 5 for additional information.

of poor women, but fails to provide medical backup that is both quantitatively and qualitatively adequate. Nurse-midwives know when to involve a physician. If no physician comes when she calls, or if the physician's response is inadequate, nurse-midwives, who cannot abandon their patients, may be forced to provide care to women with complications that are beyond their scope of practice. Midwifery services that provide care to poor women in some of the nation's beleaguered inner-city public hospitals have had to deal with this situation. Many fear that this problem will become worse as state and federal funding become more limited.

A 1995 *New York Times* exposé of "mismanaged care" in New York City's public hospitals focused on problems related to maternity care—hospitals inundated with high-risk patients, overcrowding, understaffing, lack of access to necessary drugs, and heavy reliance on nurse-midwives backed up by too few physicians. Many of the physicians who were available were young, inexperienced residents working with little guidance from senior physicians, doctors from developing countries who were unfamiliar with modern technology and treatments, or medical school graduates who had either failed or had not yet taken their licensing examinations (Fritsch & Baquet, 1995). Although the hospitals were supposed to provide "attending physicians" (fully qualified senior obstetricians to supervise the inexperienced, less qualified doctors), studies have shown that residents in most of the New York City public hospitals were largely unsupervised. Specific tragedies reported in the series included two instances in which nurse-midwives identified severe fetal distress but could not get a doctor to come in time. In one case, two of the three physicians assigned to the delivery suite were performing a cesarean section and one was in the emergency room.

The *New York Times* series focused on the North Central Bronx (NCB) Hospital, which serves some of New York's poorest areas—neighborhoods afflicted by high rates of AIDS and other sexually transmitted diseases, domestic violence, drug and alcohol addiction, unemployment, and despair. NCB functioned with too few doctors for the number of patients. Nurse-midwives provided most of the care to most of the pregnant women (Fritsch & Baquet, 1995; Haire & Elsberry, 1991; Clark-Coller, 1995). An earlier publication described maternity care and outcomes at NCB in 1988, when the obstetric staff consisted of twenty CNMs and fourteen obstetricians. Although 70 percent of the mothers were "high risk" (which does not mean that all of them had actual complications), it was run as a nurse-midwifery service. CNMs saw every patient at her first prenatal visit and made the initial assessment and triage decision regarding every woman admitted to the hospital during labor. The service's midwifery model of care made it popular among the poor and racial/ethnic minority women of the Bronx. Women who wanted to deliver their babies at NCB soon learned that they would not be transferred to another hospital if they were in labor when they arrived at NCB. Although the service was designed to care for 2,200 mothers per year, more than 3,500 babies were born there in 1988; 86 percent of the deliveries were managed by nurse-midwives (Haire & Elsberry, 1991).

The head of the Health and Hospitals Corporation of New York City concluded that the midwives at North Central Bronx "may have taken on too much." The Chief of Obstetrics at NCB blamed an exhausted system—year after year of too many patients and too few doctors—and described the labor and delivery suite as functioning like "a war room" (Fritsch & Baquet, 1995). The New York State Health Commissioner said that "We should not have instances in which nurse-midwives are desperately seeking the assistance of physicians in crisis situations, with no help arriving" (Linden & Urang, 1995).

Letters flowed to the editor of the *New York Times*. The chairman of the New York

State section of the American College of Obstetricians and Gynecologists affirmed ACOG's support for a collaborative team approach to maternity care but warned against overreliance on midwives as a way for underfinanced health care systems to save money (Boyce, 1995). A letter from a World Health Organization physician and a letter from seven family physicians who had received part of their obstetrical training from CNMs at North Central Bronx urged that the problems be resolved by strengthening the obstetric support without undermining the essential role of certified nurse-midwives (Wagner, M., 1995; Soloway *et al.*, 1995). The result was new regulations that detail what midwives may and may not do on their own, demand that senior physicians assume responsibility for the care of women with serious complications, and require the doctors to be available and respond when they are summoned by midwives (Fritsch, 1995).

Role of Physicians in a Medical/Midwifery Partnership or Team

The other major model for MD/CNM collaboration involves midwives and physicians working together as an interdisciplinary partnership or team that has joint responsibility for the care of a group of patients. The Department of Obstetrics and Gynecology at Kaiser Permanente Medical Center in Anaheim, California, is organized according to this model. Physicians concentrate on the care of women with medically complicated pregnancies, consult with the midwives, and participate in comanagement of some patients. Midwives concentrate on the care of women with normal, uncomplicated pregnancies but comanage the care of some patients and provide education and support to all. It is not necessary to make very clear distinctions between consultation, comanagement and referral; other than the general principle that physicians focus on complications and pathology and midwives concentrate on women who are normal, the workload can be divided in any way that suits

the group. In a joint practice, a physician must always be available for labor and delivery backup, but the midwives do not necessarily have to provide around-the-clock coverage. This model provides maximum flexibility and is very efficient, for example, making it easier for obstetricians to schedule uninterrupted office visits and to have uninterrupted sleep the nights before they are scheduled to perform surgery. The cost is less continuity of care and dilution of the one-to-one relationship between an individual midwife or doctor and a client.

Medical/midwifery collaboration in a joint practice contains the potential for medical infringement on midwifery practice decisions, either by inappropriate demands regarding general policies (such as imposition of a rigid rule against eating during labor), or by always resolving interdisciplinary disagreements about the care of particular patients by accepting the judgment of the physician (such as when a physician thinks the situation requires a cesarean section, but the midwife thinks the woman may be able to deliver vaginally, but needs to rest or sleep for awhile to regain her energy and establish more effective labor). Some disagreements are to be expected, especially because of the philosophical differences between midwives and physicians described in Chapter 6—differences in beliefs about the nature of pregnancy and birth and the appropriate role of clients in relationship to health professionals. The use of differing criteria for considering a particular woman's condition as "normal" (i.e., appropriate for midwifery care) or "abnormal" (i.e., pathologic and thus requiring *medical* expertise) is probably the most difficult problem to resolve.

Effective collaboration between midwives and physicians requires prevention or appropriate resolution of such disagreements. Conflict can largely be prevented when the physicians and midwives have compatible beliefs and values, when there is good communication, and when the medical and other institutional leaders have a genuine understanding of the nature and purpose of midwifery—that it is a separate profession, with its own philosophy and expertise, and that, although it overlaps with medicine, it is not part of the medical profession and much of its expertise and role are unique. Fortunately, this circumstance is becoming increasingly common, as more and more physicians have experience with CNMs. Where this is not the case, physicians are apt to have authority over most clinical matters. If the situation plays out so that every conflict is automatically resolved by accepting a physician's judgment or decision over that of a midwife, midwives cannot function as professionals. Such a practice can provide only a compromised and diluted form of midwifery care.

Some confusion can arise from the fact that nurse-midwives are nurses as well as midwives and function under the nurse practice act in many states. They may be seen as nurse specialists, rather than as midwives, in services where they play a significant role in the care of women with serious complications. In those instances, CNMs may combine or move back and forth between the role of a nurse providing medical care to a sick person under the authority of a physician and the role of a midwife providing midwifery care to normal women under her own authority. It is not surprising that people get confused.

ACNM's Agreements and Disagreements with ACOG

The following is a summary of key points in the *Joint Statement of Practice Relationships Between Obstetrician-Gynecologists and Certified Nurse-Midwives* regarding collaboration:

- Appropriate CNM practice includes the participation and involvement of an ob-gyn.
- There should be mutually agreed on written guidelines or protocols that define the individual and shared responsibilities of both the CNM(s) and the

ob-gyn(s), provide for ongoing communication, and define the circumstances that require consultation.
- The CNM(s) and ob-gyn(s) should participate in joint evaluation of their practice or service through periodic chart reviews, case reviews, evaluations of patients, and review of outcome statistics.
- Clinical care provided by the maternity care team should be directed by a qualified ob-gyn. This does not imply that the physician must be physically present when the CNM is giving care to a patient.
- All administrative relationships should be mutually agreed on by the participating parties.

In 1995 ACOG developed a new document entitled *Guidelines for Implementing Collaborative Practice* (ACOG, 1995). Although there was a CNM on the committee that developed the guidelines, ACOG did not seek input from the ACNM. The guidelines were written to assist an obstetrician–gynecologist who is considering or has decided to develop a collaborative practice with one or more clinical nurse specialists, CNMs, nurse practitioners, or physician assistants. Most aspects of the document deal with all four kinds of "nonphysician providers" as a group and are not specific to the collaborative relationship between ob-gyns and nurse-midwives. In addition, it focuses on interdisciplinary collaboration within a practice that is *directed* by a physician who *employs* the other professionals according to his need: An obstetrician who needs assistance with deliveries, on-call schedules, or in-hospital obstetric care is advised to hire a CNM. Nurse practitioners are recommended "if the practice specializes in high-risk obstetrics" and has many patients on bed rest who require close monitoring and psychosocial support. A gynecologist who does a lot of surgery should consider a physician assistant, who can assist the surgeon during operations and help with preoperative and postoperative patient management. A clinical nurse specialist is recommended "if the practice includes a subspecialty such as infertility and has increased needs for patient counseling and education." Although other kinds of collaboration (i.e., in which the ob-gyn is not the employer) are not described, the preface explains that the guidelines "should not be construed as excluding other acceptable . . . practice variations" (ACOG, 1995).

The ACOG guidelines are very positive about the benefits of multidisciplinary practice, noting that bringing health care professionals with different but complementary knowledge and skills together increases access to services, as well as their scope and quality, for instance, by providing "greater opportunities to educate and counsel patients with the goal of preventing disease, promoting wellness, and increasing compliance with treatment regimens during illness" (ACOG, 1995). Nevertheless, CNMs and the ACNM are critical of some aspects of the ACOG document, especially because its description of nurse-midwifery practice omits the word "independent," which is a critical part of the ACNM definition, and its statement that obstetrician–gynecologists are "ultimately responsible" for care provided by the "nonphysician providers" with whom they collaborate. The ACNM retorted that some aspects of the guidelines "are antithetical to the concept of collaboration, discount the distinct professional and legal status of the nurse-midwife," and would increase the cost of providing care. Implementation of those concepts would make physicians ultimately responsible for the content of nurse-midwifery care, tending to obviate the important differences between nurse-midwifery care and medical care (Roberts, 1995a, 1996a).

Collaboration with Family Physicians

Although most CNMs collaborate with obstetrician–gynecologists, some, especially those who work in rural areas, collaborate primarily with FPs or general practitioners. Despite the American Academy of Family Physicians' hostile official position on nurse-

midwives (see Chapter 5), the AAFP "strongly endorses the newer concepts in family-oriented obstetrics such as bonding and alternative settings while in hospitals," and the general philosophy and orientation of family physicians has much in common with that of midwives. Both disciplines are family-centered and holistic, focus on the pregnant woman within the context of her family, and value and use knowledge from the behavioral, as well as the biological and clinical sciences. Both emphasize the preventive aspects of health care, foster self-determination, and focus on helping clients take responsibility for their own health (Carr, 1986). Although family physicians tend to use fewer interventions than obstetricians use during normal labor and delivery (Rosenberg & Klein, 1987; Reid *et al.*, 1989), their practice is closer to that of obstetricians than to the practices of midwives (Rosenblatt *et al.*, 1997). Nurse-midwives observe that this is probably because FPs have not learned midwifery interventions; lacking them, they have to fall back on obstetric procedures (Howe, 1995).

Like CNMs, FPs mainly care for women whose pregnancies are within the range of normal and involve obstetricians in the care of women with serious complications. Of course, the actual scope of practice of individual FPs and CNMs varies. Although the American Board of Family Practice requires only three months of obstetrics and gynecology training during a family practice residency, FPs with a special interest or need to practice obstetrics can obtain additional training and experience. Some CNMs have more expertise in obstetrics than most FPs, and some FPs have more expertise in this area than most CNMs. The appropriateness of collaboration can only be addressed within the context of a specific situation. Most FPs who practice obstetrics can perform cesarean sections and use forceps, both essential capabilities for a physician who backs up a midwife, and, unlike CNMs, FPs are not restricted in the medications they can prescribe. However, nurse-midwives who practice with family physicians or use them for consultation and referral also need to have a collaborative relationship with an obstetrician, who may live further away. The practices in Morehead, Kentucky, and Wolf Point, Montana, described earlier in this chapter, provide examples of how rural practitioners build networks that utilize available resources to meet their patients' needs.

Although there are positive aspects to having a more similar philosophy and practice style, nurse-midwives need to collaborate with physicians who have a *different* scope of practice—physicians who can do what CNMs cannot. However, many CNMs and FPs enjoy working together, and there are advantages to the arrangement. In 1986 an FP in the Department of Family Medicine at the State University of New York proposed that FPs could overcome barriers to providing maternity care and become more involved in the care of children and families by allying themselves with CNMs (Feinbloom, 1986). Although malpractice concerns were thought to be the main reason for declining FP participation in obstetrics, other factors contribute to this trend: the large proportion of rural women who are indigent, some FPs' insecurity about the adequacy of their obstetric training, the difficulty of maintaining office hours while attending women in labor, and being on constant call for births (Hueston & Murry, 1992; Carr, 1986). Bringing nurse-midwives into the program developed to care for Medicaid-eligible women at St. Claire Medical Center in Morehead, Kentucky, provided some relief to all of those problems for family physicians in the area (Hueston & Murry, 1992). Collaboration with FPs also holds a particular advantage for rural CNMs, who need to work with someone who can manage the many nonobstetric, nongynecologic medical problems of their patients (Carr, 1986). Potential disadvantages for FPs include eventual loss of normal obstetrics, which may be one of the most rewarding parts of their practice. In addi-

tion, if the nurse-midwife takes care of all the normal pregnancies, the family physician may lose his skills in that area. In the long run, that becomes a problem for the midwife, as well as the physician.

Supervision and Vicarious Legal Liability

Collaboration does not imply supervision. Avoiding supervisory language in documents defining the relationship between CNMs and MDs can relieve physicians of the need to cosign the written record of the history and physical examination performed by a nurse-midwife when a woman is admitted to a hospital in labor. It also protects physicians from vicarious liability for the acts or omissions of nurse-midwives. Requirements that nurse-midwives be supervised by physicians are based in part on the assumption that physicians who work with CNMs and hospitals that grant privileges to CNMs can be held liable for injuries resulting from errors—malpractice—committed by a midwife. A 1994 review of case law found no reported cases to support that assumption (Jenkins, 1994). "Vicarious liability" arises from the relationship between two parties and is based on the nature of that relationship. Employers are almost always liable for the actions of their employees. A physician who employs a nurse-midwife is liable for her actions. However, a physician who collaborates with a nurse-midwife but neither employs nor supervises her should not be liable for damage resulting from her actions, unless she was acting on his advice. He would also be responsible for damage resulting from his failure to provide collaboration that he had contracted or was otherwise obligated to provide. The underlying principle of vicarious liability is control. Control results in liability, and supervision implies control (Jenkins, 1994).

Barriers and Supports to Nurse-Midwifery Practice

The fifteen-year period encapsulated in this chapter started and ended with crises that had deep effects throughout the entire health care system. The 1980s started off with the malpractice insurance crisis; the first half of the 1990s brought the promise (and threat) of federally legislated health care reform. Although attempts at official policy changes fizzled, the system began its own rapid devolution toward a system of competing managed health care corporations.* Nurse-midwifery is a small boat on the very large ocean of health care in this country: Although storms that roll across this ocean rock even the largest ocean liners, big boats have the weight to ride out the storm. Such gigantic waves of change may produce a frightening and sometimes fatal ride for midwifery practices, which are in smaller, much lighter boats.

In addition to dealing with large-scale changes in the health care system, nurse-midwives worked to achieve the structural supports required for nurse-midwifery practice: laws that regulate and sanction nurse-midwifery in every jurisdiction, authority to order laboratory studies and prescribe medications, affordable and adequate professional liability insurance, the ability to admit patients to hospitals, third-party payment for nurse-midwifery services provided to women covered by health care payment plans, and effective working relationships with physicians—anesthesiologists and pediatricians, as well as obstetrician–gynecologists and family physicians. Unavailability of any of these supports may constitute a complete or relative barrier to nurse-midwifery practice. Most of them have been more accessible to CNMs who are employed by physicians, hospitals or other organizations, and less available to nurse-midwives who establish or try to establish practices of their own.

Findings from National Studies

A study published by the General Accounting Office (the "watchdog" agency of the

U.S. Congress) in 1979 identified several obstacles to wider utilization of nurse-midwives (General Accounting Office, 1979). The government was primarily concerned with barriers limiting the ability of CNMs to provide care to indigent women (Tom, 1982). The major obstacles identified from that perspective during the period leading up to the 1980s included a limited supply of nurse-midwives, relatively few training programs, resistance from physicians, inability of some CNMs to find obstetricians to work with them, reluctance of some nurse-midwives to practice in rural or other undesirable areas, restrictive state licensing laws, and limitations on coverage of nurse-midwifery services by third-party health care payment plans. Two other national studies have been conducted since then, one in 1985 and one in 1990.

Most of the 280 nurse-midwives surveyed during a 1985 ACNM Foundation study of factors that influence the level of success of individual CNMs perceived themselves as quite successful (Haas & Rooks, 1986). None of the individual characteristics measured in the study (e.g., age, level of education) was associated with level of success. The nurse-midwives rated their practices highest with regard to staff skills and lowest regarding financial success. Nurse-midwives who owned or were financial partners in their practices tended to give their practices lower financial ratings. Practices without direct physician involvement were least able to attract an adequate number of clients. Regardless of their own level of success, the nurse-midwives identified suitable physician collaboration and philosophical agreement between members of the practice as the most important factors for success. Nurse-midwives who had the most successful practices said that it was very important for the physicians with whom nurse-midwives collaborate to be part of the "mainstream" medical community (Haas, 1986). Opposition from physicians, public ignorance about nurse-midwifery, and public confusion

---

*See Chapter 5 for discussions of the effects of both changes on the U.S. health care system.

about the differences between lay midwives and nurse-midwives were identified as the most important problems (Haas & Rooks, 1986).

A study conducted by the Office of the Inspector General of the Department of Health and Human Services was motivated by government concern about access to prenatal care, especially for women on Medicaid (Kusserow, 1992). Data were collected through questionnaires completed by 338 CNMs,* by reviewing the practices of twenty-six CNMs working in five settings, by interviewing knowledgeable people, and by use of published papers and documents. The CNMs surveyed cited the attitudes and perceptions of the medical community as the most important barrier to their profession. Other barriers included limitations on prescriptive privileges, restrictive hospital admitting privileges, attitudes and perceptions of the general public, and lack of access to malpractice insurance. The researchers concluded that the attitudes and perceptions of physicians may contribute to some of the other barriers, especially lack of authority to write prescriptions and inaccessible or restrictive hospital admitting privileges. CNMs who were closely affiliated with physicians or organizations controlled by physicians experienced fewer barriers.

Professional Liability Insurance

Securing adequate, affordable professional liability insurance was the most demanding challenge faced by nurse-midwives during the 1980s. The development and effect of the medical (and midwifery) malpractice liability insurance crisis was described in Chapter 5. The cost of liability insurance purchased through a program sponsored by the ACNM

---

*Surveys were mailed to a random sample of ACNM members living in the United States; 462 responded; 124 were excluded from the analysis because they were not in practice or because they worked for the federal government (for instance, in the military or the Indian Health Service).

rose from a flat premium of $38/year in 1980 (a flat premium means that everyone paid the same amount) to between $2,132 and $13,500 in 1995 (depending on region of the country and the number of years the CNM had been covered by the policy). The ACNM had to arrange new insurance programs twice between 1980 and mid-1985, when it became unable to offer any policy to its members. That condition continued for a year. Lack of insurance forced some CNMs to stop practicing or to leave private practice and take jobs in which the employer provided the insurance. Since 1993 the ACNM has endorsed a program that offers policies that provide the necessary level of protection (payment of up to $1 million per claim and $3 million for all claims in one year). The policy does not cover home births attended by CNMs. Another policy is available, but it is very expensive and does not provide the necessary level of coverage. As a result, CNM participation in home births has dropped by almost two-thirds (see Table 7). The company that provides the ACNM-endorsed insurance program also writes policies for accredited free-standing birth centers.

The policies and practices of some insurance companies impede nurse-midwifery practice by making it impossible or impractical for physicians to collaborate with nurse-midwives.

Prescriptive Authority

As of June 1995, the laws of thirty-nine jurisdictions (thirty-eight states and the District of Columbia) gave nurse-midwives legal authority to prescribe drugs and other treatments. These authorizations vary in the degree of independence they afford and in the kinds of drugs and devices nurse-midwives are allowed to prescribe. Some states maintain formularies that list specific drugs that can be prescribed by CNMs. The State of Oregon is considering the opposite approach—allowing CNMs to prescribe all drugs except those on a limited list. In addition to state statutes, the federal Rural

Health Services Act of 1989 provides prescriptive privileges to CNMs who work in medically underserved sites and are licensed as advanced registered nurse practitioners (ARNPs). A few states limit prescription privileges to nurse-midwives who have master's degrees or, more commonly and more logically, require a certain number of hours of course work in pharmacology.

In some states the laws that give prescriptive authority to nurse-midwives conflict with parts of the medical practice act or with the laws that regulate pharmacists. Some pharmacists have refused to fill prescriptions signed by CNMs (Moon, 1990).

CNMs who practice in states that do not provide prescriptive authority work out some way to provide necessary medications and prescriptions under the authority of the physicians with whom they collaborate—for example, by using prescription forms that have been presigned by the physician, by calling prescriptions into a pharmacy under the physician's name, by asking the physician to sign prescriptions that were written by the nurse-midwife, by using standing order protocols, or by distributing stocked medications (Moon, 1990). Some of these practices may be legally precarious. However, the vast majority of prescriptions are for a relatively small number of frequently used drugs, and the arrangements require the full approval of physicians, who may delegate many aspects of medical practice to nurses. Despite the lack of prescriptive authority in the laws of some states, a survey conducted in 1993 found that virtually all practicing nurse-midwives (99 percent) write prescriptions for medications. More than half of the respondents (51 percent) had full legal authority to write prescriptions. Another 32 percent could write prescriptions for a preapproved list of drugs, but had to obtain a physician's signature on the form. Sixteen percent recommended prescriptions that had to be authorized by a physician (Franklin Communications, 1994).

The most restrictive aspect of prescriptive authority for nurse-midwives is prescrip-

tion of "controlled substances," i.e., narcotics and other psychotropic drugs, the prescribing and administration of which are controlled by federal law. All practitioners who dispense controlled substances are required to register with the Drug Enforcement Agency (DEA) of the U.S. Department of Justice (Fennell, 1991). The ACNM, working with other groups, was successful in reversing a DEA proposal that would have tied a nurse-midwife's authority to prescribe controlled substances to a physician. In 1993 the DEA published a *Midlevel Practitioner's Manual* that covers CNMs (Williams, 1994a).

Hospital Privileges

Hospital privileges give a health professional authority to admit patients to a specific hospital, to provide care to patients who have been admitted to that hospital, to access the hospital's services on behalf of patients, and to discharge patients from the hospital. Hospital privileges did not become an issue until nurse-midwives began to take care of private patients. Before that most nurse-midwives who provided care to women in hospitals were direct employees of either the hospitals in which they practiced or institutions affiliated with those hospitals. The employing institution paid the nurse-midwives' salaries, absorbed income generated by their services, and accepted liability for the care they provided. Patients cared for by nurse-midwives were admitted and discharged under the authority of the chief of the obstetric service. The employer–employee relationship between the hospital and the CNM avoided the issue of hospital privileges (Rooks & Schmidt, 1980). Nurse-midwives (and physicians) who are not employed by a hospital must have explicit permission to admit and provide care to patients in that hospital. Even midwives who attend births in birth centers and homes need hospital privileges so that they can accompany women who develop complications into the hospital—to provide continuity of care and enable the nurse-midwife to collaborate with the physician who assumes some or all of the responsibility for the patient's care.

Hospital privileges come under the jurisdiction of the hospital's medical staff bylaws. The Joint Commission on Accreditation of Healthcare Organizations (JCAHO) is a private, not-for-profit national organization that has primary responsibility for the accreditation of hospitals.* JCAHO requires the hospital medical staff to exercise care and responsibility in granting hospital privileges. Hospitals are also subject to tort laws and can be sued for providing credentials to practitioners in a negligent way. JCAHO standards specify professional criteria such as "evidence of current licensure, relevant training and/or experience, current competence, and health status," as well as "other reasonable qualifications," such as evidence of adequate liability insurance (Burst, 1986). The standards require that every patient admitted to a hospital must be under the care of an MD, doctor of osteopathy (DO), doctor of dental surgery or dental medicine, doctor of podiatry, doctor of optometry, or a chiropractor. However, JCAHO gives hospitals discretion in deciding whether to extend privileges to practitioners other than MDs and DOs.

There are two basic types of hospital privileges—admitting privileges, which are generally held only by physicians, and practice privileges for other professionals. Full membership in the medical staff, and thus the power and control that come with voting, is usually restricted to those with admitting privileges, that is, physicians. A nurse-midwife with practice privileges but no admitting privileges has to admit patients to the hospital under the name of a physician with admitting privileges (Burst, 1986).

During the 1980s, "the granting or withholding of hospital privileges became a battlefield where the economic, power and control issues between nurse-midwives and physicians" were fought (Burst, 1986). It is not a level battlefield. The medical staff of some hospitals have used their power to deny hospital privileges to prevent CNMs from establishing practices in their area or have required nurse-midwives to accept restrictions that are not related to the quality of patient care as conditions for granting hospital privileges. Examples include denial of privileges unless the CNM is employed by a physician (an economic relationship that is separate from the need for a nurse-midwife to have a clinical practice relationship with a physician), requiring a physician to be present for all deliveries conducted by the CNM, limiting privileges to CNMs with master's degrees, prohibiting CNM involvement in out-of-hospital births, or requiring a physician to cosign the nurse-midwife's entries on medical records (Burst, 1986). Thirty-six percent of the CNMs who participated in the 1982 ACNM survey reported that their "backup" physician had to be in the hospital when they were attending a birth; 6 percent said that a physician had to be in the delivery room. These are interesting requirements considering that few private obstetricians remain in the hospital throughout the labors of their own patients. Although they arrive at the hospital in time for the delivery, many rely on obstetric nurses who are not midwives to manage their patient's labors under standing orders augmented by telephone communication.

In 1985 the ACNM created an ad hoc committee to investigate the hospital privileges issue. The committee mailed a questionnaire to every nurse-midwifery service listed in the *1985 ACNM Service Directory*; data were collected from 361 practices. The CNMs in one-fourth of the practices did not

*To participate in the Medicare and Medicaid programs, hospitals must meet the Conditions of Participation specified by the Health Care Financing Administration (HCFA) or be accredited by either the JCAHO or the American Osteopathic Association (AOA). The Medicaid Conditions of Participation and the JCAHO and AOA standards all include requirements related to the granting of hospital privileges. All three sets of rules are similar in regards to hospital privileges for midwives.

have privileges at any hospital; CNMs working in two-thirds of the practices had privileges at one hospital; CNMs in 8 percent of the practices had privileges at more than one hospital. Those who had hospital privileges identified ninety-six different titles under which hospital privileges had been extended to them. Most were referred to as "associate medical staff," "allied medical staff," "affiliated medical staff," or "adjunct medical staff." Some had to live with titles such as "dependent practitioner," "CNM physician extender," or "physician's personal employee." Nurse-midwives in ninety-three of the ninety-six practices that had no hospital privileges had requested privileges at some point in time. Their requests had been denied for a variety of reasons, most frequently because the nurse-midwife was not *employed* by a physician or because there was "no need for a nurse-midwife in the community." Other reasons included the belief that having a CNM on the medical staff would increase what the hospital would have to pay for malpractice insurance, no mechanism for granting privileges to a CNM within the medical staff bylaws, and dislike of the CNM's involvement in an out-of-hospital birth center or home births (Burst, 1987).

The situation is improving. Five jurisdictions (the District of Columbia, Florida, Ohio, Oregon, and Virginia) have passed laws that prohibit hospitals from discriminating against nurse-midwives as a class in the granting of admitting privileges. Some hospitals in these and other states have rewritten their medical staff bylaws to include nurse-midwives who practice in that hospital in the definition of the "medical staff" (Oregon Health Sciences University, 1994–95). CNMs who practice at those hospitals now have the same privileges and responsibilities as other members of the medical staff. Such statutes and bylaws are possible only in states in which nurse-midwives are licensed to practice without medical direction or supervision (Williams, 1994). There have also been legal battles

about hospital privileges for CNMs in several states and the District of Columbia. The Federal Trade Commission (FTC) has challenged medical staff control of hospital privileges as a means to obstruct competition from health care providers who are not physicians. In 1993 the FTC notified the Georgia Hospital Association that the model medical staff bylaws developed and endorsed by the Medical Association of Georgia were anticompetitive and could result in antitrust liability for hospitals and their medical staffs (Horoschak, 1993).

JCAHO standards require that a history and physical examination be performed and recorded on the clinical record soon after a patient is admitted to the hospital. Except for patients admitted for the sole purpose of dental surgery, the admitting history and physical must either be performed by an MD or DO, or an MD or DO must cosign the other care provider's written record of the admission history and physical. Because JCAHO understands that normal births are physiologic events (i.e., not illnesses), it allows an updated prenatal record to take the place of an admitting history and physical for women admitted to hospitals with the expectation of a normal, vaginal delivery. However, the prenatal record must be "authenticated" (cosigned) by a physician within a short period after the patient is admitted. The only exception may occur in states where CNMs are licensed as independent practitioners. Hospitals in those states may give CNMs privileges to conduct or document the admitting history and physical of a woman admitted for normal childbirth without the requirement of a physician's signature (Williams, 1994). JCAHO's cosignature requirement is an important issue because it forces physicians to spend time on a nonproductive task, making collaboration with a nurse-midwife unnecessarily burdensome to physicians. Eliminating this burden is an important benefit of writing the laws that regulate nurse-midwifery practice without reference to medical supervision.

Third-Party Payment for Health Care

In 1979 Congress passed laws that require two federal health care financing programs to pay for services provided by nurse-midwives: Medicaid (the program that provides health care to indigent pregnant women) and CHAMPUS (the program that pays for health care provided to civilian dependents of members of the military services). By 1982 eight states had passed laws to require all third-party payers to reimburse for nurse-midwifery care, and many private insurance companies had voluntarily decided to pay for nurse-midwifery services (Tom, 1982). In 1982 the Government Accounting Office (GAO) estimated that the health care financing plans of more than 90 percent of government workers included coverage for nurse-midwifery services (Tom, 1982). A 1982 American Foundation for Maternal and Child Health survey of more than 300 U.S. health insurance companies also found that most private health insurance companies paid for care provided by CNMs. Blue Cross/Blue Shield companies were somewhat less likely to do so than the other companies surveyed; the president of the foundation hypothesized that this reflected "the fact that the policy boards of many of the 'Blues' are heavily weighted with physicians, many of whom see nurse-midwives as an economic threat" (Haire, 1982).

Although some state Medicaid programs pay CNMs the same amount they pay physicians for the same service, some states pay nurse-midwives only 70 to 90 percent of the fee paid to physicians. This is a significant issue because full Medicaid payment in many states is less than private practice fees for maternity care and Medicaid clients often have more nutritional, social, behavioral, and medical problems than other patients and need more intensive education, counseling, and other services. Even full Medicaid payment does not cover the actual cost of providing care to many of the multiproblem women on Medicaid. Nurse-midwifery services that receive 70 percent of the usual Medicaid fee can go broke by providing the care these women need. In some places the amount paid to a nurse-midwife to care for a woman on Medicaid is less than half the fee most physicians charge for care of private patients. Paying less for services provided by a CNM than for the same services provided by a physician provides strong incentives for CNM/MD teams to bill for all care under the names of the physicians.

In 1994, Medicare, the federal program that pays for care provided to elderly and disabled women, has set nurse-midwifery fees at 65 percent of the fees established for the same services provided by physicians. Unlike Medicaid, which uses both state and federal money and is managed by the states, Medicare payment policies are established at the federal level. Although relatively few women obtain nurse-midwifery services that are paid for by Medicare, it is a very large and influential program whose payment structure is copied by many other third-party payers. CHAMPUS adopted Medicare's payment policies in 1993 (Fennell, 1994).

As of 1995, thirty-one states required all third-party health care plans to pay for care provided by nurse-midwives. On the other hand, a few states do not permit third-party payment or reimbursement for nurse-midwifery care, and third parties in some states pay at a very low level. In states where covering nurse-midwifery services is permitted but not required, most private insurance plans pay for CNM care. Some companies cover CNM services but require subscribers to obtain special authorization prior to receipt of the services. Some have structured their reimbursement to encourage use of nurse-midwives, providing full reimbursement for their services, while requiring subscribers to pay additional costs of physician care out of their own pockets.

Relationships with Physicians

All studies of barriers and supports to nurse-midwifery practice have noted the importance of physicians. CNMs from both the most successful practices and the least successful practices identify good working relationships with physicians as the most important factor for success (Haas & Rooks, 1986). In addition to problems discussed in the section on collaboration with physicians, there are a variety of other problems: Some anesthesiologists have refused to give epidurals to patients who are under the care of a nurse-midwife; others enter the rooms in which nurse-midwives' patients are in labor to urge them to ask for epidurals. Some pediatricians have refused to examine babies delivered by CNMs. Some physicians have demanded excessive payments to provide backup to a CNM; one asked for 75 percent of the nurse-midwife's fees, even if he was not consulted and never saw the patient. Medical opposition has prevented many nurse-midwives from obtaining hospital privileges or has resulted in hospital privileges for CNMs that are burdened with untenable conditions. Some physicians have been threatened with loss of their own hospital privileges unless they stopped providing backup to a nurse-midwifery service or individual CNM. Physicians who support midwifery are sometimes forced to do battle with those who do not.

Several studies have identified lack of physicians who are available and willing to work with CNMs as a particular barrier to greater utilization of nurse-midwives in rural areas. A study conducted in North Carolina in 1991 cited a nationwide shortage of CNMs, a lack of physicians in rural areas to provide needed backup, and the unwillingness of some physicians who could provide backup to CNMs to do so as the three most important factors limiting nurse-midwives' contributions to care of women in rural parts of the state (Taylor & Ricketts, 1993). In a study of obstetric practices in Washington State, the primary reason CNMs gave for not locating in rural areas was the lack of physicians to work with them (Rosenblatt & Detering, 1988).

Despite these problems, all CNMs collaborate with physicians, and most of those collaborations either begin with or develop into good relationships and mutual respect. Although some physicians oppose nurse-midwives and speak and write against them, published harangues against nurse-midwives come almost exclusively from physicians who have not worked with CNMs, and they have had no impact on the American College of Obstetricians and Gynecologists' official position of support for nurse-midwifery practice. Most of the opposition arises from lack of experience with nurse-midwives, lack of accurate information about their education and practice, and concerns about competition. As these factors are overcome, opposition lessens or dissolves. Some physicians who have opposed nurse-midwives' efforts to establish their own midwifery practices have welcomed the same nurse-midwives into their medical practice. Many medical students and residents now receive at least part of their training in hospitals in which nurse-midwives practice. CNMs are on the faculties of an increasing number of medical schools, where they give lectures on breast-feeding, the social and psychological needs of pregnant women, and management of normal labor and delivery; teach medical students to conduct pelvic examinations; and serve as clinical preceptors for medical students and residents who are having experience in labor and delivery. As a result, a growing proportion of physicians understand and respect midwifery and enjoy working with nurse-midwives.

Antitrust Issues

The Federal Trade Commission (FTC) enforces the consumer protection and antitrust laws of the United States. Health care did not come under the regulatory authority of the commission until 1975. During the first years after that change, the FTC took actions aimed at increasing competition among health care providers and fought the American Medical Association (AMA) policy against physician advertising (Bailey, 1986). In 1982 the AMA spent millions of dollars in an effort to convince Congress to remove medicine from the jurisdiction of the FTC. An ACNM-led coalition of consumer, labor, business, and professional organizations convinced Congress that competition in the delivery of health care fosters innovations that provide consumers with a choice of treatment alternatives—probably at lowered cost and without any adverse effect on the quality of care—and that such competition is in the public interest (Bailey, 1986; Tom, 1983). The FTC's 1983 intervention in a case involving two CNMs who attempted to establish a practice in Nashville, Tennessee, was described in Chapter 5.

The commissioner of the FTC spoke at the opening session of the ACNM's 1984 convention regarding the Federal Trade Commission's interest in nurse-midwifery. The FTC is not interested in midwifery per se, or even in better care for mothers and babies; it is interested in competition and promoting an open and fair society. The FTC's involvement with nurse-midwives has centered on hospital privileges, malpractice insurance for physicians who work with CNMs, and third-party reimbursement for nurse-midwifery services (Bailey, 1986). Its objectives are to prevent hospitals, physicians, insurance companies, and other entities from excluding CNMs in ways that are arbitrary, unreasonable, unjust, maintain an unnecessary monopoly, prevent competition, and restrict consumer choice. Concern for these values is also played out at other levels of government. In 1992 the insurance superintendent for the District of Columbia ordered officials of a company that imposed a $13,000 malpractice insurance surcharge on obstetricians who work with nurse-midwives to drop the surcharge.

The Mass Movement to Managed Care

Chapter 5 described the growth of HMOs during the 1980s, the rapid movement to managed health care during the first half of the 1990s, the effects of these changes on state Medicaid programs and public hospi-

tals, the "gatekeeper" role of primary care physicians and other primary care providers in managed care, concerns about the effects of managed care's domination on choice, quality, and access to health care, and the effects of the transition to for-profit managed care on indigent pregnant women. The turmoil resulting from all of these changes has induced insecurity and enhanced turf-guarding throughout the health care industry.

Such systemic changes have effects on midwives. Differences between HMOs and other kinds of managed care organizations seem to affect their actions regarding CNMs. All health care professionals who work for HMOs are salaried employees whose job security and pay are dependent on the financial well-being of the entire HMO. HMOs have incentives to keep costs low while providing services that maintain the health of their subscribers over time—the reason they are called health *maintenance* organizations. HMOs have been more likely than other health care organizations to invest in health education and other programs to help subscribers adopt healthful lifestyles, and they have been leaders in the use of midwives. During the first years of the transition to managed care, there was a large and growing demand for nurse-midwives to work in HMOs. Other managed care organizations (preferred provider organizations, or PPOs) are mainly local coalitions of health care providers who agree to charge less for care provided to people who pay monthly premiums to the managed care organization. In return, the subscribers agree to obtain all of their care from the physicians, hospitals, and other providers associated with the PPO. Although gatekeepers try to avoid unnecessary use of services, the constituent parts of the organization retain their individual identity and are paid on a fee-for-service basis. This kind of managed care organization has tended to exclude nurse-midwives while enrolling many of the medically indigent women who had previously received their care from nurse-midwifery services in large, inner-city medical centers and specially designed community-based programs.

The following is a summary of some *short-term* negative effects on nurse-midwives from changes in the health care system during the first half of the 1990s:

- Physicians who were disinterested in taking care of poor pregnant women have become more willing. When Medicaid increased its fees to match those of most other third-party payers, this patient population became more attractive to private physicians. The development of Medicaid managed care plans contributes to this trend, because physicians who are part of managed care organizations that contract with Medicaid must provide care to Medicaid patients. This has caused drastic reductions in patients at many of the large CNM services based in publicly supported academic medical centers that serve residents of the racial and ethnic minority inner-city ghettos of the nation's largest cities. Because many of these services are run in association with nurse-midwifery education programs, loss of patients at public hospitals has an effect on nurse-midwifery education.

- Although federal law requires all state Medicaid programs to pay for care provided by nurse-midwives, some states have been given "waivers" from all federal Medicaid mandates in order to allow them to experiment with managed health care and other approaches to reducing the cost of providing care to Medicaid-eligible women. In states with waivers, managed care plans that contract to provide care to Medicaid-eligible women do not have to provide access to nurse-midwifery care (Jenkins & Fennell, 1994).

- Many new CNM services were developed during the second half of the

1980s, as hospitals, community health centers, and county health departments sought nurse-midwifery solutions to local access-to-care problems. Increased physician interest in caring for women on Medicaid has resulted in withdrawal of previous physician support for some of these services.

- The development of large organizations that monopolize health care in some geographic areas provides new opportunities for the exclusion of midwives. The insecurity associated with rapid, uncharted change in the system provides motivation to eliminate potential competition. The situation extant during the mid-1990s provides both the motivation and the opportunity to exclude midwives from managed care organizations directed by physicians.

- In areas where a large proportion of the people are enrolled in managed care organizations, midwives who are not part of a managed care organization become less accessible to women who want midwifery care. A woman may also be unable to obtain care from a particular physician of her choice. However, every woman enrolled in a managed care plan can obtain care from *some* physician; under current circumstances, women enrolled in some managed care plans may not be able to obtain care from *any* nurse-midwife (unless she is willing to pay for it in addition to her monthly prepaid health care premium).

- For a woman to have access to midwifery care, her entire family may have to enroll in an organization that provides it. This can be a problem if the family of a woman who wants to use a midwife prefers an internist or pediatrician who is in a different plan.

- Directors of large managed care organizations tend to focus on the bottom line—how to cut costs—and many do not understand the nature and role of midwifery. Nurse-midwives are finding themselves under pressure to see more patients faster. This is unacceptable to many midwives and ignores lessons learned during the last twenty-five years about the kind of care that can reduce the incidence of poor pregnancy outcomes among low-income, socially distressed women.

- Although all managed care organizations must offer maternity care, some small managed care organizations are not particularly eager to attract childbearing families, who tend to use more health care than subscribers who are not in the midst of having babies and raising children. This may be a disincentive to hiring or including CNMs in the organization, because CNMs tend to attract pregnant women.

- Small managed care organizations need generalists and are encouraging family physicians to reenter obstetrics (Skubi, 1994). Nurse-midwives who are in these organizations may be under pressure to expand their scope of practice—by taking care of patients with a wide range of complications and by expanding the range of services they provide.

- Some birth centers are contracting with or being bought out by managed care organizations. This will compromise their autonomy and thus may threaten their ability to maintain a noninterventionist approach to childbirth (Roberts, 1996).

Many more changes, *even in the opposite direction,* can be anticipated as the system continues to evolve. Despite trauma and insecurity during this period of upheaval, managed care may promote midwifery in the long run. The need to become involved in care of the poor makes some physicians want to bring midwives into their practice. In some places, physicians are taking the initiative to seek administrative support for recruiting CNMs and establishing a nurse-midwifery service. The focus on cost effectiveness also favors midwifery.

Mutual Support, But Significant Disagreements with Nursing

Nurse-midwifery is based in nursing. All nurse-midwives have completed a nursing education program and are licensed as registered nurses; most of them had years of experience as nurses before they became CNMs. Most nurse-midwifery education programs are in departments, divisions, colleges, or schools of nursing. Most CNMs have master's degrees in nursing; some have doctoral degrees in nursing. Thus most nurse-midwifery students study the history and major concepts and theories of nursing. Nurse-midwifery faculty are colleagues of nursing faculty and are identified as professors of nursing. Most federal funding for nurse-midwifery education is authorized under the Nurse Training Act and comes through the Division of Nursing. Most nurse-midwives practice under state nurse practice laws and are regulated by state boards of nursing. The American Nurses' Association, at the national level, and state nursing associations, at the local level, have provided critical support for the legislation needed to support nurse-midwifery.

Nurse-midwives have also supported nursing. Nurse-midwives have made major contributions to the development of maternal and child health nursing in this country—as educators, theoreticians, exemplars, and a source of inspiration. CNMs have been particularly important as models for development of the nurse-practitioner role. The easy-to-understand role of the midwife, the well-documented excellent outcomes of nurse-midwifery care, public apprecia-tion for nurse-midwives' long-standing commitment to providing care to medically indigent women, the cost advantages of nurse-midwifery care, and the enthusiastic support of former clients have made it possible to pass supportive legislation that has included nurse practitioners in many states.

There are, however, some important disagreements. Leaders of major nursing organizations define nurse-midwifery as an advanced specialty practice of nursing. They want all basic nursing education to lead to a baccalaureate degree in nursing. Although they have been unable to achieve that goal, they are adamant in insisting that the education of advanced practice nurses occur in programs that lead to a master's degree in nursing. They have recommended to all state boards of nursing that nurse-midwives, nurse practitioners, clinical nurse specialists, and nurse-anesthetists be required to have an additional license as "advanced practice registered nurses" (APRNs), and that a master's degree in nursing be a requirement for this license. Because they see nurse-midwifery as part of nursing, they believe that it is within their province and presume the right to speak for nurse-midwifery.

The ACNM defines nurse-midwives as educated in *two separate* professions, nursing and midwifery. Nurse-midwives think of themselves as nurse-midwives, or simply as midwives. Few are happy to be legally defined as "advanced practice registered nurses." Nurse-midwifery education is actually midwifery education for people who are already nurses—*beginning-level* midwifery ed-

ucation, rather than specialty education. Although it makes sense to give master's degrees to individuals who already have bachelor's degrees and undertake another arduous eighteen- to twenty-four-month program, it is not "master's education" in the sense of building on the base of a bachelor's degree in the same field. The ACNM does not require master's degrees and will not require bachelor's degrees until 1999, having designed and implemented other, more effective means to ensure the quality of nurse-midwifery education. Due to these quality assurance mechanisms, nurse-midwifery education can be successfully implemented in diverse educational environments, including programs leading to a master's degree in public health, a master's degree in nursing, a master of arts degree, a baccalaureate degree, or no degree at all. The ACNM has represented and spoken for nurse-midwifery since its incorporation in 1955. The vast majority of practicing nurse-midwives are members of the ACNM, which maintains multiple means of communication with its members and is responsive to their concerns. Less than one-fourth of CNMs are members of the ANA (Adams, 1989), which is an enormous organization in which they have no organized voice. The ACNM asserts that it and it alone can represent and speak for nurse-midwifery.

Chapter 9
Development of Direct-Entry Midwifery, 1980–1995

This chapter describes the development of direct-entry midwifery in the United States between 1980 and 1995. At the beginning of this period most midwives who were not nurse-midwives were referred to, and referred to themselves, as "lay midwives." As time progressed, the women who had become lay midwives during the 1970s became more experienced and more involved in midwifery, and some of them became deeply committed to developing lay midwifery into a professional form of midwifery. Most of this chapter is devoted to describing their accomplishments and progress. As a result of the accelerating changes described here, a large and dynamic segment of this group of midwives is evolving into a distinct arm of professional midwifery.

The current form of direct-entry midwifery in this country developed as part of the social and cultural ferment of the late 1960s and 1970s—the feminist and consumer critique of obstetrics and obstetricians; childbirth educators and the disappointed couples who prepared themselves for normal births but got obstetric interventions; La Leche League; and the "hippie" counterculture, antiauthority movement. It is also strongly associated with religious conviction that emphasizes the sanctity of the family and the home. Focusing on home births, it developed purposefully outside the matrix of mainstream medical institutions and authority. Midwives invented themselves in rural communes, religious communities, and the nooks and crannies of urban counterculture enclaves. Most functioned as individuals or members of small, informal, local groups. Many practiced illegally, and thus clandestinely; most simply worked without reference to the law. Some accepted no money for their services, which were given as part of their membership in a particular community. Lay midwives were renounced by the American College of Obstetricians and Gynecologists; members of local medical associations encouraged police and prosecuters to arrest and indict them. Entering the "system" was not even a consideration for most of them for many years. Although a few training programs were developed, most were short lived, and there were no widely accepted educational standards. By the late 1970s there may have been several thousand lay midwives practicing on their own or as members of local groups.

The 1980s were the beginning of a new era—the development of a national organization, passage of laws that sanction and regulate direct-entry midwifery in an increasing number of states, new schools, and intense discussion about the pros, the cons, and the process of evolving into a profession. The Midwives' Alliance of North America (MANA), started in 1982, welcomed and hoped to unite all kinds of midwives. Although one-third of its members are certified nurse-midwives (CNMs), it has focused on direct-entry midwives. During its first thirteen years, MANA created an organizational structure; developed written statements of midwifery ethics and values, standards, and core competencies; and launched separate organizations to develop processes to accredit direct-entry midwifery educational programs and examine and certify direct-entry midwives. Progress was slowed by internal disagreement about the desirability of national standards and concern that accreditation and certification processes would discriminate against apprentice-trained midwives. Direct-entry midwifery developed outside the system, and some midwives want to keep it that way. They feel that nurse-midwives compromised too much in order to enter and survive in the system, and they fear that setting standards will lead to "professionalization" that will create artificial distances between women and their midwives. The functional unit for midwifery is the woman and the midwife; they perceive everything extraneous to that unit as a barrier.

Direct-entry midwifery developed as the mirror image of nurse-midwifery, which started small, grew slowly, and developed a strong national organization and enforceable national educational and practice standards while there were still few nurse-midwives. Nurse-midwives assumed the necessity of formal education, defined "nurse-midwife" in a way that limits its application to individuals who have completed a recognized educational program, and struggled to develop a place for midwifery within the established health care system and within universities, which are the usual institutions for preparing health practitioners. Nurse-midwifery was started and supported for the purpose of providing care to the poor; thus nurse-midwives themselves were usually of a different social class than their clients.

Direct-entry midwifery, in contrast, seemed to either start large or grow fast, bursting on the scene during a period of powerful social and cultural change. Although the social movement that called them into practice was national in scope, most lay midwives experienced their transition into this role as unique and embedded in a particular community. Although the actual number of lay midwives was unknown, there may have been more than two thousand by 1980; yet there were few schools, no national organization, no standards, and no commonly accepted definition. In the beginning of this movement, most midwives and the women they took care of were members of the same small social groups. There was no widely accepted way to determine who was a midwife, or when one became a midwife (as compared to being a woman who was still learning to be a midwife). Sometimes it was a designation conferred by one's social group. Women who evolved into the role gradually were often hesitant to assume the title. There was little desire to become part of the system; the goal was to allow women to experience natural births in their own homes, to keep the system out.

Nurse-midwives had their structure well in place by 1980 and used the next fifteen years to grow in number. Direct-entry midwives used that time to evolve and develop structure. In the process, many no longer fit the concept or title of a midwife who is "lay." Even at the beginning of this period there was great variation. A study conducted at the University of Washington in 1980 found some midwives who were entirely self-taught, "having done little more than attending births periodically (with or without an experienced partner) and reading a book or two on the birth process." The report described them as "the real 'lay midwives'." But the investigators also found some midwives who had completed several years of special training, including structured theoretical preparation and supervised clinical instruction (University of Washington, 1980). As time passed, there were fewer "real lay midwives," and people became uncomfortable with the term.

During the 1980s the term *direct-entry midwife* was introduced as an appellation for midwives who are not nurse-midwives but have achieved a level of professionalism by having completed a formal midwifery educational program or by having met criteria allowing them to be licensed to practice in a specific state or local jurisdiction or to be certified by a state or local midwifery organization. Before long the distinction between lay and direct-entry midwives was dropped, and "direct-entry" was used in reference to all midwives other than CNMs. During the first half of the 1990s, much effort was directed toward developing a process to distinguish fully qualified direct-entry midwives from those who are still learning to be midwives or who cannot or choose not to meet educational and other standards. This has been hard to accomplish with large numbers of diversely prepared, increasingly experienced midwives already in practice.

There may have been little or no growth in the number of direct-entry midwives during this fifteen-year period. A 1981 issue of *Mothering* magazine estimated the number at between 2,000 and 3,000 (Sallomi *et al.*). In 1982 MANA estimated it at 6,000 to 10,000 (Flanagan, 1990). In 1988, the executive director of the Seattle Midwifery School estimated that there were several hundred "direct-entry" midwives (who had completed requirements for licensure or certification) and perhaps several thousand "lay midwives" (who had not) (Myers-Ciecko, 1988). *Mothering* magazine's 1990 update did not provide an estimate for the entire country, but gave exact numbers or well-based estimates of the number practicing in each state (Becker *et al.*, 1990). Based on that information, between 1,600 and 1,900 direct-entry midwives were practicing in 1990—at least one in every state except Maryland and South Dakota. Three states—Texas (estimated to have 450 midwives in 1990), California (200 to 400) and New York (100)—accounted for about half of the total.

The number of births for which the birth certificate names a direct-entry midwife as the attendant is very stable—between 11,500 and 12,500 births per year during 1989 to 1994, as shown in Tables 2 and 3 in Chapter 7. However, births attended by "other midwives" are underreported in many states, especially where their practice is illegal. For example, "other midwife" was not indicated as the attendant for *any* births in New York state in 1994! Some of these births may not be registered at all; in that case, the infant will not have a birth certificate unless and until someone goes through a special process for retrospective registration of the birth. If the birth is registered several years after it actually occurred, it will never be included in most reports based on birth certificate data for the actual year of the birth.

Some births attended by direct-entry midwives may be counted as births that occurred in nonhospital sites with "other" or "unspecified" listed as the attendant. There were 11,664 such births in 1994. This number includes births attended by practitioners other than physicians or midwives (e.g., naturopaths), unplanned out-of-hospital births (which occur at home for various reasons), and home births for which there is no trained attendant. Table 2 in Chapter 7 presents an estimate that accounts for underreporting of births by direct-entry midwives. It is based on the assumption that "other midwives" attended half of the out-of-hospital births with "other" or "unspecified" indicated as the attendant. Applying this assumption to the data for 1994 increases the number of births attended by direct-entry midwives by almost 50 percent—from 11,846 to 17,678; the actual amount of underreporting is probably not that great.* Based on this high-end estimate of the number of births, if the estimate of 10,000 direct-entry midwives were accurate, each midwife would have attended, on average, fewer than 2 births in 1994. If the actual number of direct-entry midwives is 1,600 (the lower estimate of the state-by-state count made by *Mothering* magazine), the average would have been slightly more than 11 births per midwife in 1994. Some direct-entry midwives report that they attend 2 to 10, or even 20 births per month. Either the estimated number of midwives is exaggerated or many of the midwives included in the estimate attend very few births. Direct-entry midwifery practice remains entirely out of hospital, with an emphasis on home births, the demand for which has been relatively steady, but small as shown in Table 3 in Chapter 7

The high estimates from the early 1980s included some women with marginal investments in midwifery, who have since dropped out. Some direct-entry midwives were nurses

who enrolled in nurse-midwifery education programs and became CNMs. Others completed nursing programs in order to enter nurse-midwifery programs. Women who were lay midwives in the early 1980s and were still practicing in 1995 had learned much from their experience, and most had taken advantage of various educational opportunities. In addition, new people entered the field through apprenticeships with established midwives and a small but growing number of organized educational programs. More than 100 midwives have graduated from the Seattle Midwifery School, which was in constant operation throughout these fifteen years.

Because of the history and culture of the direct-entry midwifery movement and the locale-specific circumstances of direct-entry midwives, the most rapid process toward establishing standards occurred within specific states through the work of local midwifery organizations, some of which developed their own certification processes. The standards developed by state midwifery associations vary with local circumstances, including licensing laws in states that have them. Thus the standards behind a licensed or state-certified direct-entry midwife are not the same from state to state.

In addition to the need for standards for educational programs for people entering the field, there is a strongly felt need to provide means for experienced midwives without formal training to demonstrate their competence in order to become credentialed. Midwives who have been practicing for fifteen to twenty years are not looking for education so much as a way to document their experience and demonstrate their current knowledge as being equivalent to what other midwives have achieved through formal education. Their objective is to obtain the credentials necessary to practice legally and to be able to bill Medicaid and other third-party payers for the services they provide.

Two organizations created by MANA are developing national standards and processes

---

*The data on which this estimate is based are laid out in Table 2. Findings from studies that have measured underreporting in specific places and times are described in Chapter 7.

for accrediting direct-entry midwifery educational programs and examining and certifying direct-entry midwives. The first written examination to test the knowledge needed for safe beginning-level direct-entry midwifery practice was offered in 1991. The North American Registry of Midwives (NARM) began to implement a process to certify experienced direct-entry midwives in 1994. It expanded the process to include entry-level midwives in 1996. The Midwifery Education Accreditation Council (MEAC) is pilot-testing a process to accredit education programs; it will be possible to accredit a single midwife who teaches apprentices as a midwifery education program through this process. In the meantime, the American College of Nurse-Midwives (ACNM) has developed a process to accredit direct-entry midwifery education programs that are taught at the baccalaureate or postbaccalaureate level; the ACNM Certification Council (ACC) will examine and certify graduates of direct-entry midwifery education programs accredited by the ACNM. The MANA-derived organizations are developing standards for a professional direct-entry midwife whose scope of practice is similar to that of licensed direct-entry midwives in states with progressive laws; the object is to develop professional standards for midwives practicing in out-of-hospital birth sites. The ACNM is developing standards for direct-entry midwives who will be similar to CNMs in all ways except that they are not nurses. The first direct-entry education program to receive preaccreditation status from the ACNM was developed by CNMs.

Women becoming direct-entry midwives during the 1970s and 1980s were self-selected and not motivated by the usual career choice considerations. Since training programs were scarce, most had to forge their own path. Many who thought they wanted to become midwives did not complete the process. Changes during the past fifteen years may make direct-entry midwifery a more attractive prospect for young women

seeking a career. This will change the dynamics of recruitment, selection, and retention, perhaps drawing a different kind of woman into the rapidly changing profession.

The direct-entry midwifery community retains a strong commitment to education through apprenticeship; a preference for experiential learning; belief in the validity of intuition and intuitive knowledge; confidence in private, tuition-based midwifery schools that are free-standing and under the control of midwives; and a general distrust of universities. A combination of lack of training in statistics and epidemiology and skepticism resulting from historical medical misuse of statistical information has reinforced a tradition of heavy reliance on anecdotal information and teaching by recounting personal birth experiences. Many feel that the medical literature reflects values, assumptions, and practices that are irrelevant to their practice (Gaskin, 1996). There has been very little research on the methods used by direct-entry midwives.

Despite extreme variation in the preparation and circumstances of this broad category of midwives, they are psychologically and politically bonded by their common history, by out-of-hospital births as their mode of practice, by opposition to typical medical obstetric care, and by the dichotomy between CNMs and all other midwives. Although individual midwives may increase their level of training or become licensed by their states or certified by midwifery organizations other than the ACNM, they remain members of this category unless they become certified nurse-midwives or ACC certified midwives (CMs).

Some of the erstwhile "lay" midwives remain philosophically opposed to the professionalization of midwifery. Some are not members of any midwifery organization and practice without reference to any standards other than their own. The lack of uniformly defined, widely accepted terms to distinguish easily between lay midwives and professional direct-entry midwives is a barrier to further development of this arm of midwifery.

Most of MANA's formal documents refer to direct-entry midwives simply as "midwives." This generic term, which includes CNMs, does not distinguish between midwives who have met professional standards and those who have not. In this chapter I use the term *direct-entry midwife* except in reference to laws or circumstances that refer specifically to lay midwives. Direct-entry midwives themselves use a variety of terms, including *community midwives, traditional midwives,* and *independent midwives.*

The past twenty-five years have brought remarkable change in the legal status of direct-entry midwifery in many states. California provides a sharp example: More than 40 midwives were investigated, arrested, and prosecuted for practicing midwifery in California during a twenty-year period between the early 1970s and 1993, when a law intended to legalize direct-entry midwifery in California was passed. Nevertheless, direct-entry midwifery practice remains illegal in some states; a law meant to support direct-entry midwifery resulted in unprecedented arrests of midwives in New York State. Consumer support has been a hallmark of the direct-entry midwifery movement; the threat, image, and reality of midwives being arrested has been a major stimulus of this support.

Legal Status

The legal status of direct-entry midwives varies greatly from state to state, and there have been many recent changes. Midwifery practiced by anyone but a CNM is clearly illegal in some states, is neither legal nor illegal in some states, is legal but not regulated in some states, and is regulated under old or new laws in others. Some recent laws continue a long tradition of bringing lay midwives under the control of state public health authorities; such statutes tend to specify components of a training program or the kinds and amounts of clinical experience needed to qualify to take a state licensing examination. Other states passed laws that provide for licensing lay midwives but have no educational requirements, and in 1991 Illinois enacted a law that makes midwifery illegal if practiced by anyone but a CNM or a physician. At the other end of the continuum, between 1981 and 1993 four influential states passed laws requiring at least three years of formal midwifery education (the standard for direct-entry midwives in Europe) or a baccalaureate degree. The great variation in state laws both reflects and perpetuates the polymorphic nature of this category of midwives.

Some states that do not recognize or regulate midwives other than CNMs in their laws are, nevertheless, permissive toward practice by other midwives. But midwives in some states with vague laws have been subjected to random or selective prosecution for practicing medicine, midwifery, or even nursing without a license. A few states regulate certified or licensed midwives but allow those who choose not to be licensed to practice as lay midwives.

Despite ground-breaking new laws in several states, there has been no unanimity among direct-entry midwives regarding the desirability or wisdom of seeking legal sanction through attempts to change state laws. Some individuals want to continue to practice as lay midwives—desiring only to be left alone and for midwifery to be decriminalized but not regulated or licensed by the state. Midwives in some states have experienced negative consequences from efforts to increase standards by certification and licensing. A rule requiring licensing of birth centers in Texas resulted in closure of at least ten centers run by midwives (Harper, 1995). Some midwives in states that provide for licensing do not seek licenses and are adamant in their belief that midwives should be able to practice without legal restraint. Some midwives disagree with statutory restrictions that disallow home births for women who have had previous cesarean sections or are carrying twins or babies in breech position, based on their belief that they can handle such births and that women have the right to choose their place of birth and birth attendant without reference to a law (Becker *et al.*, 1990). Sociologists studying the effect of government regulation on lay midwives in Arizona found that licensure did not generate backup and other support from the medical community and resulted in unwanted medicalization and practice restrictions (Weitz & Sullivan, 1985). There is controversy about not only the risks and benefits of laws that provide regulation along with explicit legal sanction, but also about the ethical appropriateness of midwifery licensing laws (DeVries, 1985).

Nevertheless, the field has been moving toward professionalization, especially during the 1990s. Most recent law changes have been supportive. By the end of 1994, six states required their Medicaid programs to pay licensed direct-entry midwives for care provided to eligible women (MANA Legislative Committee, 1987). Some states have amended their laws several times, with each amendment requiring higher standards while giving direct-entry midwives greater status and authority.

Summary of State Laws Affecting Direct-Entry Midwives

The following summary is based on information published between 1990 and 1994.* The changes described earlier should be expected to continue—due not only to passage of new laws, but also to changes in the rules and regulations used to implement current

laws, particularly in response to the very new and evolving processes for accrediting direct-entry educational programs and certifying direct-entry midwives. The descriptions provided in this section were accurate when written, but some may be out of date by the time this book is published. The information is useful, however, as a general picture of the wide variety of legal status of direct-entry midwives in the United States during the early and mid-1990s.

- Seventeen jurisdictions either limit the practice of midwifery to CNMs, considering all other midwifery practice to be illegal, or require a license or permit that is no longer available: Alabama, Delaware, the District of Columbia, Georgia, Hawaii, Illinois, Indiana, Iowa, Kentucky, Maryland, Missouri, New Jersey, North Carolina, Ohio, Rhode Island, Virginia, and West Virginia. Direct-entry midwives in some of these states practice covertly. Under that circumstance, their clients come from word-of-mouth recommendations, little or no physician consultation is available,[†] and in some instances, midwives do not accompany women or infants who need to be transported to a hospital. They may also be less likely to carry emergency drugs and equipment, which can be used as evidence of their intention to commit a crime and so exposes them to risk (Becker *et al.*, 1990). However, direct-entry midwives in some of these states practice openly, even signing birth certificates. Much seems to depend on the history, personalities, relative supply versus demand for maternity care, and politics of each specific state. Many midwives who practice illegally do go to the hospital with women

---

*This summary is based primarily on information published by *Mothering* magazine in 1990 (Becker *et al.*, 1990), information published by the ACNM Political and Economic Affairs Committee in 1992 (Barickman *et al.*, 1992), an article published in the *Yale Journal of Law and Feminism* in 1993 (Suarez, 1993), and information compiled by the Legislative Committee of MANA as of the end of 1994.

---

†Some physicians who believe in midwifery provide covert backup; they are available, but the relationship is not acknowledged to other health professionals (Gaskin, 1996).

and infants who need medical care and most carry emergency equipment regardless of possible legal risk to themselves (NARM, 1996).

- Direct-entry midwifery is neither clearly legal nor illegal in eight states, either because the laws are silent, vague, or internally inconsistent: Idaho, Kansas, Nebraska, Nevada, North Dakota, Oklahoma, South Dakota, and Wisconsin. Some midwives practice openly and have good relationships with physicians in certain communities within many of these states.

- Direct-entry midwifery is legal but not regulated in nine states due to attorney-general or case law decisions that midwifery does not constitute the unlawful practice of medicine (or nurse-midwifery) and thus does not require a license or laws that legalize midwifery but have not yet been fully implemented with regulations and procedures: Connecticut, Maine, Massachusetts, Michigan, Mississippi, Pennsylvania, Tennessee, Utah, and Vermont.

- A 1987 opinion of the attorney general of Missouri allows registered nurses (RNs) who are not CNMs to practice midwifery due to a statement in the nurse practice act that "a licensed professional nurse may practice to the extent of her training." But it is illegal for midwives who are not nurses to practice in Missouri.

- Some states make exceptions to their rules to allow unlicensed lay midwives to provide care to members of particular subcultures. Washington does not require midwives who serve members of their religious communities to be licensed if they do not advertise and are not paid for their service. A lay midwife who serves a Mennonite community has a permit to practice in Delaware. Alaska's licensing requirement excludes midwives whose cultural tradition includes the use of midwives. Virginia requires all midwives to be RNs, but

defines a "midwife" as someone who assists during deliveries *for compensation.* Taking advantage of this language, some direct-entry midwives advertise their services and charge $600 to $800 for the educational services they provide to women whose deliveries they attend without charge. Twenty unlicensed direct-entry midwives were practicing in Virginia in 1990 (Becker *et al.,* 1990).

Thirteen states license lay or direct-entry midwives but do not require extensive formal midwifery education. Some of these states revised old laws that had been enacted as public health efforts to upgrade the practice of rural "granny" midwives. Some were old laws that had fallen into disuse and were discovered by lay midwives during the 1970s; their applications for licensure often led to new rules and regulations. However, some of the laws are new, including several passed since 1990. These laws tend to include detailed specifications regarding subjects to be covered in courses, numbers of supervised clinical experiences required to apply for a license, practices that must be carried out, practices that are prohibited, and requirements for the involvement of physicians.

Some states have established regulatory boards, which usually include physicians and CNMs, as well as licensed midwives, and require applicants to pass a state-administered examination. Although the licensing requirements vary, all seem to be predicated on the assumption that the practice of licensed midwives is confined to out-of-hospital births. Licensure or certification is optional in some of these states; e.g., Oregon licenses direct-entry midwives, but does not prohibit unlicensed midwives from practicing. Although these laws began as efforts to license *lay* midwives, the requirements for licensure have become more arduous in some of these states over time. In addition to the nine states whose laws are described below, Louisiana, Minnesota, Montana, and New Hampshire also fall into this category:

Alaska: In 1985 Alaska passed a law to recognize midwifery as a legally sanctioned profession and regulate it under the Department of Health and Social Services. Passage of the law was followed by five years of wrangling over the rules and regulations. The regulations that were presented in 1991 reflected input from the Alaska Medical Association but none from the Alaska Midwives Association, which predicted that restrictions in the rules would virtually eliminate direct-entry midwifery in Alaska (Kanne, 1992). In 1992 the midwives obtained support for new legislation, which called for a midwifery board that is responsible for implementation of the law.

Certified direct-entry midwives may assist the deliveries of women with specified complications (twins, breech presentations, previous cesarean sections, or pregnancies greater than forty-two weeks gestation) and may own and operate birth centers without the involvement of CNMs or physicians. Services provided by direct-entry midwives are covered by Alaska's Medicaid program.

Arizona: A 1957 law gives the Arizona Department of Health Services responsibility for licensing and supervising lay midwives. Approximately twenty-five women were licensed soon after the law was enacted, but only four were licensed between 1959 and 1977. A rise in requests for licensure during the mid-1970s prompted the adoption of new rules and regulations in January 1978 (Sullivan & Beeman, 1983). Licensing requires completion of a course of instruction covering specific content and experiences; passing written, oral, and clinical examinations; having a formal arrangement for consultation with a physician; examination of all clients by a physician during the third trimester, and conducting specified laboratory tests on every pregnant woman. Midwives may not use drugs or herbs except for a medication to prevent eye infections in the newborn.

Arkansas: Although licensed midwives must submit an emergency backup plan for each client, practice by unlicensed midwives is not illegal. Many direct-entry midwives do not participate in the licensing procedures. Nearly as many unlicensed as licensed midwives were practicing in 1990.

Colorado: A 1993 law requires direct-entry midwives to be registered based on passing a nationally accepted examination that is administered by the state. Qualifications to take the examination include graduation from high school, observing at least thirty births and serving as the primary attendant at thirty others. It is necessary to complete some kind of formal midwifery education, including a minimum of 430 hours of "theory" instruction. Hours of independent study count as hours of instruction; apprenticeship is recognized as a mode of midwifery education (Richardson, 1996).

Although the law requires use of a national examination, Colorado is using its own revision of a test developed by the Tennessee Midwives Association. The law is based on home birth practice and specifies that licensed midwives are not to be considered professional. Nineteen direct-entry midwives had been licensed as of April 1, 1994.

New Mexico: Licensure is overseen by a board that includes a physician, a CNM, a representative of the health department, a consumer, and two licensed midwives. Qualifications include completion of high school; specified courses and clinical experiences; certification in cardiopulmonary resuscitation (CPR); and satisfactory references from a physician or CNM, a midwifery instructor, a consumer, and a person from the applicant's community. Apprenticeships, self-study, and formal education are all acceptable. State regulations govern standards of practice, use of medicines and procedures, record keeping, continuing education, and consultation with physicians. Licensed midwives may use pitocin, cut episiotomies, and start intravenous infusions during emergencies. All third-party payers, including Medicaid, must pay for care provided by licensed midwives to residents of New Mexico.

The state's licensure program is so appealing to direct-entry midwives that many who practice in other states go through the process to become licensed in New Mexico. Of 120 midwives registered with the New Mexico Department of Health and Environment in 1988, all but 35 were practicing in other states.

Oregon: A 1993 law establishes a mechanism to license direct-entry midwives who meet criteria regarding experience (100 prenatal visits, 25 deliveries as an assistant, 25 deliveries as the primary care provider), have a written plan for emergency transport, and pass a written and oral examination. The law is implemented through a board composed of four licensed direct-entry midwives, two CNMs, and an obstetrician–gynecologist. Applicants for licensure must document that they have had learning experiences that could reasonably be expected to lead to development of the core competencies for basic midwifery practice as defined by MANA.*

Guidelines specify equipment that must be carried, absolute contraindications to home births, and conditions that require consultation. The law was passed to allow midwives to be paid through Medicaid and other third parties; it does not require midwives to be licensed. According to an attorney general's decision, anyone can practice midwifery legally in Oregon.

South Carolina: Registration as a direct-entry midwife requires completion of a correspondence or approved self-study course; apprenticeship with a CNM, physician, or registered direct-entry midwife; and passing a written and oral examination. The registra-

tion process is overseen by a Lay Midwifery Advisory Board that includes two CNMs, a physician, an attorney, three registered direct-entry midwives, and two consumers.

Texas: A 1956 Texas attorney general's opinion declared that midwifery does not constitute the practice of medicine. A 1983 law required midwives to identify themselves with the local county clerk annually, to give clients "disclosure" forms which explain that they attend only normal births and are not supposed to administer medications or perform procedures (including episiotomies), and to not refer to themselves as "certified" or "registered" midwives. A Lay Midwifery Board was established in 1987, and the law was amended to allow use of medicine to prevent newborn eye infections.

A 1991 amendment dropped "lay" from the title. The Midwifery Board (three direct-entry midwives, a CNM, an obstetrician-gynecologist, a pediatrician, and three consumers) established a basic midwifery training course, issued a training manual, and prepared an examination. The Department of Health issues a "letter of completion" to midwives who pass the exam. Because neither the training nor the examination were mandatory at first, some municipalities established their own requirements. Training and examination became mandatory throughout Texas in 1993.

Wyoming: A law that went into effect in 1989 allows lay midwives to attend home births but does not allow them to take care of women during either the prenatal or the postpartum period.

Laws That Require Three Years of Formal Midwifery Education

Four large, influential states have passed laws that require at least three years of midwifery education (the standard called for by the International Confederation of Midwives and the World Health Organization) or a bachelor's or higher degree. The law

---

*See section on "MANA Core Competencies for Basic Midwifery Practice" on page 246.

passed in New York State in 1992 is the first intended to cover CNMs and licensed direct-entry midwives under the same set of regulations. Implementation of the law has had a negative effect on direct-entry midwives in New York.

Washington: A 1917 law required the Department of Licensing to administer a midwifery test to anyone who had graduated from a midwifery school that met certain specifications and to license anyone who passed the test. It was revised in 1981. The revision provides for licensure based on graduation from a state-accredited three-year educational program. The clinical component of the program must include assisting at 50 births and acting as the primary attendant at 50 births, under supervision. The program may be shortened to two years for students with prior midwifery or relevant nursing experience. The presence of the Seattle Midwifery School was an important factor in passage of this law. Naturopaths who attend births must meet the same requirements and hold midwifery licenses.

The law does not prohibit unlicensed persons from attending births if they do not advertise as midwives or collect fees for their services. This provision was intended to enable the practice of lay midwives who serve particular religious communities; unlicensed midwives are the only persons available to attend home births in some parts of the state.

Licensed midwives must submit a plan for medical consultation and emergency transfer of clients. They may administer oxytocic drugs, local anesthetics, and intravenous infusions and carry and use certain emergency equipment. Although the law permits them to work in homes, clinics, or hospitals, none have received hospital privileges. A bill authorizing continuation of the 1981 law was passed unanimously in 1987.

Florida: Florida revised its midwifery law three times between 1982 and 1992. The law

passed in 1982 recognized "the need for parents' freedom of choice in the manner of, cost of, and setting for their children's births"; established a Lay Midwifery Advisory Committee within the Department of Health and Rehabilitative Services (DHRS); and required DHRS to license midwives based on an examination. DHRS was directed to administer the examination to any applicant who was a high school graduate in good health and had completed "an approved program for the preparation of midwives" and to develop and promulgate standards by which it would approve a midwifery training program. Such programs must be associated with a state-accredited educational institution and include three years of course work and clinical training. The program could be reduced to two years for students who were registered nurses or registered practical nurses or had practical midwifery experience.

A "sunset" provision required legislative review of the effects of the new law by October 1984. Two schools designed to meet the requirements of the law opened in 1984. Review of the law that fall resulted in an amendment that limited additional midwifery licenses to students already enrolled in those two schools.

In 1990 the legislature requested the staff of the Senate Committee on Health and Rehabilitative Services to study and prepare a report on the practice of licensed midwives in Florida between 1984 and 1990. The report, issued in 1991, documented a crisis in maternity care and infant mortality in the state of Florida, a doubling in the percentage of births attended by CNMs during the 1980s, and the inability of existing graduate nursing programs to train enough CNMs to meet the need in Florida. To help alleviate this crisis, the report recommended reinstating the 1982 law with changes to strengthen the educational requirements and mandate accreditation of midwifery schools. It also recommended that licensed midwives be trained and then permitted to administer certain prescription drugs, that the Florida Medicaid program pay for prenatal and post-partum care provided by licensed midwives, and that publicly funded hospitals and birth centers be required to provide clinical experience to midwifery students. New legislation was written to incorporate these recommendations. A Friends of Midwives organization lobbied for the bill, focusing on access to care and cost containment. (It did not hurt that two of the governor's grandchildren had been delivered by licensed midwives.) The law passed in 1992.

New York: The Professional Midwifery Practice Act that was signed into law in July 1992 and became effective in February 1995 is described in Chapter 8. The law provides a single legal standard for all midwives and recognizes midwifery as a profession that is separate and independent from nursing. CNMs were the only midwives who could practice legally in New York before this law was enacted. Under the new law, one does not have to be a nurse to be licensed to practice midwifery in New York. Although the intent was to expand the profession, so far the law has had the opposite effect (Behrmann, 1996). Before the new law was enacted, practicing midwifery without a license was a misdemeanor; direct-entry midwives practiced without fear and were not arrested. Under the new law, practicing without a license is a felony. Direct-entry midwives have been arrested; one was taken from her premises in handcuffs. Midwives are afraid and angry, and feel that they have been betrayed.

The legislation that eventually resulted in the new law was initiated by nurse-midwives. Several direct-entry midwives had begun to work on their own concept of ideal midwifery legislation, even before the nurse-midwives had begun to work on theirs. Thus at one point there were two midwifery bills in the New York legislative hopper. When their own bill died in committee, the direct-entry midwives began to lobby to be included in the bill being promoted by the CNMs. They were given reason to believe that at least one seat on the Midwifery Board to be established under this legislation would be reserved for a non-CNM midwifery educator and that there would be a mechanism by which the approximately 100 direct-entry midwives practicing in New York at that time could apply for licensure. But, as the bill worked its way through the legislative process it was altered, perhaps due to the influence of obstetricians, in ways that had a negative impact on direct-entry midwives (Davis-Floyd, 1997).

The law calls for midwifery to be regulated by a Board of Midwifery that consists primarily of midwives. Although midwives appointed to the board should represent "a broad range of midwifery practice and education," all midwives appointed to the board as of the end of 1996 were nurse-midwives. This occurred in part because the law requires midwife board members to be licensed and CNMs were the only midwives licensed by the State of New York when the first board members were appointed.

The rules and regulations for implementation of the Midwifery Practice Act were written by the Board of Midwifery and the staff of the New York State Education Department (NYSED). Licensure as a professional midwife requires (1) completion of a midwifery education program that leads to a baccalaureate or higher degree and has been registered by the NYSED or has been determined to be equivalent to a program registered by the NYSED and (2) passing a professional licensing examination that is acceptable to the NYSED. With the exception of the mandatory baccalaureate degree, the educational standards established in the regulations are similar to those of the ACNM. The ACNM Certification Council examination was adopted as the state licensing exam. The scope of practice authorized in the law is similar to that of a CNM.

As of February 1995, all midwives practicing in New York were required to apply for licensure under this law. CNMs who had been authorized to practice in New York under the previous arrangement were grandmothered into the new law. Direct-entry midwives were encouraged to apply, and thirteen did. The only practicing direct-entry midwife who was allowed to take the exam was accepted because she had completed a nursing course and had received formal midwifery education in England (Davis-Floyd, 1997). The applications of all other direct-entry midwives were rejected, usually because their midwifery education did not lead to a bachelor's degree (Burkhardt, 1996).

Home births have become less available in New York as a result of the new law. Few physicians are willing to provide the backup required for CNMs to attend home births, and some direct-entry midwives who had been attending home births in New York for many years have left the state, gone further underground, or stopped practicing.

In 1996, the State University of New York Health Science Center at Brooklyn and the North Central Bronx Hospital jointly opened a postbaccalaureate direct-entry midwifery education program designed to meet the requirements of the New York law (Shah & Hsia, 1996). Applicants must have a baccalaureate degree; must have completed college-level courses in biology, chemistry, microbiology, anatomy and physiology, human development, psychology, sociology, epidemiology or statistics, pathophysiology, and nutrition; and must have had prior experience in women's health care. Five students were accepted into the first class—a physician assistant, a direct-entry midwife who had completed some nursing education, two former nursing students, and a licensed practical nurse (LPN). The State University of New York Health Science Center at Brooklyn has operated a certified nurse-midwifery education program since 1973. The North Central Bronx Hospital has operated a long-standing, high-volume nurse-midwifery service. The new direct-entry program was developed and is being taught by nurse-midwives. It has received preaccreditation status from the ACNM Division of Accreditation.*

California: A law to legalize direct-entry midwifery in California was passed in 1993. Opposition from the California Medical Association had prevented passage of other bills during five previous sessions of the legislature. The new law is administered by the Division of Allied Health Professions of the California Board of Medicine, which decided the rules and regulations; there are no midwives on the committee. The rules and regulations for implementation were not approved until late 1995. Disagreements between midwives and the Board of Medicine regarding supervision by physicians and which examination to use caused considerable delay. In 1996 the board agreed to use the examination developed by the North American Registry of Midwives (described later in this chapter) as a basis for the license in California. More than forty California midwives were investigated, arrested, and prosecuted by the California Board of Medical Quality Assurance between 1974 and the signing of the new law in September 1993 (Becker *et al.*,1982; Wykes, 1993). In 1993, the state agreed to cease legal action against midwives until the new rules are in place.

The two requirements for licensing are: (1) completion of a midwifery education program that meets specified requirements and (2) passing of an examination. Criteria for both were based on the ACNM core competencies. Although the rules do not require an educational program that leads to an academic degree, the program must continue over at least three academic years, which can

---

*This program was the first direct-entry midwifery education program to receive preaccreditation status from the ACNM. See the section on the ACNM's role in direct-entry education and certification later in this chapter for additional information about this program and ACNM's involvement in the credentialing of direct-entry midwives.

be compressed into slightly more than two calendar years. Supervision by an obstetrician–gynecologist (ob–gyn) is required; the ratio of midwives to ob–gyns cannot be greater than four to one. Midwives must practice under a protocol approved by the supervising physician. The scope of practice authorized by the law is similar to that of a CNM, including elements, such as prescription of hormonal contraception, that no direct-entry midwives in California had included in their practice prior to passage of this law. There are three ways to meet the educational requirement:

1. Complete a three-year midwifery education program that has been accredited by a national accrediting agency recognized by the U.S. Department of Education (USDOE). As of the end of 1996, no direct-entry midwifery educational program in California met those criteria. However, two schools in other states did—the Seattle Midwifery School and a program run by Miami Dade Community College, in Miami, Florida. Both of these schools are accredited by USDOE-recognized national accrediting organizations that have expertise in education and curriculum, but not in midwifery. A process for accrediting direct-entry midwifery programs has been developed by the Midwifery Education Accreditation Council (MEAC).* As of the end of 1996, the Seattle Midwifery School had been accredited by MEAC, and the Miami Dade Community College program was going through the accreditation process. A three-year direct-entry program was started in San Francisco by the Midwifery Institute of California in 1996. It was one of ten programs included in the pilot test of MEAC's new accreditation process. Although it re-

ceived preaccreditation status from MEAC, because MEAC is not yet eligible for recognition by the USDOE, the Midwifery Institute of California program does not meet that requirement of the California law.

2. Have or acquire a license from another state with standards that have been determined to be comparable to California's. As of September 1995, Washington and Florida were the only states determined to have comparable standards.

3. Experienced midwives may challenge individual courses or the complete curriculum of an educational program that meets the standards specified in the law. The challenge process requires applicants to provide evidence of having had specified numbers of clinical experiences, to complete written examinations, and to undergo clinical examinations. The California Board of Medicine has approved challenge mechanisms submitted by the Miami Dade Community College program and the Seattle Midwifery School (SMS) . Although SMS has a mechanism by which its own students can challenge particular courses, the SMS challenge mechanism approved by the California Board of Medicine was developed specifically for experienced midwives seeking licensure in California. SMS agreed to make this mechanism available for two years—1996 and 1997. Approximately thirty California midwives successfully completed the SMS challenge process during 1996. It was developed as a means to test the knowledge and clinical skills of experienced midwives who need to be "grandmothered" into the new law and is not intended to serve as an alternative to a formal educational program for inexperienced people who want to become midwives.

The state of California will administer the NARM examination for the first time in

---

*Development of the MEAC accreditation process is described later in this chapter.

1997. The only licenses granted during 1995 and 1996 were to midwives who were already licensed in Washington or Florida. The law will "sunset" in 1998. An assessment will be conducted at that time.

State Midwifery Organizations

Lay midwifery arose as a local phenomenon created by individuals or small groups of people working within their own communities, and it developed as part of a social movement that was distrustful of centralized authority. Many direct-entry midwives continue to prefer individual or local responsibility over national-level authority regarding midwifery. For these reasons, and because of great variation in the legal and practice circumstances of midwives in different states, local midwifery organizations were started many years before the development of a national organization for direct-entry midwives. Some CNMs, especially those with home birth practices, also belong to some of these organizations.

State midwifery associations often began as informal meetings organized for the purpose of sharing information and developing opportunities for learning. Some of them developed into formal organizations and began to develop standards. For example, during the late 1970s the Cascade Midwives Association (CMA), based in Portland, Oregon, developed practice standards that all members agreed to uphold. Each member of the association was expected to take an examination to demonstrate her abilities, to file a synopsis of each case with the CMA, to participate in at least twenty hours of continuing education workshops or classes each year, to maintain current certification in infant and adult CPR, to attend all CMA peer review meetings, and to be thoroughly familiar with the organization's practice guidelines. The guidelines covered informed consent; obtaining the woman's medical, family, and obstetric history; a prescribed schedule of prenatal visits; some clinical "dos

and don'ts," including circumstances in which the midwife must notify a physician; being available twenty-four hours a day for three weeks before a client's due date; aspects to consider in making plans for a home birth; information to provide to the parents; and having at least two midwives at each birth, with the two together representing experience with one-hundred or more home births.

Every CMA meeting began with case reviews, during which each midwife discussed any pregnant woman under her care who had a risk factor, complication, or other unusual circumstance and reported on all births she had attended since the last meeting, giving the name of her assistant at each birth and stating what could have been done differently or better. Every meeting included an educational session. Every member was also required to participate in peer review meetings that were held every six weeks. Everyone participating in peer review was encouraged to point out any deviation from a guideline. When that occurred, the group was required to come to one of four conclusions: (1) The midwife disagreed with the guideline and convinced the other members of the group to change it. (2) The midwife disagreed with the guideline and ended her membership in CMA. (3) The midwife convinced the group that she followed the spirit, if not the exact wording, of the guideline. (4) The midwife agreed with the guideline and agreed to follow it in the future.

The CMA later merged with groups in other parts of the state to become the Oregon Midwifery Council. In 1982 the Oregon Midwifery Council became the first state midwifery organization to develop a process to certify local midwives based on written and oral examinations. The CMA may have been ahead of the curve in developing and implementing standards. However, direct-entry midwives throughout the country were (and are) serious, responsible people. Although many came into midwifery almost accidentally, those who stayed and grew to love it were deeply committed to the well-being of the women and families they served. They needed and sought ways to overcome isolation and their lack of formal training. Many were motivated to create the structure needed to provide safety for their clients, themselves as individuals, and the vulnerable profession they were building.

Direct-entry midwifery organizations were functioning in at least thirty-six states in 1994. Many of them published newsletters; at least twenty had their own process for certifying midwives. In at least eight states, certification by the midwifery organization required passing a written test; some also required an oral and/or clinical examination (MANA, 1993). Although the certification standards vary widely, some state midwifery organizations require more training than the minimum specified by the regulatory agencies in their states. As of 1990, forty-three local midwifery organizations offered peer review (Becker *et al.*, 1990). This also varies widely. Some state midwifery organizations mandate a highly structured form of peer review; for others, peer review is an informal process that is offered, but not required. Peer review contributed to the development of a concept of acceptable practice; thus it has played an important role in the development of direct-entry midwifery (Myers-Ciecko, 1996).

Consumer Support

In the early days, there was only a fine distinction between lay midwives and the women who used their services. Some women became midwives after having had a home birth. Explaining how she became a midwife in the 1970s, a midwife in northern California replied, "How could I stop it? I had a home birth, everyone heard, and they all wanted me at their births. I couldn't stop it" (Osborn & Esty, 1995). Most women who had home births during that period had done a lot of reading in the course of reaching a decision to have a home birth and had

to search to find someone to help them. A woman who asked a relative, friend or neighbor to attend her birth was likely to know as much about it as the person she asked for help; the "midwife" differed from the mother only in having had some experience. There was not a clear distinction between midwives and the women they assisted; they were part of the same social group and thought of themselves as members of a movement, not as professionals and clients. Mothers became midwives; midwives became mothers. As a result, lay midwives never thought of the women they took care of as "patients." They are often referred to simply as "women" or as "mothers." Home birthing was a philosophy and way of life shared by friends and neighbors; midwifery was not originally thought of as a career.

Nevertheless, some women had a special interest in birth and sought more knowledge and experience. Eventually they were recognized as becoming midwives. But the distinction was gradual, and midwives and their clients continued to be bonded in a concept of childbirth that was outside the system. These bonds were especially strong in states where midwives were persecuted and arrested (McIntyre, 1982). Activists among the clients found ways to contribute to the cause. Thus as midwifery organizations formed, many included consumers, some of whom helped to start the organizations. Consumers serve on the boards of some state midwifery associations and play important roles in MANA.

Consumers in some areas formed separate "Friends of Midwives" support and advocacy groups. These groups consist primarily of people interested in preserving home birth as an option, including midwives' clients and childbirth educators who have lost faith in the ability of hospitals and physicians to provide the kind of care sought by the people who take their courses. Some medical writers, anthropologists, sociologists, feminists, and others who support midwifery and home births for philosophical reasons are also active in these groups. Some midwifery support groups were formed in response to a crisis involving threats to an individual midwife (sometimes including arrest) or threats to all home birth practice in a particular community. Other groups developed to support legislation designed to sanction midwifery practice in a state. Some are informal and disband after the specific threat or opportunity has passed; others develop a formal structure and continue. Although most of these groups are especially interested in preserving home birth as an option for women in their area, some groups have broadened their focus to include active support of nurse-midwives and midwifery care in hospitals (Brodsky, 1996).

Six women who were members of midwifery support groups in Georgia, Kansas, and Kentucky founded Citizens for Midwifery, a nonprofit, grass-roots volunteer organization of midwifery advocates in the United States and Canada, in February 1996. A grant from a small, private trust assisted in the development of the organization, which facilitates networking and provides education and resources to individuals and groups trying to promote universal availability of the midwifery model of maternity care. Despite its name, which focuses on midwifery, the organization supports the efforts of all who promote or put into practice a "woman-centered, respectful and holistic way of being with women during childbirth, whatever their title," recognizing "that a variety of health care providers can deliver this model of care in a variety of settings" (Citizens for Midwifery, 1996). Nevertheless, the organization believes that midwives are the best qualified to do so and should be independent professionals to assure availability of this kind of care (Hodges, 1997). A number of other national organizations focus on midwifery as part of a broader agenda of education and support for home births and other alternatives to mainstream medical obstetrics, for example, the National Coalition for Birthing Alternatives, which focuses on public education.

The Midwives' Alliance of North America

An "open forum" discussion during the ACNM's 1981 convention focused on whether the college should expand its focus to include other midwives. Although there was no consensus on that issue, there was wide agreement that nurse-midwives and the ACNM should be in dialogue with other midwives.

The ACNM president who took office at that meeting was from Texas—the state with the largest number of direct-entry midwives. Once in office, she was approached by many nurse-midwives who wanted to open a dialogue with direct-entry midwives. She was also approached by a representative of the American College of Obstetricians and Gynecologists (ACOG), who complained that ACOG needed a way to communicate with direct-entry midwives but did not know how, because the ACNM was the only national midwifery organization and represented only CNMs.

That autumn, ACNM President Sister Angela Murdaugh invited representatives of the Seattle Midwifery School and the Farm (in Tennessee), a few other direct-entry midwives, and several CNMs who had started as lay midwives to a meeting to discuss these issues (Murdaugh, 1992). The midwives who participated in that meeting made plans to organize an "American Midwifery Guild" that would expand communication between all types of midwives in the United States; set educational guidelines; establish competency standards for practicing midwives, perhaps leading to some kind of national certification; and form a more inclusive midwifery organization (Shah, 1982; Ventre & Leonard, 1982). A follow-up meeting held during the next ACNM convention led to the founding of the Midwives' Alliance of North America (MANA). All midwives in the United States, Canada and Mexico—actually, anyone with an interest in midwifery—were welcome to join. This inclusivity was in purposeful contrast to the ACNM's exclusivity and rigid eligibility requirements. The ACNM's organizational structure and key documents were used as models, however, in part because the founders hoped the two organizations might merge at some point in the future (Stallings, 1992). One of MANA's major goals is to develop unity among all midwives.

More than a hundred midwives from all over the United States and Canada attended MANA's first annual meeting in October 1983. Two of the most difficult issues discussed at that meeting were a process to develop practice standards and the concept of educational criteria as a basis for certification (Schlinger, 1992). Many factors made it hard for MANA to move in the direction of creating definitions and processes to distinguish categories of midwives based on education and other criteria—the organization's embrace of anyone who considers herself a midwife; its intention to represent midwives in Mexico, as well as Canada and the United States; a commitment to affirmative action to achieve racial, ethnic, and cultural diversity; and a desire to honor the "granny" or "Grand Midwives."

The international aspect of the organization has been an important source of support to midwives in all of the countries included in MANA. The 1991 convention was attended by more than four hundred midwives and people who support midwifery, including individuals from Argentina and Germany, as well as the three countries of North America. In one of the educational sessions, licensed traditional midwives from Mexico used an interpreter to explain how they move babies from the breech to the head-down position and assist women at birth without performing any vaginal examinations.

MANA's annual conferences are preceded and followed by workshops, and its newsletter carries information on workshops offered by other organizations. A periodically updated "Information Packet for Aspiring Midwives" that lists and describes books, audiovisual learning tools, networking contacts, schools, apprenticeships, and learning resources has been available since 1990.

Despite its many accomplishments, less than half of all direct-entry midwives are members of MANA. About one-third of MANA's 1,400 members are CNMs; one-tenth of ACNM members are also members of MANA. Some direct-entry midwives belong to a state midwifery association but do not belong to MANA. Perhaps three-fourths of all practicing direct-entry midwives belong to either MANA and/or a state midwifery association (Stallings, 1994).

Membership in the International Confederation of Midwives

Acceptance into the International Confederation of Midwives (ICM) was another of MANA's original goals. Its initial application was rejected because its membership included persons who do not meet the international definition of a midwife, which requires successful completion of a recognized midwifery educational program and acquisition of the qualifications required to be registered or legally licensed to practice midwifery.* In response to MANA's unusual situation, ICM changed its bylaws to make it possible to accept a *branch* of an organization if all members of that part of the organization are midwives "recognized by their government or professional organizations as being competent to practice midwifery" (Cowper-Smith). In response to that change, MANA formed an "International Section" that includes only CNMs and direct-entry midwives who are licensed in their states or graduated from a state-approved midwifery education program or a midwifery school with standing in another country. The International Section of MANA was accepted into the ICM in 1984. The existence of the Inter-

---

*See the international definition of a midwife in Chapter 1.

national Section gave impetus to MANA's Certification Committee, which began to examine the circumstances in states where a local midwifery association had developed a certification process. If the certification procedure of the state midwifery association was determined to be acceptable, members of MANA who had been certified by their state association were considered to be eligible for membership in the International Section of MANA, and in the ICM.

Having a special section for midwives who meet certain criteria was controversial within MANA because it is not consistent with the organization's emphasis on unity and equal status (Patkelly, 1992). However MANA members who attended ICM Triennial Congresses reported that MANA's participation in ICM is important to midwives throughout the world. MANA members were welcomed by midwives from other countries, who feel that knowing about the home birth practices of direct-entry midwives in North America is helping to keep a pure form of midwifery alive for midwives in Europe, Australia, and New Zealand. Although midwifery is part of the system in those countries, some midwives fear that they have "lost their soul" and "look at MANA as the soul of midwifery" (Stallings, 1992).

Development of Standards and Qualifications

A Standards and Practice Committee was started in 1983. Initial discussions focused on whether it is possible to develop any kind of practice standards that are not exclusive. Standards were a "touchy subject" because of the wide variety of practice circumstances of MANA members; some feared that any standards would be so elitist or exclusionary that they would be left out (Leonard, 1992) or that the adoption of standards would mean that midwives "will never be able to step outside of 'accepted practice' and would result in "more transports, less autonomy and the erosion of consumers' rights" (Hobbs,

1992). There was great concern about adopting a medical model with a list of "dos and don'ts" or adopting standards with which midwives who practice illegally could not possibly comply. Progress was made based on the concept that midwives need to define their own practice, and that someone else would do it if they did not.

A statement on the *Standards and Qualifications for the Art and Practice of Midwifery* was adopted in 1985 and revised in 1991. It recognizes that childbearing belongs to women and encourages active involvement of family members. It outlines necessary midwifery skills and affirms the role of intuition. It describes the need to carry and maintain appropriate equipment, to keep accurate records of the care provided to each woman, and to comply with local public health requirements. It requires the midwife to "assess each woman for initial and continuing eligibility for midwifery services" and to "make a reasonable attempt to assure that her client has access to consultation and/or referral to a medical care system when indicated" and asserts her right and responsibility to refuse or discontinue services and make referrals when indicated "for the protection of the mother, baby, or midwife." The standards do not oblige midwives to actually arrange for medical consultation and referral; the responsibility to do so resides with the pregnant woman. Each midwife is expected to assure informed consent for her care by presenting accurate information about herself and her service, including her midwifery education and experience, protocols and standards, financial charges, the services she provides, and the responsibilities of the pregnant woman and her family. Midwives are expected to update their knowledge and skills, participate in peer review, and develop appropriate practice protocols.

MANA's *Statement of Values and Ethics*

MANA developed a *Statement of Values and Ethics*, which was formally adopted in 1992.

It describes beliefs that permeate and energize this arm of midwifery in the United States. The following are the major precepts regarding values:

- *Valuing women* as individuals with unique worth, who have creative, life-affirming and life-giving powers and the right to make choices regarding all aspects of their lives.
- *Valuing the inseparability and interdependence of the pregnant mother and her unborn child;* the integrity of a woman's body, which should be supported to achieve a natural, spontaneous vaginal birth; the baby's right to be born in a caring and loving manner, without separation from mother and family; the sentient and sensitive nature of the newborn, and breast-feeding as the ideal way of nourishing and nurturing the newborn.
- *Valuing pregnancy and birth* as an essential mystery; as natural processes that technology will never supplant; as integrated experiences in which the physical, emotional, mental, psychological, and spiritual components are inseparable; as personal, intimate, internal, sexual, social events to be shared in the environment and with the attendants a woman chooses; as experiences from which we learn, and as processes that have lifelong impacts on a woman's self-esteem, health, ability to nurture, and personal growth.
- *Valuing the art of midwifery and the right to practice it* as an ancient vocation of women; as expertise that incorporates academic knowledge, clinical skill, intuitive judgment, and spiritual awareness; as the art of nurturing the intrinsic normalcy of birth; as a way of empowering women in all aspects of life, particularly as their strength is realized during and as a result of pregnancy and birth; as the art of encouraging women to express their strength so that they can give birth unhindered, with confidence in their abilities and the support of midwives; as including skills that help a complicated pregnancy move to a state of greater well-being or to the most healing conclusion, accepting death as a possible outcome of birth, focusing on supporting life rather than avoiding death. Holding these values leads to valuing all forms of midwifery education and acknowledging the ongoing wisdom of apprenticeship as the original model for training midwives and to valuing midwives standing for what they believe in in the face of social and political oppression.
- *Valuing women as mothers;* a mother's intuitive knowledge of herself and her baby before, during and after birth; her innate ability to nurture her pregnancy and birth her baby; the power and beauty of her body, the awesome strength summoned in labor; the mother as the only direct care provider for her unborn child; pregnancy and birth as rites of passage integral to a woman's evolution into mothering; the potential of a woman's partners, family, and community to support her in all aspects of birth and mothering. Holding these values leads to supporting women in a nonjudgmental way, regardless of their physical, emotional, social, or spiritual health; broadening available resources when possible so that women can realize the desired goals of health, happiness, and personal growth according to their needs and perceptions; and valuing each woman's right to choose a caregiver who is appropriate to her needs and compatible with her beliefs.
- *Valuing relationship;* believing that the quality, integrity, equality, and uniqueness of personal interactions affect individual choices and decisions; valuing honesty in relationship; caring for women to the best of one's ability without prejudice; exercising personal responsibility; honoring individuals' rights to make choices according to what they

think is best for themselves, to true informed choice, not merely informed consent to what the midwife thinks is best; providing access to readily understood information, including the midwife's knowledge and understanding about birth; valuing the midwifery community as a support system and essential place of learning and sisterhood, diversity among midwives, mutual trust and respect, making decisions and acting ethically.

- *Valuing a relationship to a process larger than themselves*; recognizing that birth is something midwives can seek to learn from and know, but never control; retaining humility in their work; recognizing their own limits and limitations.

Ambivalence About Certification

An open forum on certification during MANA's 1985 annual meeting focused on whether the organization should get involved in certification and, if so, whether certification should be mandatory or voluntary, whether a certification examination should test for entry -level or more advanced skills, and how certification would be used by states, provinces, and MANA's International Section (Spindel, 1992). It was a contentious issue, with strong arguments and feelings for and against (Schlinger, 1992).

Arguments against certification were based on deeply held philosophical convictions: Some midwives saw testing, standards, licensing, and certification as tools that physicians and others have used to monopolize health care and prevent consumers from having access to alternatives. Midwives who believe "that the midwife's ultimate responsibility is to the people of her community, not to a midwifery licensing board" argued against allowing state governments to regulate midwifery (Vogler, 1992). Pointing out that some licensed professionals are incompetent, many believe that quality of care is best assured by giving women real options,

information, and choice (Kingsepp, 1992). Each woman has the "right and responsibility to study the birth process and to make an informed choice regarding the type of birth attendant and environment" she believes to be most suited to her needs. Certification is "fundamentally inconsistent with each individual being *truly* responsible for their own experience" and maintains an artificial separation between professionals and laypersons. "To certify ourselves, even with the best of intentions, we would run the risk of merely creating a new class of birth professionals, and quickly lose sight of the very things which most require transformation," that is, "putting the power of the birthing process back into the hands of women" (Frye, 1992a). Arguing that the licensed professions "have virtually excluded low-income, minority groups, and those persons lacking 'test-taking' skills," one midwife expressed concern about having "our granny midwives passed over or condemned as 'ignorant' simply because her cultural and educational background is different from our own" (Vogler, 1992).

In 1986 MANA decided to defer action on certification in favor of developing a national registry of midwives who pass a voluntary examination developed to test midwifery knowledge. The decision to defer action on certification was based on several considerations—a desire to be fair to rural midwives, many of whom have too few births to meet standards for national certification; a desire to encourage states to develop their own certification processes; and concern about legal liability. A registry examination was thought to be less threatening. In the words of one participant in the debate, "All we're really saying is, 'This person has passed a national exam.' We're not saying anything about their competency, because we're not testing it" (Davis, 1992). MANA established the North American Registry of Midwives (NARM) to develop an examination and registry. Over time, support for national certification grew among the members of MANA, and NARM was given a mandate to develop and implement a national certification process. By late 1994, the pilot phase of this process was in place. A group of midwifery teachers formed another separate organization for the purpose of developing a process for accrediting educational programs. Requirements for discipline, continuing education, peer review, and so on, have been left to NARM and local jurisdictions (*MANA News*, 1987). All processes developed by MANA itself are voluntary. MANA supports processes intended to unite midwives, and any midwife can join. MANA does not want to be a gatekeeper or fence builder.

MANA Core Competencies for Basic Midwifery Practice

MANA developed its own core competencies statement, which was formally adopted in April 1990. An early draft listed midwifery tasks in great detail but was too specific to be applied across the broad range of cultural, ethnic, and philosophic differences and countries represented in MANA. It was revised to further demedicalize its language, articulate the midwifery model of care more clearly, and respect and encompass the diverse midwives within MANA, while setting minimum standards. References to specific contraceptive methods were dropped in deference to midwives whose religious beliefs preclude a role in con-traception. Requirements for pharmacologic competencies were not included because the use and prescription of medications are not a recognized part of direct-entry midwifery practice in many jurisdictions.

After a list of guiding principles, the document lists skills and areas of knowledge from the social and health sciences that are relevant to midwifery and describes competencies required to provide midwifery care during each phase of the maternity cycle, including care of the newborn, family planning and well-woman care, and competencies related to the legal and other professional

aspects of midwifery. The section on family planning and well-woman care is optional; although "the entry level midwife *may* provide well woman gynecological and family planning care," knowing how to do so is not an essential competency.

Data Collection and Research

MANA's Statistics and Research Committee spent several years developing a form for routine prospective collection of uniform data on midwifery clients and care. This was a challenging assignment because, although detailed information is needed, the form should be short enough that midwives would be willing to fill it out on a continuing basis. In 1989 the committee began to work with a Canadian epidemiologist to test and revise a form that had been developed for use in Ontario (Daviss-Putt, 1992). The form is now in use for both prospective and retrospective studies.

This unique database should contribute to our understanding of normal pregnancy, labor, and birth, as well as information allowing objective evaluation of certain midwifery methods. Because midwives tend to have greater comfort, respect and patience with variations in the way individual women labor, this data set will provide an opportunity to document some of these variations and their effects on outcomes. MANA provides an ideal base for conducting this research because it has no disciplinary function. The midwives are encouraged to report the process and outcomes of their care without fear of repercussion or disciplinary action (Johnson & Daviss, 1996). See Chapter 6 for additional information.

Seminars and an Interorganizational Work Group on Midwifery Education

In 1989 the Carnegie Foundation for the Advancement of Teaching convened a seminar on midwifery education. Stimulated by a crisis in the provision of maternity care to women throughout the country, the meeting was intended to define the extent to which midwives could reduce the shortage of professionals to provide maternity care and deliver babies, and to examine the recruitment and education of midwives. The foundation was especially interested in the potential impact of further development of direct-entry midwifery education on recruitment into the profession. In 1990 the Carnegie Foundation convened a second seminar to further explore the feasibility of establishing one standard for professional midwifery while recognizing multiple routes of entry. The thirty participants included officers and key committee chairpersons from the ACNM and MANA. It was clear that the two organizations had many common objectives and needed to have better communication. At the end of the second seminar the foundation agreed to support meetings of an Interorganizational Work-Group on Midwifery Education (IWG) that would include representatives of the ACNM and MANA, as well as consumers, and would function for the purpose of developing core competencies and a core curriculum for professional midwifery and work needed to unify the profession.

During the first seminar, Dr. Ernest Boyer, who was president of the foundation, asked what it would take for the ACNM to accredit an educational program for direct-entry midwives. Since the ACNM accreditation process is based on the ACNM core competencies, nurse-midwives at the meeting realized that in order to accredit an education program for midwives who are not nurses, "the ACNM would need to identify all of the relevant knowledge, skills and competencies that nurses are presumed to bring to nurse-midwifery education and then require that those essential competencies be acquired by the completion of a midwifery education program" (Roberts, 1996). The ACNM responded by requesting its Division of Accreditation to define the "core health skills" needed by midwives who are not nurses.

The IWG met five times between 1991 and 1994. It focused exclusively on professional midwifery, deciding not to deal with midwives who do not seek legal recognition (Katz-Rothman, 1992). That issue in itself was problematic, because "professionalism" had negative connotations for some members of MANA.

As a consequence, the definition of a "professional midwife," developed by the IWG was not approved by MANA. It was replaced with an IWG statement on midwifery certification that recognized the diversity of midwifery education and practice in the United States and defined a certified midwife (either direct-entry or nurse-midwife) as a person who has successfully completed prescribed studies in midwifery, has met the requisite qualifications to be certified, and is qualified to be legally authorized to practice in at least one state. The statement described the qualifications and standards of both a certified midwife and a certified nurse-midwife and designated the ACNM as the organization with authority to certify nurse-midwives and MANA as the organization for certification of direct-entry midwives. During nearly four years of work the IWG reviewed both organizations' documents on core competencies, standards of practice, philosophy, ethics, and values. However, the statement on midwifery certification and a statement on Grand Midwives were the only documents produced by the IWG that were approved by the board of directors of both organizations. The recurrent sticking point was disagreement about the need for professional midwives to undergo a formal educational process. The ACNM is committed to formal education. MANA is committed to preserving multiple educational routes to midwifery, including apprenticeships. The ACNM representatives rejected apprenticeship as a valid educational approach, in part because there were no mechanisms for evaluating the skills of an apprentice-trained midwife.

The Evolution of a Process to Certify Professional Direct-Entry Midwives

The IWG process moved the direct-entry midwifery community toward accepting the need for a process to certify professional direct-entry midwives and resulted in initiation of some of the necessary steps. The ACNM's plan to identify the knowledge and skills from nursing education that provide a base for nurse-midwifery put MANA and NARM on alert; if direct-entry midwives did not identify their own entry-level midwifery skills, they would be forced to accept a midwifery skills list that was based on nursing and developed by nurse-midwives. When a skills list drafted by the ACNM was circulated at an IWG meeting, the MANA representatives recognized the need to develop a list of midwifery and general health care skills that reflects the perspective of the direct-entry midwifery community. In 1992 the IWG funded MANA and NARM to carry out a skills/task analysis for the purpose of identifying midwifery skills. The IWG process also identified the need for a formal means to assess the competence of an apprentice-trained midwife (Sammon, 1996).

The need to create a way to validate the knowledge and skills of practicing midwives became increasingly acute as the 1980s progressed, in part because midwives were becoming more experienced and more invested in midwifery as a career and because midwives in some areas continued to be prosecuted and, in a few cases, jailed. One jailed midwife has a huge impact on all others. Other things also brought these issues to the fore. One was the need to identify which members of MANA meet the educational and other criteria inherent in the international definition of a midwife (in order to qualify for membership in the International Section). Another was state legislators' demands that some kind of standards and quality assurance be written into laws that give midwives other than CNMs authority to practice in their states. The standards developed in individual states were very different, and the level of respect and clout flowing from certification based on such disparate standards was relatively low. Midwives lobbying for legislation in California were asked about accreditation of educational programs and saw that legislators wanted a *nationally* recognized certification process (Davis, 1992). MANA's participation in the Carnegie Foundation seminars and Interorganizational Work Group intensified the discussions and provided an understanding of the quality assurance processes used by the ACNM.

The North American Registry Exam for Midwives

In 1986 MANA established an Interim Registry Board for the purpose of developing and administering a written test of basic, entry-level knowledge essential to responsible midwifery practice and establishing a registry for listing the names of midwives who pass the exam. MANA did not intend for the exam to test competencies other than knowledge and did not plan to provide any kind of credential to midwives who passed it. Nevertheless, MANA leaders hoped that being listed on the registry would help individual midwives establish themselves as recognized practitioners (Frye, 1992b).

The test was to be based on MANA's core competencies; it was to be offered to midwives of all educational backgrounds. Anyone who passed it would be listed in a Registry of Midwives to be maintained by the Registry Board. Registration was to be voluntary, to avoid stigmatizing those who did not choose to take the test.

The group appointed to the Interim Registry Board included four direct-entry midwives and a CNM. They began by stating the principles that would guide them—many different styles of practice and kinds of training can and do lead to safe, competent midwifery care; experienced midwives from many backgrounds and philosophies should be involved in defining the body of knowledge essential for entry-level midwifery practice; an entry-level exam should emphasize normal pregnancy, not complications (Sullivan, 1994). They wanted to test practical knowledge, not sophisticated vocabulary, and wanted a test that any modern, entry-level midwife "who really knows what she is doing can sit down and pass without special studying" (Frye, 1992b). A test expert proposed a sequence of activities (Frye, 1992b; Sullivan, 1994):

1. *Gather test questions from any organizations willing to share them with MANA.* Four state midwifery associations, two state licensing bodies, and three midwifery training programs contributed more than two thousand questions.

2. *Make a list of questions.* Nearly 600 questions were selected for the first level of review. Some were rejected as being beyond entry level, a few new questions were added, and some questions were revised based on information in reference textbooks* or to conform with the rules of test construction. Multiple-choice format was favored; whenever possible, items in other formats were rewritten as multiple-choice or true/false questions. The first revision included 570 multiple-choice and true/false questions and 11 essay/case history questions.

3. *Ask "expert midwives" to review the questions for clarity, relevance to entry-level practice, and reflection of the midwifery model of care.* Thirty midwives with various back-

grounds were chosen for this task, including CNMs; a grand midwife; a shamanic midwife; midwives practicing in homes, in small and large birth centers, and in hospitals; midwives who had founded midwifery schools and training programs, who had written midwifery books, and who had never attended a midwifery school; midwives practicing in a wide range of urban and rural settings; representatives from Canada; Spanish-speaking midwives serving Mexican women; and midwives of color. All were widely regarded as experts in midwifery. Each reviewer was sent a random selection of half of the multiple-choice and true/false questions and all of the case history/essay questions. They were asked to assess the accuracy and clarity of each question, to rank it on a five-point scale between essential and unnecessary (or outside the midwife's scope of practice), and to suggest changes in content and wording.

4. *Revise the questions based on the experts' comments.* If any reviewer indicated that a question was too medical or criticized it for any reason, it was discarded. About two-thirds of the questions were discarded, and fifty-three new questions were written to address topics that were not sufficiently covered and to test more practice-oriented knowledge.

5. *Pilot-test the exam on two groups of midwives—some who have taken other midwifery exams and some apprentice-trained midwives who have not taken other tests.* The revised questions were organized into an examination that was administered to midwives in five states.

6. *Ask for feedback from the first groups of midwives who take the exam and use it to refine the test.* Midwives who pilot-tested the exam were asked to fill out a questionnaire and comment on each question and the exam as a whole. Their input was used in revising the exam.

Myles Textbook for Midwives (the classic British midwifery textbook); *Nurse-Midwifery,* by Varney (the classic U.S. nurse-midwifery textbook); four books written by and for American direct-entry midwives (*Heart and Hands,* by Elizabeth Davis; *Helping Hands: The Apprentice Workbook,* by Carla Hartley; *Becoming a Midwife,* by Carolyn Steiger; and *Spiritual Midwifery,* by Ina May Gaskin); *Dorland's Illustrated Medical Dictionary,* the *Physiological Basis of Medical Practice,* by Best & Taylor, and *The New Our Bodies, Ourselves,* by the Boston Women's Health Collective.

A passing score of 75 percent was established, based in part on the pilot test, during which a group of experienced midwives answered between 79 and 92 percent of the questions correctly (Sullivan, 1994).

With completion of the exam, the Interim Registry Board became incorporated as the North American Registry of Midwives (NARM), an entity separate from MANA (Sullivan, 1994). NARM is an independent, not-for-profit corporation administered by an eight-member Registry Board appointed by MANA's board of directors.

The North American Registry Exam for Midwives (NAREM) was administered for the first time in October 1991. Nineteen experienced midwives took it during 1991. The test was further revised based on their comments and suggestions. Only one person failed (with a score of 37 percent). Excluding that one score, the average was 84.5 percent (Sullivan, 1994).

By the end of 1992, eighty people had taken the test and an alternate equivalent exam had been developed for security reasons and for candidates who might want to retake the exam after a failure. A study guide with reference texts and sample questions was written (Sullivan, 1994).

Results of exams taken by ninety-four experienced midwives during 1992 and the first half of 1993 were analyzed. No one failed, and both the mean and median scores were between 86.3 and 88.6 percent. Little or no correlation was found between the exam scores and the number of years of experience of the midwives who took the exam. Because the exam was designed for entry-level midwives, the more difficult questions, which might have distinguished between more and less experienced midwives, had been omitted (Sullivan, 1994).

The early forms of the exam were criticized by many CNMs and some direct-entry midwives because they seemed too easy and because they were not based on a systematic analysis of the knowledge, skills, and abilities required for actual current midwifery practice—that is, a task analysis similar to those conducted by the ACNM Division of Examiners in 1984–86 and 1993 (see Chapter 8). In addition, although the high scores and pass rate seemed to make the issue irrelevant, there was no limit on the number of retakes.

NARM took the criticism to heart; each new form of the exam improved its psychometric defensibility. The revision that created the third version of the exam (Form C) included topics identified by the 1993 skills/task analysis funded by the IWG.* In addition, the Minnesota Board of Medicine funded an Angoff cut-score study to determine a legally defensible passing score. By early 1996, Form C of the NARM exam was being used as the basis for certifying or licensing midwives in thirteen states and one Canadian province, and documentation had been provided to validate the correct answer to each question. The next revision, Form D,

---

*NARM began to plan the skills/task analysis survey in 1992. Florida offered technical assistance because of its interest in using the NARM exam for state licensure; state requirements specified that certain psychometric procedures be performed to improve the validity and reliability of the test (Myers-Ciecko & Stallings, 1994). During 1993 a list of skills required for entry-level midwifery practice was developed with assistance from the Psychometric and Research Unit of the Florida Department of Business and Professional Regulations. The skills-list survey form was developed in sequenced steps: A master skills list was compiled based on lists provided by three schools and two state midwifery certification programs; all five lists were based on MANA's core competencies. After approval by the MANA Board, the list was presented at a meeting of the IWG. Skills included on at least three of the five lists were categorized as either basic or expanded-performance skills. Forty-two experienced, practicing midwives and midwifery experts in the United States, Canada, and Mexico gave their opinions on whether each skill should be on the final list. The revised list was published in the MANA newsletter and *Birth Gazette,* a quarterly journal published by Ina May Gaskin (of the Farm community, in Tennessee), with a request for feedback. Responses from 125 people were tallied and considered in revising the list. The final version included 130 entry-level midwifery tasks and seven categories of skills that are beyond entry-level. The skills list was ready for use in October 1993 (NARM, 1994).

reflects the results of the midwifery job/task analysis conducted by NARM in 1995, which was developed under the supervision of a testing company following the guidelines of the National Organization of Certifying Agencies. The exam is offered twice a year; tight test security is maintained. The pass rate for those who took form C or D during 1996 was 76 percent. The reduction in the pass rate reflects improvements in the exam and examination of a more diverse, less experienced group of midwives (Sammon, 1996).

Use of the NARM examination for purposes of the registry was terminated at the end of 1995, when NARM shifted its focus from registration to certification. More than four hundred midwives had been registered. As of 1996, the examination is used only as part of either a state or provincial licensing process or the multistep NARM certification process.

The Decision to Develop a National Certification Process

In August 1993 MANA requested NARM and the Midwifery Education Accreditation Council (MEAC) to establish a Certification Task Force to advise the NARM Board and assist it in developing a national certification process that would include a hands-on skills assessment. Because of sensitivity about certification, it was important that the task force include representation from the wide spectrum of midwives in MANA. The approximately eighty midwives and consumers who served on the task force came from forty states and diverse backgrounds, including CNMs and direct-entry midwives working in states where their practice is illegal (Sammon, 1996).

The task force met for the first time in September 1993. It decided to make all decisions through the development of consensus. There was consensus that national certification should be available to midwives of any educational or cultural background, that methods used to evaluate midwives for certification must be culturally unbiased, that there should be no restrictions on the

time needed for individuals to complete their education and pass the certification examination, and that midwives must be the primary educators of midwives. The task force met four times between 1993 and 1995. One of its purposes was to define the midwifery model of care as the standard to be reflected in the NARM certification process (Sammon, 1996).

Job and Task Analysis and Development of a Manual Skills Exam

In January 1995 the Certification Task Force reached an impasse over whether to include certain medical skills in the midwifery skills exam. This led to recognition of the need for a more substantial job analysis. In February 1995, NARM hired a testing company to conduct a survey to identify the tasks that practicing midwives consider important for competent entry-level practice. The survey was mailed to 2,869 midwives on a mailing list compiled by merging MANA's membership list with the list of midwives kept by *Midwifery Today* (a midwifery magazine) and the Christian Midwives Coalition. The number of CNMs on the list was adjusted to make it proportional to the percentage of CNMs among MANA members (one-third). Completed forms were returned by 817 practicing midwives, a response rate of 29 percent (NARM, 1996).

Minor revisions in the NARM examination were made to reflect the results of the job and task analysis. The results were also used to create an examination to test the manual skills considered necessary on the basis of the survey (NARM, 1996).

NARM's Certification Processes

In late 1994 NARM began to implement a process for certifying experienced direct-entry midwives as "certified professional midwives" (CPMs). After the skills examination was field tested, certification was expanded to include entry-level midwives in May 1996.

The certification process for entry-level midwives has three phases: (1) Establishing eligibility to take the NARM examination, (2) taking and passing the exam, and (3) taking and passing the hands-on skills assessment. Eligibility to take the examination requires the following:

- *Verification of experience,* which must include having attended at least 40 births as an active participant, including 20 births at which the applicant served as the primary midwife, under supervision. At least 10 of the 20 must have been out-of-hospital births. The applicant must have provided complete care (prenatal, birth, examination of the newborn, and postpartum examination of the mother) for at least 3 of the 20 births attended as the primary midwife. Minimum numbers of other clinical experiences are also specified.
- *Verification of practical skills* listed in the *Practical Skills Guide for Midwifery.* The entire set of skills must be verified by a responsible person involved in the applicant's midwifery education, for example, a member of the faculty of a school or the senior midwife/preceptor. In addition, a NARM qualified evaluator assesses the applicant's performance of selected skills at an appropriate clinical site. (NARM qualified evaluators are experienced CPMs who have been trained in practical skills assessment.)
- *CPR certification.* Verification of current American Heart Association certification in cardiopulmonary resuscitation of adults and newborns or infants.
- *A copy of the applicant's informed consent statement.* Guidelines for developing an informed consent statement are included in a packet of information sent to midwives who apply to take the test.
- *Practice guidelines.* The applicant must submit a signed statement that asserts that she has developed practice guidelines. Guidance for developing practice guidelines is included in the applicant packet.

- *Three letters of reference.* One must be from a client, one from a health care professional, and one from a personal friend.

Midwives with at least five years of unsupervised clinical experience who cannot verify some of the required clinical experiences have been offered a limited window of opportunity for special consideration. They must document having been the primary midwife at 75 or more births within the previous 10 years, including at least 3 births for which they provided care during the complete maternity cycle, 20 out-of-hospital births, and 10 births involving a complication or other challenging situation. In addition, the applicant must provide a notarized, written account of how she acquired the skills included in the *Practical Skills Guide for Midwifery.* A committee reviews each application individually. All other eligibility requirements are the same as for entry-level midwives. Midwives who want to use this process had to apply for certification as an experienced midwife by the end of 1996. One hundred and twenty-three experienced direct-entry midwives had been certified as CPMs as of the end of November 1996.

Other special processes have been developed for other kinds of midwives. Midwives who are certified, registered, or licensed in states where the NARM examination has replaced the state examination or the state examination has been deemed equivalent to the NARM examination do not have to take the current NARM examination. Certified nurse-midwives can obtain NARM certification by providing evidence of current ACNM certification and documenting having served as the primary midwife for ten births in nonhospital settings, including at least three for which the CNM provided care during the entire maternity cycle. The practical experience and clinical skills of graduates of midwifery education programs accredited by MEAC are verified by their educational program. Grand Midwives only need to provide the references in order to establish their eligibility to take the examination. Certification under any of these processes will lead to designation as a certified professional midwife.

CPM certification must be renewed every three years. Renewal requires evidence of annual renewal of CPR certification and 10 hours of continuing education during each year of the three-year period, for a total of 30 hours.

Informal Educational Opportunities

Although a few schools were in operation by 1980, most women who became direct-entry midwives during the 1970s and 1980s pieced their preparation together on their own. The northern California midwife referred to earlier (who became a midwife because women who knew she'd had a home birth asked her to attend theirs) said that she "learned by doing. After a few years, there were so many of us that we would gather together in study groups. It's not the most formal way to begin—but that's how it happened" (Osborn & Esty, 1995). Most midwives augmented "learning by doing" by studying books on their own, participating in some kind of apprenticeship, and taking advantage of any other opportunities that became practically available. The possibilities included home-study correspondence courses, local study groups, workshops, conferences, continuing education sessions presented during meetings of a state or local midwifery association or MANA, and short, intensive organized apprenticeships in high-volume birth centers. Sympathetic CNMs, physicians, hospital labor-and-delivery-room nurses, and experienced direct-entry midwives contributed to creating educational opportunities.

In addition, many women come to midwifery with relevant prior training and experience—as nurses, emergency medical technicians (EMTs), or childbirth educa-

tors. Others have had special training as homeopaths, herbalists, or practitioners of other nonallopathic healing traditions.

Study Groups

Study groups were particularly important when the lay midwifery movement was just getting started and there were no training programs. These groups led to the development of some of the earliest training programs.* Study groups were a natural model for that time, when the women's movement arose from the work of local "consciousness-raising groups" and the Boston Women's Health Book Collective, authors of *Our Bodies, Ourselves,* provided a model for women getting together to learn about their own bodies and health. Study groups for women who wanted to become midwives generally resulted in something akin to a class, with everyone studying one or more basic midwifery textbook and taking turns researching and presenting information on specific subjects. Study groups for women aspiring to be midwives also needed sustained input from experienced midwives or physicians and opportunity to attend births, first as observers and assistants (Beauchamp, 1992). Nutritionists, herbalists, lactation consultants, nurses, La Leche League leaders, and childbirth educators were often also asked to share their knowledge (Tritten, 1992).

Apprenticeships

In 1990, a group of midwife educators defined midwifery apprenticeship as the self-directed study of midwifery under the supervision of a person recognized in his or her community as a midwife or under the supervision of an obstetric-care provider who is not a midwife but is interested in midwifery (National Coalition of Midwifery Edu-

---

*See descriptions in Chapter 4 of the development of the Birth Collective at Fremont Women's Clinic in Seattle (the origin of the Seattle Midwifery School) and the Birth Center of Santa Cruz.

cators, 1990). Women who want to direct their own education are attracted to apprenticeships, which may be formally or informally organized by either the senior midwife or the apprentice and are individualized, local and diverse. Apprenticeships should provide one-to-one discussion of case management and the rationale behind the care provided to individual women, teaching of the basic manual and technical skills required to provide midwifery care, instruction on the circumstances that require referring a woman for medical care, training in management of emergencies, experience in counseling and referring women to community resources, exposure to the administrative and financial management of a midwifery practice, and access to textbooks and other relevant sources of information (National Coalition of Midwifery Educators, 1990). Self-study using books and other references is an integral part of an apprenticeship, which may be enriched by attending workshops and conferences.

Some women become childbirth educators or *doulas** before entering a midwifery apprenticeship, which usually continues for two to four years—however long it takes the apprentice to feel competent. Some places that provide apprenticeships require a certain number of clinical experiences; for example, the Farm in Tennessee requires attendance at one hundred births. An individual may apprentice with more than one midwife or combine an apprenticeship with experience in a high-volume service where she is likely to see a wider range of clinical conditions.

The direct-entry midwifery community is highly motivated to retain apprenticeship as a viable, bona fide form of midwifery education and has conducted an extensive dis-

cussion and analysis of its strengths and weaknesses (Steiger, 1987; Parra, 1995; Gilmore, 1990; Osborn & Esty, 1995; Frye, 1995b; Hodges, 1992). Some advantages are that apprenticeships are self-paced, provide immediate exposure to the realities of practice, and make the developing midwife aware of nuances in the intense, one-to-one relationship with clients. Most apprentices have time between births to reflect on their experiences, and opportunities to develop personal relationships with the women they take care of. Clinical experience and didactic learning are integrated in time; a student who sees a certain complication can read about it and discuss it with the senior midwife. Teachers can pass on the "spirit" as well as the knowledge and skills of midwifery, teaching their students to approach each woman with a loving touch and to use their intuition as well as their hands, senses, and intellect. The student's personal growth can be nurtured. If the preceptor is honest, humble, compassionate, and patient, the apprentice will experience these qualities and tend to develop them herself.

Teaching can be individualized to meet the needs of each apprentice. A preceptor who does not have a classroom of students can tell when her apprentice does not understand something. The close, continuous interaction makes it easier to identify a student who is not cut out for midwifery. Apprenticeships may be better suited than other teaching methods to some women's most effective method of learning.

Apprenticeships potentially enable a more diverse group of women to become prepared as midwives. Apprenticeships are actually or potentially available in many communities, and they can be woven into the other aspects of a woman's life. Many women become interested in midwifery in response to their own birth experiences, at a time when they are caring for young children. Apprenticeships make it less likely that a woman would have to leave her home and family in order to achieve her goal of be-

---

*A doula is a woman trained or experienced in childbirth who provides continuous emotional, physical, and informational support to women before, during, and just after childbirth (Douglas of North America, 1995). A doula is not responsible for managing the birth and does not take the place of a midwife or physician.

coming a midwife. Because there is relatively little exchange of money between an apprentice and her mentor, it is less costly than going to a school. Because formal educational credentials are not required, apprenticeships open midwifery to capable women who would otherwise be excluded from midwifery training (Gaskin, 1996).

Disadvantages include variation in the quality of the experience, inability to control the sequencing of learning experiences, and the possibility of personality conflicts. The preceptor may have no aptitude for teaching, and, unless she has an unusually busy practice, the student may have relatively limited experiences. What the apprentice learns is limited by the preceptor's knowledge and skills, as well as her scope of practice. For example, if the preceptor does not provide care to women who are not pregnant, the apprentice will have no experience in well-woman gynecology. There is no structured curriculum, and some vital experiences may not arise or may not be available through a student's initial preceptor. Apprenticeship is unlikely to provide exposure to the full variety and variance that occurs during even normal, healthy pregnancies. Obtaining enough experience may take an unreasonably long period of time; even after a long period of apprenticeship, there are likely to be gaps in the learning. It is up to the student to understand what she needs to complete her training; if she overestimates her abilities, she may not recognize what is needed. Students have little opportunity to learn more than one way to do something and thus tend to copy their mentors' practice styles. Although most eventually develop their own styles and remain open to new ideas and methods, some apprentices admire their preceptors so much that they become blocked from further learning (Steiger, 1987; Parra, 1995; Gilmore, 1990; Osborn & Esty, 1995; Frye, 1995b). The apprentice and preceptor have to negotiate the changing role of the apprentice and how long the apprenticeship should last; if they

disagree, the apprenticeship may be terminated prematurely (Reid, 1986).

Such analysis led to efforts to address the weaknesses of this method. In 1987 Carolyn Steiger, an experienced midwife practicing in Portland, Oregon, published *Becoming a Midwife* primarily for midwifery apprentices and their teachers. In addition to an abundance of midwifery wisdom and insight, the book provides a detailed, three-phase curriculum for midwifery apprenticeships. Each phase includes reading and skills lists, required learning activities, a list of necessary equipment and supplies, and forms to facilitate evaluation and assessment of progress. Several other books and aids have been developed to provide structure and support—curriculum guides, evaluation guides, a practical skills guide, forms for keeping records of the apprentice's clinical experiences, and an apprentice workbook. Certification programs run by state agencies and state midwifery associations provide structure for apprenticeships, as do state laws that require applicants to document having had a certain number of specific kinds of clinical experience. Eventually programs were developed to provide structure and oversight of midwifery apprenticeships, especially for the purpose of documenting that an individual apprentice covered the content and had the clinical experiences required for certification by a particular midwifery association or the legal status required to practice in a particular state. With the development of these programs, it has become difficult to draw a clear distinction between an apprenticeship combined with a correspondence course and a formal "at-a-distance" educational program.

Workshops, Conferences, and Seminars

Continuing education is offered at MANA's annual meetings, at regional conferences put on by Midwifery Today (a midwifery and childbirth education organization based in Eugene, Oregon), by basic direct-entry midwifery educational programs (e.g., the Seattle Midwifery School), and by other organizations, as well as individuals, on an ad hoc basis. Midwifery Today has offered a three-day conference in four or five different locations each year since 1991. Lectures and full-day workshops are presented by direct-entry midwives, CNMs, and physicians. Although each conference has a unique theme, the most popular sessions focus on the substance of midwifery care, such as identification of risk factors, methods to assess fetal well-being, and neonatal resuscitation.

Books and Other Learning Materials

Books are an important source of information for direct-entry midwives, who have, in the past at least, relied heavily on independent study. In addition to several books written by and specifically for direct-entry midwives,* they use American obstetric, nurse-midwifery, and nursing textbooks, a British midwifery textbook, and books for childbirth educators. A British midwife who observed and interviewed forty-nine American direct-entry midwives during the early 1980s found that most studied several books, including at least one that presented orthodox obstetric theory and practice and at least one that focused on midwifery care during home births (Reid, 1986). She was struck by a practice that she referred to as "dipping into the books," in which the independent student would look up the same subject in all of her books in order to "hear

it in different ways," noting that some books included information that others did not and that there were different theories, perspectives, and approaches (Reid, 1986). This method is also used in some current midwifery education programs, which encourage students to read about the same subject in several sources in order to discover the truth for themselves. However, some midwives may use a book written and published by a single direct-entry midwife as their main source of information.

Several periodic publications are available, including the *Birth Gazette*, produced by Ina May Gaskin, and *Midwifery Today*. Although neither of these could be classified as a professional journal, a question and answer article called "Ask the Midwife" is a regular feature of each issue of the *Birth Gazette*, and every issue of *Midwifery Today* includes informative articles and a one-page feature called "Tricks of the Trade," which passes on suggestions contributed by readers. Both publications usually include first-person "birth stories"—narratives of the sequence of events during particular births, which are used as a way to share and, thus, pool experience. These are often examples of home births that involved unexpected complications. Each issue of *Midwifery Today* also includes abstracts of recent articles from obstetric journals and other sources. A randomly selected single issue of *Midwifery Today* (Winter 1992–1993) included articles on the following subjects:

- Methods a home birth midwife can use to induce labor (written by a direct-entry midwife who was studying to become a CNM)
- A homeopathic remedy (herb) that may make it easier for a baby in breech presentation to move into the normal, head-down position (written by a midwife who is a homeopathic educator and owns a store that carries homeopathic remedies)

---

*For example, Baldwin's *Special Delivery* (1986), Daviss' *Heart and Hands: A Guide to Midwifery* (1987), Steiger's *Becoming a Midwife* (1987), Hartley's *Helping Hands: The Apprentice Workbook* (1988); Gaskin's *Spiritual Midwifery* (1991), and several books by Anne Frye, including *Understanding Diagnostic Tests in the Childbearing Year* (1993), *Healing Passage: A Midwife's Guide to the Care and Repair of Tissues Involved in Birth* (1995a), and the first volume (on prenatal care) of *Holistic Midwifery: A Comprehensive Textbook for Midwives in Homebirth Practice* (1995b); the second volume will be on care during labor and birth, the third will be on care during the postpartum/postnatal period.

- A description and discussion of the advantages of group prenatal care (written by a CNM)
- How to prepare clients for the possible need to transport them to a hospital during labor and how to reduce the trauma of an actual transport for everyone involved (written by a practicing midwife)
- A midwife's description of her approach to providing prenatal care in women's homes
- Methods to relieve pain without using drugs (written by a home birth midwife)
- Detailed instructions on how to use a fetoscope to monitor the fetal heart beat (written by a midwife who is an RN but not a CNM)
- Methods to determine if the fetus is not getting enough oxygen during contractions (written by another midwife who is an RN but not a CNM)
- Prenatal risk assessment (written by a physician who is head of a hospital fetal diagnostic center)

The same issue included five "birth stories"—a midwife's first solo birth, which turned out to be twins; a birth in which the newborn had seizures and needed to be transported to a hospital; a birth that occurred during a snow storm (the midwife asked the woman's husband to plow the driveway in case they needed to take the mother to a hospital); a successful breech delivery in which the woman labored at home in a large tub of warm water; and the successful vaginal birth of twins to a woman with three previous cesarean sections—one twin was born at home and one at a hospital twenty-two hours later, after a sonogram and external version of the fetus, which had been in transverse position.

Most direct-entry midwifery education programs and some individual direct-entry midwives subscribe to the *Journal of Nurse-Midwifery* (the official journal of the ACNM) and *Birth* (a professional and scientific jour-nal that addresses issues related to perinatal care). Some schools also subscribe to MIDIRS, (Midwives Information and Resource Service), a British clipping and reprint service that sends three packets of excerpts and reprints to subscribers every year. Information gleaned from hundreds of publications is arranged by subject for easy access, including complete articles, abstracts, book reviews, interviews, and case study questions answered by a variety of authoritative midwives.

Videos, audiotapes, and other learning materials produced by direct-entry midwives are also important. Gaskin's videos on assisting vaginal breech delivery and shoulder dystocia are widely known and used, as is Frye's video on the anatomy of the perineum and methods of suturing.

There are both strengths and weaknesses to the books and other publications written by and for direct-entry midwives. Most of the books are written by a single midwife and produced by a small-scale local printer. They are as good as the author's personal knowledge base and research and writing skills. They do not go through the kind of review and editing that occurs when books of this kind are written by mainstream health professionals and are published by mainstream publishing houses. Nor are the authors members of multidisciplinary health science universities, whose work is subjected to the critique of members of related professions, as well as their intraprofessional peers. Nevertheless, direct-entry midwifery books are valuable sources of information, ideas, interpretations, approaches, perspectives and experience that are relatively uninfluenced by the medical care system and are not available anywhere else (Gaskin, 1996). They are best when they stick to normal pregnancy and the care of the normal pregnant woman. Some present theories as facts, especially regarding pregnancy complications. Although there are several newsletter-type publications, there is no strenuously edited, refereed professional journal.

In addition, few direct-entry midwives are oriented toward the generation and use of statistics as a major means to discover the best ways to take care of pregnant women—the effort to discover truth through analysis of controlled observation or measurement of a limited aspect of a large number of pregnancies. Valuing the particularity of each individual woman and the uniqueness of each birth conflicts with the idea of basing an individual woman's care on generalizations derived from the experiences of many women, such as advising against a home birth because of a circumstance that has been shown to be associated with a higher-than-average rate of serious problems. All current midwives know about the misuse of statistics—used to falsely blame earlier midwives for the high rates of maternal and infant mortality in the United States during the early 1900s, and later to provide a faulty rationale for using invasive medical procedures during every birth. But few direct-entry midwives have more than a rudimentary knowledge of statistics, or the combination of opportunity and motivation required to learn more. As a consequence, there is little demand for information to be presented in the form of *rates*—for example, how frequently does this happen, in what percent of cases does this treatment work?

The critical analysis applied to mainstream medical approaches seems to mellow when applied to alternative methods. The ethic that values accepting others uncritically may extend to theories and treatment modalities offered by nonallopathic practitioners who are friendly to midwifery. For example, an article promoting a homeopathic treatment to turn babies in breech presentation states that the treatment works and provides a fascinating biological explanation: Pulsatilla stimulates the uterine muscle to grow more evenly; in response, the baby assumes the most advantageous position willingly and naturally. But the article provides no data from a series of situations in which this treatment was tried. It just says that giving pulsatilla is "always worth a try . . . . Since you are

giving a dose that can do no harm, the worse that can happen is that she simply will not respond to, or resonate with, the remedy. If the baby needs to remain in this present position for mechanical reasons, such as the location of the placenta, or a tight cord wrap, the remedy will have no effect" (Brennan, 1992-1993).

Schools and Organized Courses

A wide variety of courses have been conducted, including courses centered around local study groups, correspondence courses for midwifery apprentices, short but intensive courses associated with high-volume birth centers, and others. Some courses have had a special emphasis and flavor: A group of black women focused on traditional childbearing practices; a course in traditional midwifery and woman-craft emphasized the potential for spiritual transformation associated with pregnancy and birth (Myers-Ciecko & Stallings, 1994). In addition, the passage of state laws with specific educational requirements stimulated the development of programs designed to meet requirements for licensure in specific states. Not all programs continued. Most that have continued have evolved over time.

Many women who became lay midwives during the 1970s and early 1980s were college graduate. Delivering babies outside of hospitals, illegally in many places, at a time when some physicians were dropping obstetrics because of fear of legal liability, is not for those with faint hearts or weak minds. However, *lay* midwifery is *lay*—not professionalized and not part of the system. Just as direct-entry midwifery practice developed outside the regular health care system, direct-entry midwifery education developed outside the regular system for training health professionals. There was distrust of universities and a strong preference for schools that were under their control. Direct-entry midwives see many weaknesses in universities and are concerned about laws that could force the preparation of midwives into institutions in which they might be subjected to overly medicalized training. Many widely respected leaders—intelligent, experienced women now in their forties or fifties, "master" midwives who outwitted or outlasted powerful opposition to bring direct-entry midwifery this far—lack the degrees required to teach in mainstream institutions of higher learning. Most also lack experience in dealing with the academic world, and the skills, habits, and values needed to survive in it. Today's direct-entry midwives are part of a movement that has spent a quarter century developing support for midwifery outside "the system." As midwifery has gained respect, direct-entry midwives feel more secure and have become more successful and comfortable in their alternative world. Few are eager to leave their own institutions to move into educational institutions that are part of a system they see as rigid, contrary to their model of care, and sometimes hostile.

The standard for professional direct-entry midwifery education in Europe is three years of postsecondary education. That is the standard written into the laws of Washington, Florida, and California. New York is the only state that requires direct-entry midwifery programs to lead to a baccalaureate or higher degree; the degree requirement was written into the regulations, but is not in the law itself. Although direct-entry midwives in New York originally supported passage of the law, they were opposed to changes made late in the process and were unable to influence the rules requiring a bachelor's degree and completion of a state-approved midwifery education program.

Training Programs Available in 1995

The early 1990s brought increasing interest in developing new direct-entry midwifery education programs. This arose in part as a response to the widely publicized maternity care crisis of the late 1980s, during which many statements were made and articles published expressing concern about the nation's inability to provide effective health care to all of its pregnant women. Passage of new direct-entry midwifery laws in several states, the Carnegie Foundation seminars on midwifery education, the ACNM/MANA Interorganizational Work Group on Midwifery Education, and the prospect of processes to accredit direct-entry midwifery education programs and certify direct-entry midwives also fueled interest in starting new educational programs. These factors have also played a role in generating new interest in midwifery among young women in search of careers.

A list of direct-entry midwifery education programs compiled by MANA provided the name and address but, in most cases, no other information on forty programs in operation as of November 1995. *Getting An Education: Paths to Becoming a Midwife,* a 1995 publication of *Midwifery Today,* lists thirty-nine programs and provides brief descriptions of most of them. Twenty-three programs were on both lists. One of them was not planning to open until autumn 1996, no descriptive information was provided for three of them, two of the programs that were described have closed, and the telephone numbers for two programs had been changed or disconnected. Excluding those eight programs and assuming that other programs included on both lists are relatively substantial and stable, the following summary is based on them. Most of these fifteen programs are in the Western United States. Three are in California, three in Oregon, one in Washington, one in New Mexico, one in Colorado, three in Texas, one in Oklahoma, and two in Florida.

These fifteen programs are categorized and described briefly based on information in the *Midwifery Today* publication, catalogs or other materials provided by some of the programs, and telephone interviews with the director or other staff of some programs. Several of the schools are quite new, and some of the newest schools are among the most substantial. The closure or inability to contact or obtain information about seven of twenty-three programs included on both 1995 lists suggests that weak schools may be closing. Things are in flux.

The list provided by MANA is introduced with a reminder that there was no process for national accreditation of direct-entry midwifery education programs and that, while some programs are recognized by specific states, some had not received any official recognition. However, an accreditation process is being pilot tested, as discussed later in this chapter. Many schools are making changes in order to meet the standards that will be required for accreditation. In addition, each school's curriculum is designed to meet the requirements of the law of the state in which the school is located. Programs also tend to be as long as required by the state law. This is somewhat confusing, however, because some "three-year" programs are full time and some are only part time. In addition, the length of many programs is flexible. Although the average time to complete the National College of Midwifery program is twenty-four months, a student from California, which requires a three-year program, can take three years to complete the program.

The prospect of accreditation is causing many programs to become more substantial, reducing the differences between programs to some degree. However, the range remains wide, and each program is unique. Some have substantial libraries, require students to study medical obstetric textbooks, as well as books written by and for nurse-midwives and direct-entry midwives, use a variety of professional journals, and make good use of experts from related fields. Others use only midwifery textbooks and do not subscribe to professional journals. Some are virtually a one-woman operation; other somewhat larger programs may be strongly imbued with the perspective of a single strong, sometimes charismatic leader. Students may be exposed to the perspective of only one or very few midwives, and the teacher(s) may be iso-

lated from advances being made in other fields.

One of the purposes for developing an accreditation process is to make the schools eligible for federal financial assistance and to make their students eligible for scholarships. Some programs already have varying amounts of state financial support. A program in a community college in Miami is tax supported. About one-third of Seattle Midwifery School students receive scholarships through a program to prepare health care providers to work in medically underserved areas of Washington State.

The following information is intended to provide a general understanding of the variety of direct-entry midwifery education programs available in mid-1995. It may not be a complete list, the categories are somewhat arbitrary, and the amount and kinds of information included in the descriptions are not the same for every program. Thus this information should not be thought of as an adequate catalog of programs.

Schools That Provide a Comprehensive Three-Year Midwifery Curriculum: Three programs meet the standards established by the International Confederation of Midwives, the International Federation of Obstetricians and Gynecologists, and the European Economic Community, as well as the education and experience requirements for licensure in Washington, Florida and California. The laws call for a curriculum of three *academic* years, which can be compressed into two-and-a-half *calendar* years, if the program continues without long breaks. All of the schools described here are operated so that students can graduate in that length of time. Students must be high school graduates. The curricula are designed, in combination with prerequisite courses, to lead to development of the MANA core competencies. All programs in this category give students some experience in local hospitals, mainly for observation, and utilize some clinical placements with CNMs or physicians. Two of the programs rely on high-volume maternity hospitals in Caribbean Island countries to provide part of the necessary clinical experience for most of their students. The hospitals provide large numbers of births and valuable experience with complications during births. Nevertheless, the primary focus and intention of these programs is to produce midwives for practice in out-of-hospital settings.

Two of these programs are in free-standing schools, and one is in a community college. However, both of the schools in Florida offer associate degrees. The Florida Department of Education went through a process to determine the appropriate level for educational programs designed to meet the requirement of the state's direct-entry midwifery law and determined that they should be at the post-secondary vocational level. The determination was made with significant input from direct-entry midwives in Florida. Postsecondary vocational programs of the length of the midwifery programs (at least three years, as required by the midwifery law) must be licensed by the state and are authorized to award a specialized associate degree (Borino, 1996).

The *Seattle Midwifery School* (SMS) was the first formally structured three-year direct-entry midwifery educational program in the United States. The organization and content of the curriculum were drawn from European models of direct-entry midwifery education. SMS admits approximately ten students each September. Students must come to the school having completed prerequisite courses in anatomy and physiology, English, math, microbiology, nutrition, and social science. During the first academic year students have three days of classroom and laboratory skills work and four-to-six hours of clinical experience each week. The first summer is devoted to intensive clinical experience. This is followed by three more months of classes, a break for the winter holidays, and a twelve-month period devoted exclusively to clinical learning.

The Washington law requires student clinical experiences to be with preceptors who are practicing legally (although not necessarily with a license). All students have their main clinical experience in an independent home birth practice or birth center, where they remain for an average of six months in order to provide the entire cycle of care to at least fifteen pregnant women. Most students are placed with licensed midwives or CNMs in Washington; physicians and physician assistants are also utilized. All students have clinical experience in at least two settings. Most work with at least two preceptors in the United States; many also go to one of the Caribbean islands or other foreign sites for one to three months of experience in a hospital staffed predominantly by midwives. Students also spend at least fifty hours in clinics that provide gynecologic and family planning services.

Miami Dade Community College in Miami, Florida offers two midwifery programs—a three-year program leading to an associate in science degree in midwifery and a four-month accelerated prelicensure course for out-of-state midwives and for physicians educated in other countries. The curriculum of the three-year associate-degree program includes one year of general education and basic science (English composition, algebra, psychology, humanities, sociology, chemistry, anatomy and physiology, microbiology, and nutrition), followed by two years of courses and experience in midwifery. Students must earn at least a C average on the general education and basic science courses and cannot have repeated any of the courses more than once in order to earn the 2.0 average.

The program opened in August 1994; it accepts a class of fifteen students each year. It takes twenty-seven months to complete the program. Faculty include licensed midwives, CNMs, a registered nurse, an obstetrician, a biologist (teaching embryology, fetal development, and genetics), and laboratory technicians. The program's siting in a community college provides access to high-tech equipment. Students have clinical experience with a variety of preceptors in hospitals, public health facilities, birth centers and home birth practices in Florida, and at a high-volume hospital in Jamaica. The program's first class of students graduated in April 1996.

The *Florida School of Traditional Midwifery* in Gainesville, Florida is a not-for-profit corporation that is licensed by the Florida Department of Education, which has authorized it to award a specialized associate degree. The curriculum takes three years to complete. Nurses receive advanced standing, which enables them to complete the program in two years (the minimum specified in the law). Students can obtain credit for courses taken at other institutions. During the first year, students are enrolled in both the midwifery school and a local community college, where they take human anatomy and physiology, chemistry for midwives, and microbiology for midwives. The faculty of the midwifery school includes licensed midwives (LMs), CNMs, and specialists in related fields (e.g., nutrition). Clinical preceptors include LMs, CNMs, and physicians. Although students have experience in hospitals, as well as clinics, birth centers, and home birth practices, the program is not designed to prepare midwives for practice in hospitals. The clinical component of the program includes observing at least 25 women during labor and birth and providing complete maternity care to at least 50 additional women under the supervision of a preceptor. The school enrolled its first class (fifteen students) in January 1995. About half of them had prior midwifery experience. The second class (nine students) enrolled in January 1996. The school plans to take one class of ten to fifteen students per year.

Academic Courses Combined with Apprenticeships: Some of these courses are taught through classes that meet weekly or less often; others are taught as distance learning programs. They vary in length and the degree to which they monitor the students' progress in both the academic part of the program and during the precepted clinical learning experience. Students in some programs have to arrange their own apprenticeship; other programs maintain a list of preceptors and offer apprenticeships to some or all of their students. Although "apprenticeship" implies a one-to-one teaching–learning relationship, many preceptors take more than one apprentice concurrently. These courses are designed to prepare students to take specific examinations and/or to qualify them for certification by NARM or for certification or licensure in specific states.

The *National College of Midwifery* in Taos, New Mexico, offers a program designed to teach the MANA core competencies and qualify graduates to take the New Mexico licensing examination. Each student must make all arrangements with her own preceptor, who could be a physician, a CNM, or a direct-entry midwife who is licensed by the state or country in which she practices or who, if unlicensed, has been certified by NARM or her state midwifery organization. The program was started in 1992. Approximately 70 percent of the preceptors have been direct-entry midwives; the others have been physicians.

The National College charges a one-time fee for the educational materials and its oversight of the student's progress, record keeping, et cetera. The major responsibility for each student's education rests with her preceptor, who must determine that the student has completed all of the learning activities called for in the curriculum. Students pay tuition directly to the preceptor. Preceptor fees recommended by the National College come to about $4,000 per year, although many preceptors ask for less, recognizing that the student's labor is also of value. Most preceptors have more than one student at a time; some have three or four. All interaction between the National College and the preceptors and students is conducted by telephone or mail. Students and preceptors send reports to the National College at regular intervals (three per year). Preceptors report on the students' progress; students evaluate their preceptors. Faculty of the National College do not visit the preceptor sites. However, the college contacts each preceptor at random times to request an hour-long video of a current teaching–learning activity. Students can enter the program at any time. Although there is a five-year time limit, students work at their own speed and can take time off or change preceptors.

The National College is licensed as an institution of higher learning in the state of New Mexico and is authorized to award both undergraduate degrees (associate and baccalaureate) and graduate degrees (masters and doctorates). As of early 1996, it had given five associate of arts (AA) degrees and two bachelor of science (BS) degrees, and had twenty-three enrolled students. People who complete the basic midwifery program earn an AA. Baccalaureate degrees are given to people who were already licensed or certified direct-entry midwives when they enrolled in the National College program. Students working towards a BS degree must write a research paper and meet all New Mexico rules for baccalaureate education, including completion of courses in statistics and writing. Both courses are available through the National College through use of videocassettes and a preceptor. Preceptors for individuals seeking any but the AA degree must have the same or a higher degree than the student is working toward.

The National College of Midwifery is associated with the *Northern New Mexico Midwifery Center,* a birth center in Taos that had been running its own midwifery training program. The birth center now accepts three to five National College students per year. It expects its own students to complete the program within twenty-seven months. The fastest student finished in twelve months; the average is twenty-four months.

The National College also enrolls all midwifery students of the *Vineyard School of Missions* in El Paso, Texas. The Vineyard School prepares people for work in Christian missions. It is associated with a large group of churches all over the world; most of its students come from those churches. In addition to a three-month general program for anyone planning to work in a Christian mission, the Vineyard School offers several advanced programs, including one in midwifery and one in primary health care. The fifteen-month midwifery program combines the three-month general mission work program with the primary health care program and the National College of Midwifery's distance learning program. All Vineyard School midwifery students have their clinical experience in birth centers and hospitals in the Philippines or Mexico. Vineyard School graduates delivered more than 300 babies in the Philippines during 1996 and expected to deliver more than 600 babies in that country during 1997. As of early 1996, the Vineyard School had ten students enrolled in the National College associate degree program. The director of the Vineyard School is one of the two people who have received baccalaureate degrees from the National College. Vineyard School students who graduate during 1997 are planning to start birth centers in Guatemala and Africa.

The *Association of Texas Midwives (ATM)* in Austin, Texas, offers a self-paced home study course to be combined with an apprenticeship. It is designed to qualify and prepare a student with no prior experience or training to take and pass the examination that is necessary to practice in Texas.

Students should be able to complete the program in three years. Students must find their own preceptors, who must be certified in Texas in order for the student's program to qualify her to take the Texas examination.

The *Ancient Arts Midwifery Institute* (previously called Apprentice Academics), in

Claremore, Oklahoma, has been providing home study midwifery courses since 1981. More than 1,200 people have taken courses through this program. Currently it offers three-year introductory courses and six- to eighteen-month supplementary courses.

The *Oregon School of Midwifery* in Eugene, Oregon, provides a two-year series of classes, with an additional year of supervised clinical training. Students must be high school graduates and complete a prerequisite course in human anatomy and physiology. Didactic classwork during the first two years is complemented by laboratory skills development, supporting women during labor in a hospital or birth center, and providing one hundred hours of service in the community. The purpose of the community service is to give students experience with the social problems that affect low-income families.

The school helps students locate clinical placements or apprentice positions for their third year of clinical experience and provides supervision during the apprenticeship. Although some students are placed with the midwifery service operated by the school or with other midwives in Eugene, most apprentice in home birth practices, birth centers, and clinics elsewhere in Oregon or in Texas or Alaska. Experienced midwives can apply for advanced placement. Preceptors are screened and approved by the school, which provides learning objectives, skill check-off lists, and an evaluation mechanism for both the student and the preceptor. An independent research project and study modules are also part of the program during the third year.

Sage Femme Midwifery School in Santa Cruz, California, and Portland, Oregon, provides an academic program in both locations, as well as a home learning program. The school was started in Santa Cruz in 1985. Over the years it evolved from a ten-week series of classes to a thirty-four-week series of classes—as required by the new California law. More than one hundred stu-

dents have completed the Santa Cruz program. The Portland campus opened in 1990. In 1996 the Santa Cruz program will be phased out and replaced with a program similar to the one in Portland.

The series of classes offered in Oregon is completed in twelve months, after which students can enroll in a one-year clinical skills course that should be taken concurrently with an apprenticeship that is structured and monitored by the school. During the twelve-month academic program, students meet for six 5-hour class days per month. Because students are expected to spend at least two hours in outside study or clinical experience for every hour in class, the total workload is the equivalent of half-time study. Sage Femme guarantees apprenticeship placement with a preceptor for students who complete all first-year requirements satisfactorily. During the first year of apprenticeship students are required to attend class once a month, submit quarterly papers, document their clinical learning experiences, and complete evaluations. Minimal time for completion of the program, including the apprenticeship, is two years; students must complete the program within five years. The program meets criteria for certification by the Oregon Midwifery Council and licensure in Oregon.

Students enrolled in the home learning program take the same content, either through once-a-month classes they attend in person or through use of videotapes. Students send completed learning assignments to the school by mail or e-mail.

Birthingway Midwifery School in Portland, Oregon, offers a three-year program of one day per week classes augmented by learning activities that the students complete at home and send to the school for grading. Class time is used for lectures, discussions, and instruction and practice in basic clinical skills. The first year of the program precedes and the second and third years are taken concurrently with an apprenticeship. The school opened in 1993; it takes one class of nine or ten students per year. The director of the school, who is both a midwife and an anthropologist, designed and teaches the entire curriculum, with help from guest lecturers and community preceptors. Students must be high school graduates and complete a prerequisite anatomy and physiology course that is offered either by the midwifery school or a course offered by a college. Some of the students are college graduates. The program is designed to qualify students for NARM certification.

The curriculum is designed to help students learn how to evaluate the validity of information from various sources. Students are expected to buy and use several textbooks—two by direct-entry midwives, the main nurse-midwifery textbook, an English obstetrics textbook, and books on nutrition and breastfeeding—and read articles and a variety of childbirth education materials. Each student is given one assignment that requires her to research a subject using journals and other resources available at the local health sciences university library. Although students are told that they will not be flunked out of the program, they must earn scores of at least 80 percent on every exam. Examinations may be repeated as many times as necessary for the student to achieve that score.

The school maintains a list of local direct-entry midwives who are willing to serve as preceptors for apprentice midwives. No money is exchanged between apprentices and their preceptors. Some preceptors take more than one apprentice at a time. The program director decides when each student is ready to begin her apprenticeship; students with significant prior experience might be able to start after the first six months of classes. Although the school provides guidelines for the apprenticeship, each preceptor is responsible for her apprentice(s); each student is responsible to her preceptor. This structure is intended to protect the true nature of apprenticeship learning. Although the classwork is completed in

three years, apprenticeships may continue as long as necessary. None of the first class of nine students had graduated by March 1996, three years after they entered the program; one had graduated by April 1997.

The *ACHI Institute for Midwifery Studies (AIMS)* in Glendale, California, (near Los Angeles), is a program of the Association for Childbirth at Home International (ACHI), which was started in Boston in 1972. It is a self-paced correspondence course program. Students are not accepted into the midwifery program until they have completed ACHI's self-study training-of-trainers course to prepare people to teach childbirth educators. It takes most people about eighteen months to complete this program, which requires students to study more than forty books and other references. Midwifery students must be high school graduates, have a current certificate in neonatal CPR, and complete prerequisite college courses in anatomy and physiology, chemistry, biology, pharmacology, and microbiology. Students use many books and other resources and are given assignments that require them to consult several sources for information on the same subjects. Academic assignments are sent to Glendale to be graded and returned.

Because AIMS students have already completed the ACHI teacher training program, they are ready to start an apprenticeship as soon as they start the midwifery program; thus the academic and clinical training are taken simultaneously. The preceptors are responsible for ensuring that students complete all clinical assignments satisfactorily. Finding clinical preceptors that are adequately prepared is a major concern. Preceptors must have attended at least 1,000 out-of-hospital births and visit the AIMS office in Glendale for a clinical skills test and interview; only eighteen preceptors have been approved. To have more control over the quality of students' clinical experiences, AIMS opened a birth center in the Los Angeles area in 1984. Although it is a distance learning program, all students go to the birth center three times a year for two weeks at a time; some go for as long as six months to a year. Preceptors may also go to the ACHI birth center for a few weeks. The birth center is run by a CNM and two direct-entry midwives, each of whom has attended more than 1,000 out-of-hospital births. There are usually five or six apprentice students or preceptors at the birth center at any given time. There were 284 births at the ACHI birth center during 1995, plus 3 or 4 home births per month—a total of about 27 births attended by the program staff and students during an average month.

The AIMS program director has been training midwives since 1975; she started the AIMS program in 1989. About 350 students have started and more than 100 have completed the program since then. Most people take two to three years to complete the program.

Resourcing Birth in Boulder, Colorado, offers a five-month Birth Overview course once or twice a year. The course, which was started in 1987, includes a series of weekly three-hour classes and out-of-class reading and other learning assignments, for example, interviewing people or making a model of a female pelvis. The course content is organized into ten learning modules. Completed learning activities are submitted to the course instructor, who returns them to the students with evaluative feedback. The course can be taken as a correspondence course; the class sessions augment the ten self-learning modules, which can stand on their own. The course was designed and is taught by one midwife. It meets the Colorado Midwives Association (CMA) Certification Program didactic learning requirements for entry into an apprenticeship. The CMA Certification Program recognizes four categories of midwives and aspiring midwives: students, apprentices, interns, and senior midwives. Individuals progressing through this sequence must meet academic and experience

criteria at each level and pass an examination to enter the next level. Resourcing Birth does not test its students because the CMA administers a test to those who want to enter an apprenticeship.

The Resourcing Birth instructor precepts some of the women who complete her course, but can take only two or three apprentices at a time. She and her apprentices attend about twenty births a year. Although they can spend a great deal of time with each client, most of her apprentices take three years to obtain enough experience to take the CMA Intern Examination. Although there are seven midwives practicing in the Boulder area, only two are certified by the CMA and thus are eligible to serve as preceptors. The other midwives were "grandmothered in" when the new law was passed in 1993. Only senior CMA-certified midwives who have received special preceptor training can take apprentices. Lack of approved preceptors creates a bottleneck for students who complete the Resourcing Birth course, many of whom cannot find local apprenticeships.

Programs Based in High-Volume Birth Centers: This section discusses programs based in high-volume birth centers that include didactic teaching as well as supervised clinical experience.

Maternidad La Luz in El Paso, Texas, offers programs of various lengths, including a six-month academic and clinical program for beginning midwifery students. The program is based in a licensed birth center that provides childbirth care to approximately fifty women per month. Most of the clients are Spanish speaking, so students must speak Spanish too. Three-hour classes are held three afternoons per week. In addition, students work three 24-hour shifts per week and are on call for another 24 hours. The students work under the supervision of midwives who have permits to practice in El Paso. The midwives and apprentices provide care to women during prenatal and postpartum clinics, teach childbirth classes, support and coach women during labor, attend births, and monitor women and newborns during the immediate postpartum/postnatal period. Seven to nine students are enrolled during each session; they are counted on to provide a considerable amount of the patient care. Medical consultation and referral for the birth center are provided in the nearby town of Juarez, Mexico. The program tries but cannot guarantee that students will have the numbers of specified clinical experiences required to take the examinations for licensure in New Mexico or for a permit to practice in El Paso.

Family Birth Services Midwifery Course in Grand Prairie, Texas, is based in a birth center. During the first nine months students meet for weekly study groups. After that, they apprentice for one or two years, either at Family Birth Services or with a preceptor approved by Family Birth Services; they can expect to attend about one hundred births during their apprenticeships. Two or three apprentices usually work with one graduate midwife during the apprenticeships. The program is approved by the state of Texas. The midwife who runs this program started to teach others even while she was learning midwifery herself. (A hospital labor-and-delivery-room nurse went with her to thirteen home births, after which she was on her own until she took an intensive one-week lecture course after having attended fifty births.) She opened her own birth center in 1982, where she and one or two apprentices attend eight to ten births per month. Although she had been conducting weekly study groups for her own apprentices before 1993, when training and examination of midwives became mandatory in Texas, she restructured the study groups into a course that meets the state requirements. The course is now open to other apprentices in the area. Eight students were taking the course in early 1996. Students use one direct-entry midwifery book, the main nurse-

midwifery textbook, and books on anatomy and breastfeeding.

Courses Designed to Meet Specific Students' Needs: *Artimis College* in Sebastopol, California, will fashion a course to meet a specific student's goals—for example, to prepare for an examination, to begin seeking an apprenticeship, or to prepare for apprenticeship. Artemis also offers a weekend-long session for experienced midwives. *Heart and Hands Midwifery Intensives* in Windsor, California, organizes intensive courses appropriate for specific students. The courses, which are generally about ten weeks in length, blend academic content with clinical experience and training in specific clinical skills.

Access to Clinical Experience

In the past, relatively few programs were designed to provide comprehensive midwifery education to a person who wants to enter the field but has no prior midwifery experience. Although this is changing, the need to provide an adequate number of birth experiences is a significant problem for schools that try to provide the clinical as well as the academic aspect of a complete midwifery education and enroll more than a very small number of students. Direct-entry schools rely on out-of-hospital births for student clinical experience, and, while the number of schools and students is increasing, the number of out-of-hospital births in the United States is stable and low. With more schools and production of more midwives, the number of births for students of some schools may be declining:

- Three hundred and fifty babies were born at the birth center associated with the ACHI Institute for Midwifery Studies (near Los Angeles) in 1994; in 1995 there were only 284 births—19 percent fewer (Brooks, 1996).
- The birth center associated with the Family Birth Services Midwifery Course in Grand Prairie, Texas, was doing fifteen to twenty births per month during

the late 1980s and early 1990s. During 1995 it did only eight to ten births per month (Jolly, 1996).

Most schools that enroll relatively large numbers of students send their students to high-volume hospitals in other countries for part of their clinical experience. The students' experience is supervised by midwives at those hospitals. The schools usually do not send their own faculty to these hospitals to assist in instructing their students.

Developing a Process to Accredit Direct-Entry Midwifery Education Programs

In June 1990 a group of educators from various direct-entry programs met in Flagstaff, Arizona, to share and explore models of midwifery education and develop a set of common terms related to midwifery education. They formed themselves as the National Coalition of Midwifery Educators, an independent organization that is not part of MANA, and drafted a statement of support for national accreditation of direct-entry midwifery education programs. Other discussions focused on the advantages and disadvantages of basing midwifery programs in universities as compared with community colleges, the need to safeguard the essence and philosophy of midwifery, concerns about the lack of access to maternity care, and the role of direct-entry midwifery education in making the midwifery profession accessible to women in underserved communities. They also considered the need to describe and validate the apprenticeship model of midwifery education and the need for midwives to be the primary educators of midwives. They saw wisdom in diverse models of midwifery education, including distance learning, the conventional classroom approach, and preceptorships combined with a university-without-walls, all of which should lead to the mastery of core competencies. MANA's core competencies statement had not yet been developed, and they were eager for this process to start.

The assembled educators also discussed the need for national certification of direct-entry midwives. They agreed that a challenge mechanism for national certification should be available to midwives of any educational or cultural background, that methods used to evaluate midwives for certification should be culturally unbiased, and that there should be no restrictions on the time needed for individuals to complete their education and pass the certification examination.

The Midwifery Education Accreditation Council (MEAC)

In April 1991 the National Coalition of Midwifery Educators created the Midwifery Education Accreditation Council (MEAC). Annual meetings held since then have focused on developing a national accreditation process for direct-entry midwifery education programs. MEAC began to work on guidelines for this process in 1992. The accreditation criteria were designed to ensure that accredited programs achieve three standards: (1) Meet all US Department of Education (USDOE) requirements for funding by Title IV of the Higher Education Act; (2) meet requirements implied by MANA's statements and policies regarding core competencies for basic midwifery practice, standards and qualifications, and values and ethics; and (3) inform applicants and students whether the program provides all of the educational experiences required for eligibility to take the NARM examination leading to designation as a Certified Professional Midwife (CPM) and explain any requirements that might not be met (e.g., requirements related to having a certain role during a specified number of births).

Accreditation will be available to educational programs that provide both academic and clinical learning experiences designed to prepare an entry-level direct-entry midwife through a curriculum that meets standards for certification or licensing by some state or national entity. As long as the accreditation criteria are met, the program can be of any size and based in any kind of institution, including a private midwifery practice. A single midwife who serves as preceptor for apprentice midwives can be eligible for accreditation as a midwifery education program if she provides learning experiences necessary to achieve all of the MANA core competencies. A program must graduate at least one person before seeking accreditation.

The accreditation process was pilot tested on ten educational programs during 1995–1996. A wide variety of programs, including an apprenticeship, were included in the pilot test. Seven programs were accredited during 1996. An accreditating agency must be in operation long enough to complete two accreditation cycles for at least one school before it can apply for recognition by the USDOE. MEAC will be eligible to apply in 1999.

Practice

Women who go to direct-entry midwives are interested in having out-of-hospital births. Seventy-one percent of the births attended by direct-entry midwives in 1994 occurred in homes; most of the rest were in free-standing birth centers, mainly in Texas, as described in Chapter 7. The proportion of home births increased and the proportion of births in birth centers declined between 1989 and 1994.

Although there are no national data to describe the practice of direct-entry midwives, more than three hundred members of MANA (CNMs as well as direct-entry midwives) are participating in a study, NARM has completed a job/task analysis, and several small studies have been published. Most studies have focused primarily on outcomes, rather than descriptions of the care.* Sakala's studies describing the practices of

direct-entry midwives working in urban areas of Utah during the mid-1980s were rare exceptions; her findings are summarized later in this section.

At the beginning of the lay midwifery, home birth movement, many lay midwives did not feel qualified to provide prenatal care. Women planning to have a midwife attend their home birth were expected to obtain prenatal care from physicians. Now most direct-entry midwives provide prenatal and postpartum care, as well as care during labor and delivery. The scope of practice for home birth midwives includes diagnosis of pregnancy; prenatal care; care during labor, delivery, and for several hours after the birth; several home visits during the first week or two after the birth; and examination and consultation at the end of the postpartum period (four to six weeks after the birth). Some midwives also provide physical examinations and health and nutrition counseling to women who are not pregnant, but that is not the norm. Most midwives have some kind of clinical office, often a separate area of their own home, where they conduct most of the prenatal visits and the four to six week postpartum examination.[†] Most work as solo practitioners, although they collaborate with others in their community. Many have apprentices.

During a recent informal poll, practicing midwives who are members of the boards of MANA, NARM, and MEAC reported that they attend between two and ten births during an average month (Sammon, 1996). Some others have very few clients. Each direct-entry midwife attended an aver-

---

*Studies of outcomes of care provided by direct-entry midwives are described in Chapter 11.

†This description pertains only to the care provided by direct-entry midwives to women who are planning to have home births, and it is very general. It is based on discussions with many direct-entry midwives; numerous books, audiovisual presentations, and articles by or about direct-entry midwives; and information and instructions in Frye's recent book on prenatal care, which was written as a comprehensive textbook for midwives in home birth practice (Frye, 1995b).

age of two to eleven births in 1994, depending on what estimate is used for the number of direct-entry midwives and what assumption is used regarding underreporting of births attended by "other midwives" in states where their practice is illegal (see discussion in Chapter 7). Licensed direct-entry midwives in Washington—a state with a supportive law and the nation's oldest existing direct-entry midwifery school—averaged about three births per month during 1987 (Baldwin *et al.*, 1992). Except under unusual circumstances, most midwives plan to provide complete care to their clients, that is, care throughout the maternity cycle. Most have working relationships with other midwives, who may be consulted and who may take calls and attend births for them when they cannot be available. However, most midwives try to avoid missing a client's birth, by planning far in advance and not accepting clients whose babies are due near the time of a long-awaited vacation.

Informed Consent

Care usually begins with a long initial consultation, during which the midwife and woman meet one another and each tries to determine if she wants to engage the other for the journey through the woman's pregnancy and birth. This is an opportunity for the pregnant woman to ask and have her questions answered and for the midwife to make an initial judgment regarding the appropriateness of a home birth for this particular woman. If the woman decides to engage the midwife, she must do so based on informed consent. To obtain informed consent, the midwife provides a description of her background and experience. She emphasizes that there are no guarantees in life or in birth, that there are risks and benefits associated with every birthing environment, and that the parents must choose which set of risks to take. She explains the midwifery philosophy and model of care and makes sure that the client understands and accepts her own responsibilities, including good nutrition, other self-care, and

establishing a relationship with a physician in case there is need for consultation or referral (Frye, 1995b).

Prenatal Care

Some midwives gather groups of clients for prenatal visits combined with childbirth education; however, most have relatively long visits—thirty minutes to an hour—with individual clients, following a schedule of visits similar to that followed by CNMs and physicians. Frye describes education and informed choice as the cornerstones of direct-entry midwifery care (Frye, 1995b). There is much emphasis on nutrition and other aspects of self-care. Most midwives recommend that their clients read several books. Clients are given a list of supplies to obtain in preparation for the birth and in preparation for the baby. Some midwives conduct series of classes for pregnant women and their partners. Others recommend classes offered by childbirth educators, or feel that classes are unnecessary because their clients are expected to read books and the midwife provides additional information and takes care to answer her clients' questions. Women are encouraged to bring husbands or other primary support persons with them to all prenatal visits, and some midwives insist on this.

Although some midwives conduct every prenatal visit in the woman's home, most do not. However, most make at least one home visit several weeks before the baby is due to make sure they know how to find the woman's house, to meet other members of the family, and to assess the adequacy of the room in which the woman plans to give birth. The midwife also checks the family's preparations for transporting the woman or infant to a hospital, if required, and makes sure that the mother has obtained the necessary supplies (Frye, 1995b).

Some laboratory tests are performed in the midwife's office, using kits or other materials that are readily available. Most midwives also want their clients to have other laboratory tests performed, including routine tests needed to provide baseline information and tests ordered because of an individual woman's history or current condition. Midwives in a few states can order laboratory work on their own. Elsewhere they have to work out an arrangement with a local physician or CNM, who agrees to see their patients for at least one prenatal visit, during which specimens for laboratory tests are obtained. Otherwise, the pregnant woman herself is expected to establish a relationship with a physician, or in some cases a CNM, to provide this and other backup care. Few direct-entry midwives have authority to prescribe or otherwise provide medications that require prescriptions.

Care During Labor, Birth, and the Postpartum Period

Most midwives work with one or more apprentices, doulas, or other assistants and thus have another trained, experienced person with them at each birth. They might also ask another midwife to attend some births with them, especially if they have some unusual concern about the possibility of complications. However, most midwives in the United States do not regularly attend births with another fully prepared midwife (whereas two midwives at a birth is required in some provinces in Canada). Some midwives ask their apprentice or assistant to go to the woman's house ahead of them. Most try to arrive at the woman's home at about the same time that a hospital-based practitioner would have advised the woman to go to the hospital. Once the midwife is at the mother's home, she will stay as long as it takes to accomplish the birth and for several hours thereafter, unless it becomes necessary for the woman or infant to go to a hospital.

Each midwife carries her own supplies and equipment, including those needed for the initial response to a medical emergency. Midwives in some states are allowed to carry pitocin (for treating postpartum hemorrhage). Regardless of the law, midwives who think it is necessary to carry pitocin obtain the drug one way or another, and carry it with their supplies. Some are confident in other methods to prevent or control hemorrhage and do not think this drug is essential.

The midwife recognizes that she is in her client's home and respects the woman's authority. She sees her role as watching, listening, and observing the woman; encouraging, comforting, supporting, and guiding her; not managing the process, unless an emergency requires her to take a more directive role. She sees birth as an intimate, sexual process that belongs to the woman and her husband or partner, often a spiritual experience, not something to be treated in a routine manner or gotten through as quickly as possible.

Her involvement with clients is intensive, requiring nearly continuous total attention and a considerable degree of physical support.

The midwife may guide the mother to place her hand on the baby's head as it is being born and may instruct and help the father "catch" his baby after the midwife has helped to ease out the head and shoulders. After the birth the baby is placed on the mother's chest while they await delivery of the placenta.* After the placenta is delivered, the midwife cleans the baby up, weighs, examines, and returns it to the father's care, and then helps the mother to the bathroom to clean up and, perhaps, take a shower. While the mother is up, the midwife changes the linens, probably starts a load of laundry in the family's washing machine, staying at the home long enough to help initiate breastfeeding and watch for complications.

Most midwives make two home visits during the first week after the birth, usually on the day after the birth or at least within

---

*This approach, as well as the attitudes described here, are descriptive of midwifery in general, and are not unique either to direct-entry midwives or home births.

the first three days, and at the end of the first week. This is usually followed by visits at the midwife's office, or additional home visits, at about two weeks, and again at six weeks (Frye, 1996a).

Midwifery Methods to Reduce and Help Women Cope with Pain

This and the next section report findings from an ethnographic study of fifteen direct-entry midwives practicing in the main metropolitan areas of Utah during a twelve-month period in the mid-1980s. The purpose of the study was to learn about midwives' understanding of birth and approach to maternity care (Sakala, 1988,1993). Five of the midwives had attended more than thirty births during the previous twelve months; all of the others had attended at least five births during that period. Thirteen of the midwives were very involved in religion; eleven of them were Mormons (members of the Church of Jesus Christ of Latter-day Saints). They had practiced as primary midwives (not apprentices) for 7.7 years on average (ranging from 1 to 35 years). The least experienced had attended ten births as the primary midwife; the most experienced had attended more than one thousand. They had fourteen years of formal education on average (ranging from 11 to 18 years). All were mothers, most with many children of their own (nearly six children on average). Three gave birth to all of their own children in hospitals; eight shifted to home births after having delivered at least one baby in a hospital. Four had all of their babies at home. All were dedicated to midwifery. The fees they charged for care ranged from nothing to $695 ($333 on average). Several subsidized vitamin and mineral supplements and other supplies needed by clients who could not afford to buy them (Sakala, 1988).

The midwives were asked to describe the care they would have given during the past year to women like a hypothetical "Mrs. Johnson," whose sociodemographic charac-

teristics, obstetric history, and experience during her current pregnancy and labor were the epitome of a low-risk woman having a normal birth. In one part of the interview the midwives were asked to describe, as completely as possible, how they "have most regularly helped women like Mrs. Johnson deal with the pain of labor and birth during the past year." Later they were asked to identify any other ways they had helped women like Mrs. Johnson deal with pain. If they did not mention prenatal care, the interviewer asked whether any aspect of the prenatal care they provide helps women prepare for and deal with the pain of labor and birth, and, if so, to explain how it has that effect (Sakala, 1988).

The midwives assumed that no woman requires analgesic or anesthetic drugs; none carried those medications, and none reported that a client had been unable or unwilling to continue labor without such medication. Although they expressed strong opposition to administration of these drugs, they defended women's right to choose medicated births. However, they believe that women make such choices out of ignorance of the risks and alternatives. They advised prospective clients who expressed strong interest in conventional pain medications to go to a physician (Sakala, 1988).

The midwives believed that preparation for dealing with pain during labor should begin during prenatal care. They believed that pregnancy and birth are potent catalysts for the expression of conflicts that a woman may have with important people in her life, such as her husband or mother-in-law, that these kinds of conflicts can interfere with efficient labor and make it difficult for loved ones to provide effective support. They also believed that fear is a significant source of pain. Based on these beliefs, they placed strong emphasis on helping women resolve conflicts with family members, developing a bond of mutual trust between the midwife and the pregnant woman, and educating the woman about labor and birth in order to reduce fear of the unknown, to help her feel comfortable with her body, and to increase her faith in her body and in the biological processes of birth. Most of their prenatal visits took at least an hour, and some took as long as three hours. The midwives encouraged their clients to read two to three books per month throughout their pregnancies, and provided exposure to pictures, films, and videotapes of births. They involved and educated the husbands, tried to help women identify and resolve conflicts in their lives, and encouraged resolution of conflicts through discussions with the midwife, work within the troubled relationship, and, if necessary, professional help. They also believed that good nutrition and exercise during pregnancy help to reduce the pain of childbirth (Sakala, 1988).

Some of the midwives also used or taught pregnant women to use specific treatments during pregnancy. A muscle therapist had taught three of the midwives to use a direct muscle-tension release technique involving use of the thumbs or fingers to apply strong constant pressure on tight, contracted muscles until the tension eases and the initial pain from the pressure subsides. Although their treatments focused on muscles in the pelvis and abdominal areas, they sometimes provided complete head-to-toe treatments, including the neck, jaw, shoulders, back, and buttocks. Six of the fifteen midwives recommended that the pregnant woman or her husband regularly massage her perineum with olive or other vegetable oil in the weeks preceding birth; some also recommended gentle stretching of the tissues. However, some of the midwives discounted the value of such massage.*

Once labor started, most of the midwives tried several methods to reduce and help women cope with pain. They would try different approaches to see what seemed to work. All but one reported regular use of physical manipulations such as application of pressure, massage, foot or hand reflexology, effleurage,[†] and other forms of touch. Thirteen midwives said that they apply pressure and that, once they begin, the mothers experience such relief that they will not allow the midwives to stop. Some used Shiatsu pressure points, some massaged acupressure points in the woman's hand. Afterward the midwives felt sore and tired from their own exertion. Many mentioned the general value of touch to make the woman know that someone cares about her and she is not alone. One midwife encouraged the women's husbands to pat their wives and hold their hands. Twelve used some form of hydrotherapy and thought it was very effective. Their clients would labor in a clean bathtub full of warm water; some added herbs to the water, some poured water on the woman's abdomen during a contraction. They reported that some women like to have warm water poured on their breasts. Although the midwives were opposed to use of conventional obstetric analgesia and anesthesia, many utilized herbs with pharmacological properties for pain relief during labor; others disapproved of this practice. There was relatively little confidence in the breathing and relaxation techniques commonly taught during childbirth education; only one-third of the midwives encouraged their clients to learn special breathing and relaxation techniques. However, five of them used formal relaxation techniques in which the midwife encourages the woman to focus on relaxing a sequence of body parts (Sakala, 1988).

---

*Data from the National Birth Center Study and preliminary analysis of data from the prospective study being conducted by MANA suggests that perineal massage is not effective and may even be associated with an increased incidence of minor lacerations (Rooks *et al.,* 1992b; Johnson & Daviss, 1996a).

---

†Effleurage involves gentle stroking of the skin. The hands conform to the surface of the body, so that the muscle mass is not compressed.

Most of the midwives emphasized the importance of the attentiveness of the midwife, her assistants, and the husband, and contrasted this focused support with the mundane chatting of hospital personnel during births. Many gave women tea to drink, to make them feel cared for and attended to. Other approaches included maintaining eye-to-eye contact, encouraging the woman, talking about the baby and the beauty of birth instead of talking about pain. Some mentioned the importance of the midwife's calm demeanor—her quiet, low, gentle voice, confidence and lack of fear. They also described techniques to distract the woman—encouraging her to walk, do the laundry, bake cookies, or visualize herself holding the baby. However, some women need silence so that they can distance themselves from the setting during strong contractions; three midwives reported that they sometimes disconnect the telephone and close the curtains or pull down the shades (Sakala, 1988).

Methods and Theories Related to Preventing and Treating Dystocia

The midwives were also asked to describe and explain what they do to prevent and treat dystocia (the medical term for unacceptably slow or absent progress in labor).* Dystocia is often diagnosed on the basis of a woman's "failure" to progress as quickly as "normal," with progress measured by cervical dilation and the descent of the baby's head through the birth canal, and "normal progress" based on data derived from observation of large numbers of woman giving birth in hospitals. Nearly 5 percent of all women who gave birth and more than 19 percent of those who had Cesarean sections in the United States in 1986 were diagnosed as having disproportion

---

*Dystocia is the most common reason for cesarean sections. Various medical approaches to reducing the cesarean section rate by better prevention and treatment of dystocia are described in Chapter 5.

between the dimensions of the mother's pelvis and the size of the fetal head, a condition that is sometimes called "inadequate pelvis" (Placek & Taffel, 1988).

The mainly Mormon direct-entry midwives practicing in urban areas of Utah during the 1980s were not concerned about the rate of progress or length of labor and disapproved of telling women that either their pelvis or the progress of their labor was inadequate. In their belief system, "As long as the mother and baby are stable, patience and faith in the mother's ability to give birth vaginally are fundamental" (Sakala, 1993). Comparing the midwives' beliefs and practices on dystocia to orthodox medical knowledge and practice, the researcher concluded that "the midwives offered a substantially different yet plausible and coherent system." They felt that it is very rare to encounter an "inadequate pelvis," that slow or absent change in cervical dilation is not a problem in and of itself, and that the range of normal is wide enough to encompass much variation.

Like physicians, the midwives did try to assess the dimensions of the space enclosed by the bones of a pregnant woman's pelvis. Although several reported that they use the formal measurements of clinical pelvimetry to make this assessment, most stated that they "get a 'feel,' a 'sense,' or an 'intuition' about this" while performing a regular vaginal examination or by watching how the woman walks. Questioned about the precision of clinical pelvimetery and the ability of these measurements to predict whether the woman can deliver her baby, the midwives commented on the ability of a hormone produced during pregnancy to cause the ligaments that hold the bones of the pelvis together to relax, allowing the pelvis to expand, and the ability of the bones in the baby's head to overlap and mold to fit through the pelvis. They said things such as, you can "get a baby through a knothole," "I've never seen [a pelvis] that isn't large enough", "I know how to get [babies] out," and "women are built to open up there" (Sakala, 1993). A midwife who had attended more than one thousand births said that she had seen five cases of fetopelvic disproportion in her practice, a rate of less than 0.5 percent; the national rate was 4.7 percent in 1986 (Placek & Taffel, 1988).

The midwives stressed the importance of preventive work during prenatal care —nutrition, exercise, and avoiding harmful substances, in addition to judicious use of interventions during the labor and birth (Sakala, 1993). Five of the midwives gave women herbal preventatives and remedies during the prenatal period. One said that she asks each woman to take one or two herbal formulations during the last month of pregnancy and bases the concoction on the mother's characteristics. Two midwives asked their clients to take a combination of ten herbs during the last five or six weeks of pregnancy—a specific mixture developed by local midwives to facilitate birth, shorten labors of women who tend to have long labors, lengthen labors of women who tend to have rapid labors, and enhance postpartum recovery. Others recommended other herbal combinations to soften and prepare the cervix, prepare the glands, provide minerals, and remove toxins (Sakala, 1988).

During labor the midwives placed emphasis on having the woman move around, encouraged her to maintain her energy by taking light nourishment, tried to help her relax so that she could "open up" and "let go," and assisted her in the use of a variety of positions (Sakala, 1993). One emphasized the importance of having the woman urinate frequently, so that she "doesn't worry about holding something in while trying to let something out." The midwives who had learned muscle tension release techniques from a muscle therapist used intensive pressure applied to certain muscles to help women "open up" and "to decrease resistance to the descending baby" (Sakala, 1988).

The Holistic Health Care Model

Frye's textbook for home birth midwives is entitled *Holistic Midwifery* (Frye, 1995b). In the introduction to the first volume, Robbie Davis-Floyd, an anthropologist studying direct-entry midwifery practice as a participant observer, defined the "holistic model of care" and distinguished it from the "technocratic model" and the "humanistic model," which, Frye believes, are generally descriptive of the care provided by physicians (the technocratic model) and nurse-midwives (the humanistic model). Davis-Floyd and Frye believe that the holistic model is the philosophical and conceptual base for direct-entry midwifery practice in the United States.

Davis-Floyd identifies separation as the basic principle of the technocratic model, for which she listed nine major characteristics: (1) mechanization of the body; (2) isolation and objectification of the patient; (3) focus on curing disease and repairing dysfunction; (4) aggressive, interventionist approaches to diagnosis and treatment; (5) alienation of practitioner from patient; (6) reliance on objective findings as the basis for diagnosis; (7) supervaluation of technology; (8) hierarchical organization, with the patient subordinate to both the practitioner and the institution; and (9) authority and responsibility inherent in the practitioner. The technocratic model defines the core beliefs operating in most American hospitals and sets the standards used by insurance companies, et cetera (Davis-Floyd, 1995).

Respect and connection are identified as the basic principles underlying the humanistic model, for which she listed six basic precepts*: (1) The individual is to be valued as unique and worthy. (2) The body is an or-

---

*In the introduction to *Holistic Midwifery*, Davis-Floyd identifies respect as the main principle underlying the humanistic model and connection as the basic principle of the holistic model. The conceptual framework described here was revised, based on her subsequent work.

ganism, not a machine. (3) The whole person should always be considered. (4) The needs of the individual and the institution should be balanced. (5) Information, decision-making, and responsibility should be shared between patient and practitioner. (6) Empathetic communication, including eye contact and touch, is essential to healing. This paradigm is also known as the *bio-psycho-social model*. While it requires communication and offers rich opportunities for patients and practitioners to work together, many midwives think it does not go outside of the technocratic model far enough to make a critical difference. The example provided is holding a laboring woman's hand and whispering loving words of encouragement to her as she is being hooked up to an unnecessary intravenous infusion and electronic fetal monitor (Davis-Floyd, 1995).

The basic principle of the holistic model is integration—connection so profound that the care provider becomes integrated with the person receiving the care. Davis-Floyd describes the holistic model as presenting a radical, even subversive, challenge to the dominant technocratic health care model. For example, it would urge the laboring woman to avoid the hospital altogether. For this model, which she believes to be the basis of home birth midwifery, she provided more information about the primary underlying principles (Davis-Floyd, 1995):

1. The body is an energy system that is interlinked with other energy systems. This belief is so central that "energy medicine" is a common synonym for holistic medicine. "This view acknowledges the possibilities that a pregnant woman's health can be influenced by such subtleties as the 'bad vibes' generated by anger or hostility. . . . It is the reason why midwives pay attention to their body wisdom as they sense the energetic rhythms of a woman's pregnancy and birth, and why, like other holistic practitioners, midwives work with the invisible sub-

tleties of energy flow, blockage, and release."

2. Total healing requires attention to the body, mind, spirit, emotions, family, community, and all other aspects of the environment. This principle contradicts the idea that any one diagnosis, drug, or therapeutic approach is sufficient to address a woman's health problems, which must be addressed in terms of the whole person in the context of the whole environment in which she lives.

3. Focus on creating and maintaining health and well-being, instead of reducing symptoms and curing disease.

4. Approach diagnosis and treatment through a nurturant relationship. Examples of applying this approach include asking a woman who loses her urge to push if she is afraid to let the baby be born, asking the mother-in-law who seems terrified of birth to leave the room because the midwife knows the woman's labor may be affected by this fear, agreeing to attend births in the environment chosen by a pregnant woman because the midwife knows that women give birth most easily wherever they feel the safest and most nurtured.

5. The essential unity of the practitioner and the client is vital. Deepak Chopra, a physician, author, and primary spokesperson for the holistic health movement, insists that the best way to diagnose is to "become one" with the client.

6. Respect the value of inner knowing. Midwives' "deep trust in the body and in their ability to connect psychically and spiritually with the women they attend makes them willing to consciously rely on intuition for decision-making during childbirth." This does not mean that they devalue logical, linear thought, but that they also listen to their inner voice, which "can only be heard if the midwife remains connected, not only to the mother and child, but also, and most importantly, to herself. . . . Independent midwives are

often willing to expand protocol parameters to reflect their intuitions, their body knowing, about the actual circumstances of individual labors. . . ."

7. Use technology in the service of the individual. This requires refusal to subordinate the mother to a machine. Although midwives use technical equipment and procedures, these things are not allowed to dominate a birth.

8. Use a lateral, webbed organizational structure (i.e., the opposite of hierarchical).

9. Authority and responsibility are inherent in the individual. Midwives see their proper role as nurturing and supporting. They seek to empower birthing women by giving them as much information as possible, believing that the woman herself has ultimate authority and responsibility for making decisions about her care.

Davis-Floyd goes on to describe new research she is conducting on holistic physicians, whose very existence demonstrates that it is not possible to fit all physicians into her technocratic model (David-Floyd & St. John, 1997). Likewise, her model cannot be applied to all CNMs or direct-entry midwives.

Some individuals in each group could be characterized as adhering primarily to each of these models. Most individual practitioners participate in all three models to some degree, moving between them depending on circumstances and the individual's ability and willingness to deal with the ambiguity and conflict inherent in valuing aspects of all three models. However, Davis-Floyd is probably generally correct in associating physicians with the technocratic model, nurse-midwives with the humanistic model, and direct-entry midwives with the holistic model. Although there is a continuum, her descriptions reflect differences in the weight of the influence of each model on the cultures of these three groups.

Use of Intuition and Other Subjective Knowledge

In 1993 a professor in the Department of Community and Preventive Medicine at the Medical College of Pennsylvania published a paper on the home birth movement in the United States. It was based on interviews conducted in 1981 with twelve couples who had experienced at least one home birth with the assistance of a lay midwife. The paper included an extensive review of the literature and a general description of the home-birth movement. "Valorization of subjective knowledge, which is accepted as having equal or greater authority than objectively derived knowledge in certain circumstances" was identified as a central feature (O'Conner, 1992). Personal experience and the testimonial accounts of others were said to carry the greatest authority, with a body of knowledge about the variations and possibilities in childbirth emerging from informal exchanges of ideas and narratives. "Decisions are made and conclusions reached by the use of ordinary inference, introspection, reflection, comparative and probabilistic reasoning, and occasionally as the result of a direct apprehension of knowledge," which members of the movement refer to as "just knowing" (O'Conner, 1992).

Intuition is the word that means "just knowing." MANA's official statements on core competencies, standards and qualifications, and values and ethics all affirm intuition as a valid, important part of midwifery practice. "Respect for the value of inner knowing" is also identified as a basic construct of holistic health care.

During the early 1990s, anthropologist Davis-Floyd teamed with Elizabeth Davis, a respected home birth midwife, to explore the use of intuition as authoritative knowledge in midwifery and home birth (Davis-Floyd & Davis, 1996). The introduction to the paper in which they report their findings synthesizes current thinking on the meaning of intuition (Davis-Floyd & Davis, 1996). The 1993 edition of the *American Heritage Dictio-*

nary defines intuition as "the act or faculty of knowing or sensing without the use of rational processes; immediate cognition." A 1982 book on the subject characterized intuition as a confident form of knowing, involving a sense of certainty about the truth of one's insights, sudden and immediate awareness of knowing, with an association between affect and insight; the nonanalytic (nonrational, nonlogical) appreciation of the whole, integrated nature of an experience, knowledge that cannot be explained. Intuition plays an essential role in any creative activity. However, "knowledge" apprehended through intuition is not always correct (Bastick, 1982).

To study midwives' use of intuition, Davis-Floyd and Davis interviewed twenty-two midwives, whom they characterized as highly literate, competent in technological skills and biomedical diagnosis, and keenly aware of the cultural and legal risks they run when they cannot justify their actions during a birth in logical, rational terms. Seventeen were direct-entry midwives who attended primarily home births. Five were CNMs, three of whom attended births in both homes and hospitals; two were hospital-based CNMs. All were attending MANA conferences when they were interviewed. The purpose of the interviews was to elicit personal stories about the midwives' experiences with intuition. Additional stories were gathered during a workshop that drew midwives with a special interest in this subject.

The midwives said that they "listen to and follow their 'inner voice' during birth, rather than operating only according to protocols and standard parameters for 'normal birth,'" and that being "connected" to the woman and her birth is a prerequisite to hearing their inner voice. The midwives placed great value on physical, emotional, intellectual and psychic "connections" linking the midwife with the mother, the mother with the child, and, in a web-like pattern, the mother, child, father, and midwives, each with the others. To achieve the necessary connection, the midwives reported that they must arrive at a birth

"open." If they are closed—"shut down," "disconnected"—they cannot hear their inner voice and must rely on their intellectual knowledge and accumulated expertise. While they see nothing wrong with this, they said that it results in a qualitatively different kind of care. All of the midwives interviewed considered being connected to the birth process as the primary ingredient of their success—more important than their technical knowledge and skills. One (a CNM) said that intuition is really all that's needed: "I listen to the baby's heartbeat . . . but I don't really care about it, because I have this inner knowing that everything's fine." She also knows when everything isn't fine, because "you know, there's an energy there."

A midwife who works in a collective provided an example: Members of the collective had noticed that if one of the midwives at a birth developed diarrhea, it was a message that they should look at things closer; the midwife's gut knew that something wasn't right. Co-author Davis offered a story of her own: Before going to a birth she often lies down for a few minutes to unwind, let go of her other concerns, and open herself up to herself, so that she can be open to the woman and her birth. While she was doing this prior to a particular birth, she heard a voice say that, after the birth she was about to attend, the placenta would separate only partially, a situation that can cause serious postpartum hemorrhage. She went over the woman's history in her mind, could find no reason to anticipate this kind of problem, and thought, "Well, that's okay, because I've handled this before—I've done manual removals [of the placenta]." But the voice insisted that this would be worse than Davis had ever experienced. When she got to the birth, she told her partner about it, encouraged the woman to drink plenty of fluids, drew up a syringe of pitocin in advance, and rehearsed in her mind what she would need to do if some of the placenta adhered to the uterine wall and she had to remove it manually during a heavy hemorrhage. When the woman did start to bleed after the birth,

Davis was able to do exactly what was needed, as though she were "on automatic pilot"; everything happened as she had foreseen it (Davis-Floyd & Davis, 1996).

Many opposite examples were also given—when the midwife "knew" the baby would be all right and the birth would be normal, despite the presence of complications. In one example the woman involved had at least five "risk factors"—both of her previous births had been complicated, she had a vertical cesarean section scar on her uterus (the kind of scar that is most likely to rupture during a subsequent labor), her membranes had been ruptured for four days before she went into labor (a risk factor for infection), the baby was in breech position and did not turn after several attempts, and she was in strong labor for about eighteen hours. The baby was ultimately born vaginally, without problems. The midwife attributed her willingness to stay the course with this home birth to the strong intuitive certainty, felt by both the midwife and the mother, that the baby was healthy and safe. The authors explained that home birth midwives often "normalize uniqueness"; that is, instead of insisting that labor fit narrow protocol parameters, they are willing to expand the parameters to encompass each woman's unique rhythms and needs. In this case, the midwife felt that a three-day labor was safe and not inappropriate for this particular woman, who needed time to work through the legacy of fear left by her prior birth experience. The midwife's willingness to normalize uniqueness in a given birth often depends on the degree of intuitive connection she feels with the mother and child. If there was no such connection, midwives would transport a woman in this situation; when the connection and inner sense of safety are strong, they will "go the extra mile" to stay at home (Davis-Floyd & Davis, 1996).

Christian Midwives

A segment of direct-entry midwives and their clientele are members of fundamentalist Christian denominations. Religion and values related to their religious beliefs play a strong role in calling many midwives to midwifery and in the commitment of both the midwives and their clients to home births. There is a desire to keep birth within the province of the family and the church and out of the control of the state and large bureaucratic institutions. It is also important to protect women from immodest exposure to men and to avoid obtaining health care from anyone who plays a role in the performance of abortions. Birth has great religious importance, and all persons attending the birth, and the laboring woman herself, invoke God's help in protecting the mother and the baby. Prayer is a complement to the other aspects of the care provided by the midwife. For a few, prayer may be the main way the midwife tries to help a woman experiencing a problem during childbirth. In some cases the pregnant woman and family may refuse to take a woman or baby to a hospital in the event of a life-threatening complication.

Controversy About the Need to Refer Women with Certain Complications

Midwifery is conceptualized as a profession and discipline that is not part of medicine because its focus—pregnancy and childbirth—are normal physiologic processes that are a basic part of human experience and are not inherently pathologic. Pathologies, including those that affect the pregnant woman or fetus and pathologic abnormalities of labor and delivery, are the focus and responsibility of physicians. But there is a "range of normal," and its boundary with pathology is not precise. There is controversy about whether midwives should take care of or refer women who have conditions that are not diseases but are associated with an increased incidence of poor pregnancy outcomes. This controversy focuses on issues such as multiple gestations (e.g., twins), breech births, labor that does not start until more than two weeks after the woman's "due date" (i.e., "post-term" or "postdates" deliveries), and pregnancies that continue without labor even though the bag of fluid surrounding the fetus is leaking or has ruptured. Each of these conditions or circumstances is associated with an increased risk of serious complications and perinatal mortality (death of the fetus shortly before or during labor or of the newborn during the first hours or weeks after birth). Perinatal mortality from these causes is thought to represent only "the tip of an iceberg," so to speak, with the larger, underwater part of the iceberg being sublethal, but sometimes permanent damage to the fetus. Although the likelihood of bad outcomes is higher than usual under these circumstances, the vast majority of the births have good outcomes; thus they can accurately be described as both "risky" and "safe."

The "risk approach" to maternity care (described in Chapter 4) introduced the idea that women should be referred to sophisticated perinatal care centers based on high-risk status alone, rather than waiting to see if the women developed actual complications. Ultimately the idea got out of control, with the development of risk assessment tools that assign risk points to an extensive list of conditions that are statistically associated with higher-than-average perinatal mortality and formalized risk assessment processes that assign a risk score to women based on the sum of the points assigned to all of their high-risk factors. Women with scores above a certain number are designated "high risk" and referred to obstetric units in tertiary hospitals. Because socioeconomic factors are associated with varying levels of perinatal risk, they are included in the risk assessment systems, some of which designate more than 80 percent of pregnant women as high risk. The major benefit of this effort has been the development of a nationwide network of neonatal intensive care centers able to provide life-saving care to very low birth weight babies. The many negative things that also resulted are described in Chapter 4. Despite many limitations and

problems, the concept has achieved widespread acceptance.

One apparently long-lasting effect of the risk approach to maternity care is confusion and lack of precision in distinguishing between risk factors and actual complications. As a result, women with risk factors are treated as though they have real complications. Although the risk approach is now being criticized and reassessed (Rooks & Winikoff, 1992; Fortney, 1995), it has long been criticized by home birth midwives, whose experience testifies to the fact that the vast majority of high-risk women have normal births. Home birth midwives' lack of faith in obstetrical pronouncements about high risk meld into a controversy about whether they should retain or refer women with conditions such as twins and babies in breech position. This issue is further complicated because high-risk conditions, such as multiple pregnancies (twins) and breech births, are associated with increased mortality even when they are attended by the most skilled obstetricians. The mortality rate is twice as high for babies in breech presentation, even when they are delivered by cesarean section (Cunningham *et al.*, 1993). Each of the conditions mentioned earlier is associated with a significantly increased risk of death or damage to the baby, if not also to the mother. Yet most women with these conditions who give birth at home have healthy babies. Midwifery newsletters and journals publish many inspirational stories about such successful home births.

This controversy is one of many divisive issues between direct-entry midwives and CNMs. Nurse-midwives have created a significant niche for midwifery in the regular health care system. To do so, they zealously created and have jealously guarded a record for excellent pregnancy outcomes. Most of them carry heavy clinical case loads; their salaries, for the most part, are not dependent on the number of births they attend. They want to protect their excellent record, and most accept the medical consensus that conditions such as breech presentation and twins constitute forms of pathology that make births inappropriate for midwifery care and require management by a physician. Their circumstances and approach to these controversies is in stark contrast to those of most direct-entry midwives, who have relatively few clients, who are critical of an approach to maternity care that focuses primarily on "risks" and identifies women with even minor risk factors as so high risk that they should have their babies at tertiary medical centers, and whose income is affected by the number of births they attend. In addition, MANA's statements regarding standards, values, and ethics direct them to inform the woman of the risks and allow her to choose which risks she prefers to take. Direct-entry midwives are concerned about iatrogenic risks associated with the kind of care women with these complications often encounter in hospitals, including unnecessary cesarean sections and trauma to both the mother and infant due to use of forceps. In addition, MANA's statement of values and ethics specifically affirms the value of accepting death as a possible outcome of birth and urges a focus on supporting life rather than avoiding death.

Medical Care for Women and Newborns with Serious Complications

All midwives know that even the healthiest pregnant woman can develop unforeseen serious complications that require medical intervention. Due to their very different histories and roles in the American culture and health care system, nurse-midwives and direct-entry midwives have developed different approaches to meeting their clients' needs for rapid access to medical care. The ACNM's core competencies statement identifies collaboration with and referral of clients to physicians and other members of the health care team as major components of nurse-midwifery care. Nurse-midwives must be able to demonstrate a safe mechanism for obtaining medical consultation,

collaboration, and referral; every nurse-midwifery practice or service must have written policies or practice guidelines that outline the parameters for seeking medical collaboration or referring a woman or newborn to a physician. As discussed in Chapter 8, the requirement for medical collaboration in a nurse-midwifery practice has made it impossible for CNMs to establish practices in some areas. Direct-entry midwives have been critical of the ACNM's willingness to allow physicians to exert this kind of veto over midwives. In a 1983 letter to the editor of the Journal of Nurse-Midwifery, the president of MANA pointed out that the ACNM had placed nurse-midwives in a vulnerable position by making alliance with a physician a standard for nurse-midwifery practice. "We . . . need to be careful," she wrote, "that our ability to practice is not . . . contingent on our competitor's approval" (Charvet, 1984).

MANA's statements identify midwives as autonomous practitioners who collaborate with other health and social service providers when necessary; the midwife should "make a reasonable attempt to ensure that her client has access to consultation and/or referral to a medical care system when indicated." Given the vituperative early history of the relationship between direct-entry midwives and obstetricians, including the executive director of ACOG's characterization of lay midwife-attended home births as "maternal trauma" and "child abuse" (see Chapter 4) and the continuing illegal status of direct-entry midwives in many states, it would have been suicidal for MANA to adopt standards that require its members to have working relationships with physicians. Nevertheless, many "lay midwives" have evolved into "direct-entry midwives" and have now been part of the maternity care scene for more than twenty years. They have undergone significant change, and there have been changes in medicine too. Some direct-entry midwives have developed effective working relationships with obstetricians, family physicians, and pediatricians. Many have not been able to because of physicians' refusal to work with them. A few have chosen not to have any association with physicians or the established medical care system.

Some direct-entry midwives consider establishing a relationship with a physician to be a responsibility of the pregnant woman. When medical input is needed during prenatal care, the midwife advises the woman to see a physician; however, it is the client's responsibility to follow the midwife's advice. When the need for medical care arises during labor, midwives practicing in urban areas may call for an ambulance or drive the woman or newborn to a hospital. If a private car will not be available, some midwives ask the pregnant woman to notify the closest ambulance service about her plans to give birth at home and to make sure they know how to find her house.

The enormous variation in state laws and other local circumstances create enormous variation in the degree, tone, arrangements, and effectiveness of medical backup. Some states that regulate direct-entry midwives require them to have written collaborative agreements with physicians. Some states simply require the midwife to have a plan; her plan may be to take the woman to the nearest hospital. Even Washington State does not require a doctor or hospital to have agreed to the midwife's plan. The Oregon law only requires the midwife to provide a detailed description of her backup arrangement to women who seek her care. Nevertheless, some midwives have developed good consultation and referral arrangements with physicians who share the midwives' criticism of mainstream obstetric care, with physicians who have social relationships with the midwives, and with physicians who believe that providing medical care to midwives' clients is part of the responsible role of an obstetrician. Some physicians back up direct-entry midwives covertly, due to harrassment by their colleagues (Gaskin, 1996). Some refuse to consult but invite midwives to refer women to them—a good business practice for an obstetrician who needs more patients.

As a result of efforts to implement regionalization of perinatal care, many urban academic medical centers function as the level III perinatal referral center for large areas, in some cases an entire state.* Obstetric faculty, residents, and other staff at those centers expect to provide consultation and referral services for less sophisticated maternity care providers in their region. Obstetricians with a public health orientation and desire to improve the health of mothers and babies realize that they need to reduce barriers to emergency obstetric care for any woman who needs it; those in states with substantial numbers of home birth midwives realize that reaching out to the midwives will result in better outcomes when emergencies occur. Thus, although there is a long history of mutual disrespect and anger between obstetricians and direct-entry midwives in many states and communities, responsible physicians and midwives have turned this around in some areas. For example, the obstetrician who sits on the Board of Direct Entry Midwifery of the State of Oregon is on the faculty of the Department of Obstetrics and Gynecology at Oregon Health Sciences University (OHSU). He has invited every direct-entry midwife in the state to call him when she has a question. In fact, the obstetric department at OHSU gets two or three calls from direct-entry midwives every month. Some direct-entry midwives have asked to receive announcements of the Department of Obstetrics and Gynecology's "grand rounds" (weekly early morning continuing education sessions). The midwives are welcome at the grand rounds, and a few have attended some sessions (Nichols, 1996).

Despite some improvement, effective collaboration between direct-entry midwives and physicians is insufficient in general, and

---

*See discussion of regionalized perinatal care systems in Chapter 4.

this compromises the safety of the care provided by some midwives. A study of professional relationships between midwives (CNMs, licensed direct-entry midwives, and unlicensed lay midwives) and physicians (family practitioners and obstetricians) in Washington—the state with the longest modern experience with a supportive law and a formal, three-year direct-entry midwifery school—concluded that "only CNMs have forged mutually satisfactory relationships with the physician community. Increased hospital-based training and practice opportunities are needed before licensed midwives can improve their professional relationships with physicians" (Baldwin *et al.*, 1992). The study was conducted by public health-oriented family physicians. Their conclusions were based on data from questionnaires completed by 50 ob–gyns, 180 family physicians (FPs), 29 CNMs, 34 licensed midwives (LMs), and 16 lay midwives who were providing care to pregnant women in Washington during 1988.

In the Washington study, two-thirds of the ob–gyns and 44 percent of the FPs had consulted with or received a referral from a midwife at some time during their medical practice. More than half of the ob–gyns and one-third of the FPs received a referral from a midwife during 1987. Although most of the physicians felt that midwives can provide an acceptable alternative to physician care for low-risk pregnant women and half of the physicians who had no experience with midwives said they would be willing to establish a referral relationship, none were willing to attend a home birth (Baldwin *et al.*, 1992).

All of the CNMs, 97 percent of the LMs, and half of the lay midwives had referral relationships with physicians. CNMs mainly consulted with and made referrals to ob–gyns. About two-thirds of the licensed direct-entry midwives consulted with ob–gyns; the others consulted with FPs. Half of the unlicensed lay midwives had referral relationships—three with ob–gyns, three with FPs, and two with naturopaths. Almost 70 percent of the CNMs were satisfied with their referral relationships; 62 percent had written contracts, and 52 percent met with the doctors on a regular basis. Only 6 percent of the licensed midwives had written contracts, none had regular meetings, and virtually all wanted to establish more formal referral relationships with physicians. They also wanted more respect, appreciation, and communication from the doctors to whom they made referrals, and greater integration into the mainstream health care system, including hospital privileges, more physicians willing to back them up, and insurance coverage for home births (Baldwin *et al.*, 1992). Some of these problems have since been mitigated in Washington state to some degree, as discussed later in this chapter.

Many barriers continue to prevent effective working relationships between direct-entry midwives and physicians. Because the midwives are not in the regular health care system, most doctors never see them or get to know them socially. Physicians are most likely to become aware of direct-entry midwives when the doctors become involved in the care of women or newborns who are brought to hospitals because of complications. Some deaths and serious damage result from the inability to access medical care quickly. Doctors tend to focus on these without realizing that they are seeing only the problems and none of the much larger number of healthy home births; that is, they see only the cases in the denominator, and none of those in the numerator of a serious complication rate that may be quite low.* Physicians are busy and, aside from those with a public health concern, most have little motivation to become involved with care providers whose approach is very different from their own. Doctors are used to having

---

*Some bad outcomes also result from unnecessary use of interventions in hospitals. Evidence regarding the safety and risks of midwife-attended home births is presented and analyzed in Chapter 11.

their professional authority accepted as authentic, to having the last word in clinical controversies based on the assumption of superior knowledge. Many have little tolerance for dialogue with a care provider who challenges the validity of their supremacy in the care of normal pregnant women. Even physicians who enjoy this kind of challenge can be deterred by pressure from their peers, including, in some cases, the threat of losing their hospital privileges or malpractice insurance. In states where direct-entry midwifery is illegal, that is the greatest barrier to collaboration with physicians.

Some direct-entry midwives have to use backup from physicians who treat them or their clients with contempt. The only physician who is willing to backup a direct-entry midwife working in a certain area may disapprove of home births and express his disdain by treating patients transferred to his care because of a labor crisis with contempt for their "stupidity" or by subjecting them to unnecessary procedures, such as episiotomies, which he knows the women do not want.

Recruitment, Selection, and Retention

Recruitment, selection, and retention are as critical as education to the quality of service provided by most professions. In the case of direct-entry midwifery, the circumstances have been unique: Most direct-entry midwives in practice during the 1990s became midwives despite lack of supportive laws, threat of arrest and imprisonment in some states, disdain and disparagement from physicians, few organized educational programs, and no societal support in the form of third-party payment for their services. After entering the field, they were sustained and invigorated by their attraction to the practice itself, the support and gratitude of their clients and others who value home birth, pride in their growing skill and competence, determination not to let this form of midwifery die, the exhilaration of fighting for a good cause, and the sense that they

were gaining ground. Many would not articulate these reasons, but would say simply that they were "called" by some higher value or authority—religion, for some; reverence for the power, beauty, and sanctity of birth for many others. In any case, their decisions to become midwives were not based on calculated assessments of the monetary or prestige advantages of lay midwifery compared with other potential careers.

Although many women have wanted to become midwives, relatively few completed the process, and of those who did, many "burned out" and left the field after only a few years (Tritten, 1992). Without schools, the transition from aspiring to be a midwife to actually becoming a midwife was a long road that had to be traversed with little structural support. In addition, many dropped out once they understood the demands and gravity of the responsibility of the role. There is a large dropout rate even among students enrolled in organized training programs:

- Birthingway Midwifery School, in Portland, Oregon, admitted its first class of nine students in March 1993. Since it is billed as a three-year program, these students should have been expected to finish in March 1996. None of them did. As of March 1996, five of the nine were in extended apprenticeships, one had decided to enroll in a nurse-midwifery education program, one decided to become a naturopath, one took the course because she was pregnant and never planned to become a midwife, and one who had wanted to become a midwife had changed her mind (Sholles, 1996).
- About half of the women who complete the five-month Resourcing Birth course in Boulder, Colorado, do not enter an apprenticeship immediately after completing the course. Some get an apprenticeship in another place or at another time; some decide not to become midwives. Many use their training in a related

or similar field, becoming childbirth educators, massage therapists, or doulas who provide labor support in hospitals (Richardson, 1996).

Heretofore direct-entry midwifery has depended on self-recruitment, self-selection, and individual women's personal decisions to continue or discontinue the self-study and informal training that could lead to becoming a midwife. The ethic was for all involved in midwifery to be mutually supportive. A senior midwife might try to discourage an apprentice who seemed unsuited for midwifery, but the apprentice–preceptor relationship may be very personal and there are no objective criteria for failure or success. An apprentice discouraged by one mentor can seek another. Although a testing and certification process has been developed, it is primarily intended to reward those who pass the hurdles, not to prevent practice by people who fail or do not choose to take the test. Discussions of the development of a national examination were originally couched in terms of "validating" the knowledge of the midwife taking the test, not in terms of determining whether she actually had the requisite knowledge.

Developments during recent years have begun to change this picture—supportive laws, more physicians who are willing to cooperate, coverage of direct-entry midwifery services by Medicaid and other third-party health care financing plans in some states, malpractice insurance available through joint underwriters' agreements in Washington and Florida, strengthening of the exam, and a certification process. Midwives practicing under supportive laws buy listings in the *Yellow Pages* and run ads in local papers. Midwives in areas where there is a substantial demand for home births can make a good income.* These factors are generating new

interest in midwifery among young women in search of careers. There are schools to apply to now; the steps required to become a midwife are becoming clearer, more definite, and more expensive. All of this affects recruitment, selection, and retention.

What Kinds of Women Apply to Direct-Entry Midwifery Schools?

For many years most of the applicants were women who were already practicing midwifery and needed to complete a formal program in order to obtain a license. This was the situation of virtually all students in the first classes admitted to the Seattle Midwifery School. The proportion of experienced midwives in each class has decreased over the years; about one-fourth of the women enrolling in SMS during the 1990s had previous midwifery experience (Myers-Ciecko, 1996). This change has an impact on the educational experiences required by students. SMS has begun to require students to have some labor support experience before they enter the program; it offers a course for doulas and is considering making experience as a doula a requirement. Twenty percent of the first 71 SMS graduates were nurses.

Most SMS students are in their early thirties, although there has been a wide age range (from twenty-one to sixty-five years). The proportion who are younger is increasing. Two-thirds to three-fourths of the students in each SMS class are mothers; many SMS students have had at least one home birth of their own. (One of more than one hundred students admitted to SMS during the past eighteen years was a man.) Most students of the Birthingway program in Portland have been in their late twenties to early forties. More than half were mothers when they entered the program. Some had completed some college courses, but none had graduated from college.

Most women who became lay midwives during the 1970s entered the field almost by accident; those who remained to become leaders of the new direct-entry midwifery

---

*A letter from the head of one of the new educational programs in Florida informs prospective students that midwives in that state can earn from $20,000 to $50,000 a year, depending on the circumstances.

movement are extraordinary women, survivors of an extraordinary time, pioneers who became dedicated to midwifery. Recruitment and selection for new three- or four-year educational programs offered to persons without previous midwifery experience will be different; the effect of that difference on the group as a whole is not yet known. The Seattle Midwifery School is beginning to get applications from young women who became interested during college women's studies courses (Myers-Ciecko, 1996).

Barriers as Well as Increasing Support for Practice

As direct-entry midwifery becomes more professionalized, more direct-entry midwives are pursuing it as a career and basis for earning a living. But there are still many constraints, even where the environment is relatively supportive.

The most obvious constraint is the limitation to out-of-hospital practice; the proportion of out-of-hospital births has remained at one percent for nineteen years, including births attended by physicians and CNMs and births that occur out of hospital by accident, as well as those attended by direct-entry midwives. The fact that the rate has not increased does not mean that it would not grow if the circumstances were different. The percent of births attended by direct-entry midwives is much higher in some communities—for example, about 4 percent in Boulder, Colorado (Erickson, 1997). A 1995 survey of members of the largest HMO in Washington found that 8 percent were interested in the idea of a midwife-attended home birth and might use such a service if the cooperative would provide the same benefits for a home birth that it provides for a birth in one of the HMO hospitals (Spencer, 1996).

As a result of this survey, home births attended by licensed direct-entry midwives (LMs) became available to members of the Group Health Cooperative of Washington in January 1996. The cooperative functions as an assemblage of semiautonomous regional units, each of which has agreed to contract with at least some LMs in its geographic area. Members of the coop can seek the services of an LM directly, that is, they do not have to be referred by the primary care provider assigned to them by the HMO. To be eligible for a contract, a midwife must be licensed by the state and have professional liability insurance (Spencer, 1996). Professional liability insurance is available through a joint underwriting agreement in which all liability insurance companies operating in Washington have to participate. The state organized the joint underwriting agreement. LMs covered by the insurance policy must participate in a program of quality assurance that includes a practice review and continuing education. The obstetrics department of the local Group Health hospital provides the medical backup. All of these components—licensure based on education and examination (as per Washington's 1981 Midwifery Act), coverage by third-party payers, professional liability insurance, participation in a quality assurance program, and medical backup—need to be in place in order for any latent demand for home births to materialize. Until they are in place, we do not know what proportion of American woman might want to use this kind of service.

Unless these supports become available, it is unlikely that the number and proportion of births attended by direct-entry midwives will increase significantly. The number has remained between 11,500 to 12,500 births per year, 0.3 percent of all births in the country, for as long as the data have been available. The "market" for home birth midwifery services is becoming saturated in some places, making established midwives less than welcoming to new ones (Osborn & Esty, 1995).

ACNM's Role in Direct-Entry Midwifery Education and Certification

Lay and direct-entry midwives have always presented a dilemma for nurse-midwives and the ACNM. Both the common ground and differences are profound. Nurse-midwives appreciate and respect the contributions of direct-entry midwives but have been gravely concerned about the lack of universal standards for education and practice and inadequate collaboration with physicians. They have also been critical of the care provided in some situations, and concerned about confusion among the general public and other health professionals regarding the education, practices, and outcomes of direct-entry midwives as compared with CNMs.

The turmoil began as soon as lay midwives became a visible part of the obstetric care scene during the 1970s. Although both groups were midwives, their experiences, perspectives, situations, and needs could not have been more different. Although most nurse-midwives educated during the 1940s and 1950s had experience with home births and were confident that they could be safe when part of a system that provides access to medical care when needed, most CNMs in practice during the 1970s had not had that experience. They had learned midwifery by taking care of indigent women, who have a relatively high incidence of problems during childbirth, in institutions dominated by obstetricians who believed in the efficacy and necessity of a variety of invasive techniques for monitoring and managing labor and delivery. Nearly three-fourths of nurse-midwives surveyed in 1982 had no out-of-hospital birth experience during their nurse-midwifery education program (Adams, 1984). Although private sector nurse-midwifery was growing, most CNMs in practice at that time were employees who had limited control of patient care policies. Their standards required them to work in collaboration with physicians, and few physicians were willing to work with them except under those conditions. Most were not free to develop and implement their own style of practice. Although many tried to change practices they disagreed with, they were pushing against the grain within institutions in which they had limited influence.

Nurse-midwives began to be criticized in the lay midwifery/home birth literature as "compromised," "co-opted by medicine," "too quick to intervene," and "not much better than physicians." They were described as not being "real" midwives, of having "sold-out" to medicine and the health care system, probably due to their "socialization" as nurses. Barbara Katz Rothman, a sociologist with a special interest in midwifery, wrote that "nurse-midwife" may be a contradiction in terms: "Nurses, in our medical system, are defined by their relationship to doctors," whereas midwives are supposed to be "with the woman" (Rothman, 1981). The accusations made many nurse-midwives feel belittled, unappreciated, hurt, angry and bitter (Burst, 1990). Nevertheless, many CNMs concurred, at least in part, with the critique.

Working outside of the mainstream system, lay midwives were unfettered by the fears and constraints experienced by nurse-midwives. Lay midwives had no need to compromise and thus were free to develop their own style of childbirth care. Nurse-midwives were well aware of the lay midwives' beautiful home births and were challenged to examine their own practices. In 1980 the ACNM developed guidelines for establishing "alternative" birthing services and dropped a negative home birth statement (originally approved in 1971) in favor of a statement that endorsed practice in all settings (ACNM, 1971, 1980).

The 1978 annual meeting and convention of the ACNM included an open forum discussion about what, if any, involvement the college should have with lay midwifery education, certification, and licensure and whether the ACNM should have an official liaison relationship with lay midwifery groups. ACNM members voting during a business meeting held as part of the 1980 convention recommended that the board of directors "study the philosophical and practical implications of any change in the title and education" of nurse-midwives. Committees were charged to study this issue, and local chapters and all members were invited to provide input for presentation at another open forum discussion of this issue during the 1981 annual meeting and convention (Burst, 1995a). That fall, the ACNM president convened a meeting at the ACNM's office in Washington, D.C., for the purpose of establishing dialogue between CNMs and "non-nurse-midwives." It was this meeting that led to the founding of MANA in 1982. The internal debate about how the ACNM should relate to other midwives continued. Similar discussions went on in MANA, which established a long-term goal of unifying midwives of all kinds under a single organization.

The seminars on midwifery education convened by the Carnegie Foundation for the Advancement of Teaching in 1989 and 1990 were intended to create an opportunity for constructive dialogue between both kinds of midwives. Participants of the 1990 Carnegie Foundation seminar included officers and key committee chairpersons from the ACNM and MANA. Although all factions of midwifery were represented, the seminar focused on professional midwifery. With the exception of a statement on the scope of practice for professional midwives, there was no attempt to achieve formal consensus. However, there was agreement on some important points:

- Although students may enter midwifery education programs with a variety of identities and prior experiences, all should have the same minimum knowledge, skills, and competencies when they graduate.
- Individualized assessment and learning programs should be developed to assist already practicing or credentialed midwives to meet new standards.
- Midwifery must be a credible profession, with high standards leading to clinical competence and safe practice.

The Carnegie Foundation Seminars on Midwifery Education, and the Interorganizational Work Group that followed, encouraged MANA to deal with the issues of educational and practice standards, stimulating the initiation of steps that led to the development of the MEAC process for accrediting direct-entry midwifery education programs and the NARM process for certifying direct-entry midwives. It also stimulated the ACNM to initiate a process to identify the knowledge, skills, and competencies nurse-midwifery students obtain during nursing education and experience that provide a necessary base for their midwifery education. These nursing competencies were assumed, but not explicitly identified in the ACNM core competencies document (Roberts, 1996b). In 1989 the ACNM directed its Division of Accreditation (DOA) to investigate means to assess non-nurse professional midwifery education. The DOA determined that the first step was identification of the nursing competencies that provide a base for nurse-midwifery education.

The DOA planned to use a consensus-building strategy to identify which aspects of the preparation of nurses need to be incorporated into the education of professional midwives who are not nurses; it estimated that it would take two to three years to define these "core health skills" and develop criteria for evaluating direct-entry educational programs. While the DOA worked on that task, the general membership of the college continued to grapple with the question of how the ACNM should deal with other midwives, some of whom seemed eager to develop professional standards and some of whom did not, and questions about nurse-midwifery's relationship to nursing. Although some CNMs identify strongly with nursing, many see themselves mainly as midwives. Some became nurses only as a necessary step to becoming a nurse-midwife. Although valid arguments were made about the contribution of nursing education and experience for midwives who take care of many of the nation's most socioeconomically high-risk pregnant women, the costs of nurse-midwifery's educational and political association with nursing were also becoming apparent. Many nurse-midwives bridled at the American Nurses' Association's claim to represent CNMs and its demand that nurse-midwives be licensed as "advanced practice registered nurses" and that a master's degree in nursing be a requirement for this license.*

As the dialogue progressed, it became clear that the most important difference between nurse-midwives and other midwives is not that CNMs are nurses; in fact, some direct-entry midwives are nurses too. Instead the critical difference arises from the quality assurance that clients, physicians, others in the health care system, and the public, as represented by government, have learned that they can rely on when they are dealing with a CNM. Because of the ACNM's clear definitions and exclusive criteria, the standards for a certified nurse-midwife are the same throughout the country. The care provided by midwives who meet those standards has been carefully and redundantly evaluated and found to be safe and effective. It is those standards, and the research-based record of safe, effective care by midwives who meet those standards, that have made it possible for nurse-midwives to have a growing role in the American health care system—the standards, not the fact that they are nurses.

This became even more clear as nurse-midwives became aware that a growing number of physician assistants (PAs) were practicing as "midwives," in some cases without any additional obstetric training, and that a direct-entry school in Florida was developing a special track to prepare foreign-trained physicians to take the Florida exam

for licensure as midwives. By the spring of 1994, nurse-midwives knew of five states that were seeking educational standards and mechanisms to use for credentialing PAs, nurse practitioners, physicians, or others as midwives (Burst, 1995a).

In addition, nurse-midwives who followed NARM's progress in developing an examination for direct-entry midwives were alarmed about the process that had been used—pooling items from a variety of local tests and throwing out questions that anyone objected to. And they were skeptical because virtually everyone who took the early version of the NARM exam passed it.† Some members of MANA had similar concerns; NARM has since taken important steps to improve the test, including a recent substantial job and task analysis. Nevertheless, the NARM examination had developed a poor reputation among many CNMs, and use of a written test, unsupported by educational requirements or any means to assess clinical judgment and skills, did not strike most nurse-midwives as an adequate way to determine a midwife's competence. Nurse-midwives faced the possibility of PA-midwives, naturopathic-midwives, and foreign-trained physicians being licensed as midwives in Florida. Many were fighting local battles for hospital privileges and a role in managed health care and feared the effect of confusion between CNMs and direct-entry midwives certified by state and local governments, state midwifery associations, and NARM.

In 1990 the ACNM board of directors approved a set of *Guidelines for Experimental Education Programs*. The guidelines included the Education Committee's proposed criteria for accreditation of direct-entry midwifery education programs (Burst, 1995a).

---

*See the section "Mutual Support, But Significant Disagreement with Nursing" in Chapter 8.

†Almost all of the first people who took the examination were experienced midwives. See section on the North American Registry Exam for Midwives earlier in this chapter.

Nevertheless, in April 1993 the ACNM board of directors approved the Interorganizational Work Group on Midwifery Education's statement on *Midwifery Certification in the United States*. It defined a *certified midwife* as someone who has "completed prescribed studies in midwifery accomplished through a variety of educational routes . . . has demonstrated competency in the skills required for midwifery practice and passed the MANA Registry Exam" (i.e., the NARM exam). A *certified nurse-midwife* was defined as someone who has completed the education and certification requirements of the ACNM and the ACNM Certification Council (ACC).

The 1993 ACNM convention was held one month after the College endorsed the Interorganizational Work Group statement on midwifery certification. During the business meeting, two ACNM members made a motion which recommended that the College appoint a commission to "develop standards and credentialing mechanisms for professional midwifery in the United States, make recommendations for implementation of one Standard of Professional Midwifery, and explore the impact of other professionals on midwifery practice" (Burst, 1995a). Discussion of the resolution focused on the role of PAs, FPs, and other health professionals in the care of pregnant women, as well as the role of direct-entry midwives. The motion was passed on the vote of the members who were present at the meeting. At its postconvention meeting, the ACNM board of directors responded to this motion with actions that resulted in (1) the development of a "preliminary study group" to investigate ramifications of expanding the ACNM's credentialing and standard-setting functions to include all forms of professional midwifery and (2) planning for yet another open forum discussion of the issue, to be held during the 1994 convention (Burst, 1995a).

Presentations and discussion during the open forum on this subject at the 1994 convention highlighted concerns among both members and leaders of the College about the effect on the profession of the proliferation of state-generated standards for professional midwives. A motion recommending that the Division of Accreditation (DOA) "immediately establish and implement" an accreditation process for "non-nurse professional midwifery programs" and that the ACNM, in cooperation with the ACNM Certification Council, create a "certified professional midwife" (CPM) credential for graduates of those DOA-accredited programs was passed during the business meeting that followed the open forum. The motion also recommended that the board of directors survey the full membership on these issues if it decides that it cannot take this action without giving all members an opportunity to express their opinion. A by-mail opinion survey of all ACNM members was conducted in June 1994. Forty-four percent completed and returned the survey. Of those who responded, 73 percent thought the College should accredit non-nurse professional midwifery education programs, "using, at a minimum, the same criteria used in accrediting nurse-midwifery education programs;" 71 percent thought the College should create a program to credential "certified professional midwives"(Burst, 1995a).

In July 1994 the ACNM board of directors voted "to support the use of ACNM credentialing mechanisms to set the standard for professional midwifery in the United States." In pursuit of that objective, the board asked the DOA to establish and implement mechanisms for review and accreditation of non-nurse professional midwifery education programs and recommended that the ACNM Certification Council (ACC) explore creation of a certification examination for graduates of direct-entry education programs that are accredited by the ACC (Burst, 1995a).

Many members of MANA felt that the ACNM's decision to create a route to non-nurse midwifery certification was intended to undermine NARM's progress toward developing a certification process that would be controlled by direct-entry midwives. In August 1993 NARM had appointed a certification Task Force to advise its board of directors about certification and to make plans for a national certification process. In October 1994 the NARM task force announced its intention to initiate a credentialing process for a certified professional midwife. Because of NARM's use of the term "certified professional midwife," direct-entry midwives certified by the ACC will be referred to as ACC "certified midwives" or "CMs."

Later in the same month, October 1994, the ACNM Division of Accreditation published its criteria for accreditation of a "basic" midwifery (i.e., direct-entry) education program. No direct-entry midwifery school in existence at that time could meet all of the DOA criteria (Rooks & Carr, 1995). The criteria included the following requirements, among others: (1) All students must have experience in hospitals; (2) programs must either require a baccalaureate degree as a prerequisite or award a baccalaureate degree for work done in the program; and (3) all faculty, including the program director, must be midwives who have been certified by the ACNM or the ACC. No "grace period" was allowed for meeting this requirement (Burst, 1995a).

In the autumn of 1996, the State University of New York (SUNY) Health Science Center at Brooklyn and the Midwifery Education and Service Division of the North Central Bronx Hospital, both located in New York City, opened the first "basic" midwifery education program designed to meet the requirements of the ACNM Division of Accreditation. The program was also designed to meet the requirements of the new Professional Midwifery Practice Act in New York State. The SUNY Health Science Center at Brooklyn is a public university located in a densely populated, medically underserved, inner-city area with many minorities and first- and second-generation immigrant families. It has had a nurse-midwifery educational program since 1973. The North Central Bronx Hospital has operated a nurse-midwifery service since 1978. CNMs attended 86 percent of the 3,287 deliveries at the North Central Bronx Hospital in 1988 (Haire & Elsberry, 1991).

Although considered a basic (i.e., direct-entry) midwifery program, all students must be college graduates who have completed the biologic and behavioral science courses required for most health professions, and must have had some women's health care experience before entering the program.

With the exception of two courses designed especially for them, the basic midwifery students take the same midwifery courses as students enrolled in the nurse-midwifery program at SUNY Health Science Center at Brooklyn. One of the two special courses is a ten-day basic health-skills course during which the students are updated and checked out on all manual skills included in a list of skills specified by the ACNM Division of Accreditation as necessary for entry-level midwifery practice. The other is an integrated medical science course covering general knowledge in psychiatry, pediatrics, medicine, and surgery (as required by the New York Midwifery Practice Act). Students with sufficient prior education and experience can challenge either or both of these courses (Shah, 1996).

Faculty of this program plan to develop a true "direct-entry" midwifery education program—one that does not require prior education or experience in women's health care. They hope to accomplish this within three years (Shah, 1996).

At least three other universities that currently operate nurse-midwifery education programs are considering the development of separate direct-entry midwifery tracks. The ACNM anticipates that most of the first students to apply for these programs will be physician assistants who have experience in obstetrics, direct-entry midwives who have completed a midwifery education program in other countries (e.g., Denmark, France), and informally prepared direct-entry midwives who have been practicing in the United States.

Challenges for Direct-Entry Midwifery in the United States

More than 25 years after women with no formal training began to practice midwifery in some communities during the late 1960s and early 1970s, direct-entry midwifery is recognized as a distinct form of American midwifery and has developed many of the quality control processes that are essential to an autonomous profession. During that period direct-entry midwives have had a significant effect on maternity care in the United States—because of their strong connection with a highly motivated, activist group of consumers and the appeal of the uncompromised form of midwifery care they have modeled. They have challenged assumptions; demonstrated new methods; presented a consistent, strong, articulate critique of mainstream obstetrical care, and generally pushed the envelope of midwifery in this country, even in our "peer countries". Their example may have contributed to a reassertion of direct-entry midwifery in some countries. While they have done this primarily from outside the system, they have developed a foothold within the system in a few states with favorable laws.

Practicing outside the system, often outside the law, has been a critical factor in their evolution—allowing direct-entry midwives to develop in many positive ways that would not have been possible while meeting the demands, expectations, and constraints exerted within the system. At the same time, being outside the system has deprived them of supports they need; they have been held back by that deprivation. A dozen years ago a sociologist at a small college in California published a book about the costs and benefits of regulating midwifery—making it legal, bringing it into the system (DeVries, 1985). He presented a paradox: Not being licensed by the state makes lay-midwives vulnerable to legal action for practicing medicine without a license and limits the availability of this kind of care; regulation by the state would

change it and, eventually, ruin it—making it, in his opinion, no better than nurse-midwifery, which he considered to be seriously compromised. The tension and conflict of this dilemma continued to be played out in both the external forces and internal politics affecting direct-entry midwifery as it has evolved during the intervening time. The following paragraphs present some of the major challenges that continue to face this still vulnerable and limited form of midwifery:

- *Despite many new, mostly favorable laws, direct-entry midwifery is still illegal in many states.* Their continuing illegal status in some states and the fact that direct-entry midwives have been arrested, handcuffed, jailed, and tried for "crimes" including illegal practice and manslaughter (sometimes because of an unavoidable infant death) has had a deep impact on the development of this form of midwifery in the United States. Because of a law passed in 1993, midwives are no longer being arrested in California. But because of a law passed in 1992, midwives who used to practice without fear in New York are now being arrested. Direct-entry midwifery cannot progress beyond a marginal status where it remains illegal.

- *Licensing standards, where they exist, vary from state to state, and there are no mandatory national standards for entry into practice.* As a result, there is no clear definition of a "midwife" as a person who has met widely accepted educational and competency standards. The combination of MEAC's new process for accrediting direct-entry education programs and NARM's new experience- and competency-based testing and certification process—both based on MANA's core competencies statement—have created a means by which individual direct-entry midwives can demonstrate and document their adherence to national standards established by their peers. The development of these processes was an enormous accomplishment and may be a pivotal turning point in the evolution of direct-entry midwifery in the United States. However, one does not need to be a CPM in order to be accepted as a midwife or to practice as midwife. Less than half of all direct-entry midwives are members of MANA; many will not even attempt to become certified through NARM. Although some uncredentialed midwives are excellent practitioners, there is no minimum standard and no systematic way to exclude those whose preparation and practice are inadequate.

• *The new MEAC and NARM processes are competency based; neither requires completion of a specified number of years of formal professional education or requires an academic degree.* MEAC's and NARM's adherance to standards that measure experience and the demonstration of competence is appropriate given the existence of many highly experienced, competent, informally trained direct-entry midwives in our country. Competency-based standards are more valid than degrees as a means to measure learning required for performing a particular role. Most Americans, however, assume that formal education is necessary to prepare professionals, especially health professionals who perform a role that is usually filled by physicians. The standard for direct-entry midwifery in Europe is three years of formal professional education and training. All American nurse-midwives have a minimum of three-and-a half years of professional training (at least a two-year associate degree in nursing followed by a nurse-midwifery program that is at least eighteen months in length), and 70 percent have master's degrees. In addition, a baccalaureate degree will be required for certification as a nurse-midwife beginning in 1999.

Graduates of direct-entry midwifery education programs accreditated by the ACNM must have at least a bachelor's degree. Four states now require three years of formal midwifery education or a baccalaureate degree for direct-entry midwifery licensure. It is likely that this standard will be adopted more widely as a criterion for licensure, third-party payment, malpractice insurance, et cetera.

• *Americans generally associate an "apprenticeship" with preparation for a craft or trade, rather than a profession.* Direct-entry midwives' loyalty to the concept of apprenticeship, and to use of that term, may prejudice some people, making it difficult for them to assess a midwife's clinical learning experiences objectively. Nevertheless, there are significant similarities between an apprenticeship and the precepted clinical training that is part of the preparation of all health professionals. When "apprenticeships" are structured, monitored, and directed towards the attainment of clearly specified competencies, the difference may disappear.

• *The MEAC/NARM accreditation and certification processes are new, and the examination is an improved, strengthened iteration of an earlier examination, which was known by the same name and did not receive a positive response.* Neither process is well known beyond the MANA community, although a growing number of states have adopted the NARM exam. It will be necessary for the processes to become better known. The certification process will ultimately earn a reputation based on the judgments others make about the process itself, and on judgments they make about the performance of midwives who have been certified by those standards, that is, "certified professional midwives," or "CPMs." Development of a good reputation on this basis will require consistent use of this term and a willingness to distinguish between CMPs and other direct-entry midwives.

- *There is very little reliable data about direct-entry midwives and their practice. It is impossible even to state with accuracy and confidence either the number of direct-entry midwives who are practicing or the number of births they attend.* The lack of these most basic facts undermines efforts to move this form of midwifery ahead.
- *Direct-entry midwives' sharp criticism of the medical profession combined with their physical isolation from the mainstream health care system have made it difficult or impossible for many of them to acquire adequate medical backup.*

Direct-entry midwives attend only about one of every two hundred births in the United States, including a significant adjustment for undercounting. This proportion has not increased during the past fifteen years, despite significant advancements in the field during that period of time. To some extent this reflects the limited demand for home births. However, the proportion of women who would like to give birth at home or in a free-standing birth center may be significantly larger than the proportion who actually do so. Licensure based on education and examination, coverage by third-party payers, professional liability insurance, participation in a quality assurance program, and medical backup—all need to be in place for any latent demand for home births to materialize. Direct-entry midwives practicing in Boulder, Colorado, have experienced many changes as a result of the law passed in 1992:

Whereas they were merely tolerated before the law change, they are now well received when they take women or newborns to local hospitals because of complications. The doctors and nurses treat them more professionally. Hospital support for home births is now a legitimate part of local obstetrics, and some hospitals are competing for this business. If the complication is not an emergency, the midwife may call more than one hospital to see which doctors are on call. If there is a choice, they use the hospital whose doctors are friendlier and whose nurses are nicest to their clients. Some nurses try to comfort the pregnant woman and support the midwife. The midwives also report that they are taking care of a wider group of women—mainstream women who were unwilling to consider a home birth when the midwives' practice was illegal. Midwives in Boulder are advertising in the *Yellow Pages* now, which they could not do before (Erickson, 1997).

With two new programs to certify direct-entry midwives—one operated by NARM and one operated by the ACNM—the country will soon have even more classifications of midwives and even more confusion: certified nurse midwives (CNMs, certified by the ACNM), certified professional midwives (CPMs, certified by NARM), certified midwives (CMs, certified by the ACNM Certification Council), direct-entry midwives who have been certified by local midwifery organizations but not by NARM, licensed midwives (LMs, direct-entry midwives who are licensed by specific states, who may or may not also be certified by NARM or the ACNM), and midwives who are neither licensed nor certified.

Chapter 10
The Quality, Safety, and Effectiveness of Midwifery as Practiced in the United States

Chapters 10, 11, and 12 deal with the outcomes and benefits of midwifery as practiced in the United States during the past fifteen years. By far the largest part of that practice is care provided by nurse-midwives who attend births in hospitals. Chapter 10 focuses on the outcomes of midwifery care in general, but does not address the safety of out-of-hospital births, which is the subject of Chapter 11. Chapter 12 focuses on the effect of midwifery care on health care costs and the particular contribution nurse-midwives have made by providing effective care to low-income, special-needs women. In all three chapters, the information on midwifery care is based on a comprehensive review of research on the subject.

To assess the quality of care provided by midwives, it is necessary to have something with which to compare it. In addition to research on midwifery care and its outcomes, Chapter 10 provides information on how nurse-midwifery care stands up to the American College of Obstetricians and Gynecologists' standards for prenatal care, research describing the labor and delivery care provided to low-risk women by physicians and nurses, and research findings that explain the importance of breast-feeding, maternal–infant bonding, and care that supports a healthy transition into motherhood during the period surrounding birth.

The Primacy of Safety

The main concern about midwifery has always been whether midwives can provide care that is as safe and effective as care provided by physicians, whose education and training takes place over a much longer period of time. For most people, all other considerations—including costs and women's preferences—pale beside the importance of effectiveness and safety.

295

Although pregnancy is not inherently pathologic, pregnant women and their fetuses and newborns are susceptible to potentially lethal diseases that arise from pregnancy itself, as well as potentially lethal problems during childbirth. When these problems occur, timely medical and/or surgical intervention may make the difference between life and health versus death or lifelong impairment, which sometimes seems as bad as or worse than death. However, the vast majority of pregnancies do not result in any serious problems. When problems do not occur, there are many benefits to the kind of care provided by midwives. Midwives may prevent some poor pregnancy outcomes by helping women make lifestyle changes needed to improve their health and avoid some kinds of complications and by supporting the natural powers of labor in a way that facilitates the process of birth. In addition, midwifery care can prevent some serious complications, even deaths, by avoiding iatrogenic problems caused by unnecessary use of obstetric interventions during labor and birth.* Ideally, all pregnant women should have midwifery care. Those with diseases or complications should also have medical obstetric care. And, because complications can arise with very little warning, all pregnant women should have quick, easy access to medical obstetric care. This is the way it works in most European countries—in which the infant mortality rate is, for a variety of reasons, much lower than ours. That is not how it works in the United States, although it has become or is becoming the way it works in some parts of our health care system. This chapter summarizes the results where this approach has been implemented and examined.

Most of the information in this chapter comes from research conducted in the United States between 1980 and 1995, as well as a few studies conducted during ear-

lier periods and research from other countries that is relevant to the situation in the United States. Some of the information and many of the conclusions are based on evidence summarized in the second edition of *A Guide to Effective Care in Pregnancy & Childbirth*, by Murray Enkin and his colleagues, whose work was introduced in Chapter 6 (1995). The guide is based on systematic review of the evidence resulting from well-controlled evaluations of the effectiveness of various approaches to the care of pregnant women. The greatest weight is given to findings from randomized controlled trials reported in journals published in many countries. The Cochrane Pregnancy and Childbirth Database conducts an ongoing systematic critical review of this literature.

Nurse-midwives account for nearly 95 percent of the births attended by midwives in the United States. Most of the information on midwifery care and its outcomes is based on studies of nurse-midwifery care.

Outcomes of Midwifery Care When the Births Occur in Hospitals: Overview

Nurse-midwifery care has been carefully documented. Mary Breckinridge's expectation that Frontier Nursing Service midwives keep careful records of their practice outcomes has been inculcated in all subsequent generations of nurse-midwives. Later development of nurse-midwifery within academic health science centers facilitated and ensured a thorough and virtually continuous evaluation of the safety and effectiveness of nurse-midwifery practice.

Results of some of the earliest studies are summarized in Chapter 4. Most of the women cared for through the first nurse-midwifery services were poor and lived in rural areas with few or no doctors or inner-city areas served by public charity hospitals. The women tended to be poorly nourished and poorly educated. Most were black, Hispanic, or Native Americans. Many were unmarried

---

*Iatrogenic problems are those that are inadvertent effects of medical treatment.

adolescents. Many of the married white women were of very high parity. The earliest studies were based on nurse-midwifery services in which most of the births occurred in women's homes. Many of the studies compared outcomes for the nurse-midwifery service to data on all births in the county, state, or country during the same time period, or compared outcomes for women in the same population before and after the nurse-midwifery service started. Some compared pregnancy outcomes for women cared for through a nurse-midwifery service with those for women using the regular care available to women in that area. Although each study examined a different set of outcomes, every study reported improvements associated with nurse-midwifery care: increased attendance at prenatal clinics; increased weight gain and fewer cases of preeclampsia and anemia among pregnant adolescents; a lower incidence of preterm births, higher average birth weight and a lower incidence of low birth weight babies; reductions in maternal, perinatal, neonatal, and infant mortality; reduced expenditures for personnel and for prolonged hospitalization of the mother or infant; and reduction in the birth rate due to better use of family planning.

Most of the improvements came from providing care to women who had little or none before. But this was not true in all cases. Outcomes for pregnant adolescents served through special nurse-midwifery programs were compared with outcomes for teenagers served through other clinics. The evaluation of the nurse-midwifery project in Madera County, California, analyzed data for periods of time before, during, and after closure of the demonstration project. Large reductions in prematurity and neonatal deaths during the project were reversed when the nurse-midwives left, even though additional physicians had moved into the area and were providing services.

In 1980, Albert Gore, Jr., then a congressman from Tennessee, held hearings on obstacles to nurse-midwifery practice. The hearings were stimulated by a situation in which CNMs who had been providing care to poor women in Nashville were denied access to every hospital in the city when they sought privileges that would allow them to admit private patients. During the hearings Dr. C. Arden Miller, chairman of the Department of Maternal and Child Health at the University of North Carolina School of Public Health and a past-president of the American Public Health Association, testified that "If one looks for reasons why this country is deprived in many areas of the services of midwives, one has to look in the political and economic arenas. The answer is not to be found in terms of health outcomes. All of the studies I know confirm that the health benefits rendered by nurse-midwives stand up to scientific scrutiny exceedingly well" (House Committee on Interstate and Foreign Commerce, 1980).

Studies conducted during the 1980s continued to find good outcomes associated with the care provided by nurse-midwives. There were no studies in which the outcomes were worse. New studies began to look at additional variables, including patient satisfaction.

In 1986 the director of the nurse-midwifery program at the University of Pennsylvania published a critical examination of nurse-midwifery research conducted in the United States between 1925 and 1984. None of the studies were able to control for all factors that influence pregnancy outcomes. Nevertheless, the studies were consistent in finding lower maternal and infant morbidity and mortality rates when nurse-midwives began to provide care to women who had lacked sufficient care before the midwifery service started and similar or better outcomes when nurse-midwifery care was compared with care provided by physicians. The studies also found exceptionally high rates of kept appointments and women who returned for postpartum follow-up and high levels of patient satisfaction (Thompson, J.E., 1986).

During the same period of time, the congressional Office of Technology Assessment (OTA) conducted its own review of published data relevant to the safety and effectiveness of nurse-midwifery care. *The OTA concluded that nurse-midwives manage routine pregnancies safely and as well as, if not better than, physicians.* The OTA report cited studies that found that CNMs were more likely than physicians to test their prenatal patients for urinary tract infections and diabetes, but were less inclined to prescribe drugs; that CNMs were less likely to rely on technology, but interacted more intensively with their patients; and that nurse-midwives' patients spent less time waiting for visits, had shorter hospitalizations, and were more likely to feel satisfied with their care. "The weight of evidence indicates that, within their areas of competence, . . . CNMs provide care whose quality is equivalent to that of care provided by physicians. Moreover, . . . CNMs are more adept than physicians at providing services that depend on communication with patients and preventive actions. . . . Patients are generally satisfied with the quality of care provided by . . . CNMs, particularly with the interpersonal aspect of care . . ." (Office of Technology Assessment, 1986).

During seventy years of practice, only one negative report has been published—the 1995 *New York Times* exposé of "mismanaged care" in New York City's public hospitals described in Chapter 8. This was shocking, because it was the first time anyone had reported a higher incidence of bad outcomes associated with nurse-midwifery care. Later review of the situation at the New York City hospitals described in the "exposé" found that the two hospitals most indicted in the *New York Times* articles had a lower rate of adverse outcomes than the average for all public hospitals in New York City and that the average for all public hospitals was about the same as for private hospitals affiliated with the New York City Health and Hospitals Corporation—3.0 percent for the public hospitals compared with 2.8 percent for

affiliated private hospitals (Burkhardt, 1996a).

During the early 1990s, the American Nurses' Association commissioned a meta-analysis of research comparing outcomes of primary health care provided by nurse practitioners or CNMs with outcomes of care provided by physicians (Brown & Grimes, 1995). Meta-analysis is a research method that allows synthesis of quantitative conclusions from a large body of diverse research. The first step is a thorough search for both published and unpublished studies. The researchers conducting the meta-analysis used a computerized database that references articles published in journals indexed by the National Library of Medicine and another that provides information on unpublished studies conducted by graduate students. Unpublished studies were also requested from educational programs that offer graduate degrees in nursing, schools of public health, and relevant professional and health care organizations.* The search for studies was conducted during 1991 and 1992.

Although many studies of nurse-midwifery care had been published, the meta-analysis search yielded only fifteen studies that used acceptable research methods to compare the outcomes of care provided by CNMs and physicians. Seven had been published in the *Journal of Nurse-Midwifery*, three in medical journals, two in nursing journals, and one in a multidisciplinary perinatal health care journal; two of the studies were unpublished graduate student theses. Nine studies excluded women who would not have been eligible for nurse-midwifery care (i.e., higher risk women) from the physician care comparison group. Meta-analysis of the data from those nine studies found many differences in the care provided by CNMs as compared with physicians, but relatively few

---

*Unpublished studies are included in meta-analyses in an effort to overcome an assumed bias against publication of negative findings (Glass *et al.*, 1981).

differences in outcomes. The most important difference in outcomes was a reduced low birth weight rate for babies born to women whose prenatal care was provided by nurse-midwives. The two groups of women and babies were equivalent in measures related to fetal distress and in the incidence of low one-minute Apgar scores (scores based on systematic observation of the newborn's heart rate, breathing, color, and other signs of well-being at one and five minutes after the baby is born).

There can be little doubt about the safety of nurse-midwifery care when the births occur in hospitals. Bad outcomes would be difficult to hide in these settings; any pattern of untoward effects would surely have come to light during forty years of experience and well over fifty published studies. Instead of finding problems, the data suggest that nurse-midwifery care may result in better outcomes—less maternal morbidity and probably a lower incidence of low birth weight and fewer cesarean sections. In addition, there are many benefits related to maternal–infant bonding, breast-feeding, and other more subtle or longer term effects on the well-being of the family. Last, but not least, most women who experience midwifery care are highly satisfied with it. Information on these outcomes is provided later in this chapter.

Methodologic Problems in Looking for Causes of Better or Worse Outcomes

Many studies have found reduced rates of low birth weight and cesarean deliveries associated with nurse-midwifery care. If these associations are valid, they are extremely important: Low birth weight is the leading cause of infant mortality and the reason why the infant mortality rate is higher in the United States than in virtually all other wealthy, industrialized countries. The United States also leads almost all countries in the rate of cesarean sections. The cesarean delivery rate is widely acknowledged to be too

high and a problem that should be fixed. In 1985 the highly esteemed Institute of Medicine (IOM) recommended that the nation rely more heavily on nurse-midwives to provide care to "hard-to-reach" high-risk women and that state laws be amended to support nurse-midwifery practice (IOM, 1985). Those recommendations were based on studies that had found that fewer low birth weight babies were born to socioeconomically high-risk women who had received their care from nurse-midwives (Levy *et al.*, 1971; Piechnik & Corbett, 1985). In 1995 an independent consumer advocacy group published *Encouraging the Use of Nurse-Midwives: A Report for Policymakers*. It recommended expanding nurse-midwifery education with a goal of gradually adjusting the ratio of CNMs to obstetricians so that nurse-midwives become the primary provider of care to low-risk pregnant women. The report and recommendations were based on a Public Citizen Health Research Group study of 41 nurse-midwifery practices with in-hospital births and 41 nurse-midwifery practices in freestanding birth centers. A major finding of the study was lower cesarean delivery rates associated with care by nurse-midwives (Gabay & Wolfe, 1995).

The conclusions reached by these influential institutions were based on many studies that have found better outcomes and fewer cesarean deliveries among women cared for by CNMs. It is very difficult, however, to determine if these benefits are due to the care provided by the midwives or to inherent differences between women who get their care from midwives and women who get their care from doctors. Women receive care from midwives because they choose to or because they are identified as appropriate for midwifery care. Both circumstances introduce *selection bias*. The effect of selection bias is obvious when high-risk women are assigned to physicians and low-risk women are assigned to midwives, who refer women who develop serious complications back to the physicians. Because the physicians take care of the high-risk women and the low-risk women who develop complications, we should expect their patients to have a higher incidence of poor pregnancy outcomes. Although less obvious, selection bias may also influence the results when only low-risk women are included in the physician-care comparison group.

Many factors affect pregnancy outcomes. Low birth weight rates vary with maternal age, marital status, parity, race, socioeconomic status, education, and prepregnancy weight, and are affected by smoking, weight gain during pregnancy, drug use, physical abuse, genitourinary tract infections, stress, and the mother's attitude toward her pregnancy (IOM, 1985; Fiscella, 1995). This is not a complete list of relevant factors, and we do not know what triggers most cases of preterm labor, which is the most important proximal cause of low birth weight. Cesarean delivery rates vary with maternal age, parity, education, and socioeconomic status, and with health system factors, including financial incentives and disincentives, what kind of hospital the birth occurs in (i.e., level I, II or III), and whether it is a teaching hospital. Cesarean delivery rates are different in different parts of the country and have changed over time. None of these factors are equally distributed between women cared for by CNMs and women cared for by physicians.

Even when studies measure and take account of factors such as age, race, marital status, and the results of psychological tests, women who choose midwives are likely to be different from women who choose doctors in ways that have not been taken into account. The practice of midwifery is relatively small in this country and is seen as an "alternative" to regular, that is, physician, care. Women have reasons for choosing midwives; those who make that choice are different from those who do not. Those differences are difficult to measure and may affect the outcomes of their pregnancies.

The only way to avoid selection bias completely is to assign women who are eligible for midwifery care to a midwife or physician randomly. This is hard to accomplish. Most women who want midwifery care are adamant about it; few would be willing to have their childbirth experience determined by a coin toss. There have been few randomized trials. Those few have found less effect of CNM care on the incidence of low birth weight and some have found no effect of CNM care on the rate of primary, i.e., first cesarean sections.

When a study finds a significant difference in outcomes between groups that are different in one characteristic, we say that there is an *association* between that characteristic and the outcome. However, the association is not necessarily one of cause and effect. For example, early studies of birth control pills found an association between use of pills and cervical cancer. We now know that cervical cancer is caused by a sexually transmitted virus; women who begin sexual activity at a young age and have many sexual partners are more likely to encounter the virus and are more likely to develop cervical cancer. And, of course, women who are sexually active are more likely to use birth control pills—thus the association between oral contraception and cervical carcinoma. The association is due to *selection bias* and *confounding*. Women who are more likely to develop cervical cancer are more likely to choose to use birth control pills—an example of selection bias. Oral contraception and cervical cancer are both associated with sexual activity; as a result, observational studies find an association between oral contraception and cervical cancer—an example of confounding. In a randomized trial, women would be assigned to the oral contraception group or the no oral contraception group on a random basis. This would break the confounding connection between pill use and sexual activity, which would be randomly distributed between the two groups of women in the study. Such a study would not find an association between oral contraception and the development of cervical cancer.

Prenatal Care

This section is the first of several that describe the sequence of maternity care: prenatal care, care during labor and delivery, and care during the postpartum period. In each section, the content and purpose of care provided to women during that phase of the maternity cycle is described and explained in order to provide context for information on the effectiveness and outcomes of the care provided by midwives.

Routine prenatal care is a relatively new tradition. Since its introduction, prenatal care has contributed to preventing and treating illnesses in mothers and their babies, for example, by preventing death or brain damage of Rh-positive fetuses carried by Rh-negative mothers, by controlling the glucose metabolism of pregnant women who are diabetic, and by treating infections and hypertension. Prenatal care can also play a preventive role by educating women in ways to avoid health risks and maintain or improve their health and by helping to prepare them for both the birth and the baby. In addition, the development of a relationship between a pregnant woman and the person who provides her prenatal care over the many months of pregnancy offers a unique "window of opportunity for preventive health care" (Merkatz & Thompson, 1990). Prenatal care provides an opportunity to provide counseling about family planning and to link women with other services, such as nutrition supplementation and counseling; legal, social service, and drug abuse programs; assistance for physically abused women; and parenting support and education. Many of these opportunities are missed, however, due to the "routineness" of most prenatal care.

In 1986, the U.S. Public Health Service assembled a multidisciplinary panel of experts and asked them to examine the content of prenatal care and its effectiveness in promoting the health and well-being of women and their infants. The expert panel prepared a report, which was published in 1989 (DHHS, 1989). On the first page of the report the obstetrician who chaired the panel noted that prenatal care appears to lead to healthier pregnancies even in the absence of disease. "We often cannot explain why a mother who enters a prenatal health care system early in pregnancy appears to have improved pregnancy and newborn outcome, compared with a similar mother who receives little or no prenatal care" (Rosen, 1989). Selection bias is part of the reason. Well-organized, well-educated, middle-class women who want to have babies tend to go to their doctors or midwives at the first sign of pregnancy and follow whatever advice they are given regarding diet, resting, not smoking, et cetera. Most of them are healthy to begin with, and they are relatively unaffected by the bevy of social, economic, environmental, and lifestyle stresses that are associated with poor reproductive outcomes. Women who lack access to prenatal care or do not come to care early or consistently even if they have access are often of low socioeconomic status, have little social support, have negative or ambivalent feelings about their pregnancy, and are highly affected by the life stresses associated with poorer outcomes (IOM, 1985). It is exceedingly difficult to untangle the real benefits of prenatal care from the effects of selection bias.

The expert panel recommended that prenatal care be enriched in order to make it more effective, and that more emphasis be given to the period before conception and during the early months of pregnancy. Other recommendations included broadening the focus to include attention to other aspects of the woman's health before, during, and after pregnancy and promoting healthy child development, positive family relationships, and family planning. The panel's report emphasized that prenatal care cannot be effective unless it is available and used. Prenatal care providers were advised to expand the traditional medical model of prenatal care to give new emphasis to the psychological and social aspects of the woman's life and concerns (DHHS, 1989).

The report of the expert panel was titled *Caring for Our Future: The Content of Prenatal Care*. Some studies have been conducted to measure the extent to which its recommendations regarding enhanced efforts to educate women during the early months of pregnancy have affected practice:

- A study conducted in New York City found that women using public clinics received more information during prenatal care as compared to women who received their prenatal care from private physicians (Freda *et al.*, 1993). Fewer than half of the private patients reported having received information about acquired immunodeficiency syndrome (AIDS), sexually transmitted diseases, prevention and early detection of preterm labor, postpartum family planning, and violence within the family. These findings may be based in part on differences between the patients: The women who attended the public clinics were more likely to be having their first baby, Hispanic, unmarried, younger than 25 years, and not educated beyond high school. More of the private patients were non-Hispanic whites who were married, were at least 25 years old, and had attended college. Nevertheless, many of the private patients indicated that they were not satisfied with the amount of information they received during prenatal care, but had felt embarrassed to ask questions.
- Another study described the prenatal care provided by a stratified random sample of physicians practicing obstetrics in an area of North Carolina that includes several major universities and two of the nation's leading academic medical centers. Most of the women were white, married, and privately in-

sured. The study aimed to determine the extent to which the care conformed to the recommendations in *Caring for Our Future*, especially with regard to risk assessment and education conducted early in each woman's pregnancy— when changed behavior could have the greatest impact on the pregnancy. Sixty percent of the practices had a nutritionist on staff, and 91 percent of the women received nutrition counseling at some time during prenatal care. But only 61 percent received nutrition counseling during their first visit, when there is the greatest amount of time to interrupt or correct practices and circumstances that could endanger the health of the mother or fetus. This pattern was true for many of the recommended kinds of counseling and education: Although most of the women were counseled about smoking, drinking, drug use, and general self-care at some point during their pregnancies, except for nutrition counseling, only about half of the women received this information and counseling during their first prenatal visit. Although more than 17 percent of the women smoked, fewer than 1 percent were referred to any kind of behavior modification or treatment program (Peoples-Sheps *et al.*, 1996).

Prenatal Care Provided by Midwives

Prenatal care provided by midwives is consistent with the recommendations of the Public Health Service Expert Panel on the Content of Prenatal Care. Chapter 6 explained how midwifery care differs from care provided by physicians; Chapters 8 and 9 described how some of those differences play out in the prenatal care provided by CNMs and direct-entry midwives.

A few studies have actually measured differences between prenatal care provided by nurse-midwives and physicians. The 1986 report by the Congressional Office of Technology Assessment (see earlier section on "Outcomes of Midwifery Care When the Births Occur in Hospitals") cited findings from early studies of prenatal care provided by nurse-midwives. In addition, at least two studies have compared the extent to which prenatal care provided by nurse-midwives and physicians complies with medical standards.

A study conducted in Canada in 1984 evaluated the prenatal care provided to forty-four low-risk women by nurse-midwives and a matched two-to-one sample of low-risk women who obtained prenatal care from family physicians (Buhler *et al.*, 1988). The women were matched for the date of delivery, age, socioeconomic status, and numbers of previous pregnancies, abortions, and births. Evaluation criteria consistent with standards published by the organizations that represent obstetrician–gynecologists (ob-gyns) in Canada and the United States were used to assess the quality of prenatal care provided to both groups of women based on information in their clinic records. The evaluation looked for recorded observations that are essential for adequate monitoring of a woman's progress during pregnancy, evidence of sound clinical judgment and decision making, and recognition of symptoms, signs, or laboratory findings that could affect the pregnancy outcome. The care provided to each woman was rated as superior, adequate, or inadequate. Eighty-four percent of the nurse-midwives' charts were rated as superior or adequate, compared with only 40 percent of the family physicians' charts. Indications of superior care were more than twice as frequent among the nurse-midwife charts; omissions that indicated inadequate care were more than four times more frequent among the family physician charts.

A similar study used information from the prenatal records of low-risk women whose care was provided by randomly selected samples of ob-gyns, family physicians (FPs), and CNMs practicing in Washington State during 1988 and 1989 (Baldwin *et al.*, 1994). The prenatal care recorded in the patient records was compared to standards recommended by the American College of Obstetricians and Gynecologists (ACOG). Although the care provided by all three kinds of practitioners adhered closely to the published standards, the records of CNM clients matched the ACOG standards more closely than those of either type of physician. Standards for which there were significant differences between the CNMs and physicians included completeness of the information obtained during the initial history taking, especially information on smoking and prepregnancy weight; recording results of urine tests, increases in uterine size, and the mother's report of fetal activity at every prenatal visit; determining fetal presentation during the eighth month of pregnancy; and use of screening tests for diabetes, cervical cancer, and a certain kind of fetal defect.

The study was conducted by faculty of the Department of Family Medicine at the University of Washington. Although the research team thought that many of the physician lapses in compliance with the standards were not very important, they were concerned about poor adherence to the standard that calls for recording the fetal presentation during the eighth month. Making this determination before labor begins makes it possible to try to turn a baby in breech position (Baldwin *et al.*, 1994). External cephalic version at term reduces breech presentations at birth by more than 80 percent (Enkin *et al.*, 1995). Analysis of data from twelve studies resulted in an estimate that failure to attempt external version of babies in breech presentation increases the cesarean section rate by 1.9 additional cesarean sections per 100 births (Baldwin *et al.*, 1994).

Effect of CNM Care on the Incidence of Low and Very Low Birth Weight

The evidence to date suggests that nurse-midwifery care may decrease the low birth weight (LBW) rate for women who are at the very highest risk of giving birth to low-weight babies, and that it may be especially effective in preventing very low birth weight (VLBW)—babies born weighing less than 1,500 grams (about three and one-third pounds), whose chances for healthy survival are the very worst. Nevertheless, this issue is confounded by the biases that are part of virtually all studies of prenatal care. In addition, it requires that we answer a series of questions: Does regular prenatal care reduce the incidence of low birth weight? Are special programs that provide some kind of enhanced prenatal care more effective than regular prenatal care? Does care provided by CNMs make a particular contribution?

The answer to all of these questions should change as we learn more about the etiology of preterm labor. All LBW prevention efforts are limited by our incomplete understanding of the pathophysiology that culminates in early labor. Recent studies suggest that maternal infections may play an important role in initiating many cases of preterm labor, including infections of the gums (periodontal disease), as well as chronic subclinical intrauterine infections and bacterial vaginosis (Offenbacher *et al.*, 1996; Hillier *et al.*, 1995; Goldenberg & Andrews, 1996; Novy *et al.*, 1995). This research should lead to effective strategies to prevent some cases of low birth weight. For instance, a randomized trial of the use of antibiotic treatment of pregnant women considered high risk for LBW because of low maternal weight or because they had experienced previous preterm births resulted in a significant reduction in the incidence of preterm deliveries, with all of the reduction coming from women who had bacterial infections of the vagina during the second trimester of their pregnancies (Hauth *et al.*, 1995). All studies and conclusions discussed in this section predate this research. *Low birth weight* is, however, a catch-all descriptive term, not a diagnosis; there are probably several, if not many distinct pathologic pathways. Each

may be susceptible to different prevention and treatment strategies.

The 1985 Institute of Medicine report on *Preventing Low Birth Weight* acknowledged the effect of selection bias on studies of the association between prenatal care and LBW but concluded that there was "substantial evidence that prenatal care begun early in pregnancy can lower the incidence of low birth weight" (IOM, 1985). In response to that report concerted efforts were made to remove barriers to prenatal care, especially for socioeconomically high-risk women.

The results of increased use of prenatal care were not impressive, especially for black women, whose LBW rate is consistently twice as high as the rate for white women. The proportion of black women beginning prenatal care during the first trimester of pregnancy increased by 40 percent during the 1970s, but the incidence of very low birth weight (VLBW) infants born to black women did not decrease at all, and there was only a slight reduction in the overall LBW rate (Fiscella, 1995). Use of prenatal care increased between 1991 and 1994 for American women in general—the first improvement in more than a decade. The low birth weight rate increased during that period.

Attention was also directed at improving prenatal care in order to make it more effective in reducing low birth weight. Special prenatal care programs focused on nutrition, efforts to help women stop smoking, monitoring cervical changes that precede the onset of preterm labor, and ways to help women cope more effectively with stress. Stressful life changes during pregnancy are associated with preterm birth and low birth weight (Newton & Hunt, 1984; Williamson *et al.*, 1989; Hedegaard *et al.*, 1993). Several studies have evaluated special programs intended to help women cope with stress. None of these programs has achieved a statistically significant reduction in low birth weight among a heterogeneous group of pregnant women. However, some studies have found significant improvement among a particularly high-risk subset of the women in the study, especially teenagers who are having their first child (Olds *et al.*, 1986 Spencer *et al.*, 1989).

In 1995 Dr. Kevin Fiscella, from the Department of Family Medicine at the University of Rochester, published a critical review of studies of the effect of prenatal care on low birth weight (Fiscella, 1995). He reviewed all articles published between 1966 and October 1994 that reported the results of studies that met certain research methodology criteria. Most of the studies evaluated the effect of prenatal care that had been enhanced in an effort to make it more effective. Although a large number of studies were identified, only fifty met the research methodology criteria for inclusion in his analysis; there were only eleven randomized controlled clinical trials. Based on those fifty studies, Fiscella determined that "prenatal care has not been demonstrated to improve birth outcomes conclusively." He noted that it is difficult to draw confident conclusions because the results of many of the studies are confounded by selection bias. In addition, only a small proportion of low birth weight is due to factors that could be changed through prenatal care, for example, risk factors such as smoking and poor nutrition. "Although it is biologically plausible that prenatal care reduces rates of preterm delivery through the modification of risk factors, the magnitude of this effect is limited by the rate of modifiable risk factors in a given population and by the existence of effective interventions." As a result, Fiscella concluded that the effect of intervention programs is too low to make them cost effective and too low to result in statistically significant differences without very large studies. "Among populations with higher rates of modifiable risk factors, greater reductions may be possible" (Fiscella, 1995).

Four of the fifty studies in Fiscella's review (including three of the eleven controlled clinical trials) were investigations of

the effect of prenatal care or some kind of special intervention provided by nurse-midwives. A number of other studies that had found reductions in low birth weight associated with nurse-midwifery care were excluded from the review because they did not meet Fiscella's research criteria. Among the studies not included in the review were several that found reductions in low birth weight (or reduced preterm births or increased average birth weight) among infants born to teenagers who attended special nurse-midwifery clinics (McAnarney *et al.*, 1978; Doyle & Widhalm, 1979; Chanis *et al.*, 1979; Corbett & Burst, 1983; Beal, 1984; Piechnik & Corbett, 1985; Brucker & Muellner, 1985) and a study that found a much lower rate of very preterm births (and thus very low birth weight) among twins whose mothers attended a special preterm birth prevention clinic in which the care was provided by a CNM (Ellings *et al.*, 1993).

Of the four studies of care provided by nurse-midwives included in Fiscella's analysis, all found positive effects for at least some component of the study population—usually a particularly high-risk group. However, three of the four studies failed to prove the main hypotheses being tested—that the overall LBW rate would be significantly lower or would fall by a predetermined percentage in the group of women who received the special (i.e., nurse-midwifery) care. The studies are summarized here:

1. The evaluation of the nurse-midwifery demonstration project in Madera County, California (Levy *et al.*, 1971), was cited as one of two time series, both of which reported improved population birth outcome statistics, including declines in fetal mortality or neonatal mortality, after implementation of prenatal care programs in previously underserved areas. "In both studies, outcomes worsened after the services were discontinued." But provision of prenatal care was not discontinued when the nurse-

midwives were forced to leave Madera County.* More physicians moved into the area to provide services after the nurse-midwifery project ended. *Thus the rebound in the incidence of prematurity and neonatal deaths was associated with discontinuation of prenatal care provided by nurse-midwives, not discontinuation of prenatal care per se.*[†] Fiscella (1995) discounted the importance of both time-series studies in reaching a conclusion about the effectiveness of prenatal care in general, because "not all studies of expanded access to prenatal care have reported improvements in birth outcomes." Yet, both of these studies found effectiveness. *Studies that reach positive conclusions should not be given less weight than studies that reach negative conclusions.* Inconsistent findings may simply reflect the complexity of the situation being studied, in this case, including qualitative differences in the interventions.

2. A study conducted in South Carolina during 1983–1987 randomized 1,458 pregnant women judged to be high risk for having LBW infants to an experimental group that received prenatal interventions provided by CNMs and a control group that received standard high-risk prenatal care provided by obstetricians (Heins *et al.*, 1990). The prenatal care tested during the randomized trial combined the interventions that had been found to be successful in two earlier studies—a South Carolina study that had found a large reduction in LBW associated with nurse-midwifery services provided to pregnant teenagers[‡] and the evaluation of a successful preterm birth prevention program developed in Haguenau, France (Papiernik-Berkhauer, 1980; Herron *et al.*, 1982). The randomized trial (1983–1987) was designed to test the effectiveness of having nurse-midwives provide some of the interventions developed in Haguenau—teaching pregnant women to identify and report increased uterine activity and other signs and symptoms of early preterm labor, frequent vaginal examinations to monitor cervical changes, social support, nutrition counseling with emphasis on weight gain, and substance-abuse counseling. The trial would be considered a success if the LBW rate among babies born to the women who received the special care from CNMs was significantly lower than the rate in the control group.

There was no meaningful difference in the LBW rate between the two groups of women. However, *there was a significantly lower incidence of very low birth weight among babies born to black women in the experimental group (2.6 percent) versus the control group (6.7 percent).* Although the majority (53 percent) of women in the study were black, and very low birth weight is a much more serious problem than LBW in general, the hypothesis be-

---

*Although midwifery was illegal in California, a special law allowed nurse-midwives to practice in a state-supported project designed to alleviate chronic physician shortages in Madera County. Although the project resulted in improved pregnancy outcomes, the special law was rescinded and the project was terminated in 1963.

†The LBW rate decreased from 11.0 to 6.4 percent and the neonatal mortality rate decreased from 23.9 to 10.3 per 1,000 live births during the three-year project. After the nurse-midwifery service closed, the LBW rates increased to 9.8%, and the neonatal mortality rate increased to 32.1 per 1,000 live births. The methodology and other findings from this study are described in Chapter 4.

---

‡This study had found a 28 percent reduction in LBW among infants born to poor, mainly black adolescents cared for by a multidisciplinary team (medicine, midwifery, nursing, nutrition, and social work), with CNMs providing primary patient care management, as compared with a matched control group whose care was provided through state-supported clinics (Piechnick & Corbett, 1985). The methodology and findings of this study are also described in Chapter 4. Although this study was cited in the Institute of Medicine report on *Preventing Low Birth Weight*, it was not included in the fifty studies analyzed by Fiscella.

ing tested related to the entire group of study subjects and to LBW in general. This study was not planned to test a hypothesis about very low birth weight. Because the hypothesis under study was not proven, the study was said to have negative findings. As a result, *many people have overlooked the positive findings—reduction in the worst kind of low birth weight among the highest risk group of women.*

3. A study conducted in Australia hoped to test the effect of emotional/social support provided by nurse-midwives on the preterm birth rate of women considered high risk for preterm birth because of problems during previous pregnancies (Bryce *et al.*, 1991). High-risk women were randomized to the midwife support group or a control group. Women in both groups obtained their prenatal care from physicians. The midwives' role was limited to telephone calls and home visits. The midwives were instructed to provide emotional support in the form of sympathy, empathy, understanding, affection, acceptance, and being a confidante. They were not supposed to give the women information, advice, or other substantive aid. Thirteen percent of the 983 women in the midwife-support group did not have any contact with the midwife prior to their delivery but were retained in that group during the analysis. The preterm birth rate was 12.8 percent for women in the midwife-support group and 14.9 percent for the control group, a reduction of 14 percent. Although the difference was statistically significant, the researchers had determined that a 25 percent reduction would be necessary for them to consider the intervention a success. There was a 25 percent reduction in the rate among women who were carrying only one fetus and had a previous preterm birth. There would have had to be almost twice as many women in each group for the study to have a reasonable chance of finding a true 25 percent reduction. In addition, the midwives felt very constrained at being unable to offer other kinds of assistance to these women.

4. A study conducted at Metropolitan Nashville General Hospital assigned 428 low-income women predicted to be at risk of maltreating their children to routine care or comprehensive care on a random basis (McLaughlin *et al.*, 1992). Women assigned to comprehensive care received prenatal care from a multidisciplinary team including nurse-midwives, social workers, a nutritionist, paraprofessional home visitors, and a psychologist. The team focused on psychosocial support for the mothers, education about self-care, and promotion of healthful behaviors during pregnancy, including advice about nutrition, smoking, alcohol, and drugs. The control group had standard prenatal care provided by obstetric residents. Comprehensive care was not associated with a reduced incidence of low birth weight, although the mean birth weight was significantly higher for infants born to women in the comprehensive care group who were having their first baby.

None of these studies failed to find some association between nurse-midwifery care and improved birth weights. Three of the four studies found reduced LBW or VLBW only in the highest risk groups—exactly what Fiscella said we should expect. The other study failed to find a reduction in LBW but observed an increase in the average birth weight of babies born to first-time mothers in the nurse-midwifery care group. In addition, two of the randomized trials were not evaluations of nurse-midwifery care per se but of nurse-midwives' implementation of a set of specific interventions. At least four other randomized trials have failed to find a benefit associated with the French preterm birth prevention program tested in the study from South Carolina (Main *et al.*, 1985, 1989; Goldenberg *et al.*, 1990; Collaborative Group on Preterm Birth Prevention, 1993)*. There is some concern that the frequent cervical examinations that are part of this set of interventions could stimulate preterm labor in some women. Vaginal examinations increase the level of a hormone that plays a role in the onset of labor (Mitchell *et al.*, 1977), and vaginal, cervical, and intrauterine infections play an etiologic role in some cases of preterm birth. Frequent cervical examinations could trigger release of prostaglandins (the hormone that stimulates contractions) or introduce infection (Murphy, 1993).

In his discussion of selection bias in studies of prenatal care, Fiscelli noted the importance of *compliance* as a factor that may affect pregnancy outcomes. Prenatal care cannot be effective unless women keep their appointments and follow the advice they receive during care. Unusually high levels of kept appointments were found during the Madera County study, and "overcompliance" by nurse-midwife clients was one of the differences found during an early randomized controlled comparison of care provided by nurse-midwives and ob-gyn residents at the University of Mississippi Medical Center during 1972 and 1973 (Slome *et al.*, 1976).

The high and *increasing* incidence of low birth weight in the United States has been a challenge for obstetricians, midwives, nurses, and public health scientists. Efforts to re-duce the rate by getting more women into early prenatal care have not had the desired effect. Obstetricians have focused on the development and use of equipment to enable home monitoring of uterine activity in high-risk women and of pharmacologic agents to inhibit labor. Midwives have focused on counseling and assistance to help women stop smoking, improve their diets, and cope with social and emotional stress more effectively. All have been hampered by inadequate knowledge of the pathogenesis of preterm labor (in fact, we also do not understand what controls the timing of labor at term). When the etiology is better understood, both doctors and midwives will be able to develop more effective methods to both prevent and intervene in the pathologic chain of events. Special characteristics of the care provided by midwives may be effective means to prevent or intervene in some of the causes.

MD and RN Care During Labor and Delivery in Hospitals

To understand the benefits of midwifery care during labor and birth, it is necessary to have some knowledge of the alternative. This section summarizes research-based information on the alternative—the care provided to low-risk women by physicians and nurses. In most hospitals nurses play a major role in the care provided to women during labor. A doctor or nurse may make the initial assessment of the woman when she arrives at the obstetric unit. If she is in active labor and there are no apparent problems, the woman's care is likely to be managed primarily by nurses in private hospitals (and obstetric residents in teaching hospitals), under "standing orders" provided by private physicians or protocols that reflect the clinical guidelines and policies of the leaders of the hospital's department of obstetrics and gynecology. Private obstetricians try to visit their patients in labor if possible, but direct most of the patient's care through tele-

---

*It has been virtually impossible to adequately replicate this very successful French program in the United States. A critical component of the program as it is implemented in France is medical prescription of reduced physical efforts for women determined to be high-risk for preterm labor, including modification of the jobs of employed women and substantial paid sick leave. French obstetricians are expected to work closely with "occupational physicians," and all pregnant women are informed in writing that they have a right to these accommodations if they are judged to be high risk (Papiernick, 1997). American efforts to replicate the French program have tended to emphasize only the clinical aspects, especially frequent cervical examinations.

phone communication with a nurse or obstetric resident, who is expected to keep the responsible physician advised of his patient's progress, alert him to any problems, implement his instructions, and provide the information he needs to plan his arrival at the obstetric suite in time to deliver the baby.

Support for Women in Labor

Providing consistent social and psychological support to women during labor results in measurable health benefits and may affect their perception of labor, especially their feelings of competence during labor, their success in breast-feeding, and their confidence in adapting to parenthood. Support can be provided by the professionals who are responsible for the woman's clinical care, by someone who is trained and hired specifically to provide support, or by a family member or friend of the woman in labor. The effect of providing a special person to support a woman throughout labor has been assessed in randomized, controlled trials conducted in a variety of settings in several countries. Most of the studies have examined the effect of a doula or monitrice rather than a family member or friend. The results have been consistent. The following summary is taken from the second edition of *A Guide to Effective Care in Pregnancy and Childbirth.*

> Regardless of whether or not a support person of the woman's own choosing could be present, the continuous presence of a trained support person who had no prior social bond with the labouring women reduced the likelihood of medication for pain relief, of operative vaginal delivery, and of a 5 minute Apgar score below 7. In settings which did not permit the presence of significant others, the presence of a trained support person also reduced the likelihood of cesarean delivery (Enkin *et al.*, 1995).

Support in these studies was defined as physical contact, such as rubbing the woman's back or holding her hands, conversing, walking with her, maintaining eye contact during painful contractions, making sure that she understands the purpose of every procedure and the results of every examination, keeping her informed of her progress, encouraging her, and assuring her that she will not be left alone. Advocacy may also be part of the role. Advocacy requires knowledge of the woman's plans and expectations for labor and delivery (Enkin *et al.*, 1989). Other benefits include a better subjective experience of childbirth for women, who are less likely to feel very tense or to indicate that labor was worse than they had expected. Individual studies have found fewer episiotomies and perineal lacerations and fewer women who stop breast-feeding early or have difficulty mothering (Enkin *et al.*, 1995). The length of labor is reduced, with a consequent reduction in the use of oxytocin. "The main questions about these randomized controlled trials are the mechanisms of action and the generalizability of the results. . . . The investigators believe that the most important factor is a reduction in fear, pain, and anxiety when women have a supportive companion, and they link these possible changes with effects of catecholomines on uterine contractions and uterine placental blood flow"* (Enkin *et al.*, 1989).

Although obstetric nurses are heavily involved in the management of labor, studies suggest that they provide relatively little comfort and support. Observational work-sampling studies documented and analyzed the on-duty activities of registered nurses working in the labor-and-delivery units of some Canadian hospitals during the late 1980s and early 1990s. One study recorded 616 randomly scheduled observations of eighteen nurses employed in the labor-and-

---

*Catecholamines are hormones released by the body in response to stress. They cause significant decreases in the flow of blood to and through the uterus and placenta.

delivery unit of a teaching hospital in Toronto (McNiven *et al.*, 1992). Most of the patients were low-risk (60 percent), Caucasian, well educated, and socioeconomically advantaged. Approximately 80 percent had continuous epidural anesthesia during labor. All of the nurses observed were assigned to patient care, generally on a one-nurse-for-one-patient basis. The research team described "support" as "verbal and nonverbal behaviors that convey caring and understanding to enhance an individual's ability to cope." Supportive care was defined to include emotional support, physical comfort measures, instruction or information, or advocacy on behalf of a patient. On average, the intrapartum nurses at this hospital spent slightly less than 10 percent of their on-duty time providing supportive care. Most of the nursing activities included in that 10 percent involved providing information or instruction (41 of 616 observations, or 6.7 percent). The nurses provided care intended to increase the patient's comfort during only 2 of the 616 observations (0.3 percent); in both instances the activity observed was a reassuring touch.

A similar study was conducted at a university hospital in Montréal in 1994 (Gagnon & Waghorn, 1996). The maternity unit of this hospital consisted of five private labor and delivery rooms, a high-risk labor unit with four beds, two delivery rooms for vaginal births, a room for cesarean sections, and a recovery room. Nurses working in this unit were in a patient's room during only one-fourth of the observations and spent only 6 percent of their work time providing support to women in labor. They were off the unit during 27 percent of the observations and were in the unit but not in a room with a patient during 48 percent of the observations. As in Toronto, more than half of the activities classified as "support" involved providing instructions or information. Women having their first baby received somewhat more support than women who had given birth before. But whether or not

the woman had an epidural did not affect the amount of support she received. Half of the nurses had worked in labor and delivery less than seven years. Nurses with more than seven years of intrapartum nursing experience spent even less time providing supportive care to women in labor.

Other Canadian studies have found that women who received continuous support during labor used less analgesia and anesthesia, had fewer episiotomies (Hodnett & Osborn, 1989), and that women's satisfaction with their care increased with the amount of time nurses spent with them during labor (Klein *et al.*, 1981). In most hospitals in North America, the professional who has the most contact with women during labor is a nurse. Yet nurses at the hospital in Montréal spent no more than a fourth of their work time with patients and less than 10 percent of their time providing support to women in labor. In hospitals where most women have epidural anesthesia, nurses spend much of their time dealing with intravenous infusions, catheterization, electronic fetal monitoring, and oxytocin. To provide adequate care in this setting, nurses need to have considerable technical expertise, as well as the skills required "to care for women during unmedicated painful contractions and to encourage, praise, and reassure them during long labors" (Gagnon & Waghorn, 1996). The nurses who conducted these studies believe that the technical expertise is more valued by the people with the most status in hospitals, and that the need for technical care results in deemphasis and devaluing of the supportive care needed by women in labor.

Most hospitals now allow, and even encourage, the presence of the pregnant woman's husband or other support person during labor and delivery, in part to fill the gaps in nursing care. There is growing recognition that women need psychological support during labor and that nurses are too busy to provide it. There has not been adequate research to assess the impact of the presence of the woman's husband or partner (Enkin *et al.*, 1995). Although most women appreciate the support provided by their husbands, the presence of a labor partner who has relevant knowledge and skills makes an additional contribution. In a study of women having their first births, the presence of a labor partner who could provide specific encouragement in pain-control techniques was associated with less use of epidurals and fewer women who later described their experience as involving panic, exhaustion, or being overwhelmed by pain (Enkin *et al.*, 1989).

Frequent Use of Technical Procedures and Obstetric Interventions

Chapters 2, 4, and 5 describe the long history of overuse of technical procedures and interventions during childbirth in the United States. Criticism of intervention during childbirth has existed just as long, as has evidence of morbidity and mortality associated with many routine maternity care procedures—for example, puerperal fever caused by infection introduced during vaginal examinations of women during labor (Roush, 1979), and a 44 percent increase in birth injury-related infant mortality in the United States between 1918 and 1925. The increase was attributed to an "orgy" of medical interference (Devitt, 1979; Loudon, 1992).

Criticism of overuse of obstetric interventions broadened during the 1970s, with publication of books that questioned the medical profession's view of childbirth, new organizations devoted to developing "safe alternatives in childbirth," congressional hearings on obstetric practices, and government analysis of the benefits and risks of obstetric interventions. The critique begun by lay midwives (Arms, 1975), aggrieved parents (Haire, 1972), and childbirth educators (Simkin, 1984) was strengthened as obstetricians began to conduct objective evaluations of routine use of continuous electronic fetal monitoring (Haverkamp *et al.*, 1979; Leveno

et al., 1986), episiotomies (Banta & Thacker, 1979), and epidurals (Thorp *et al.*, 1993). Despite evidence of lack of benefits, high financial costs, and health problems caused by overuse of these interventions, episiotomies are the only procedure for which actual use has begun to decline. Use of oxytocin to strengthen contractions and speed labor is also at issue. As with electronic fetal monitoring (EFM) and epidural anesthesia, its use has continued to increase.

Many factors drive continued and expanding use of obstetric procedures. Although nature designed childbirth well, the process is not perfect; these interventions were invented to make childbirth safer for the fetus, to make it shorter, to avoid damage to the woman, and to make it less painful. Each procedure accomplishes its intended purpose in some instances, especially when it is applied to address an actual complication. But each procedure carries some risk to the well-being of the mother or the fetus. Some of the risks are known and have been measured. Studies document declining benefits and increasing risks as procedures originally designed to address specific complications have been applied more and more widely. In addition to the known risks associated with each procedure, their use affects the intricate physiologic dynamics of labor, the environment in which women labor and give birth, and, ultimately, the experience and meaning of labor and childbirth for the mother.

Induction of Labor

"The decision to bring pregnancy to an end before the spontaneous onset of labour is one of the most fundamental ways of intervening in the 'natural history' of pregnancy and childbirth. The indications for such 'elective deliveries' (which may be achieved either by inducing labour or by elective cesarean section) range from those that are life-saving, to those that are trivial" (Enkin *et al.*, 1989). Although labor has been induced electively (for the convenience of the mother or physician) in the past, the use of oxytocin for elective induction has been disapproved by the U.S. Food and Drug Administration (FDA). The medical reasons for inducing labor include postterm gestation (when the baby is "overdue" by one or two weeks), leaking or rupture of the membranous sac of fluid surrounding the fetus for more than twelve hours with-out spontaneous labor, and any condition in which continuation of the pregnancy might threaten the health of the mother or baby.

"Postdates" or "postterm" pregnancy is the most common reason for inducing labor. Randomized trials have found small reductions in cesarean deliveries and perinatal deaths* when labor is induced after forty-one weeks (Hannah *et al.*, 1992; Enkin *et al.*, 1995). Nevertheless, most pregnancies that continue beyond forty-one weeks are normal and result in good outcomes (Enkin *et al.*, 1995). Although the edges of a normal curve are furthest from the mean, normal curves describe normal variation; divergence from the mean is not necessarily an indication of pathology. One problem with a policy of inducing all women at forty-one weeks gestation is that the "due date" is not always an accurate reflection of the true length of the pregnancy†. The "due date" is determined by applying a formula that assumes that all women have menstrual cycles of the same length and that 280 days is the mean length of gestation for all groups of women. In fact, there is a great deal of variation in the length of the menstrual cycle (Munster *et al.*, 1992), and the average number of days of gestation seems to be longer for some groups of women and shorter for others (Mittendorf *et al.*, 1990). Because of these differences, and special problems in establishing the time of conception for many women, some pregnancies assumed to be postterm may not even be at term. In addition, it is very difficult to identify which fetuses are likely to have problems if left in utero; the great majority of them will be fine, and induction of labor is not always successful (Cunningham *et al.*, 1993).

Rupture of the sac that contains the amniotic fluid and fetus, in the absence of labor, is another common reason for inducing labor. The sac usually remains intact during the prenatal period and ruptures during labor. The intact amniotic sac creates a barrier that protects the fetus and uterus from contamination by bacteria in the mother's vagina. The longer the period of time with ruptured membranes, the greater the chance that the fetus and mother will become infected. Many physicians induce labor if it does not start on its own within twelve hours after the membranes have ruptured. Despite many studies, it is not clear whether better outcomes are obtained by inducing labor or waiting for labor to start on its own. If there is no evidence of infection or any other kind of fetal or maternal pathology, the results of studies published through about 1994 suggest that continuation of the pregnancy is likely to result in better outcomes than inducing labor (Enkin *et al.*, 1995). It is, however, a matter on which equally expert obstetricians have differing opinions. Induction of labor under these circumstances is associated with a higher rate of cesarean deliveries.

Because of these uncertainties, there is more than one acceptable approach to managing several situations that occur rela-

---

*Perinatal deaths include fetal deaths during the last weeks of pregnancy or during labor and infant deaths during the first twenty-eight days after birth.

†The "due date" is forty weeks from the first day of the woman's last normal menstrual period, which is abbreviated as the "LMP." A pregnancy is considered to reach term at thirty-seven weeks from the LMP. Labor that begins earlier than that is "preterm" labor. A pregnancy that continues beyond forty-two completed weeks from the LMP is considered "postterm" or "postdates". Use of "postdates" instead of "postterm" conveys our understanding that we are not always sure when conception actually occurred and that the "due date" is really just an estimate.

tively frequently near the end of pregnancy. Some physicians are more likely than others to induce labor in those situations.

Induction forces a very complex system into action before it is really ready to begin. When labor starts spontaneously, some of the changes that need to occur during the process happen before the woman is aware of being in labor. When labor is forced through the use of oxytocin, this preparation is not in place. As a result, more labor is needed to accomplish the work. The various changes may not take place in the right sequence; for example, the uterus may begin to contract strongly while the cervix is still thick and closed. In addition, the individual contractions tend to arise more sharply; this makes them more painful, and harder for women to cope with. There is always an increased risk of fetal distress with use of oxytocin; EFM is necessary, and an intravenous infusion is required.

The proportion of all U.S. births in which labor was induced increased from 9.0 percent in 1989 (NCHS, 1992) to 14.7 percent in 1994 (Ventura *et al.*, 1996). The proportion increases every year.

Continuous Electronic Fetal Monitoring
EFM was developed for use during complicated births. The primary objective for its use is to detect "fetal distress" (fetal heart rate reactions to an inadequate supply of oxygen) early enough that "physicians could rescue the fetus immediately by cesarean section or instrumental delivery" in time to prevent death or permanent brain damage (MacDonald, 1996). The belief that most cases of cerebral palsy are due to fetal hypoxia (lack of oxygen) during birth was first expressed in 1862. Early proponents of EFM suggested that the incidence of cerebral palsy could be halved by the continuous use of EFM (MacDonald, 1996). The alternative to continuous EFM is listening to the fetal heart beat intermittently—usually at fifteen- to thirty-minute intervals during early labor and following every contraction during the expulsive phase.* EFM has the advantage of detecting fetal distress on a continuous basis. It also provides a continuous record of the fetal heart rate; this has the advantage of making it possible to observe changes over time. In addition, the EFM signal can be monitored by a person who is not in the same room with the woman. Thus one nurse can monitor several patients from a central nurses' station—much easier than the alternative, which requires the nurse to go into each patient's room frequently, to actually touch and spend time with each patient. As discussed earlier, it is important for women to have the touch and presence of a supportive person during labor. Enabling nurses to monitor the fetal heart rate from a distance may be convenient, but is an inferior approach to the care of women during labor.

Use of continuous EFM has increased steadily since it was introduced. The first expansions included women who did not have actual complications but were at higher-than-average risk of developing a complication. However, because we cannot predict all complications, every woman is potentially at risk; ultimately it seemed reasonable to incorporate EFM into routine labor and delivery care, including the care of low-risk women. Arguments that the efficacy of using EFM for low-risk women should be proved were met with arguments that its benefit is so obvious that it would be unethical to withhold monitoring from any woman in order to conduct a randomized trial.

---

*Other ways to monitor the fetal heart rate include use of a fetoscope (an instrument somewhat like a stethoscope), or a hand-held instrument that simulates the sound of the fetal heart beat when it is held against the mother's abdomen. EFM is continuous and does not require the person who is using the information to be in physical contact with the woman in labor. Neither of the other methods of monitoring is continuous and both require frequent close physical contact with the pregnant woman.

We now know that birth outcomes for low-risk women who have continuous EFM are not better than for those who do not. The problem is that we cannot distinguish between fetal heart rate changes that reflect damaging fetal distress and those that reflect fetal responses to other circumstances, that is, fetal heart rate changes that are part of normal labor. In addition, it is not clear that rapid delivery by cesarean section is able to protect the brain of a fetus who experiences severe distress. These pessimistic conclusions were highlighted by a study based on the EFM records of 95 children with cerebral palsy (cases) and 378 normal children (controls) drawn from a large set of data on children born in northern California during 1983 to 1985 (Nelson *et al.*, 1996). Although the investigators identified two abnormal EFM patterns that were more frequent among the children with cerebral palsy (CP), the EFM records of many healthy children showed the same abnormalities. Among the babies who had ominous fetal distress, those delivered by cesarean section were no less likely than the others to develop CP. Based on the frequency of EFM during the births of all the children in the data set ($N = 155,636$), the investigators determined that nearly 11,000 of these children would have had EFM records that showed one or both abnormalities associated with increased risk of cerebral palsy. But only 0.2 percent of those children would actually develop CP; 99.8 percent of the children with ominous EFM records would be normal nonetheless. For every child whose EFM record showed serious fetal distress and developed cerebral palsy, 499 babies had equally ominous EFM patterns that caused no ill effect.

Severe fetal distress is vastly overdiagnosed on the basis of EFM, and when it is diagnosed accurately, the usual treatment may not be effective. Although the study described in the previous paragraph was published in 1996, many earlier studies came to the same conclusion. Twelve prospective, randomized controlled trials involving more than 55,000 births in many countries have found higher rates of cesarean sections and forceps deliveries but no fewer fetal or neonatal deaths associated with electronic monitoring. In the largest study there was a statistically insignificant trend toward fewer deaths due to "asphyxia,"* but this was compensated for by more deaths from trauma (related to the higher rate of forceps deliveries associated with use of EFM). EFM was associated with a reduction in the rate of neonatal seizures, but the kind of seizures prevented by EFM are not the kind that result in long-term impairment of the newborn (Enkin *et al.*, 1995). In a study published in 1993, two obstetricians reviewed ten studies and analyzed the fetal heart rate patterns of fifty-five brain-damaged infants in an effort to identify a fetal heart rate pattern or group of patterns that leads to neurologic injury if no effective intervention is taken (Rosen & Dickinson, 1993). They could not find any such pattern. They also noted that increased use of EFM has not been associated with reduction in the overall national incidence of CP in infants born at term and explained that most cases of infant brain damage are not related to events during labor. In 1995 epidemiologists at the U.S. Centers for Disease Control published results of a meta-analysis of data from twelve randomized controlled studies of EFM published between 1966 and 1994; they found little benefit from routine use of EFM (Thacker, *et al.*, 1995).

These findings and conclusions are counterintuitive to most pregnant women. How can it possibly not be better to be able to hear the baby's heartbeat? Most mothers and fathers and doctors and nurses feel insecure without electronic monitoring. If it is possible to hear and watch the baby's heartbeat

---

*Fetal asphyxia is a lack of oxygen or excess of carbon dioxide resulting from inadequate oxygenation of the mother's blood or inadequate delivery of oxygenated blood to the fetus. The concern is that inadequate oxygen supply to the fetus will result in neurological damage.

throughout labor, many feel compelled to do it. The possibility of an unnecessary cesarean section seems a relatively small price to pay *if* the alternative is increased risk to the life and full neurological functioning of the baby. The problem is that the "if" clause is not true.

Between one in four and one in five American women have their babies by cesarean section; most experts agree that at least one-fourth of the cesarean sections performed in the United States are not necessary. However, it is a rare woman who thinks that *her* cesarean section was not essential. Doctors may be sued because of complications or maternal deaths from cesarean sections or for "not having done everything possible" if the fetal monitor indicated distress and they didn't do a cesarean. But if the mother and baby are fine after a cesarean, it is assumed they are fine *because* of the cesarean. Despite a well-documented incidence of unnecessary cesareans caused by inaccurate fetal monitoring, doctors are never sued for having performed a "successful" cesarean unnecessarily.

In addition, the price paid for unnecessary cesareans is not always small. It is, of course, very large financially, but that is not the end of the story. The health costs include maternal deaths, a significant incidence of maternal morbidity, and a higher rate of newborn complications, including an increased rate of low five-minute Apgar scores compared with babies delivered vaginally, even among babies born after repeat cesarean sections (when there was no known complication during the current pregnancy). This finding has been repeated in studies conducted in several countries over a period spanning more than thirty years. The results of these studies suggest that the process of natural, vaginal childbirth affects the fetus in ways that help to prepare it for successful extrauterine life.*

---

*See Chapter 5 for further information and references regarding the financial and health costs of unnecessary cesarean sections in the United States.

In addition, unnecessary cesareans are not the only negative effects of routine use of continuous EFM. Establishing the monitoring setup requires an invasive procedure that is painful to both the mother and the baby. It may require early artificial rupture of the sac of fluid that protects the infant and umbilical cord from harmful pressure during labor. It forces bacteria into the uterus and involves screwing an electrode into the baby's scalp. Tethering the mother to a monitor with electronic leads makes it harder for her to change positions, and makes it impossible for her to distract herself or ease her pain by taking a walk or a bath. In addition, the monitor distracts attention from the mother herself. She becomes another observer, as everyone is drawn to the ongoing auditory and visual representation of the fetal heartbeat.

A positive benefit of not using EFM is that other methods of monitoring the fetal heart rate require a nurse or midwife to be with the patient frequently, if not constantly, and the instrument used to listen to the fetal heart rate requires close physical contact with the woman. In the first randomized controlled study of EFM, nurses used fetoscopes (similar to a stethoscope) to monitor the fetal heart rate for one group of women and the other group had EFM. However, women in the nurse-monitored control group were also attached to EFM machines. Information about the fetal heart rates for women in the nurse-monitored group was recorded but was not accessible to the doctors and nurses who took care of the patients. When the information was analyzed later, the investigators found a much higher incidence of fetal heart rate patterns indicating fetal distress among the women being monitored by EFM. The researchers suggested that the lower rate of fetal distress for women in the control group may have been due to the constant presence of a nurse at the bedside of each woman (Haverkamp *et al.*, 1979).

The proportion of all U.S. births in which EFM was used increased from 68 percent in 1989 (NCHS, 1992) to 80.3 percent in 1994 (Ventura *et al.*, 1996). The proportion increases every year.

Epidural Anesthesia

The situation is equally complex regarding the risks and benefits of epidural anesthesia. Many women experience extreme pain during some part of their labor. Women fear the pain of labor, and most women cannot count on truly effective support from either nurses or doctors during childbirth except for systemic analgesics, which can depress the neurological functioning of the fetus and newborn, or epidurals, which are much more effective. During the last decade epidurals have gone from a form of anesthesia "reserved for particularly prolonged or difficult labors or cesarean sections—when they are, indeed, a godsend—to the norm for American deliveries" (Goer, 1995). The American Society of Anesthesiologists distributes a brochure that presents epidurals as part of the modern form of "natural childbirth." But epidural anesthesia introduces risks and reduces the efficacy of labor. The need to deal with those realities converts normal labor into a "high-tech event" (Goer, 1995). The mother's pulse and blood pressure must be monitored frequently because epidurals tend to cause maternal hypotension (a sharp fall in blood pressure), which reduces the flow of blood to the fetus, and because, if the epidural is placed incorrectly or too much anesthetic medication is given, the mother may have convulsions or develop respiratory paralysis or cardiac arrest. An IV must be started and kept running to provide a way to administer fluids and drugs in case of an emergency. EFM is necessary because of the increased risk of fetal distress. Trained personnel and resuscitation equipment and medications must always be immediately available.

Epidurals increase the need for use of oxytocin, episiotomies, forceps, and catheterization of the mother's urinary bladder. Each of these procedures is associated with certain risks. Women having their first babies are more likely to have a cesarean section if they have epidural anesthesia. A randomized trial to observe the effect of epidurals on the labors of nulliparous women was discontinued earlier than planned, because the effect of epidurals on the cesarean section rate was so great that it would have been "unethical to continue randomization" (Thorp *et al.*, 1993). The earlier in labor the epidural was started, the greater the likelihood that the woman would have a cesarean. The cesarean section rate was 50 percent if the epidural was started when the cervix was only dilated to two centimeters; it decreased to 33 percent for women whose epidurals were started when their cervix had dilated to three centimeters, and fell to 26 percent if the epidural was started when the cervix was dilated to four centimeters. There was no effect on the cesarean section rate if the epidural was started later, nearer to the time of the delivery (Thorp *et al.*, 1993). A meta-analysis that pooled data from six studies found that the cesarean delivery rate was 10 percent higher for women with epidurals (16 percent) compared to those without (6 percent). The difference was even greater when the analysis was limited to randomized studies—21 percent versus 7 percent (Morton *et al.*, 1994).

Women who had epidurals during labor may experience urinary incontinence, muscle weakness, abnormal sensations, and excruciatingly painful headaches during the postpartum period. They may also develop *chronic* backaches and headaches. Work is being done to improve the technique for administering epidural anesthesia, including use of a lighter dose, called a "walking epidural." "Walking" is a very generous description of the quality of ambulation allowed by the new method.

Other effects of epidurals include increased body temperature of the mother, fetus, and newborn, perhaps due to the mother's reduced ability to dissipate the body heat generated by the intense activity of labor. Fever increases the metabolic rate and thus the need for oxygen. In addition, because fever is often the first clinical sign of infection, fever during labor cannot be assumed to be benign. Because epidurals tend to increase the length of labor, they may also contribute to the incidence of fever caused by infection, which is more frequent when labor is prolonged. Because of the importance of diagnosing and treating infections, maternal fever may stimulate a number of diagnostic and therapeutic interventions during and after labor and delivery. The "fever workup" for a newborn is expensive, time-consuming, and involves painful, invasive procedures, sometimes including a lumbar puncture (in which fluid is removed from the space around the spinal cord). The baby may have to remain in the hospital for several days, often longer than the mother. Fourteen percent of the nulliparous women who had epidurals at Brigham and Women's Hospital in Boston between May 1990 and October 1994 developed fevers of at least 100.4 degrees. Thirty-four percent of their babies were tested for infection, and more than 15 percent were treated. In contrast, only 1 percent of the women who did not have epidurals developed fevers, 10 percent of their babies were tested for infection, and less than 4 percent were treated (Lieberman *et al.*, 1997).

Authors of the 1995 *Guide to Effective Care in Pregnancy and Childbirth* note that there are few experimentally derived data on the effects of epidurals on infants or the long-term effects of epidurals on women (Enkin *et al.*, 1995). There are no national data to quantify the use of epidural anesthesia during all births in the United States; however, they have become all but universal at some hospitals. In the study conducted at Brigham and Women's Hospital during the early 1990s, 63 percent of the women who were giving birth for the first time received epidural analgesia (Lieberman *et al.*, 1997).

Routine Intravenous Infusions and Withholding Food and Fluid

Most hospitals in the United States prohibit eating during labor. About half allow no oral intake except for sucking ice chips. Virtually none allow women to eat and drink as they wish (Enkin *et al.*, 1995). These policies date from the 1949 report of an influential study which examined data on maternal morbidity and mortality from aspiration and the effects of aspirated gastric fluid in the lungs of rabbits (Mendelson, 1949; Broach & Newton, 1988). The possibility of aspiration of gastric contents arises as a risk of anesthesia, especially deep general anesthesia, which was in common use for second-stage labor during the 1940s and 1950s. Now that general anesthesia is not used for normal childbirth, the possibility of needing anesthesia in order to perform a cesarean section has become the greatest concern. Because of these concerns, American obstetric textbooks written during and since the 1950s have advised increasingly strict prohibitions on the intake of food and fluids during labor (Broach & Newton, 1988). Although pulmonary aspiration is rare, it is a devastating event that can lead to the death of a previously healthy woman (Douglas, 1988).

A number of improvements in anesthetic techniques have been introduced in attempts to avoid aspiration. Failure to apply them is the major reason that deaths from aspiration of gastric contents still occur (Enkin *et al.*, 1995). Requiring a woman to fast during labor does not ensure that her stomach will be empty if she needs anesthesia for a cesarean section; the fluid that is left in the stomach of a person who is working hard (i.e., in labor) for many hours without food becomes very acidic, and acidic stomach contents are the most dangerous if aspirated during anesthesia (Goer, 1995). In England and Wales, the number of maternal deaths from acid-aspiration rose after they began to withhold food from women during labor (Crawford, 1984).

Restricting food and drink during labor may cause dehydration and ketosis (resulting from metabolism of fat to meet the body's need for immediate energy). The effects of ketosis on laboring women and their fetuses is not known. Blood studies conducted during a 24-hour religious fast concluded that the effects could impair blood supply to vital organs, which could have serious implications for the fetus of a pregnant woman with marginal placental function (Broach & Newton, 1988). Although there have been many studies of the nutritional needs of athletes, there have been no published studies of the nutritional needs of women in labor (Enkin *et al.*, 1995).

Intravenous fluids containing glucose are given as a substitute for food and fluid taken by mouth. Studies to evaluate this practice have found a number of negative effects, including an insulin response in the fetus that is followed by hypoglycemia (low blood sugar) in the newborn. Irregular administration of intravenous fluids can cause serious hyponatremia (salt deprivation) in both the mother and the fetus. *A Guide to Effective Care in Pregnancy and Childbirth* warns that the use of intravenous infusion of glucose and fluids to combat ketosis and dehydration in the mother may have potentially serious unwanted effects on the baby. Withholding food and drink from women in labor and routine intravenous infusions during labor are classified as forms of care that are unlikely to be beneficial. The guide suggests that potential hazards might be avoided by allowing women to eat and drink during labor (Enkin *et al.*, 1995).

Oxytocin Augmentation and Amniotomy: Birth by the Clock

Prolonged labor has been recognized as a problem for centuries. Truly prolonged labor endangers both the mother and the fetus, with the severity of the risk increasing with greater extensions in the duration of labor. Risks to the mother include uterine rupture, lacerations, hemorrhage, infection, exhaustion, and shock; risks to the baby include asphyxia, cerebral damage, and infection. Both are at higher risk of dying. The desire to avoid these consequences has led to efforts to diagnose the problem earlier in order to intervene in time to prevent complications. Cesarean section is, of course, the ultimate solution. Other reasons for concern with the timing and speed of labor are to avoid the need for cesarean sections and to shorten the suffering of women during labor.

Chapter 5 provided a brief description of "active management of labor" as a means to reduce cesarean sections for dystocia among women having their first births. As originally designed (at the National Maternity Hospital in Dublin, Ireland), active management of labor includes the use of strict criteria for diagnosing labor and admitting women to the labor unit of the hospital, early artificial rupture of the membranes (amniotomy), encouraging women to walk during labor, continuous one-to-one care by a midwife, avoiding routine use of EFM and epidural anesthesia, and administering oxytocin if cervical dilation does not proceed according to a rigid schedule. It was not originally developed as a way to reduce cesareans, but as a way to shorten the suffering of first-time mothers and increase physicians' control of childbirth. Women were promised that their babies would be born within twelve hours after they were admitted to the hospital. If they could not deliver vaginally in that period of time, they were delivered by cesarean section. Nevertheless, the cesarean section rate for the National Maternity Hospital was much lower than for almost all hospitals in the United States.

The idea of shortening and controlling labor, especially for women having their first baby, found fertile ground among American obstetricians, who have definite criteria for what is "normal," and thus allowable, regarding the length of each phase of labor. The seminal work in this area was done by Dr. Emanuel Friedman during the 1950s and 1960s (Friedman, 1954; Friedman & Sachtleben, 1965). By collecting and charting information on the labors of a large number of women, Friedman developed two graphs—one that shows the average degree of dilation of the cervix* in relation to the number of hours a woman has been in labor, and one that depicts the baby's progress through its mother's pelvis, also in relation to time. Friedman's graphs showed the average speed of these changes for nulliparous women (having their first babies) and for parous women (having second or higher order babies) and described an upper range of the acceptable duration of each phase of labor for both groups of women. Labors that take longer to achieve a particular amount of cervical dilation or fetal descent are diagnosed as "protracted" or "arrested." Women given either diagnosis are more likely to have cephalopelvic disproportion (when the baby's head is too large to pass through its mother's pelvis). Armed with information on the average speed of cervical dilation and the "upper limit of normal" for each phase of labor for both nulliparous and parous women, physicians were prepared to intervene on behalf of the woman and fetus endangered by cephalopelvic disproportion or some other barrier to a normal, spontaneous birth.

Friedman's work has been improved and expanded by others, but the underlying concern with the pace of labor has been consistent. The usual treatments are amniotomy (rupturing the bag of fluid surrounding the fetus) and/or administration of oxytocin to make the contractions stronger and more effective. "Active management of labor" represents a systematic and aggressive form of intervention, in which treatment is started before the problem has a chance to develop. Active management of labor requires frequent vaginal examinations to determine the degree of cervical dilation and fetal descent, and results in high rates of use of oxytocin. Oxytocin augmentation is used in about 40 percent of nulliparous births at the National Maternity Hospital in Dublin (Boylan, 1989).

The 1995 *Guide to Effective Care in Pregnancy and Childbirth* categorizes early use of oxytocin to augment slow or prolonged labor and "active management" of labor as forms of care for which the effectiveness is unknown (Enkin *et al.*, 1995). It is clear that this approach results in administering oxytocin to a large number of women who would have had normal labors without the treatment.

Using oxytocin to strengthen contractions makes labor more painful and stressful to the mother and can endanger the baby. The blood vessels that supply the placenta are squeezed during contractions. If too much oxytocin is administered, the blood supply to the fetus can be seriously impaired. As with use of oxytocin to induce labor, EFM is necessary, and an intravenous infusion is required. A 1995 book entitled *Obstetric Myths Versus Research Realities* lays out research findings that argue against administering oxytocin to a high proportion of women during labor (Goer, 1995):

- *The diagnosis of dystocia is highly subjective. Many labors that are on the slow side of the normal curve are given this diagnosis based on overly rigid time criteria and obsession with the clock.* More than 30 percent of first-time mothers at four Canadian hospitals were given this diagnosis. With such a high proportion, the researchers wondered "whether the criteria used to define 'normal' adequately reflect the actual variations in labour patterns among women" (Stewart *et al.*, 1990).
- *Although cephalopelvic disproportion (CPD) is thought to be the cause of many cases of dys-*

---

*The cervix, which should be tightly closed until shortly before the onset of labor, softens, thins out and opens as a result of a combination of chemical changes and the contractions of labor, including some that occur during several weeks before the onset of the regular, forceful contractions that are defined as active labor. The degree of cervical dilation is measured (or estimated) in centimeters. Ten centimeters of dilation is usually complete dilation.

tocia, the diagnosis is often inaccurate. Most women are capable of delivering even very large babies vaginally, if they are given time and adequate support. Women giving birth in the United States during 1980 to 1982 were six times more likely than Irish women to be diagnosed as having CPD (Sheehan, 1987).

- *Most cases of "prolonged" or "arrested" labor do not result in fetal distress except as an effect of the use of oxytocin.* In one study, 97 percent of 4,573 women who were diagnosed as having "arrest of labor disorders" but had no medical complications gave birth vaginally. There were no infant deaths and no association between low Apgar scores and "arrest disorder." Use of oxytocin to treat the "arrest disorders" was associated with an increased rate of admission to the neonatal intensive care unit (Bottoms *et al.*, 1987).
- *Women who have experienced oxytocin augmentation say that it makes labor more stressful and more painful.* Most would not want to have it done to them again (Simkin, 1986b).

Hospitalization itself may slow labor down. In a study conducted in Finland, women who arrived at the hospital during early labor were more likely than those who came later to be diagnosed as having dystocia, to receive oxytocin, and to have a cesarean section for "protracted labor," even when differences in the intrinsic speed of their labors when they were admitted to the hospital were taken into account. For women whose labors were progressing rapidly, it did not matter whether they arrived early or late. But early admission seemed to have a negative effect on labor for some women (Hemminki & Simukka, 1986). Perhaps contractions slow in response to fear, pain, and stress caused by having an intravenous infusion started and the invasive procedures required to place the intrauterine pressure gauge and electrodes required for EFM. Perhaps women lose confidence when

they are forced to enter a race with the clock.

Research on other animals shows that labor is vulnerable to stress and disturbance. In a classic study conducted during the 1960s, Newton observed the effect of disturbance on the length and outcomes of labor in mice. Parturient mice in the experimental group were picked up and held gently for one minute after they had given birth to two pups, and again after the birth of every subsequent pup; mice in the control group labored without disturbance. The mice that were disturbed during labor took longer to expel their pups, and the incidence of dead pups was 56 percent higher than for the mice who labored in peace. The experiment was repeated with variations in the kind of disturbance. In each experiment, the disturbed mice took longer to deliver their pups, and a higher proportion of the pups died (Newton *et al.*, 1966, 1968). Studies involving humans also find slower labor associated with stress. A study published in 1978 correlated maternal anxiety and high levels of hormones produced during stress with slow progress during labor (Lederman *et al.*, 1978).

Other aspects of usual hospital care may also contribute to slow labor. Continuous support speeds up labor; lack of continuous support slows it down. Walking, standing, making frequent changes in position, and lying on one's side instead of in a supine position when recumbent are all associated with more effective contractions and shorter labors, as compared with women who sit or lie on their backs. *A Guide to Effective Care in Pregnancy and Childbirth* categorizes maternal mobility and choice of position during labor as beneficial forms of care for which there is clear evidence of effectiveness based on controlled trials (Enkin *et al.*, 1995). EFM, intravenous infusions, and epidural anesthesia create relative or, in many cases, absolute barriers to ambulation and freedom of movement and position for women in labor in hospitals.

Oxytocin was used to augment labor for 11 percent of women who gave birth in the United States in 1989 (NCHS, 1992), and 15 percent of those who gave birth in 1994 (Ventura *et al.*, 1996). Its use is increasing every year.

Interventions in the Second Stage of Labor: More Birth by the Clock

The second stage of labor is the period between full dilation of the cervix and the actual birth of the baby. The average duration of the second stage is fifty minutes in nulliparous women and twenty minutes in parous women, but it can vary greatly. It may take longer due to cephalopelvic disproportion, which is more likely to become apparent during the second stage than during the period of cervical dilation, or due to the effects of epidural anesthesia or intense sedation. Current obstetric practice includes "second-stage rules" that call for expedited delivery if the second stage lasts longer than two hours in a nulliparous women who is not under the influence of epidural anesthesia, or three hours in a nulliparous woman who has had an epidural. The rules call for earlier intervention during the second stage if the woman is not having her first baby. The origin of the rules is not known, although they have been in effect since at least the turn of the century. Analysis of data on births at the Johns Hopkins Hospital in Baltimore from 1937 through 1949 showed consistent increases in infant mortality associated with increasing length of the second stage of labor. However, a similar study of births at the Beth Israel Hospital in Boston during 1977 did not show this association (Cunningham *et al.*, 1993). Nevertheless, the "second-stage rules" stand; there is a strong tendency to try to move things along during the second stage. Interventions include encouraging the woman to hold her breath while pushing and to "push!!!" during every contraction, administering oxytocin, cutting an episiotomy, and using forceps or a vacuum extractor to pull the baby out.

Many aspects of the care experienced by a large proportion of women who give birth in American hospitals contribute to slow deliveries. Epidural anesthesia reduces, delays, or abolishes the woman's urge to "bear down," to use her voluntary muscles to add to the expulsive force exerted by uterine contractions. Epidurals also make it difficult if not impossible for a woman to assume a semiupright or squatting position during second-stage contractions. Most trials have found shorter second-stage labor with upright positions, and there is evidence that women may be able to "push" more effectively in the squatting position. Squatting also increases the diameter of the pelvic outlet, reducing the tightness of the birth canal (Enkin *et al.*, 1989). Expecting a woman to lie on her back and put her feet in delivery-table stirrups is common but tends to increase the length of the second stage, reduce the amount of oxygen supplied to the fetus, and increase the rate of low Apgar scores (Enkin *et al.*, 1989).

Instrumental vaginal deliveries ("assisted deliveries") are vaginal births in which either forceps or a vacuum extractor are used to rotate the baby's head, if it is badly positioned, or to apply traction. Either method may be used for any condition thought to threaten the mother or fetus that would be relieved by delivery. The most common reasons for assisted deliveries in this country are prolonged second stage and problems resulting from epidurals (Cunningham *et al.*, 1993). Use of forceps requires more anesthesia or analgesia than vacuum extraction, but is still likely to cause more pain and carries a higher risk of injuring the mother. Use of vacuum tends to cause a blood-engorged raised area on the baby's scalp, and this results in neonatal jaundice. Forceps are more likely to lacerate the baby's face or scalp (Enkin *et al.*, 1995).

Use of forceps declined during the 1980s and early 1990s. The early part of this trend was thought to be due primarily to substituting cesarean deliveries for use of forceps in some cases (Kozak, 1989). More recent reductions seem to be mainly due to substituting use of vacuum extraction for use of forceps. Data on use of all three forms of operative delivery during 1989 through 1993 are shown in Table 8. Although less than 70 percent of all births are achieved through normal, spontaneous vaginal deliveries, the proportion is rising slowly, in response to small annual declines in the rate of cesarean sections. The overall rate of assisted vaginal deliveries was stable during 1989, 1990, and 1991, but rose slightly during 1992, 1993, and 1994. Declines in forceps deliveries have been offset by increases in vacuum extraction.

Routine or Liberal Use of Episiotomies

The practice of enlarging the vaginal outlet by cutting it (usually from the bottom of the vaginal opening toward the rectum) has a long history. There are several rationales—to avoid repeated overstretching or other damage to the muscles of the pelvic floor (a much more common problem when most women were having many babies), to prevent undue pressure and trauma to the baby's head, to hasten delivery in the event of fetal distress (or fear of fetal distress if the second stage of labor has gone on for "too long"),

and to prevent spontaneous tears, which are harder to repair than nice straight, surgical cuts. Episiotomies are sometimes required to provide space for application of forceps. Episiotomies were virtually routine, especially for women having their first babies, from the 1940s until the early 1980s, when they began to come under critical review.

An extensive review of the literature published in 1983 revealed no scientific evidence of benefits associated with routine episiotomies and significant evidence of harm, including deaths of some otherwise healthy women (Thacker & Banta, 1983). Complications include excessive blood loss, hematomas, abscesses, other forms of infection, poor healing resulting in chronic pain and dispareunia (pain associated with sexual intercourse), and damage to the anus and rectum. Once the perineal tissue has been cut, it tends to tear further under pressure; perineal tissue that has not been cut usually adapts to pressure by stretching. Tears that extend into the rectum can be serious, are rare except as an extension of an episiotomy, and are relatively frequent among women who have had episiotomies. In some studies, more than a fourth of the women who had episiotomies had tears involving their anus or rectum (Borgatta *et al.*, 1989).

Table 8
Method of Delivery, All U.S. Births, 1989–1994

Year	Cesarean Deliveries (%)	Forceps (%)	Vacuum (%)	All Assisted Vaginal Deliveries* (%)	All Operative Deliveries† (%)	Normal Spontaneous Vaginal Births (%)
1989	22.8	5.5	3.5	9.0	31.8	68.2
1990	22.7	5.1	3.9	9.0	31.7	68.3
1991	22.6	4.6	4.6	9.0	31.6	68.4
1992	22.3	4.3	4.8	9.1	31.4	68.6
1993	21.8	4.1	5.3	9.4	30.7	69.3
1994	21.2	3.8	5.7	9.5	30.7	69.3

* Deliveries assisted by use of either forceps or vacuum.

† Includes cesarean deliveries and use of either forceps or vacuum extraction.

Data are from National Center for Health Statistics reports on natality statistics for 1989 through 1994.

The epidemiologists who conducted the 1983 review commented that the risks of episiotomies are more severe than many physicians appreciate and that, although the complications are rarely life-threatening, they "can be a source of serious morbidity to young mothers who already have major personal and social adjustments to undergo" (Thacker & Banta, 1983). In randomized trials, groups of women randomized to routine or liberal use of episiotomies resume sexual intercourse later than groups of women who did not have episiotomies without a specific reason (Enkin *et al.*, 1995). Although many medical researchers had considered episiotomy "too minor an issue for serious study . . . it is almost certainly the most frequent cause of maternal morbidity associated with childbirth, it may have an impact on the woman's perceptions of her birth, and it may have long-term effects such as perineal pain or dispareunia" (Reynolds, 1993).

When episiotomies are used selectively instead of routinely, many women end up with lacerations, but most of the lacerations are superficial and do not require stitching, and many women deliver their babies over an "intact perineum," that is, no episiotomy and no laceration. Minor birth lacerations heal well, and, although it is easier to repair an episiotomy than to repair a spontaneous laceration, the postoperative pain associated with episiotomies tends to be worse than pain from lacerations (Larsson *et al.*, 1991). What is easier for the doctor is harder for the patient.

If the episiotomy extends into a third- or fourth-degree tear, it may be *much* harder for the woman, as shown by a study that followed up 59 women two to seven years after they had experienced third- or fourth-degree lacerations during childbirth (Haadem *et al.*, 1987). Two of the women had serious infections; as a result, one of them developed an opening between her vagina and rectum that allowed fecal matter to enter her vagina. The other had rerupture of the muscle that controls the anus; both women

required another surgery. Although all of the lacerations had been repaired during the immediate postpartum period, 45 percent of the women were still experiencing problems two to seven years later. Almost a third had some problem with anal incontinence, either of fecal matter or, more often, the inability to control the passing of gas. Eight percent still had pain during sexual intercourse; 7 percent still had rectal pain. The women who still had complaints were offered a medical evaluation of anal function, and half of them accepted ($N = 14$). Their anal function was compared to that of ten women of similar age and parity who had no third- or fourth-degree tears during childbirth. The women who had experienced serious tears had less muscle strength compared with the controls. The physicians conducting this follow-up felt that the damage was permanent and might worsen as the women aged (Haadem *et al.*, 1987).

A Guide to Effective Care in Pregnancy and Childbirth categorizes routine or liberal use of episiotomies as a form of care for which there is clear evidence of ineffectiveness and the likelihood of harm (Enkin *et al.*, 1995). The alternative is selective use of episiotomies. The literature review published in 1983 reported that episiotomies were being performed on nearly all nulliparous women and most parous women having vaginal births (Banta & Thacker, 1983). The practice has been declining since then. Nevertheless, more than half of all women having vaginal deliveries in the United States in 1993 had episiotomies; 1993 is the most recent year for which these data are available. Table 9 shows the rates between 1988 and 1993.

Investigators conducting a randomized trial of "liberal" versus "restricted" use of episiotomy in 1988 through 1990 found that, although there were one-third fewer episiotomies in the "restricted episiotomy" group, physicians accustomed to liberal or routine use of episiotomy had difficulty withholding the procedure (Klein *et al.*, 1992).

Table 9
Percent of Vaginal Births During Which an Episiotomy Was Performed, United States, 1988–1993

Year	Percent with Episiotomies
1988	59
1989	57
1990	55
1991	54
1992	52
1993	50

Calculated using data on episiotomies from the National Hospital Discharge Survey and national natality data on the number of vaginal births. All data are from the National Center for Health Statistics.

Effects of Midwifery Care on Labor and Delivery Interventions

Chapter 6 described many differences between midwifery care and the care provided to pregnant women by physicians. There is little "hard data" to quantify most of those differences. Quantitative comparisons of midwifery and medical care during childbirth have focused on the use of procedures, especially cesarean deliveries. Use of procedures is studied because the data are accessible (recorded on client records) and because procedures are associated with morbidity and cost. What is invisible in the data collected for most studies is the care that midwives provide instead of technical procedures—the support and comfort measures that help women go through labor without epidural anesthesia, the elements of midwifery care that help to prevent dystocia and fetal distress, the patience and skill that allow midwives to minimize the need for forceps or vacuum extraction and avoid perineal tears without cutting episiotomies. Although some of these elements of midwifery care are mentioned in the review in this section, the focus is on procedures and outcomes that are avoided.

Meta-Analysis of Comparative Studies Published Between 1969 and May 1992
The meta-analysis described in the section on "Outcomes of Midwifery Care When the Births Occur in Hospitals" used data from nine studies that compared care provided to low-risk women by nurse-midwives and physicians (Brown & Grimes, 1995). The outcomes were equivalent except for a small but statistically significant reduction in low birth weight among infants born to women who obtained their care from CNMs. The meta-analysis also used data from these studies to estimate the effect of midwifery care on use of nine labor and delivery procedures, the proportion of women having spontaneous vaginal births, and the incidence of perineal lacerations. In each study, procedures or outcomes that occurred to CNM clients who were transferred to physician care were counted as having occurred to a nurse-midwifery client. CNM care was associated with very large reductions in the use of anesthesia and IV fluids and moderate reductions in the use of narcotic analgesics, forceps, EFM, and amniotomies. CNM clients were significantly more likely to have spontaneous vaginal births (without forceps or vacuum). Although they had more perineal lacerations, the increase in lacerations was less than the decrease in episiotomies. There was no difference between the nurse-midwives' and physicians' clients in the frequency of cesarean sections. The meta-analysis did not examine the effect of nurse-midwifery care on the incidence of third- and fourth-degree lacerations.

Six Studies Published Since May 1992
At least six additional comparative studies have been published since the May 1992 cutoff for the meta-analysis—one randomized trial (Chambliss *et al.*, 1992) and five observational studies (Butler *et al.*, 1993; Davis *et al.*, 1994; Rosenblatt *et al.*, 1997; Oakley *et al.*, 1995; Schimmel *et al.*, 1994). Selected findings from these studies are shown in Table 10. Five of the six studies compared labor and delivery procedures

and outcomes for women cared for by nurse-midwives with those for women cared for by physicians. Study 6 compared labor and delivery care and outcomes for patients of a joint CNM/nurse practitioner/MD practice with outcomes for all other births in the same community. In five of the six studies, the two compared groups of women labored and delivered in the same hospital during the same period of time; the exception is study 4, which compared births attended by a random sample of all obstetrician–gynecologists, family physicians, and CNMs practicing in urban areas of Washington State in 1989. Women who had conditions that would have made them ineligible for nurse-midwifery care were excluded from the physician care group in all of the studies except study 6. In all six studies, women who selected or were assigned to midwifery care at the beginning of the data collection period (either when they initiated prenatal care or when they were admitted to the hospital in labor) were retained in the CNM care group, even if they proceeded to develop a complication that required physician care.*

All six studies found statistically significant differences in use of obstetric interventions. Every study that collected data on use of internal EFM electrodes, narcotic analgesia, epidural anesthesia, and episiotomies found differences between CNM and MD

*Women in four of the studies (1, 2, 3, and 6) selected or were assigned to midwifery or medical care when they were admitted to the hospital in labor. Women who initiated care with the nurse-midwifery service but were referred to physicians because of complications arising during the prenatal period were excluded from the midwifery care groups in those four studies. Women in study 4 and study 5 entered the midwifery care group when they began prenatal care. Women who initiated care with CNMs but were referred to physicians because of prenatal complications were retained in the midwifery group in those two studies. We can assume that the differences between the groups of women in studies (4 and 5) would have been larger if the midwifery care groups had been limited to women who were eligible for midwifery care when they were admitted to the hospital in labor.

practices that were large enough to be not only statistically but very clinically significant. Three studies collected data on use of oxytocin; two of them found significantly less use by CNMs.

All of the observational studies found statistically significant differences in the rate of cesarean sections; the single randomized trial did not. However, all six studies found significant differences in the total proportion of operative deliveries. The women attended by midwives were much more likely to have normal, spontaneous vaginal births. All studies found much higher rates of forceps deliveries among the women delivered by physicians. There was less difference in the use of vacuum extraction.

All studies that collected data on third- and fourth-degree lacerations (including the randomized trial) found significantly higher rates among the clients of physicians. The incidence of these tears varied from 6 to 23 percent among the women who received their care from physicians. There were no other consistent differences in maternal complications or in the health outcomes for the babies.

Table 10 depicts substantial variation in the utilization of labor and delivery procedures by nurse-midwives practicing in different settings. There was no apparent time trend in the frequency with which they used these procedures. However, there seems to be a relationship between the use of procedures by nurse-midwives and physicians who attend births in the same hospital. For example, the rates for all kinds of operative deliveries are lowest for both CNMs and physicians in study 1 and are highest for both CNMs and physicians in study 5. Both kinds of practitioners are probably affected by the practices and attitudes that prevail in the hospitals in which they work. The rates found in study 4 are probably most reflective of general nurse-midwife, family physician, and obstetrician–gynecologist practices, as they are based on a random sample of all members of each group of practitioners in an entire state.

Table 10

Selected Data from Six Recent Studies Comparing Labor and Delivery Care and Outcomes for Low-Risk Clients of Nurse-Midwives and Physicians

	Study 1	Study 2	Study 3	Study 4	Study 5	Study 6
Information About the Study						
Location	Los Angeles	San Francisco	Chicago	Washington State	Ann Arbor	Yolo County, CA
Data collection dates	Not stated	1981–1988	1987–1990	1988–1989	1988–1993	1990
Kind of physicians	OB residents	OB residents	Private OBs	FPs and OBs	Private OBs	Private OBs and FPs
Number of CNM clients	234	1,056	529	371	471	749
Number of women in MD care group	253	3,551	8,266	399 (FP) - 552 (OB)	710	885
Assignment to groups	Random assignment	Risk exclusions	Risk exclusions	Risk exclusions	Risk exclusions	See explanation in text, (page 325)
Labor & Delivery Procedures	CNMs–MDs	CNMs–MDs	CNMs–MDs	CNMs–FPs–OBs	CNMs–MDs	Joint Practice–MDs
	Percents	Percents	Percents	Percents	Percents	Percents
Oxytocin induction	11.7–37.2*		8.5–15.2*		15.1–17.1	
Oxytocin augmentation			23.3–35.3*		11.3–11.3	
Internal EFM	16.2–43.5*				31.0–47.9*	
Narcotic analgesia			21.0–25.2*		31.0–41.5*	
Epidural Anesthesia		17.3–32.7*	11.0–53.1*	18.4–30.8–42.1*	19.7–44.5*	
Episiotomies	10.8–35.4*				30.1–56.6*	11.4–35.4*

Operative vaginal deliveries	0–7.1	1.2–17.8*	5.3–17.1*	7.6–14.5–21.4*	7.0–15.8*	1.5–12.1*
Vacuum extraction	(0–2.0)	(0.3–5.9*)	(0.01–0.6)	(7.0–7.9–9.9)	(3.0–5.1)	
Forceps	(0–5.1)	(0.9–11.9*)	(4.2–16.5*)	(0.6–6.6–11.5*)	(4.0–10.7*)	
Cesarean sections (all)	2.1–0.4	9.75–12.3*	8.5–12.9*	8.8–15.1–13.6*	13.0–19.3*	9.3–17.7*
Repeat cesarean sections†			(5.0–23.9%*)			(33.0–73.3%*)
All operative deliveries	2.1–7.5*	11.0–30.1*	13.8–30.0*	16.5–29.6–35.0*	20.0–35.1*	10.8–29.8*
Maternal Complications						
Third- and fourth-degree lacerations	0.9–7.7*				6.6–23.3*	1.0–6.4*
Maternal hemorrhage	No difference	0.5–0.9			14.2–25.2*	
Maternal fever	2.65–4.2*				3.6–5.9	
5 minute Apgar score <7	*0.5–0*	*4.0–4.0*	*0.9–0.5*	*1.8–3.2–3.7*		*1.9–1.1*

* Difference between CNM and MD clients was statistically significant.

†Repeat cesarean sections: percent of births by cesarean section among women, who have had at least one prior cesarean delivery.

Data are from the six studies described in the section titled "Six Studies Published Since May 1992," including Butler et al., 1993; Chambliss et al., 1992; Davis et al., 1994; Rosenblatt et al., 1997; Oakley et al., 1995; Schimmel et al., 1994.

The studies shown in Table 10 reflect differences between the practices of CNMs and physicians in the United States. Although this book does not include a comprehensive review of similar studies from other countries, two recent studies of midwifery care in other countries were particularly important because the women were selected into midwifery care or the comparison group based on random allocation (Turnbull *et al.*, 1996; Harvey *et al.*, 1996). Significant findings from these studies are incorporated into the following discussion of the effect of midwifery care on the rate of cesarean sections.

Nurse-Midwifery Care and the Rate of Cesarean Deliveries

The 1994 Public Citizen Health Research Group survey of 460 nurse-midwifery practices (419 CNM practices with in-hospital births and 41 practices in free-standing birth centers) was described in Chapter 8. The nurse-midwifery practices included in the survey accounted for 50 to 60 percent of all births attended by CNMs during 1990 through 1992 (Gabay & Wolfe, 1995). Using data provided by those practices, the Health Research Group estimated an overall cesarean section rate of 11.6 percent for CNMs who delivered babies in hospitals or free-standing birth centers during 1991 through 1993. That was approximately half of the cesarean section rate for the country as a whole during that period of time. A high percentage of successful VBACs (vaginal births after cesareans) in the nurse-midwifery services contributed to the low average cesarean delivery rate: 88 percent of the nurse-midwives' clients who had previously had cesareans tried to delivery vaginally, and 78 percent of those who tried succeeded. As a result, 69 percent of the women with previous cesareans were able to give birth normally (Gabay & Wolfe, 1995). In contrast, only 21 percent of all women with previous cesareans who gave birth in the United

States in 1991 (the midpoint of the Health Research Group survey) avoided having a repeat cesarean section (NCHS, 1994). The national VBAC rate had increased to 26 percent by 1994 (Ventura *et al.*, 1996).

Authors of the studies summarized in Table 10 offered several explanations for the low cesarean section rates associated with care by midwives. Some noted that CNMs stay with their patients and cited research which has shown that constant support during labor reduces the need for cesareans. Some cited research documenting the detrimental effects of maternal anxiety on labor. Some noted that constant support from a physician was not possible at their hospitals and is inconsistent with the doctors' other responsibilities. Although not mentioned in these papers, studies described in the section on MD and RN care during labor and delivery in hospitals suggest that labor-and-delivery-room nurses are also too busy. With EFM the fetal heart rates of several patients can be transmitted to nurses who do not need to be at the women's bedsides, or even in their rooms. Authors of the study from Los Angeles pointed out that their physician service does not have enough space to allow women to walk around during labor and that, unlike women who deliver in the midwifery birth center at Women's Hospital, women delivered by obstetric residents lie on their backs on a delivery table with their feet and legs held up by stirrups. Several studies found that the physicians' higher use of epidurals was a significant factor; epidurals (and IVs and EFM) also prevent or discourage walking. The ramifications of all of these differences were discussed earlier in this chapter. Noting that physicians make the ultimate decision to perform a cesarean section on a nurse-midwifery patient, one group of authors suggested that during the time consumed by the consultation, some women may go ahead and deliver their babies vaginally or make enough progress that the decision to perform a cesarean is reversed.

Despite many reasons why midwifery care may actually reduce the chance that a low-risk woman will have a cesarean delivery, findings from some randomized trials suggest that inherent differences between women who receive their care from midwives and women who receive their care from doctors may account for much of the difference in the rate of *primary* cesarean sections,* especially in hospitals and medical centers in which the overall cesarean section rate is relatively low. The effect of midwifery care on the incidence of cesarean sections has been examined in at least four randomized clinical trials in three countries during the past twenty-five years: (1) a study conducted at the University of Mississippi Medical Center during 1972 and 1973 (Slome *et al.*, 1976), which was included in the meta-analysis; (2) the study conducted at the Los Angeles County/University of Southern California (LAC/USC) Medical Center Women's Hospital (study number 1 in Table 10), which was published in 1992; (3) a study conducted in a tertiary-care hospital in a major city in western Canada (Harvey *et al.*, 1996), which was published in 1996; and (4) a study conducted in Scotland, which was also published in 1996 (Turnbull *et al.*, 1996). Only one of the four randomized trials found a statistically significant reduction in cesarean deliveries associated with midwifery care. The study from western Canada found a large difference; although the study was small (101 women in the nurse-midwife care group, 93 in the physician care group), the difference in the cesarean rates (4 percent in the nurse-midwife care group, 15.1 percent in the physician care group) was statistically significant.

Findings from the study conducted at Ann Arbor (study number 5 in Table 10) may help to explain why some randomized trials

may not find significantly lower primary cesarean delivery rates even though CNM services almost always have cesarean section rates that are lower than the average for their locale. Because the Ann Arbor study collected data on many factors that could influence the care and outcomes of a pregnancy and collected the information prospectively, at intervals during each woman's pregnancy, it was possible to examine the influence of factors such as the women's *prenatal* preferences regarding use or nonuse of EFM and epidural anesthesia (Oakley *et al.*, 1996). In a special analysis that was done specifically for this book and went beyond the previously published analysis (presented in Table 10), the principal investigator used this rich data set to search for alternative explanations for the lower cesarean delivery rate among the nurse-midwifery clients. Women planning to have a baby at this hospital could choose whether to have a physician or nurse-midwife as their primary care provider. Women who wanted EFM and epidural anesthesia tended to choose physicians, and most women who wanted those procedures had them. As a result, women who chose physician care were more likely to have EFM and epidurals. As in many other studies, women who had EFM and epidurals were more likely to have cesareans. When a wide variety of factors including socioeconomic characteristics, the women's evolving medical condition, and their preferences regarding care were all controlled in the analysis, the difference in the cesarean section rate declined to just below the level of statistical significance, $p = .06$ (Oakley, 1996).

The two randomized trials that were conducted in the United States and did not find a difference in the cesarean section rate were based on care provided to indigent women (mainly black women in the Mississippi study, mainly Hispanic women in the Los Angeles study) in hospitals associated with medical schools. The physicians provid-

---

*Primary cesarean sections are those performed on women who have not had a previous cesarean delivery.

ing care to the women in both control groups were residents in ob-gyn specialty training programs. Other research has shown that the cesarean rate is lowest for uninsured women who attend publicly supported clinics, for women who deliver in teaching hospitals, and for women who have relatively low educational and socioeconomic status; it is especially low for Hispanic women. Other studies have found that low cesarean section rates can be achieved when leaders of the obstetric department of a teaching hospital combine a disciplined approach to managing the conditions that lead to cesarean sections with systematic peer review of the care of all women who end up with cesareans.* The cesarean section rates for both groups of women in the randomized trials that did not find a difference were much lower than rates in most other hospitals during the same time period. The rates achieved by both physicians and midwives at Women's Hospital in Los Angeles—0.4 and 2.1 percent, respectively—may be at or near the absolute minimum for low-risk women. When there are few unnecessary cesareans in the control group, there is little room for difference. It would be difficult to obtain similar results with MD care of private patients in a less controlled practice environment.

The other randomized trial that did not find a significantly lower cesarean rate for women assigned to midwifery care—the study conducted in Scotland—compared the care and outcomes for low-risk women assigned to "midwife-managed care" versus women assigned to routine "shared care," in which midwives and physicians participate in each woman's care (Turnbull *et al.*, 1996). Women who received midwife-managed care

were significantly less likely to have their labor induced by oxytocin or to have an episiotomy, were significantly more likely to deliver their babies over an "intact perineum" (no episiotomy and no tears), and were significantly more satisfied with all aspects of their care. But, there was no significant difference in the rate of cesarean sections. However, midwives provide a significant part of the routine labor care throughout Scotland and were involved in the care of women who were randomized to "shared care" in this study. Thus the comparison group also had some of the benefits of midwifery care.

Summary

Women whose hospital births are attended by nurse-midwives tend to proceed through labor and delivery with many fewer procedures than women whose care is provided by nurses and physicians. They are more likely to be given fluids to drink when they are thirsty and are less likely to have intravenous infusions. They are less likely to be tethered to their beds by electronic equipment and are more likely to walk, take baths and showers, and change their position frequently. They receive less pain medicine and are much less likely to have an epidural. They receive consistent personal attention and support, including many forms of touching, and pressure and massage to help relieve pain. They are not left alone and have a knowledgeable, skillful partner to help them cope with pain. They are less likely to receive oxytocin, and they are less likely to labor under the pressure of the clock. They are much more likely to labor and give birth in the same room and bed; they are less likely to be moved into a surgical-type delivery room, and they are unlikely to be expected to give birth while lying on their backs with their feet in stirrups. They are more likely to give birth on their own and are less likely to need to have someone pull on the baby's head with forceps or equipment applied with vacuum. They are much less

---

*Chapter 5 includes a summary of information about factors associated with higher or lower rates of cesarean delivery. Also, see the discussion of educational approaches, clinical guidelines, and peer review as methods to reduce cesarean section rates, also in Chapter 5.

likely to have a cut made in the tissue between their vagina and rectum. As a result, they are much less likely to have a serious tear involving their anus. They may avoid significant long-term problems as a result of this difference.

Women whose births are attended by midwives are less likely to experience complications requiring a cesarean delivery. In public academic hospitals that have a very low incidence of cesarean sections, the reduced primary cesarean section rate associated with midwifery care may be largely or entirely attributable to the low-risk status of the women assigned to the nurse-midwifery service. Lower primary cesarean section rates for nurse-midwifery clients in private practice settings result in part from the women's inherent low risk for the kinds of complications that lead to cesareans and their preference to avoid procedures such as continuous EFM and epidural anesthesia. In addition, midwives themselves contribute to a reduction in cesarean deliveries—by helping women who have had previous cesareans deliver vaginally and by providing care to women who want to avoid unnecessary interventions during labor and delivery but require midwifery assistance and support to forgo anesthesia. In addition, nurse-midwives who practice in academic medical centers teach medical students and model a kind of childbirth care that helps to reduce cesarean sections.

Nurturing and Protecting the Newborn and the Family

The lack of a measurable effect of midwifery care on the usual indices of newborn health—perinatal mortality, Apgar scores, et cetera—does not mean that there is no benefit to infants. Any observation or description of midwifery care demonstrates its special emphasis on supporting, promoting, and protecting breast-feeding, bonding of family members during the sensitive period after birth, and effective nurturance and

protection of the newborn within the family. This is a very strong element of the specialness of a home birth attended by a midwife and is an important part of the care provided by midwives to the families of women who give birth in birth centers. Although the environment of some hospitals makes it harder, the difference and benefit are also evident in the care provided to midwives' clients when the births occur in hospitals, even in the high-tech obstetric units in which nurse-midwives provide care to some of the nation's most high-risk, vulnerable mothers. There is relatively little quantitative data to compare this aspect of the care provided by midwives to that provided to most other women who give birth in the United States. Although providing some information on such comparisons, this section focuses on information that explains the importance and potential benefits of all midwives' emphasizing breast-feeding and the subjective experience of the mother and other family members as they welcome their newborn into a family and into the world, and nurse-midwives' additional emphasis on effective family planning.

Breast-Feeding and the Importance of the Period Immediately After Birth

Human breast milk is more easily digested than the best infant formula and is perfectly suited to the newborn's immunologic and nutritional needs. The infant is born with antibodies to the infectious agents to which its mother has become immune through contact; they are the same organisms the newborn is likely to encounter. Without its mother's breast milk, the newborn's immunologic protection declines after birth; with her breast milk, it is replenished. Baby formula based on nonhuman protein (cow milk, soy protein, et cetera) contains the wrong kinds of proteins for human babies. Babies are not able to absorb and metabolize it as well as their mothers' milk, tend to become constipated, and are more likely to have colic. Except for mothers who can afford to buy ready-to-feed baby formula, perhaps already in bottles, using formula requires preparation that offers many opportunities for introduction of pathologic organisms, especially in countries that lack safe water supplies. Formula is expensive; poor women often dilute it, filling their babies with non-nutritious, often unclean water. Breast-feeding is critically important to the health and survival of babies in the poorest countries. Nine million infants die throughout the world every year. More than six million additional deaths would occur, primarily from infectious disease, if most mothers were not breast-feeding their babies. Two million additional deaths could be averted each year if all women breast-fed their babies exclusively (with no supplemental foods or fluids) for the first four to six months and continued breast-feeding while giving supplemental foods during the rest of the infant's first year of life (Huffman *et al.*, 1996).

Although its impact on infant mortality is greatest in the less developed countries, breast-feeding also provides measurable health advantages to babies in the more developed societies. A recent detailed study conducted in Scotland followed 681 mothers and their infants for two years to look for associations between infant nutrition and gastrointestinal illness (Howie *et al.*, 1990). Only 4 percent of infants who were breast-fed for at least 13 weeks were diagnosed with gastrointestinal diseases, compared with 15 percent of infants breast-fed for shorter periods of time and 16 percent of infants who were not breast-fed at all. The differences remained highly statistically significant after adjusting the results to account for other differences between the groups of women. The reduction in infant infection was found whether or not the mother gave the baby other food, in addition to breast milk, and the protection was maintained far beyond the period of exclusive breast-feeding; it was still evident when the infants were one year old. Care was taken to make sure that there

were no differences between the groups in detection of disease. The reduction in gastrointestinal infections resulted in a lower incidence of hospital admission among the breast-fed infants (Howie *et al.*, 1990). In addition, babies who are breast-fed for at least six months have only one-third as many ear infections as babies who are bottle-fed (Oski, 1993). The incidence of sudden infant death syndrome (SIDS) may be lower among breast-fed babies, and breast-feeding may help mothers relieve stress. The blood levels of hormones that are released in response to stress decline when women start to breast-feed (Altemus *et al.*, 1995).

Breast-feeding involves an intricate interaction between the baby and its mother, whose breasts produce milk in response and in proportion to suckling and the emptying of each breast. Although breast-feeding is entirely natural and the basis for human survival and evolution to this time, it is susceptible to problems. Delay in the initiation of breast-feeding, an ineffective suckling method that irritates the mother's nipples and does not produce a good flow of milk, anything that prevents the mother from nursing her infant when her breasts are full or prevents the infant from nursing when hungry, giving the infant water or other fluids that fill its stomach and make it less interested in nursing—all interfere with the dynamic mother–baby system that is breast-feeding. Sedation and use of narcotics and anesthesia during childbirth affect breast-feeding too, as well as stress, fear, pain, and anything that interferes with immediate and prolonged contact between the mother and newborn in the period after the birth. Many routine hospital practices during and immediately after labor and delivery, as well as the mother's later postpartum hospitalization, may interfere with optimal breast-feeding. Mothers who want to breast-feed, have early contact with their babies, initiate breast-feeding during the first hour after giving birth, and keep their babies with them in the hospital breast-feed longer and have fewer problems than mothers who do not have these experiences (Klaus, 1995).

The World Health Organization (WHO) and UNICEF, the two United Nations agencies most concerned with children, have strong policies intended to encourage and support breast-feeding and discourage promotion and unnecessary use of infant formula. They have joined with other organizations in a worldwide campaign to replace hospital practices that interfere with breast-feeding with practices that promote and support breast-feeding. It is called the Baby-Friendly Hospital Initiative.

Teaching and helping mothers breast-feed is an important part of midwifery care; learning about breast-feeding is an important part of the midwifery curriculum. Researchers at the University of North Carolina recently surveyed more than 5,000 physicians who were either training to become pediatricians, obstetrician–gynecologists or family physicians ($N = 3,115$) or were already practicing one of those specialties ($N = 1,920$) to assess their knowledge of the benefits of breast-feeding and how to advise women who are breast-feeding (Freed *et al.*, 1995). Of those who responded (68 percent), most lacked both kinds of knowledge. About 70 percent of the physicians who were in the last year of an obstetrics and gynecology residency training program, and more than 70 percent of the practicing obstetrician–gynecologists said that they had received "less than adequate" or no training in how to support a woman having problems with breast-feeding. Fewer than half knew that a mother with a breast abscess does not need to stop breast-feeding. More than one-fourth did not know that exclusive breast-feeding (no other fluids or food given to the infant) is the most effective form of infant feeding available, although the professional associations for all three medical specialties have made policy statements to this effect. The authors of the research report concluded that physician knowledge deficits pose a "true threat" to successful initiation and continuation of breast-feeding (Freed *et al.*, 1995).

The U.S. Public Health Service set breast-feeding goals as part of its goals for increasing the health of the people of the United States by the year 2000. The goals call for 75 percent of mothers to initiate breast-feeding immediately after giving birth and for half of all mothers to continue breast-feeding until their infants are at least 5 months old (DHHS, 1991). Sixty percent of American women who gave birth during 1994 breast-fed their babies during the early postpartum period, and 23 percent continued breast-feeding until their infants were at least five or six months old (NCHS, 1996). Black women are much less likely to initiate breast-feeding than white women, although black women who start to breast-feed are as likely as white mothers to continue for at least three months. Teen-aged mothers are much less likely than older women to breast-feed, and are less likely to continue even if they start. In general, the duration of breast-feeding increases with maternal age and education. Among mothers who start to breast-feed, the duration of breast-feeding is shorter for women who are not married when they give birth, for women who smoke, and for women who return to work (Piper & Parks, 1996).

Midwives consistently report high levels of initiation of breast-feeding by their clients, often between 80 and almost 100 percent. Selection bias surely plays a large role in these findings for practices in which clients select midwifery care. Women who want to receive their care from midwives are likely to be particularly interested in pregnancy and motherhood, including breast-feeding. However, higher than usual rates of breast-feeding have been found even for services whose clients are assigned to midwifery care and for services that provide care to large numbers of women who are black, unmarried, and/or teenagers.

- Nurse-midwives were involved in the care of almost all women who gave birth at the North Central Bronx Hospital in New York City in 1986 (Haire & Elsberry, 1991). The hospital serves one of the poorest populations in the United States. Forty-five percent of the women were Hispanic and 35 percent were black; more than three-fourths were on Medicaid; 11 percent had no prenatal care, and many were affected by drug and alcohol addiction or infected with HIV. Most of the women gave birth in the labor bed, only 7 percent had episiotomies, the babies stayed with their mothers for at least an hour after birth unless there was an urgent medical problem, most mothers kept their babies in the same room with them during postpartum hospitalization, and breast-feeding was strongly encouraged and supported. Sixty percent of the mothers were breast-feeding when they left the hospital with their babies. They were given a special telephone number to call if they had any problem with breast-feeding after they got home. Nationwide, only 32 percent of all low-income mothers breast-fed their babies during the immediate postpartum period in 1988 (NCHS, 1996).
- In a randomized trial of comprehensive versus routine prenatal care conducted at the Metropolitan Nashville General Hospital, 33 percent of the low-income women whose care was provided by nurse-midwives breast-fed their babies, compared with only 19 percent of the women who had routine obstetric care (McLaughlin *et al.*, 1992). The difference was highly statistically significant.

A randomized trial conducted in South Africa demonstrated the effect of *any form* of consistent, empathetic support to women during labor on their ability to breast-feed (Hofmeyr *et al.*, 1991). Community volunteers were recruited to support women who were having babies in an urban community hospital that serves a low-income population. The volunteers were simply asked to stay with the women they were assigned to as continuously as possible, to support them through touch and speech, and to concentrate on providing comfort, reassurance, and praise. Women who were having their first babies, had no complications when admitted to the labor ward, and had no companions of their own were randomly allocated either to have or not to have a volunteer companion. Women in the companion-support group were significantly more likely than the mothers who had labored without consistent support to be breast-feeding their babies "exclusively" (breast-milk only, no other foods) when the babies were six weeks old. Only one-fourth as many women in the companion-support group had experienced feeding problems. Women who had stopped breast-feeding were asked to explain why they stopped. Many more women in the no-support control group stopped because they thought they were not producing an adequate supply of milk. The women who had supportive companionship during labor were also significantly more likely to report that they had found becoming a mother to be "easy" and that they were managing well.

The period immediately after birth is also important for other reasons. Anthropologist Ashley Montagu described the mother and infant during this period as needing each other as no two creatures can need each other again. He saw the infant as needing a continuation of the security it had in the womb; "the newborn and his mother are designed to continue their symbiotic relationship postnatally without the slightest interruption" (Montagu, 1977). This relationship is psychologically, physiologically, and socially beneficial to the mother, as well as the newborn. Putting the baby on the mother's abdomen causes her uterus to contract at a time when contractions are necessary to complete the birth by expelling the placenta. When the baby begins to breast-feed, its sucking continues to stimulate the contractions needed to cut off the massive supply of blood to its mother's uterus; this is very important for preventing postpartum hemorrhage. Separation of the mother and infant because of surgery, the need to repair episiotomies, or hospital routines will not usually kill either the mother or the baby, but it always represents the irrevocable loss of continuity in a precious human experience.

If the mother (and thus the newborn) were not medicated during labor, the baby is born alert and ready for active contact with its mother during the first two hours after birth. After two hours, most newborns fall asleep. But during the first two hours they are sentient and highly sensory. They can see and hear, their sense of smell is well developed, and they seem to enjoy the tactile experience of skin contact with their mothers (Righard, 1995).

In studies conducted in Sweden, thirty-eight naked newborns who had been placed on their mothers' abdomens spent the first twenty minutes resting and looking at their mothers on and off. Then they began to smack their lips, drool, and use their legs to move towards her breasts, apparently guided by the smell of her milk (Righard & Alade, 1992; Vallardi *et al.*, 1990). By fifty minutes after birth, most of the infants had latched onto a nipple and started to nurse. The control group consisted of 34 infants who were allowed to rest on their mothers' abdomens for twenty minutes, but were then removed to be measured, weighed, bathed, and dressed. This process took another twenty minutes, after which they were returned to their mothers. After the separation the infants did not perform the full sequence of behaviors demonstrated by the newborns who had uninterrupted contact with their mothers, and many did not suckle effectively. Sixty-three percent of the infants not removed from their mothers instinctively used the most effective method of suckling, compared with only 20 percent of the in-

fants returned to their mothers after the many procedures. Use of narcotic painkillers during labor also reduced the proportion of newborns who suckled effectively, regardless of whether they were in constant contact or removed from their mothers during their first hour of extrauterine life. The investigators also noted that the newborns "generally cried out loudly in protest" when separated from their mothers (Righard & Alade, 1992). Another study found that newborns can differentiate (and strongly prefer) the smell of their own mothers' milk as compared with that of another new mother, and if one breast is washed and the other isn't, most newborns chose the unwashed breast (Righard, 1995).

During the period when heavy sedation or general anesthesia was used routinely during childbirth, many babies were born too sedated to begin to breathe. Ever since then we have perceived the newborn's cry as a welcome sign of life. It may also be a sign that the infant is cold, shocked by the bright lights of the delivery room, in pain from having had an electrode screwed into its scalp, and does not want to be separated from its mother. A baby born without these traumas does not scream in the same way, and its cry may quickly dissolve into an expression of peace and security (Harper, 1994).

The lovemaking between a mother and her newborn is subtle but powerful. We are only beginning to observe it carefully enough to describe the patterns accurately and to understand the impact and implications of supporting versus disrupting this early period of bonding. The mother and baby are both active in this reciprocal lovemaking. Touch, taste, smells, sights, sounds, pressure, and warmth are all part of the experience. One study found that if a baby's hand or mouth touched its mother's nipple during the first hour after birth, the mothers kept their babies in their rooms significantly longer than mothers who did not have this contact (Widström, 1990). Another study found that healthy infants who are dried and placed on their mothers' chests, skin-to-skin under a blanket, maintain their body temperature as well as babies placed in the sophisticated warming units used in many hospitals, and that babies in skin-to-skin contact with their mothers cry less than those who are wrapped and placed in bassinets (Klaus, 1995). Skin-to-skin contact between a mother and newborn is also important because it allows the infant's skin to become colonized with the mother "normal flora" (mostly nonpathologic bacteria), to which the infant has inborn immunologic protection. This helps to protect the infant from other pathogens, which are always present in hospitals.

Do these differences matter in the long-term health and well-being of children and families? There has been research to look at the matter in the short term: Doctors and midwives in several countries have made some unexpected observations after "baby-friendly" changes were made in maternity units in some other countries (Klaus, 1995). In a hospital in Thailand the frequency of babies being abandoned by their mothers fell from 33 abandoned babies per 10,000 births to 1 per 10,000 births after rooming in and early postbirth contact with suckling were initiated at the hospital. Similar reductions in abandonment have been observed in the Philippines and Costa Rica. In a study of sixty mother–baby dyads in Portugal, extended early contact was associated with increased use of affectionate and soothing behaviors by the mothers toward their babies when they were observed together after several weeks (Klaus, 1995).

Studies conducted in the United States find similar results. In a study published in 1983, twenty-nine women who had intimate contact with their newborns during the first hour after giving birth and thirty women who received routine postbirth care (the baby was shown to the mother and then taken to the nursery) were observed with their babies two days after the birth. The mothers who had early skin-to-skin contact with their newborns smiled and talked to their babies more and were more likely to kiss them, inspect their bodies, and try to elicit a response (Anisfeld & Lipper, 1983). All of these differences between the groups were statistically significant and were greatest for mothers who had the least "social support." Social support was a composite variable in which being unmarried, being on welfare, not having graduated from high school, and not having the baby's father present in the delivery room contributed to low social support. How important is the additional touching, cooing, smiling? We don't really know. Studies with primates and World War II orphans have found physical and psychological stunting of infants who were deprived of physical contact, even though they were adequately fed and cared for in other ways; premature babies that are stroked and massaged gain weight faster than those who are not (Ackerman, 1990).

How long does the effect last? There are so many influences between the beginning and the "long term" and so many differences between women who choose to breast-feed their babies and those who do not (selection bias again) that it is almost impossible to determine whether the first experiences make a lasting difference. But we know that mothering matters, and that for many things in life, how they start sets the stage—the expectations and emotional environment—for many things that follow. This knowledge is expressed in our folk wisdom: "Getting out of bed on the wrong side" explains a bad mood that lasts all day; it's important to start a new job or relationship out on "the right foot," and we all want our team to start the game out strong. How does maternal love and commitment start, and what effect does the start have on the follow-through? A 1996 conference on "The Integrative Neurobiology of Affiliation" was devoted to the biologic underpinnings of the development of benevolence in human society. Naturally produced oxytocin, the hormone of sex, birth, and breast-feeding, was the "hormonal luminary of the conference" (Angier, 1996). In animal studies, epidural anesthesia has been found to block the sensory feedback that causes release of oxytocin; the effect is poorer maternal attachment (Kennell, 1994).

Rooming-In

It is also important to keep the mother and baby together during the mother's remaining time in the hospital, a practice known as rooming-in. Rooming-in is a component of "baby-friendly" hospital practices, because it helps mothers get a good start breast-feeding and protects infants from infections they can catch from one another in a centralized nursery. Babies who spend most of their time in central nurseries do not breast-feed as often. Human breast milk is thin and the newborn's stomach is tiny. Humans, (like monkeys and apes, whose babies cling to their mothers and nurse at will), were meant to breast-feed frequently (Konner, 1991). If newborns are kept in central nurseries and only taken to their mothers according to a schedule, they may get hungry and cry while they are in the nursery. This often prompts nurses to give them a bottle. When that happens the baby may not be hungry when it is taken to its mother, making her feel rejected or making her think that she is somehow unable to breast-feed. Mothers whose babies are kept in nurseries have to ask nurses to bring their babies to them; the baby seems to belong to the hospital, and the nurses have more authority than the mother. With rooming-in the nurses refocus their attention from taking care of the babies themselves to teaching and supporting the mothers to take care of their own babies.

Several studies have documented effects of rooming-in on mothering behavior. A study published in 1995 compared the maternal behaviors of women who had rooming-in with those whose contact with their babies was limited to feedings, which were scheduled for every four hours (Prodromidis *et al.*, 1995). Both groups were young,

ranging in age from fifteen to twenty-two years, and unmarried. Most were black and poor. All had just delivered their first baby. None had complicated deliveries, and all the babies were healthy and born at term. All of the mothers had skin-to-skin contact with their babies for an hour following the birth and remained in the hospital for two days. None of the mothers breast-fed their babies. The interaction between the mothers and their babies was observed after a feeding on the morning after the birth. Women in both groups were similar in how they held, cradled, and rocked their babies. However, there were significant differences between the groups in the attention the women gave to their babies and how they touched them. The mothers who had not been separated from their babies looked at their babies more, talked to them more, talked to others less, watched television less, and spent less time on the telephone. They spent more time touching their babies and rubbing them with the palms of their hands and were more likely to touch the baby's face and head. The limited contact mothers were more likely to tickle their babies, and to force the baby to move its limbs.

A study published in 1980 used randomized assignment to rooming-in or routine postpartum hospital care to investigate effects of rooming-in on outcomes that reflect severely inadequate parenting (O'Connor *et al.*, 1980). The study followed 301 women who delivered their first babies at Metropolitan Nashville General Hospital; 143 mothers and babies were assigned to rooming-in, 158 were assigned to routine care. Seven women randomized to the rooming-in group did not want rooming-in and received routine care but were kept in the rooming-in group for the purpose of data analysis (to avoid selection bias).

Most of the women were young, of lower socioeconomic status, and black. All had uncomplicated pregnancies and delivered healthy babies. Only 14 to 15 percent planned to breast-feed. All of the mothers got a glimpse of their babies while they were still on the delivery table, after which the babies were taken to the nursery. Rooming-in mothers got their babies back after seven hours and then had them for eight hours a day until they left the hospital. Routine-care mothers did not see their babies again for at least twelve hours, and then only during feedings. The rooming-in mothers averaged almost twelve hours with their babies during the first forty-eight hours after the birth; routine-care mothers were with their babies for a little more than two hours during that period. Outcome data were collected when the infants were between twelve and twenty-one months old. All reports of child abuse and neglect filed in the state of Tennessee during the period since the first mother and baby went home from the hospital were reviewed, as well as the medical records of all infants admitted to the hospital for physical or sexual abuse, "failure to thrive" not due to major pathology, voluntary relinquishment of parental responsibility, medical or physical neglect, or infant health problems resulting from pathology in the mother–infant relationship (O'Connor *et al.*, 1980).

Twelve infants had serious problems reflecting inadequate parenting. Ten of the twelve infants with problems related to inadequate parenting were in the routine-postpartum care group; another was the infant of a mother who had been assigned to rooming-in but refused it and had routine postpartum care. Several of these infants were diagnosed with "failure to thrive", they gained weight while under the care of nurses at the hospital but lost weight when they were returned to their mothers' care. One infant, whose mother was described as "nervous," "anxious," and "angry with the baby," had persistent vomiting while in his mother's care. Two others were hospitalized for severe dehydration. One mother complained that it was "hard to take care of this thing" and repeatedly ordered the baby to "shut up." Six infants were admitted to the hospital with injuries from physical abuse—

one had a broken bone; two had head injuries; one had multiple bruises and abrasions; two had been burned. Two infants were referred to Protective Services because their parents failed to get medical care when the child was ill. One child was placed in foster care because his mother wanted to travel and refused custody. Another mother gave her ten-month old baby for adoption. Only one case involved a woman who experienced "rooming in"—a mother who withheld water from her baby to "make him respect her" and allowed a dog to bite him because the baby had let the puppy out of its pen (O'Connor *et al.*, 1980).

Some hospitals have now adopted rooming-in as standard care. In addition to being better for the mother and baby, it is much less expensive than maintaining a centralized nursery, and avoids the risk of an epidemic of newborn infections arising in the nursery. A midwife at the Oregon Health Sciences University Hospital in Portland has noticed a reduction in babies admitted for failure to thrive since the hospital switched to routine rooming-in (Sullivan, 1996).

Support During the First Few Weeks at Home

There were several reasons for the typical three-day postpartum hospitalizations that were routine until about 1995. Obstetricians and pediatricians wanted mothers and babies to remain in the hospital long enough to make sure that they were not going to develop any significant complications. Nurses wanted them to stay long enough to make sure that the mothers knew how to take care of their babies. Many women who had other children wanted to stay in order to get some rest. But many women did not want to be separated from their families during this important period, and particularly did not want to stay in hospitals that separated them from their babies. In the past some women had to sign themselves out of hospitals "against medical advice" in order to be with their babies and other family members. That became less of a problem as accountants took over the running hospitals and determined that it costs too much for healthy mothers and babies to stay.

The length of postpartum/newborn hospitalization became a political issue during 1996, when obstetricians, pediatricians, and some consumer groups responded indignantly to some managed care organizations' new rules requiring healthy mothers to take their newborns and leave the hospital within a limited number of hours after giving birth. The American Academy of Pediatrics and the American College of Obstetricians and Gynecologists issued press releases that criticized financial coercion for short hospital stays, which became known as "drive-through deliveries." Both groups think the timing of the discharge should be decided by a doctor, not based on an arbitrary policy established by a third party, and that forty-eight hours is usually needed to fulfill all of the conditions that should be met before a mother and newborn go home. It was definitely an all-American, motherhood and apple-pie issue; Congress quickly passed and the president signed legislation ensuring two-day hospital stays for all new mothers and their babies. When the Health Insurance Association of America opposed the legislation, Labor Secretary Robert Reich, whose department is responsible for enforcing the law, responded that "Our research shows that any small additional cost in insurance will be more than exceeded by the benefits to mothers and their newborns in terms of safer and healthier deliveries" (Burns, 1996).

Although the issue was an easy political winner, the scientific data are not so clear. Relatively early postbirth hospital discharge is both safe and cost effective when accompanied by early follow-up of both the mother and the infant. Several studies (including a randomized trial) have followed outcomes of early discharge in an indigent population, a community hospital population, and a group of mothers and newborns following

cesarean deliveries (Conrad *et al.*, 1989; Welt *et al.*, 1993; Pittard & Geddes, 1988; Brooten *et al.*, 1994). The American College of Nurse-Midwives' position on the issue stresses the need to base the timing of discharge on the condition and circumstances of each individual mother and newborn, calls for flexibility in decisions about the timing of discharge, and supports payment for health care services provided in homes, birth centers, or offices to augment or substitute for hospital care. A midwifery service in Cambridge, Massachusetts, has initiated a program using doulas. Lactation consultants might also be used (Yanco, 1996). The point is to provide whatever an individual mother and baby need.

Midwives who attend births in homes or birth centers avoid the need for prolonged hospitalization by educating women in breast-feeding and newborn care during the prenatal period, teaching them to look for the signs and symptoms of common postpartum and neonatal complications, examining the mothers and babies during home visits, maintaining close working relationships and good communication with the mothers, and making sure that every mother can reach her midwife easily by telephone. Most midwives who attend home births make two home visits during the first week, usually on the day after the birth, or at least within the first three days, and at the end of the first week. This is usually followed by visits at the midwife's office, or additional home visits, at about two weeks and again at six weeks. (Frye, 1996; Morales, 1996). Many midwives who work in birth centers also make home visits, usually on the second or third day after the birth; others ask mothers to come back to the birth center with their babies during the early postpartum period. Most women who deliver in a birth center have three visits with their primary care provider (usually a midwife) during the six-week postpartum period (Rooks *et al.*, 1992c).

The issue of mothers' needs during the postpartum period go far beyond the question of early discharge. Even when mothers were hospitalized for three or four days,* many women felt underinformed and undersupported, inadequate, and overwhelmed when they got home with their new babies. Many cultures have traditions that support new mothers. A 1996 journal article described a discussion between four women who had given birth to their first babies in different countries. All of them described feelings of insecurity, confusion, and ignorance about breast-feeding and other aspects of their new responsibilities (Placksin, 1996).

- Sara explained that, in Uganda, the new mother's mother or aunties come to take care of her while she rests. "They cook special soup so that you can have milk to feed the baby. We feed whenever the baby cries. There's no time schedule."
- Gerita explained that, although middle- and upper-class women in Jamaica have their babies in hospitals and stay there for three of four days, women in more traditional settings stay in the house for nine days, and are catered to by relatives and friends. "The mom stays in bed to feed the baby. She herself is fed soups—chicken soup or vegetable soup—and special teas, mainly herbal teas. The babies are fed on demand, and sleep with the mom. That is very important. They're never separated."
- Melinda told about the "family system" in Guatemala, where for forty days the new mother has "no sex, no exercise, only take care of your new baby and adapt to the new life." Women in the family help the new mother by "doing" more than by talking. "They are helping you, teaching you how to bathe the baby, so they bathe the baby. They are

teaching you how to breast-feed. They give you hot drinks, and they rub your back with some herbs."
- Renee, a twenty-seven-year-old American professional woman, just reported being overwhelmed: "Everybody said that everything was going to come naturally. I didn't find that stuff came naturally to me."

Another article discussed short hospital stays and the ameliorating effect of home visits by midwives in England. Meg described having a midwife visit her every day for ten days after less than twenty-four hours of hospitalization when she gave birth to her first child. The midwife examined the baby and used a hand-held scale to weigh it, examined Meg, and made sure she was breast-feeding successfully. When Meg fell into a slight postpartum depression, the midwife encouraged her to talk about it. "It made a difference, because of the state I was in . . . She was solicitous and nice and very friendly, and it was lovely and reassuring when she was there. Although I think she could have done more in terms of putting me in touch with a counselor, I wanted support and comfort, and she did what she could" (Lyall, 1995). Postpartum depression (as opposed to mild, transient "blues") are thought to affect 10 to 15 percent of American mothers (Philipps & O'Hara, 1991). It generally begins about two weeks after childbirth and usually lasts for about two months, although it can last for a year or longer (Pfost *et al.*, 1990).

The usual pattern of care for childbearing women in America is to leave the hospital with knowledge of whom to call if they have a problem and appointments for follow-up care for both the mother and the newborn four to six weeks after the birth. To compensate for early discharge, some larger health care services have hired nurses to make an early postpartum home visit. However, very few American women get any kind of professional support between hospital discharge and the routine four- to six-weeks

---

*The average duration of an obstetric hospital stay in 1970 was 4.1 days. It had dropped to 2.6 days by 1992 (Centers for Disease Control, 1995).

visit. The role that was once played by the extended family has been largely lost, and many women have unmet needs for information, emotional and social support, and help solving a variety of problems. The unmet needs are greatest for women who live in poverty and have little social support.

A small study conducted by four nurse-midwifery students analyzed the content of five routine four- to six-week postpartum visits, each conducted by a different CNM (Morten *et al.*, 1991). The visits were videotaped and lasted twenty-seven minutes on average. Discussions between the CNMs and their clients covered a broad range of topics, including the woman's physical and emotional health; her other children, husband, and parents; and issues related to breastfeeding and infant care. Education merged with counseling and joint problem solving. One mother needed the nurse-midwife to support her decision to have a tubal ligation. All five visits included discussion of sexuality, contraception, exercise, and rest. Most included provision of information on signs and symptoms of physical complications the women should look for and discussion of the woman's specific concerns about herself and her infant. Most of the mothers had concerns about their adaptation to motherhood, including their experiences during labor and delivery, their feelings toward their infants, the adjustment of other family members, and stressful circumstances involving finances, physical changes or discomforts, not having enough time, and being tired. All of the visits included frequent use of affirmative, validating, reassuring, comforting, and supportive statements by the CNMs. The student researchers' identified empowering the woman as an overriding goal of the visits.

Contraception

The period of postpartum infertility associated with pregnancy may last no longer than four to six weeks in women who do not breast-feed their newborns. It may be extended to six months or longer for women who breast-feed frequently, including at night, if they do not supplement the infant's diet with other foods (Winikoff, 1990). The suppression of ovulation is associated with a neuroendocrinologic feedback mechanism triggered by the effect of suckling on the woman's nipples. Anything that reduces suckling, including use of a pacifier to meet the baby's need to suck, reduces the effect and shortens the period of postpartum infertility. Few American women want to get pregnant with another child shortly after having a baby. Unfortunately, it happens frequently. Educating women about the timing of the return to fertility and the advantages, disadvantages, and availability of all safe and effective methods of contraception is an essential part of providing adequate maternity care. In addition, the provision of family planning services to women, and sexually active girls, at other times in their lives is a critically important aspect of reproductive health care.

There is enormous evidence that these services are not being provided effectively to large proportions of the women who need them in this country (Brown & Eisenberg, 1995). Nearly 60 percent of all pregnancies in the United States are unintended. The proportion of unintended pregnancies has been increasing since the early 1980s. About three million unintended pregnancies occur to American women every year. About half of them are aborted. Women who become pregnant unintentionally are less likely to seek early prenatal care and are more likely to expose the fetus to harmful substances such as drugs and nicotine. Their babies are at greater risk of being low birth weight, of dying before they reach age one, and of being abused. Women who give birth to babies that were not planned are at greater risk of depression. Although unwanted pregnancies are most frequent among unmarried adolescents, large numbers of adult women (and men) also have difficulty preventing unwanted pregnancies. About half of all unintended pregnancies occur among women using a short-acting form of contraception, such as condoms or pills, when the method fails or is used inconsistently or improperly. The other half occur to a much smaller group of women, who do not use any method of contraception even though they are sexually active and do not want to become pregnant (Brown & Eisenberg, 1995).

The reasons for these problems are complex. As with effective prenatal care for behaviorally high-risk women, effective family planning care requires the ability to empower and support another person to decide and accomplish her own reproductive health goals. Safe provision of actual family planning methods is part of what is needed. But the greater challenge is to empower women (and men) who do not want to have a baby to make the behavioral changes necessary either to avoid sexual intercourse or use contraceptive methods effectively and consistently.

Empowering Women

Midwives perceive part of their role to be the "empowerment" of individual women. "Midwife" means "with woman"—not "for," but "with." MANA's statement of values and ethics speaks eloquently of valuing women's rights to make their own choices, supporting them in nonjudgmental ways, and making resources available to help women realize their own goals of health, happiness, and personal growth.*

The students who conducted the study described in the last section concluded that empowering the woman was the goal of the process used during the postpartum visits (Morten *et al.*, 1991). They noted a lack of authoritarianism; none of the nurse-midwives stated or implied that a client should accept the CNM's plan of care. The tone of the visits was relaxed, friendly, and supportive; the observers noted a sense of "connectedness,

empathy, mutuality, intimacy, familiarity, warmth, acceptance, and patience" in the CNM–client relationships. The researchers classified their observations of the care provided during the visits into three categories: (1) therapeutic techniques, defined as a process of communication that benefits the client or encourages growth and healing; (2) development and maintenance of a lateral relationship, defined as the CNM promoting "an interaction characterized by a sense of openness, mutual regard, and equal footing with the client, thus encouraging a sense of commonality between the two;" and (3) empowerment, defined as giving or receiving power, strength, or ego reinforcement. An interaction was described as empowering when the CNM's attitude and approach tended to enhance the client's inner energies and resources. Examples were uses of affirmation, validation, reassurance, and support (Morten *et al.*, 1991).

The student researchers felt that the therapeutic techniques and lateral relationships were used in support of empowerment, and that empowerment was the ultimate goal of the process the nurse-midwives used during the visits (Morten *et al.*, 1991). Most other studies of nurse-midwifery care focus on procedural content, health outcomes, or psychosocial issues. This study tried to analyze the process. There have been no studies to assess the effectiveness of midwifery care on actually "empowering" women—making them somehow stronger and thus better able to take care of their babies, their families, and themselves. Many studies have found high degrees of satisfaction with midwifery care, and the demand for midwifery care by women who have known it implies great satisfaction. It is important to recognize, however, that empowerment is an underlying theme and purpose of midwifery. Research is needed to identify and understand whether and how that aspect of the care provided by midwives affects the ability of women who do not want to become pregnant to avoid conception,

---

*See Chapter 9.

the ability of pregnant women to maximize their health and avoid risks to the fetuses they carry, the ability of parturient women to labor with force and effectiveness, and the ability of new mothers to take care of themselves, their babies, and their families.

The first birth center in Sweden was opened by an obstetrician and midwife, who based it on birth centers they had visited in the United States. Although it is located in a hospital, the birth center is administered independently. Compared with care provided in the regular obstetric unit at this hospital, care provided at the birth center is more personalized, there is minimal use of medical and technologic interventions during labor and delivery, it is a homelike setting, and they try to enable parents to maintain control over the childbearing process, including self-control, environmental control, and full participation in health care decisions (Waldenström & Nilsson, 1993). In a randomized, controlled study of care provided at the birth center versus the regular obstetric unit, 63 percent of women who used the birth center reported an increase in self-esteem as a result of their childbirth experience; only 18 percent of the women who delivered in the regular obstetric unit made that claim. Having more control was also associated with a lower incidence of postpartum depression.

Nurse researchers have defined four levels of empowerment by people using health care: (1) active participation in your own care, (2) exercising choices regarding your care and experiencing the consequences of your choices, (3) supporting and helping other clients or patients, and (4) interacting on an equal basis with professional staff and other clients (Connelly *et al.*, 1993). Midwifery care supports empowerment at every level: Pregnant women are taught to take their own pulse, test their own urine, and keep records of the progress of their own pregnancy. They are given the information needed to make choices about self-care during pregnancy and many aspects of their experience during labor. Many birth centers run by midwives organize support groups in which women whose babies are due at about the same time get to know one another. Such groups may continue after all of the women have given birth, providing a source of mutual support for the women as they grow into their roles as mothers. Many birth centers also ask clients and exclients to serve on advisory committees to help the birth center staff better understand the needs of women and families in the community. Birth center advisory groups have suggested important changes and improvements, making the centers better able to serve the people of a particular neighborhood (Spitzer, 1995).

These kinds of empowering activities may be especially important to young, unmarried women who live in socially distressed communities. The birth center run by nurse-midwives in the South Bronx, in New York City, has been supported by a neighborhood Council for the Empowerment of Childbearing Families. Many clients of the birth center have spoken of gaining confidence and a sense of power from their positive experiences during pregnancy and childbirth. The birth center and the Council for the Empowerment of Childbearing Families have played a role in the rejuvenation of the neighborhood (Spitzer, 1995).

Chapter 11
Safety of Out-of-Hospital Births in the United States

Ninety-nine percent of births in the United States occur in hospitals; one percent are out-of-hospital births. These proportions have remained stable for more than fifteen years. The percentages are based on information from birth certificates. The one percent of out-of-hospital births does not include births to women who intended to give birth at home or in a free-standing birth center but were transferred to a hospital during labor because of a complication. It also does not include births en route to a hospital (which are counted as births that occurred in the hospital) or home births for which no birth certificate is filed. Underregistration of home births is discussed in Chapter 7.* Although it

is assumed that home births attended by direct-entry midwives are underreported to some degree, all discussion of the number of out-of-hospital births in this chapter is based on the birth certificate-derived data provided by the National Center for Health Statistics. The true numbers and percentages of out-of-hospital births, especially home births attended by direct-entry midwives, are probably a little higher but are certainly no lower than the numbers and percentages used in this chapter.

A direct-entry midwife was listed as the attendant at 30 percent of all out-of-hospital births for which a birth certificate was filed in 1994; CNMs attended 24 percent, and

---

*Table 2 in Chapter 7 provides an estimate of the number and percentage of out-of-hospital births attended by direct-entry midwives for each year from 1989 through 1994 based on the assumption that direct-entry midwives attended half of the out-of-hospital births for which birth certificates were filed which indicated that the births were attended by someone other than a physician or a midwife or for which no birth attendant was specified.

Making this assumption increases the number and percent of births assumed to have been attended by direct-entry midwives by about 50 percent. The validity of this assumption is unknown. If it is erroneous, the error is probably in the direction of overestimating the number of births attended by direct-entry midwives. However, it has no effect on the stability of the proportion; the number and percent remain both low and stable.

physicians attended 17 percent. The other 29 percent were births that occurred in homes by accident—because the mother did not realize she was in labor or did not leave for the hospital in time—and births attended in homes, birth centers, or clinics by naturopaths, chiropractors, nurses, physician assistants, the pregnant woman's friends and family members, and lay and direct-entry midwives who do not want to be identified as such on the birth certificate. Table 3 in Chapter 7 shows these data for 1980 and for 1989 through 1994.

. Although out-of-hospital births are a small part of all births in the country, they account for all births attended by direct-entry midwives and about 5 percent of the births attended by nurse-midwives (based on national natality data for 1994). Most out-of-hospital births attended by direct-entry midwives occur in homes (71 percent), with all but a few of the others in birth centers. Most out-of-hospital births attended by CNMs occur in free-standing birth centers (69 percent), with all but a few of the others in homes. Only 0.2 percent of births attended by physicians occur in out-of-hospital settings; 56 percent of them are in homes and 26 percent are in free-standing birth centers.

Despite the small proportion, intentional out-of-hospital births arouse great emotion and controversy between those involved in them, including parents who choose to have their babies at home or in a birth center, and most obstetricians. Home births attended by midwives provide the greatest contrast to hospital births attended by physicians and are at the apex of the dispute. Home birth advocates believe in the superiority of home births and tend to be highly critical of the care available in most hospitals. Many obstetricians are equally strongly opposed to and critical of home births. The conflict draws bitterness from its origins in the early 1970s, when articulate leaders of the newly emerging women's health movement made sharp criticisms of obstetrics, displayed a startling distrust of

obstetricians, and advised women that home births attended by lay midwives were not only superior aesthetically, but were also *safer* than subjecting oneself to unnecessary procedures during a hospital birth. The American College of Obstetricians and Gynecologists (ACOG) responded by calling press conferences in which obstetricians referred to home births as forms of "maternal trauma" and "child abuse" and urged physicians to report deaths resulting from home births. State medical associations began to report deaths, or simply illegal midwifery practice, to state and local prosecutors, who began to arrest midwives, and the battle lines hardened, especially in certain states, including New York and California.

Why Do Women Have Planned Out-of-Hospital Births?

Women choose nonhospital births for many reasons, including economics, lack of reliable access to transportation for women in some rural areas, membership in certain religious communities, previous negative experience with hospital births, concern about unnecessary intervention during labor, and the desire to experience the rewards of a nurturant environment and a more gentle birth for themselves and their babies. Because the entire system is geared for hospital births, planning to have your baby elsewhere requires a clear decision and often quite strong motivation. Many women conduct significant research into the issue before deciding.

Cost is an important factor for many women. The total cost of maternity care provided by a home birth midwife may be only 30 percent of the combined cost of care provided by an obstetrician with childbirth in a hospital. Women who obtain their care through a free-standing birth center save from less than one-third to almost one-half of the cost of physician care with a hospital birth.* Chapter

---

*See Chapter 12 for more information about birth site cost differentials.

5 provided information about the ongoing problem of providing maternity care to women who have no health care insurance but are not eligible for Medicaid. Government at all levels has grappled with this problem for the past fifteen years without a long-term solution. Home births accounted for 5 percent of all births in Oregon during the early 1980s; although Oregon's home birth rate has declined since then, at 2.2 percent in 1991, the proportion of home births in Oregon was higher than in any other state (Oregon Department of Human Resources, 1993). In a study conducted during the early 1980s, two researchers asked women who had home births in Oregon if financial concerns were their primary reason for delivering at home (Curry & Brandon, 1986). Approximately half of the women had decided on home births because the cost of health insurance, hospitalization and medical care was prohibitive. Some of these women may have had other reasons also; the study did not ask (Hays, 1996). Lack of access to transportation is another reason for some home births in rural areas. This is due to rural poverty for some women, but is a religious imperative for others, such as the Amish (Armstrong & Feldman, 1986; Gaskin, 1996).

Studies of women's motivation for seeking home births have found a variety of other reasons. After reviewing studies published during the 1970s, one investigator concluded that women's birth strategies consider social and cultural risks and benefits, as well as medical risks, and found that many women's view of the medical risks are different from the judgment of physicians (McClain, 1983). Studies that allow home birth mothers to speak for themselves find that they identify the naturalness and normalcy of pregnancy and childbirth as values they are seeking, and that this "creates an aversion to the hospital milieu and medical interventions" (Hays, 1996) and "critical and skeptical views of biomedical approaches to childbirth" (Klee, 1986). Some women are afraid of hospitals and obstetric interventions; data on dissatisfaction with previous hospital experiences show that women are, "at least in part, choosing to birth at home as a way to avoid or escape a potentially unpleasant scenario" (Hays, 1996). But woman also choose home births for very positive reasons—the familiarity of the home, a relaxed, peaceful, intimate atmosphere, privacy, a feeling of safety and security, and psychological rewards, including "the continuity of birthing the baby in the same environment where it was conceived and will grow" (Hays, 1996). Studies also find that alternatives such as a birth center are not acceptable to some women, who are committed to giving birth in their own home; "the home environment itself is a unique and irreplaceable aspect of the childbirth experience to some women" (Hays, 1996).

Difficulty of Conducting Adequate Research on Out-of-Hospital Births

Women's reasons for choosing to give birth at home or in a birth center are important but are not the core element in the controversy, which focuses on safety. People who support home births believe that they are as safe, virtually as safe, or maybe even safer than hospital births for women who have no serious health problems or pregnancy complications. Those who oppose nonhospital births believe that they result in a higher rate of poor pregnancy outcomes compared to the outcomes that would have occurred if the same low-risk women had delivered their babies in hospitals. It might seem that it would be easy to collect the data needed to determine which position is correct. It is not.

The "gold standard" method to compare the safety and effectiveness of two approaches to managing any health phenomenon is a randomized clinical trial. A randomized study of this subject is probably impossible in the United States. Very few women would be willing to give birth in one place or another on the basis of random assignment. In addition, only low-risk women would be allowed into such a study, and the incidence of poor outcomes among low-risk women is low regardless of their place of birth. As a result, a very large study would be necessary. Since a randomized trial is not possible, other approaches are used. Although these methods do not provide a definitive answer to the question, they provide some idea of the safety of one birth site compared with another under specified circumstances.

However, the safety of birth sites cannot be proven in the same way that the safety of a drug can be proven. "Out-of-hospital birth" is not a standardized product; the safety will vary with the conditions. Most people agree that the following conditions are necessary to support the safety of births that do not occur in hospitals: (1) limiting out-of-hospital births to healthy women who have normal pregnancies and are unlikely to develop serious complications during labor or immediately after giving birth; (2) attendance by competent midwives or physicians; (3) the ability to transport women and newborns with serious complications to hospitals rapidly; and (4) good communication and working relationships between the midwives and physicians who attend out-of-hospital births and the physicians who take care of the women and babies who are transferred to hospitals. The incidence of poor outcomes can be expected to vary with the extent to which these conditions are in place. A study that documents good outcomes in one particular practice or service can demonstrate the level of safety that is possible, if the study is large enough to measure the incidence of poor outcomes that are rare in low-risk women. However, the conclusions from a study of one birth center or home birth practice cannot be assumed to extend to out-of-hospital birth services that do not maintain the same standards and conditions. Studies that include all or a random sample of all planned out-of-hospital births would provide a more accurate picture.

Several kinds of data can be used to study the safety of out-of-hospital births: (1) data from birth certificates and death certificates, (2) data about clients of specific out-of-hospital birth practices or services, and (3) mortality review reports (investigations of the circumstances leading to maternal and perinatal deaths). Studies based on each of these data sources have strengths and weaknesses.

Birth and Death Certificate Data

U.S. Birth certificates contain information on many demographic, behavioral and medical risk factors, some procedures used during labor and delivery, the birth attendant, and some outcomes (e.g., birth weight and Apgar scores). Infant death certificates provide information on the infant's age at the time of death and the cause of death. However, birth and death certificates are separate documents, and a complicated process is required to link them.

Data sets developed from vital records (birth and infant death records) have several advantages: Birth certificate data can be used to describe the entire population of women having out-of-hospital births in a specified geographic area. If data for the entire country are used, the number of women is relatively large; therefore the findings are stable. Any observed differences are real; they do not have to be tested for statistical significance, because they are not subject to sampling error.

Many of the out-of-hospital births that result in newborn deaths occur at home by accident, or, at least, without intention. This is especially likely for the unexpected, often precipitous preterm births of very low birth weight babies. Other high-risk births in this category include those to some mentally ill or very socially isolated women, who may not get to a hospital for their deliveries but did not consciously plan to have a home birth. "Out-of-hospital" is also the presumed place of birth for infants whose bodies are found after they were either murdered or abandoned and left to die (Burnett *et al.*, 1980). If one wants to examine the safety of planned out-of-hospital births, it is necessary to look only at births attended by a midwife or physician. Some of the others may also be planned out-of-hospital births, but it is not possible to know from the birth certificate.

Linking the data on birth and infant death certificates makes it possible to calculate neonatal mortality rates for births in hospitals, birth centers, homes, and other sites, and to subdivide births in each setting to look at mortality associated with births attended by physicians, nurse-midwives, and direct-entry midwives (for births during and after 1989). This has been done in some states, but it has not been done at the national level. However, several circumstances make it hard to draw reliable conclusions about the safety of nonhospital births from neonatal mortality rates based on data from birth and infant death certificates. There may be a great amount of error when these data are used to judge the safety of home births.

- Intrapartum deaths (fetal deaths during labor) are not included in records of live births and infant deaths,* and the intrapartum period probably accounts for a larger proportion of the deaths associated with births in nonhospital settings than of the deaths resulting from births in hospitals. (This can be seen in Table 11 in the section on "Area-Wide Data on Out-of-Hospital Births.") Comparing neonatal mortality rates for out-of-hospital births with those for hospital births distorts the true relationship between the rates, making the out-of-hospital births seem to result in fewer deaths than is true.

- Complications during a planned home birth often leads to transporting the mother to a hospital prior to the delivery. If a moribund infant is born in the hospital, its birth certificate will show the hospital as the place of birth; its death will be counted as a death associated with a hospital birth.

- Some home births that result in infant deaths may not be reported. No birth certificate is filed for some successful home births attended by direct-entry midwives. This is especially common in states where their practice is illegal; in that situation, midwives consider filing the birth certificate to be the parents' responsibility.[†] Birth registration is quite complete in general, both because of laws that require a birth certificate to be filed and because birth certificates are needed for many things of importance to parents and, eventually, to the child. This latter incentive does not exist if the infant dies. The parents and the midwife or physician who attend a home birth that results in a death may prefer to avoid making an official record of their loss. Some women who have home births are members of communities that resent government intervention in their lives in general. They may be particularly disinclined to report a newborn death following a home birth.

- Studies based on birth and death certificates filed in a particular state may either under- or overcount the deaths in relation to the number of home birth certificates filed. A newborn who is in poor condition will be taken to the nearest hospital, which may be in a different state. The vital records departments in

---

*Late fetal deaths are also supposed to be reported to the health department in each state. But fetal death reporting is very incomplete. Thus the data are very unreliable.

†Various degrees of underregistration of home births have been documented in prospective studies in which the investigator tried to identify birth certificates for infants whose births were included in the study. See Chapter 7.

some states make a concerted effort to find a birth certificate to match each reported neonatal death, and search birth certificates in adjacent states if no in-state match is found. This practice is not universal, however.

Data from Specific Out-of-Hospital Birth Practices or Services

Information contained in individual client records can be collected for use in a retrospective study, or data intended to meet the exact purposes of a study can be collected prospectively. Statistics derived from these data are often compared with similar information about women who deliver their babies in hospitals. Various methods are used in an attempt to match the hospital-birth mothers to the out-of-hospital birth mothers with regard to perinatal risk.

This kind of study can overcome the problems associated with studies based on vital data, if the study includes information on outcomes for women and babies who are transferred to hospitals during labor or soon after the birth because of complications. However, some studies of this kind do not follow all of the women and babies who were transferred. In addition, studies based on the care provided in particular out-of-hospital birth services lack the two main benefits of studies based on vital data: They usually report on a relatively small number of births and they probably reflect the outcomes of the better out-of-hospital birth practices:

- Most birth centers and home birth practices are relatively small operations. That is one of their attractions. But studies involving a relatively small number of women cannot detect differences in the occurrence of outcomes that are rare among low-risk women and their babies, regardless of their place of birth.
- Publication bias must be assumed in all retrospective studies, whether of out-of-hospital births or any other unusual health care practice. No practitioner

who has experienced a high incidence of poor outcomes is eager to amplify knowledge of that fact. Those practicing in hospitals have little control over use of the information contained in clinical records (although research ethics committees that act on behalf of the hospital do control access to the records). This, however, is different from the control exercised by individual physicians and midwives practicing in small, private out-of-hospital birth practices. Practices that have experienced poor outcomes have little motivation to compile and publish their results; they may also refuse to allow others to study their records. Every published study of a single out-of-hospital birth practice or service has either reported low mortality rates or has compared the mortality rate found during the study with an equal or higher rate for some group of in-hospital births: Mehl *et al.*, 1975; Murdaugh, 1976; Epstein & McCartney, 1977; Neilson, 1977; Estes, 1978; Faison *et al.*, 1979; McCallum, 1979; Dejong *et al.*, 1981; Cohen, 1982; Reinke, 1982; Zabrek *et al.*, 1983; Koehler *et al.*, 1984; Scupholme *et al.*, 1986; Eakins *et al.*, 1989; Acheson *et al.*, 1990; Durand, 1992.

One can overcome the small numbers problem by combining data from two or more out-of-hospital birth practices or services. Increasing the number of women in the study increases the power to detect differences, and including more practices in a study should make the findings more representative of the range of quality that exists in all health services. But unless all or a random sample of practices are included, the findings are apt to be biased by which individuals or services are included in the study. Midwives and physicians who attend home births and are known to the people conducting a study are more likely to be invited to participate, and they are probably different in some important ways from midwives and physicians who attend home births but are *not* asked to participate in a study because they are not known to the people conducting the study. Birth centers and individual home birth practitioners who are not asked to participate in such a study are less likely to be members of some kind of professional organization, or to be known because they have attended continuing education conferences or participated in peer review; individuals who practice in isolation are less likely to be invited. And, because participation in research is voluntary, services that have had poor outcomes may decline involvement. The effect is the same as publication bias. All studies of this type have also reported low mortality associated with the out-of-hospital births or lower rates compared with some other group: Mehl *et al.*, 1977, 1980; Bennetts & Lubic, 1982; Anderson & Greener, 1991; Anderson & Murphy, 1995.

Meta-analysis makes it possible to compile data from many studies, and the methodology requires a rigorous search for unpublished studies. A meta-analysis of home birth studies is under way. However, the only weakness that is overcome by a meta-analysis is small numbers. Combining many studies, each of which has significant weaknesses, may not provide much advantage.

Concern about bias involving the decision to publish data on outcomes is greatest for retrospective studies, in which all of the events to be studied occurred before the study starts. Prospective multisite studies greatly reduce the possibility of bias because the midwives or physicians involved in the study make a commitment to participate before the births to be studied have occurred. This avoids the opportunity for bias resulting from individuals refusing to participate because they have had bad outcomes. However, even in a prospective study there is likely to be bias in which practitioners' data end up in the study. In addition, there is no way to prevent a midwife or physician who agrees to participate in a study from dropping out because of a bad outcome. Bias may

be introduced by any factor that affects who is invited to participate, who agrees to participate, and how long they continue to participate in a study of nonhospital births.

Researchers have an obligation to ensure that the data they analyze are accurate; in a study of nonhospital births, it is also necessary to verify that a data form has been filled out on *every* birth in the practice. It is not easy to verify the completeness and validity of data submitted by a large number of independent out-of-hospital birth services and practitioners. An independent home birth practitioner has complete control of the documentation of the care she or he provides to clients. This contrasts with the situation in hospitals, where many people may be involved in the care of a single patient and all of them use the patient's record. Significant inaccuracies in hospital records are likely to be detected, and sophisticated systems are used to ensure that there is a complete record for every patient and that the records are kept securely and are not lost. Many home birth studies are unable to check the accuracy and completeness of the data submitted.

Researchers should try to check the accuracy of the data and should drop participants who do not meet the study's data collection standards. Unfortunately, even that action introduces bias. Experience from the National Birth Center Study* (NBCS) provides an example. The NBCS research team wanted to involve every birth center in the country in the study. They began by compiling a very complete list of birth centers and inviting every birth center on the list to participate in the study. Of 160 centers on the list, 89 agreed to participate—56 percent. A data quality control system was implemented to assess the completeness and accuracy of the data submitted by each participating center. Every record was checked for completeness and internal consistency; records with missing information or obvious errors were

---

*The methodology for the National Birth Center Study is described in Chapter 5.

returned for completion or correction. In addition, every center was visited—to evaluate their data collection procedures, correct poor practices, and gather data from client clinical records that could be compared with data submitted for use in the study. Five centers were dropped from the study because the site visits raised serious questions about the completeness and validity of the data they had submitted (Rooks *et al.*, 1992a).

The study then included 84 of the 160 birth centers on the list—52 percent of all birth centers known to be in operation during the data collection period. There were some important differences between the centers that ended up in the study and those that did not. As compared with the centers in the study, centers not in the study were more likely to serve a low-income population, were much more likely to be operated by direct-entry midwives, and were much less likely to be licensed or accredited (Rooks *et al.*, 1992). These biases in participation may have affected the outcomes of the study. As a result the conclusions can only be applied to birth centers that are similar to those in the study. Similar biases affect virtually all studies based on data from particular health services. *Any factor that influences which practitioners' data are included in a study is likely to affect the findings.*

Mortality Review Reports

Investigations of the circumstances leading to maternal and perinatal deaths or other suboptimal pregnancy outcomes can identify factors contributing to each poor outcome. Poor outcomes are usually classified as preventable or not preventable. Insights into the sequence of events leading to poor outcomes can be used to improve practice.

A problem with this approach is that it may be difficult to unravel the chain of events that lead to a bad outcome in a hospital birth involving many interventions. For instance, a bad outcome might result from use of forceps to deliver a baby that developed fetal distress subsequent to administering oxytocin to a woman whose labor stalled after receiving an epidural. The use of forceps was necessary under the circumstances. When there is a bad outcome to an out-of-hospital birth, many people assume that the outcome would have been better in a hospital. That is not always the case; however, without an electronic fetal monitoring (EFM) record and blood tests that are not available during home births, it is often impossible to determine whether the outcome could have been different in a hospital. In addition, the litigious environment of American health care creates a disincentive for open reporting and review of maternal and perinatal deaths that occur in hospitals. When tragedy strikes birth in a hospital, it tends to reinforce that assumption that birth is so dangerous that hospital care is imperative. The parents may be comforted by being told that "everything possible was done;" no one may be anxious to investigate the role of interventions.

Comparison Groups

If we want to know whether out-of-hospital births are as safe as hospital births, we need information on the safety of hospital births *for women who have the same degree of inherent risk as the women who have out-of-hospital births.* Because of the near impossibility of randomized trials, two methods have been used to try to develop appropriate control groups: excluding individuals with certain characteristics from a group of women who have had hospital births, and matching specific out-of-hospital birth mothers to specific women who have had hospital births on the basis of characteristics associated with better or worse pregnancy outcomes. It is unlikely that these methods can provide a group of women who are truly comparable to women who have out-of-hospital births. Since the vast majority of births are in hospitals, women who have nonhospital births are a distinct minority. Many struggle to find someone to attend their birth; a nonhospital birth is not something a woman slips into as the path of least resistance. Women who make and implement unusual decisions are unusual. Even if you compare them with a group of women who are matched on every factor known to be associated with perinatal risk, you cannot match them on the motivation and will required to have an out-of-hospital birth. *Maternal motivation and will are characteristics that are probably highly associated with good pregnancy outcomes.* On the other hand, some out-of-hospital birth mothers may be at particularly high risk (e.g., those having home births because they cannot afford hospital care and women who would refuse hospital care for a complication because of their religion).

Outcomes of out-of-hospital births have been compared with findings from studies of low-risk hospital births—including studies that identified a group of low-risk women for some other purpose. These hospital-based studies are also subject to a form of publication bias; statistics that describe outcomes of low-risk births in hospitals rarely come from a representative sample of all hospitals. Most are conducted at hospitals associated with universities, which is where most research-oriented obstetricians work. Pregnancy outcomes in these hospitals tend to be better than outcomes in a random sample of American hospitals. This can be seen in the data from seven studies of low-risk hospital births presented at the bottom of Table 13, pages 366 and 367 (see section on "Intrapartum and Neonatal Mortality" on page 365). Each of these studies created a data set on low-risk in-hospital births by excluding women who had repeat cesarean sections, low birth weight infants, twins, breech deliveries, or any significant prenatal complication or chronic medical condition from a larger data set. Some of the studies also excluded women with intrapartum complications and/or those with social and behavioral risk factors such as smoking or being unmarried. There was large variation in the mortality rates found during these studies of low-risk hospital births. The neonatal mortality rate found during a study that included a representative sample of all births in the United States in 1980 ("national sample") was two-and-a-half times higher than the rates found in two studies conducted at academic medical centers. Comparing nonhospital birth outcomes with outcomes from the best academic hospitals holds out-of-hospital births to a standard that many U.S. *hospitals* cannot meet.

International Data

Studies of home births in the Netherlands, the United Kingdom, and Canada are of particular interest. The Netherlands is a special case because it is the only country that has both universal access to modern obstetrics and a large proportion of home births attended by well-educated midwives. The United Kingdom is of interest because it recently reversed its anti-home-birth policy in favor of a policy intended to give every woman the right and ability to choose the type of birth care she wants, "including the option, previously largely denied to them, of having their babies at home, or in small maternity units." This policy resulted from the findings of a year-long, in-depth investigation by a parliamentary committee, which concluded that the nation's previous policy of encouraging all women to give birth in hospitals could not be justified on grounds of safety (House of Commons Health Committee, 1992). Canada is of special interest because it is our neighbor and because of similarities between the two countries in the development of a form of direct-entry midwifery that evolved from lay midwifery and is based primarily on home births.

The Netherlands
Several studies published during the 1980s and early 1990s reported excellent outcomes of Dutch home births (Damstra-Wijmenga, 1984; Treffers and Laan, 1986; Van Alten *et al.*, 1989; Tew & Damstra-Wijmenga, 1991). The largest and most recent was a population-based study that compared outcomes for all births in Holland during 1986 by the

place of birth and category of birth attendant (Tew & Damstra-Wijmenga, 1991). The perinatal mortality rate for births attended by obstetricians in hospitals was 18.9 per 1,000, versus 2.1 per 1,000 for hospital births attended by midwives and 1.0 per 1,000 for midwife-attended home births. A large difference between the rate for births attended by obstetricians and home births attended by midwives was expected, because midwives refer high-risk cases to obstetricians and women who develop complications during a home birth are transferred to hospitals. Nevertheless, the very low rate of neonatal deaths associated with this large number of home births is impressive, especially because the data reflect the home birth practices of all midwives in the country.

The United Kingdom

The place of birth has been the subject of controversy in the UK since 1970, when an influential "expert" report recommended that, for safety's sake, all births should be in hospitals. Efforts to implement that recommendation accelerated the decline in home births during the early 1970s, and elicited a reaction from women who had experienced both home and hospital deliveries and preferred to have their babies at home (Chamberlain, 1988; Campbell & Macfarlane, 1994). British epidemiologists have been deeply involved in trying to derive meaning about the safety of home births from national data—an effort that suffers from the problems explained earlier. Nevertheless, there is considerable evidence of the safety of home births (mainly attended by midwives) in England and Wales. The perinatal mortality rate for 5,917 intended home births (including those transferred to hospitals because of complications) in England and Wales in 1979 was very low, at 4.1 per 1,000 (Campbell & Macfarlane, 1986).

Canada

Prior to dramatic changes in the laws of several provinces during the early 1990s, mid-

wifery in most parts of Canada was either illegal or alegal (not illegal, but not regulated), and there were no formal midwifery education programs. Although Canada lacks a nurse-midwifery tradition (except for a few "demonstration projects"), its direct-entry midwifery practice was similar to that of the United States—having arisen as part of the cultural protests of the 1960s and 1970s and being based primarily on home births attended by midwives without formal training.* There have been at least three studies based on home births that occurred in Canada during the period from the late 1970s through the late 1980s. Together the three studies followed a total of 1,337 planned and 39 unplanned home births:

- The first study reported on 275 planned and 10 unplanned home births attended by a family physician in an urban part of Ontario between 1976 and 1986 (Schneider & Soderstrom, 1987). There were two perinatal deaths—one due to a lethal congenital anomaly and one due to meconium aspiration resulting in pneumonia.

- The second study reported on 61 planned and 29 unplanned home births in Calgary between 1984 and 1987; these included all home births that occurred in Calgary for which a birth certificate was filed during that period of time (Abernathy & Lentjes, 1989). There were no bad outcomes associated with these births. The study was conducted by staff of the health department, and it is not clear who attended the births.

- The third study reported on 1,001 home births attended by direct-entry midwives in Toronto from 1983 through the middle of 1988 (Tyson, 1991). Sixteen percent of the mothers and/or their babies were transferred to hospitals during la-

---

*This is beginning to change as a result of the new laws, which provide access to hospital privileges for midwives in some provinces.

bor or soon after the birth. The cesarean delivery rate was 3.5 percent. There were no maternal deaths, no intrapartum deaths, and only two neonatal deaths, resulting in a total mortality rate of 2 per 1,000. Ninety-nine percent of the mothers were breast-feeding exclusively (i.e., as the only source of infant nutrition) at twenty-eight days postpartum (Tyson, 1991). Although midwifery was not legally sanctioned in Ontario during the period of this study and there were no formal midwifery education programs, most of the midwives who attended these births were members of a midwifery organization that expects its members to follow guidelines regarding contraindications to home births, risk factors that require medical consultation, two midwives at each birth, and participation in peer review (Kaufman, 1991).

Limitations of the Application of Data from Other Countries

Additional information on home births in these and other countries is presented in Chapter 13. Holland is particularly important because it tells us what might be possible if home births were widely available and interwoven with other components of the maternity care system. However, that is not the case in the United States, and this chapter—Chapter 11—is about the safety of out-of-hospital births in the United States. It is necessary to assess the safety of the out-of-hospital birth practice of midwives in the United States under current circumstances.

Area-Wide Data on Out-of-Hospital Births

In 1978 the American College of Obstetricians and Gynecologists issued a press release which stated that data from eleven states showed that babies born in out-of-hospital settings are two to five times more likely to die than babies born in hospitals (ACOG News Release, 1978). Home births attended by lay midwives were the target of the message. Although the press release attracted much attention, it was scorned by individuals who were knowledgeable about the actual circumstances of deaths following out-of-hospital births.

The matter was clarified by a study of neonatal deaths associated with out-of-hospital births in North Carolina from 1974 through 1976 (Burnett *et al.*, 1980). This study looked at the circumstances behind the data cited in the ACOG press release. By calling the people who signed each baby's birth and death certificates, the investigators tried to determine whether the birth occurred in a nonhospital setting by intention or by accident, and by whom the birth was attended. There had been 63 neonatal deaths following out-of-hospital births in North Carolina during the two-year period—a rate of 27 deaths per 1,000 out-of-hospital births, compared with 12 deaths per 1,000 hospital births in the state during the same period. Thirty deaths followed births that occurred out-of-hospital unintentionally or because the mother had no alternative, a rate of 120 neonatal deaths per 1,000 unintential out-of-hospital births. Two of these births occurred at home after the mothers had been turned away from hospitals because they couldn't pay; 5 of the deaths were suspected homicides. The next highest rate was for babies born while the mother was en route to the hospital—68 deaths per 1,000 births. The next highest rate was for home births without a birth attendant—30 deaths per 1,000 births. There were 3 neonatal deaths out of 768 planned home births attended by lay midwives—4 per 1,000 births. All three were preventable deaths due to congenital anomalies. A study of out-of-hospital births in Kentucky from 1981 through 1983 also found high rates of low birth weight and neonatal mortality among unplanned out-of-hospital births and low rates among planned home births, for which the neonatal mortality rate was 3.5 per 1,000 live births (Hinds *et al,* 1985).

Statewide studies of planned home births have been conducted in at least three other states—Arizona, Missouri, and Washington—and data on outcomes of all out-of-hospital births in Vermont are available for specific years. These studies allow some examination of the outcomes of births attended by direct-entry midwives. The study from Toronto also falls into this category, which is limited to studies that include all out-of-hospital births attended by midwives in a specified geographic area during a particular period of time. The findings from these studies are summarized in Table 13 (in the section on Intrapartum and Neonatal Mortality).

Arizona, 1978–1981

Arizona adopted new rules and regulations for midwives in 1978. A study to assess the effectiveness of the new rules was based on information about 1,449 home births attended by twenty-six licensed midwives from 1978 through 1981 (Sullivan & Beeman, 1983). This is the only statewide study that provided information on both intrapartum and neonatal mortality and ascertained outcomes for women and newborns who were transferred to hospitals during or shortly after labor and delivery. Twenty-three percent of the women, or their babies, were transferred to hospitals during labor or shortly after the birth. There were two fetal deaths during labor and two neonatal deaths. Two of the deaths were due to congenital anomalies, and one was a breech birth (not allowed under the regulations). The combined intrapartum/neonatal mortality rate was 2.8 per 1,000 births (1.4 per 1,000 excluding lethal congenital anomalies). The researchers attributed a decline in complications during the four-year period to improved performance related to increased experience, close supervision, and continuing education of the midwives.

Missouri, 1978–1984

A study of home births in Missouri from 1978 through 1984 examined neonatal mortality among births attended by different categories of birth attendants (Schramm *et al.*, 1987). The highest neonatal mortality rates were for births attended by someone other than a physician or midwife (6 deaths out of 474 = 12.7 per 1,000) and births attended by midwives not recognized by the Missouri Midwife Association (6 out of 725 births = 8.3 per 1,000). The rate for home births attended by physicians, CNMs, and direct-entry midwives recognized by the Missouri Midwife Association (MMA) was 2.8 per 1,000 (5 deaths out of 1,770). Four of the deaths were infants delivered by physicians, one was an infant delivered by a CNM. There were no deaths associated with 396 home births attended by direct-entry midwives who were MMA members. The neonatal mortality rate for hospital births attended by physicians was used to calculate the expected number of deaths for each group if their outcomes had been the same as outcomes of births in hospitals. There was no effort to exclude high-risk births from the data used to calculate the neonatal mortality rate used to generate the number of expected deaths. Based on this rate, the expected number of deaths for home births attended by physicians, CNMs, and MMA midwives was 3.92. The actual number of deaths (5) was not significantly different from the expected number.

Washington, 1981–1990

A study based on linked birth and infant death certificates for Washington State compared outcomes for 6,944 out-of-hospital births attended by licensed direct-entry midwives (LMs) with outcomes for 23,596 low-risk hospital births attended by physicians, 14,777 spontaneous vaginal births attended by CNMs in hospitals, and 4,054 births attended by nurse-midwives in out-of-hospital settings (Janssen *et al.*, 1994). The low-risk physician-birth group was created by excluding from all in-hospital births attended by physicians those women who would have been ineligible for a midwife-attended home

Table 11

Outcomes for Births Attended by Midwives in Washington State, by Birth Site, 1981–1990, and for a Low-Risk In-Hospital Physician Care Comparison Group

	Low Birth Weight (per 1,000 births)	5-Minute Apgar Score <7 (per 1,000 births)	Neonatal Mortality (per 1,000 births)
All midwife births and low-risk MD births:			
MDs in-hospital	16.5	10.0	1.0
CNMs in-hospital	20.4*	10.1	1.6
CNMs nonhospital	8.9	9.9	1.7
LMs nonhospital	10.9	10.8	1.7
Reanalysis with high-risk women excluded from the midwifery groups:			
MDs in-hospital	16.5*	10.0	1.0
CNMs in-hospital	10.8	9.5	0.6
CNMs nonhospital	6.5	9.3	1.3
LMs nonhospital	9.1	10.4	1.4

*Statistically significant difference between this rate and the rate for births attended by licensed midwives.

Data are from Janssen *et al.*, 1994. Reprinted with permission.

birth due to complications noted on the birth certificate. The researchers then matched four low-risk in-hospital/physician births to every LM birth based on maternal age and the year and county in which the birth occurred. Outcomes examined were low birth weight,* low five-minute Apgar scores, neonatal mortality (death during the first twenty-eight days), and postneonatal mortality (from twenty-nine days to one year of age). Outcomes for births attended by LMs were compared with those for each other category of births.

Preliminary analysis revealed that some LMs were attending births of women with high-risk conditions, including twins and babies in breech presentation. Therefore, the comparisons were made twice. All of the midwives' clients were included in the first comparison. Women who would have been excluded from the in-hospital physician care group because of serious complications were excluded from the midwife care groups during the second comparison. Twelve percent of the in-hospital CNM births were excluded on this basis, as well as 7 percent of the LM births and 5 percent of the out-of-hospital births attended by nurse-midwives.

The findings are presented in Table 11.[†] The rates were adjusted to account for differences between the groups in maternal age, parity, smoking, county of birth, and timing of first prenatal care. Relative risks[‡]

*However, babies born before thirty-seven weeks gestation were excluded from the in-hospital physician care group.

[†]Data on postneonatal deaths were also analyzed. However, postneonatal mortality is usually associated with environmental and parenting problems, rather than problems related to the pregnancy and birth. Therefore this information is not included in Table 11.

[‡]Relative risk describes the incidence of a particular outcome in one group as compared with another.

were calculated to compare the incidence of each outcome for births attended by LMs with the incidence of the same outcome in each of the other groups. An asterisk has been placed by the rate for the other group if the difference between it and the rate for LM births met tests of statistical significance. Only two of the differences were statistically significant. Babies whose births were attended by LMs were much less likely than babies delivered by CNMs in hospitals to be low birth weight (LBW). This difference was due primarily to the large proportion of in-hospital CNM clients who have high-risk conditions; removing them from the analysis almost halved the LBW rate for CNM in-hospital births. When high-risk births were removed from the LM group, the low birthweight rate was reduced enough to make the difference between LM and physician births statistically significant (Janssen *et al.*, 1994).

A lower LBW rate for babies delivered by midwives should not be interpreted as evidence that the prenatal care provided by the midwives prevented some cases of low birth weight. Low birth weight can usually be predicted, and it is a very serious complication. Midwives should and do refer women who develop complications that retard infant growth and women who go into labor before term to physicians. Theoretically the LBW rate for midwives should be close to zero. It is not zero because some cases of borderline low birth weight may not be predicted and some babies may be so close to the 2,500 gram definition of low birth weight that a referral is not needed. In addition, many nurse-midwives who deliver babies in hospitals work in close partnership with physicians on busy obstetric units. Although the CNM may deliver the baby, the labor of a woman in preterm labor may have been managed in large part by an obstetrician, and the nurse-midwife may have handed the baby to a pediatrician as soon as it was born.

This study is limited, because we have no information on the incidence of fetal deaths during labor. Although the neonatal mortality rate for all categories of midwife-attended births was low, it was 60 to 70 percent higher than the rate for low-risk women whose births were attended by physicians in hospitals. The difference was not statistically significant. Neonatal mortality associated with all categories of midwife births was increased by the inclusion of high-risk women among their clientele. When high-risk women were eliminated from the data, the neonatal mortality rates for out-of-hospital births attended by either kind of midwife were more than twice as high as the neonatal mortality rate for births attended by CNMs in hospitals. Nevertheless, the neonatal mortality rates associated with out-of-hospital births were low and were the same whether the midwife was a licensed direct-entry midwife or a CNM.

Toronto, Ontario, 1983–1988

This study was described briefly in the section on Canada. All twenty-six midwives known to have practiced in Toronto from 1983 through 1988 agreed to participate in a retrospective study that was intended to include all planned home births attended by midwives during that period. The participants retrieved the clinical records of all clients who were under their care during that time, with the exception of women whom they had referred to other care before the onset of labor. Data were collected from the clinical records and interviews with the midwives. The study reported on more than a thousand births, and the outcomes were excellent. Although midwifery was not illegal in Ontario during the period of this study, it was not regulated by law. However, most of the midwives were members of a local midwifery association, which set and implemented its own standards. (See discussion of midwifery in Ontario in Chapter 13.)

Vermont, 1989–1994

Approximately 2 percent of births in Vermont occur in out-of-hospital locations; Vermont's rate is twice as high as the national average and was consistent from 1989 through 1994.

Almost three-fourths of the 919 nonhospital births in Vermont during the six-year period from 1989 through 1994 were attended by direct-entry midwives (Vermont Vital Statistics System, 1996). Physicians attended 9 percent, CNMs only 1.2 percent. Most of the remaining out-of-hospital births were attended by family members, emergency medical technicians, and nurses. Information on fetal deaths during labor is not available. Based on the information contained in birth and infant death certificates, there were no neonatal deaths associated with nonhospital births in Vermont during this period of time.

National Data for 1989

Information from birth certificates filed in the United States during 1989 was used to calculate the incidence of low birth weight and low Apgar scores for babies delivered by CNMs in hospitals, birth centers, and homes and for births attended by direct-entry midwives in birth centers and homes. Data from *all* births in 1989 were used for comparison (Declercq, 1995).*

The incidence of low birth weight was lower for all groups of babies delivered by midwives than for all births in the United States (Table 12). The low incidence of low

---

*An earlier paper by the same author described the demographic characteristics of the mothers (Declercq, 1993). The information is summarized in Tables 4 and 5 in Chapter 7. Almost all of the women who had out-of-hospital births attended by midwives were married and white. They were less likely than other women to be having their first baby; this was especially true for those having home births, who tended to be older, high-parity women. Nurse-midwives' out-of-hospital birth clients were relatively well educated. Most of the women who used birth centers operated by direct-entry midwives were Hispanic and had relatively little education. Nurse-midwives who delivered babies in hospitals took care of a disproportionate number of women who were black, unmarried, still in their teens, and had not finished high school (all characteristics that are strongly associated with low birth weight). Women who had given birth to a LBW baby during a previous pregnancy were most likely to have their 1989 birth in a hospital attended by a nurse-midwife; they were least likely to have a home birth attended by a direct-entry midwife.

birth weight is to be expected based on the demographic characteristics of women having out-of-hospital births, and because most midwives refer women who go into preterm labor to physicians. In considering the other outcomes shown in Table 12, we must remember that the comparison group is *all* births, including very high-risk, complicated pregnancies that are inappropriate for midwifery care and generate the most bad outcomes. "All births" also includes women who began their care with midwives but were referred to physicians prenatally or during labor because of complications. In addition, this study, like the one from Washington, dealt with low birth weight as an outcome rather than as a risk factor for low Apgar scores. *The risk of neonatal death for LBW infants is 40 times higher than the rate for infants weighing at least 2500 grams at birth* (McCormick, 1985). Therefore, we should expect the incidence of low Apgar scores to be much higher for all U.S. births, which included all of the LBW babies, than for any group of births attended by midwives.

This study can tell us something about the outcomes for births attended by different kinds of midwives in different settings. However, it can tell us little about the relative effectiveness of midwifery care versus medical care. Because the study was based on birth certificates alone (not linked with infant death certificates), it could not provide information on mortality. The incidence of low Apgar scores was lowest for CNM births in birth centers and homes. The rates for births attended by CNMs in hospitals were lower than the rates for both kinds of direct-entry births, despite a higher incidence of low birth weight.

Data on the Safety of Births in Free-Standing Birth Centers

Free-standing birth centers were developed as a place for the practice of midwifery. During the 1980s they organized in order to develop a system of supports to enhance the

Table 12
Low Birth Weight and Apgar Scores for Births Attended by Midwives, United States, 1989

Birth Site and Attendant	Number of Births	Percent Low Birth Weight	Percent One-Minute Apgar Scores <7	Percent Five-Minute Apgar Scores <7
CNMs/hospitals	122,927	3.5	7.4	0.9
CNMs/birth centers	5,680	1.3	5.4	0.4*
CNMs/homes	3,416	2.2	5.4	0.7*
DEMs†/birth centers	4,485	1.9	8.8	1.4*
DEMs/homes	8,193	1.7	8.0	1.1
All U.S. births	4,040,958	7.0	8.8	1.6

*Fewer than twenty infants had these outcomes. With such low numbers, the percentages are very unstable.
†DEMs = direct-entry midwives.
Data are from Declercq, 1995.

quality of care provided in birth centers. In the mid-1980s the National Association of Childbearing Centers conducted a large prospective study to describe birth center clients, care, and outcomes and determine the safety of birth center care. Because few poor outcomes were expected among a clientele screened to exclude women with recognizable high-risk conditions, a large study was needed. Data were collected on nearly 18,000 women who obtained care at eighty-four birth centers throughout the country from mid-1985 through 1987. CNMs provided most of the care in most of the birth centers in the study. Two-thirds of the women who started care at one of these centers were admitted to the centers in labor. Nearly half of the other third were referred to another source of care because of a prenatal complication. The others left birth center care for a variety of reasons (Rooks *et al.*, 1992a).

Almost 12,000 women were admitted to the birth centers for labor and delivery. As a group, they tended to be at lower-than-average risk of a poor pregnancy outcome based on most of the recognized demographic and behavioral risk factors. Most of the women (71 percent) had no complications or only minor complications, but 8 percent had serious complications. One woman in six (16 percent) was transferred to a hospital; 2.4 percent had transfers that were considered to be emergencies. Women having their first baby were four times more likely to be transferred (29 percent versus 7 percent), but the difference was due entirely to non-emergency transfers. Nulliparous women were no more likely than parous women to have an emergency transfer. The cesarean section rate was 4.4 percent. Although 46 percent of the women who had cesarean sections consumed nonclear fluids or solid food during labor, none of them aspirated during anesthesia* (Rooks *et al.*, 1992b). There was very complete follow-up of the women and babies who were transferred. There were no maternal deaths. There were few LBW, preterm or postterm births, but a relatively high proportion of very large babies. There were 15 intrapartum and neonatal deaths among 11,826 infants born to the women admitted to the birth centers, a rate of 1.3 deaths per 1,000 births. Seven of the babies that died had lethal congenital anomalies. The mortality rate for babies without lethal

---

†See Chapter 10 for information on the controversy regarding withholding food and fluids during labor.

anomalies was 0.7 per 1000 births (Rooks *et al.*, 1989).

The proportion of low Apgar scores and the intrapartum and neonatal mortality rates for infants born to women using the birth centers were compared to rates reported in five studies of low-risk hospital births. Each of the comparison studies created a low-risk pregnancy data set by excluding women with certain characteristics and outcomes from a large database, (e.g., twins, breech presentations, repeat cesarean sections and significant medical or prenatal complications). Some of the studies also excluded women with certain intrapartum complications. Four of the low-risk hospital birth studies reported both intrapartum and neonatal deaths. The lowest combined rate (intrapartum + neonatal deaths) was 1.0 deaths per 1,000 births, reported by an academic hospital in Dallas. The low-risk group used for that study excluded women with induced or "complicated" labors, in addition to the usual exclusions. It was the only study that found a lower rate than was found for the birth center clients. All of the other studies found mortality rates that were a little higher than the rate for the birth center mothers. The cesarean section rate for the birth center clients was very low—only about half the rates reported in studies of low-risk hospital births (Rooks *et al.*, 1989).

There was a very high degree of satisfaction with the care provided at these birth centers; 99 percent of the women who completed evaluations (76 percent of the total) said that they would recommend the birth center they had used to their friends. The researchers concluded that birth centers can identify women who are at low risk for obstetric complications and can care for them in a way that offers safety comparable to that provided in hospitals with fewer cesarean sections, lower cost, and a high degree of client satisfaction (Rooks *et al.*, 1989).

This was a very rigorous prospective study involving a large number of birth centers and women. Follow-up was very complete and the data are reliable. Studies of births in free-standing birth centers during the 1970s and early 1980s had found somewhat higher rates (Bennetts & Lubic, 1982; Eakins & Richwald, 1986). The lower rate found during the National Birth Center Study (1985–1987) may indicate a trend toward greater safety, reflecting the implementation of state regulation and licensure, accreditation, peer review, and continuing education programs during the 1980s.

Another study used the National Birth Center Study (NBCS) data collection form to collect prospective data on more than two thousand low-risk women who had babies in hospitals during the same period. The care providers for the in-hospital group were nurse-midwives and physicians who profess a supportive, family-centered, low-intervention philosophy of care. Some of them attend births in both hospitals and birth centers and were participating in the NBCS. They wanted to collect data on their in-hospital clients in order to determine whether the site of care makes a difference if the care provider has a midwifery approach to childbirth (Fullerton & Severino, 1992). Outcomes from this study were compared to findings from the NBCS. Women in both groups experienced similar rates of health problems during their pregnancies; however, there were some sociodemographic differences. Women in the hospital group were less likely to be Hispanic and more likely to be unmarried; they tended to be younger and less educated, and more of them smoked. Even when the data were controlled to account for these differences, the women cared for in hospitals received more interventions during labor and delivery compared with the women in birth centers. Women having hospital births were more likely to experience long-lasting fetal distress or cord prolapse during labor, and their babies were more likely to need assistance breathing immediately after being born. However, the incidence of low Apgar scores was low and similar to that in the NBCS. The outcomes in both studies were good.

Women cared for in birth centers achieved their good outcomes with much lower rates of intervention during labor and delivery.

Two studies have compared outcomes in specific birth centers to outcomes for a group of women who had hospital births in the same city during the same time period and were screened to exclude women who would not have been eligible for admission to the birth center (Feldman & Hurst, 1987) or were matched to the birth center clients on specific characteristics (Scupholme *et al.*, 1986). One of these studies compared the care and outcomes for seventy-seven women with normal term pregnancies who used a birth center in New York City with those for seventy-two low-risk women who delivered at a large nearby teaching hospital and would have been eligible for care at the birth center (Feldman & Hurst, 1987). Women receiving care at the hospital were more likely to have oxytocin augmentation, amniotomy, EFM, IVs, epidurals, episiotomies, and forceps deliveries. The rate of forceps deliveries at the hospital was a shocking 44 percent, compared to 6 percent for women at the birth center (actually at a hospital after being transferred from the birth center). The use of narcotic analgesia was similar in both groups. The cesarean section rate for the birth center clients (after transfers, of course) was 6.5 percent, compared with 11.3 percent for the control group. Although the womens' labors tended to last longer at the birth center, the incidence of thick meconium in the amniotic fluid (a potential sign of fetal distress) and fetal heart rate abnormalities suggesting fetal distress were much higher at the hospital, and 6 percent of the babies born to the hospital control group mothers were transferred to the neonatal intensive care unit, compared with only 1.3 percent of babies born to the birth center mothers.

In the other study, 250 women who chose to have their care at a birth center associated with a public hospital in Miami were matched with a control group of 250 women who gave birth in the hospital. The women were matched on age, parity, ethnic background, and financial status, but could not be matched on education. The birth center mothers tended to have more education. Although some birth center clients were transferred to the hospital in order to receive oxytocin, the control group women were twice as likely to receive oxytocin and were almost three times as likely to have shoulder dystocia—when the baby's shoulders get stuck after the head is delivered (Scupholme *et al.*, 1986). Shortly after this study was completed, the obstetric service at the hospital became overcrowded and began to *assign* low-risk women to the birth center. This made it possible to conduct a study to determine whether the good outcomes found during the first study were due to the tendency of better educated women to select the birth center as their source of care (Scupholme & Kamons, 1987). Outcomes for 148 women assigned to the birth center were compared to those of 148 women who had chosen to use the birth center; the two groups were matched on ethnicity, parity, financial status, and education. The researchers anticipated that the women assigned to the birth center might have more complications because they were less motivated about self-care and might be a nxious about having an out-of-hospital birth. In fact, there were no significant differences in any measure between the two groups of women. Most women assigned to the birth center returned for subsequent babies and many referred their relatives and friends.

Data on the Safety of Out-of-Hospital Births Attended by Direct-Entry Midwives

There have been few published studies of the outcomes of out-of-hospital births attended by direct-entry midwives in North America. Aside from the studies conducted in

Arizona and Toronto and studies based on birth and death certificates, all other data on the outcomes of direct-entry midwifery practice come from specific home birth services and practices, including some studies that combine data from several or many practices.

A study of 287 home births attended by midwives associated with the Santa Cruz Birth Center was published in 1975 (Mehl *et al.*, 1975), and a study reporting outcomes for 1,707 women whose care was provided by the midwives at the Farm (in Tennessee) was published in 1992 (Durand, 1992). These studies reported on two of the earliest and best known direct-entry midwife practices; the origins of both are described in Chapter 4. The Santa Cruz study reported on the first few years of a birth center that closed during the 1970s. The Farm study reported on all births at the Farm from 1971 to 1989. (The Farm is still in operation.) Two other published studies either combined data from home births attended by direct-entry midwives with data on home births attended by physicians (Mehl *et al.*, 1977) or reported on a practice in which an obstetrician and direct-entry midwife attended home births together (Koehler *et al.*, 1984). There have also been at least two unpublished studies of direct-entry midwifery outcomes (Booker, 1991; Carney, 1990). In addition, several studies have compared outcomes of births attended by direct-entry midwives and/ or family physicians with outcomes for matched control groups of similar women who had either home or hospital births attended by physicians (Mehl, 1977; Mehl *et al.*, 1980; Mehl-Madrona & Madrona, 1997). The most recent study used a large, cumulative data set, some part of which had been included in the analysis for earlier studies, to examine the effect of attending breech, twin, and postdate births on mortality associated with home births (Mehl-Madrona & Madrona, 1997).

Except for the study from the Farm and the report on the joint MD/midwife practice, all other published studies reporting outcomes of births attended by direct-entry midwives were conducted by Dr. Lewis Mehl (now Mehl-Madrona), who has published many papers based on home birth data he has been collecting since 1973. In addition to data on births attended by midwives, he collected data on home births attended by family physicians in northern California and in the area surrounding Madison, Wisconsin, during the 1970s, and data on low-risk births attended by physicians in hospitals in California and Wisconsin. He uses the hospital-birth data to form matched control groups for assessing the outcomes of home births. The same form was used for collecting all of these data. Some of the data on midwife births were recorded prospectively by the midwives who attended the births; data on some of the births were collected by retrospective chart review. The data on physician births were recorded by Dr. Mehl-Madrona or a research assistant from records in the doctors' offices or in the hospitals (Mehl-Madrona & Madrona, 1997).

The Midwives Alliance of North America (MANA) is conducting both retrospective and prospective studies of births attended by more than three hundred of its members. Data have been collected on more than six thousand births. Eighty-eight percent of the women were planning to have home births; 6 percent were planning to give birth in a birth center. Eight percent were planning to have hospital births. (Because some MANA members are nurse-midwives, the data set includes some births attended by CNMs.) A report of the findings from these studies is not available yet. See Chapter 6 for additional information on the design of these studies.

Data on the Safety of Home Births Attended by CNMs

A paper reporting outcomes from two nurse-midwifery home birth practices was published in 1991 (Anderson & Greener, 1991), and the ACNM Home Birth Committee published a large retrospective study based on data from ninety CNM home birth practices in 1995 (Anderson & Murphy, 1995). The ACNM's Home Birth Committee is also conducting a smaller, prospective study of home births attended by nurse-midwives. An intense effort to identify all CNMs who provide home birth services yielded a list of 157, including 121 nurse-midwives with solo home birth practices and 36 CNMs who are members of fifteen group practices (Anderson & Murphy, 1995). Survey forms mailed to everyone on the list were completed and returned by nurse-midwives representing two-thirds of these practices—78 solo practitioners and twelve group practices. The nurse-midwives who participated in the retrospective study were practicing in twenty-nine different states. In addition to the data describing their clients, and the care and outcomes of nearly twelve thousand home births attended by CNMs, the survey provides information on the practice protocols, risk-screening practices, and emergency preparedness of nurse-midwives who attend home births. This information is summarized in Chapter 8.

During the period of this study (1987–1991) the ninety CNM practices that participated in the study provided care to 11,788 women who were planning to have home births. Births included in the study account for 61 to 72 percent of all home births attended by CNMs from 1989 through 1991. Six percent of the women were referred to other care providers because of complications diagnosed during the prenatal period or because of preterm labor. Ninety-four percent of the women who began prenatal care with one of these practices were still intending to have a home birth when they went into labor ($N = 11,081$). Ten percent of those women, or their newborns, were transferred to hospitals during labor or shortly after the birth: 8.2 percent were transferred during labor (most frequently for failure to progress); 0.8 percent were transferred after the birth because of a problem involving the

mother; and 1.0 percent were transferred after the birth because of a problem involving the newborn. Detailed follow-up information was provided for 96 percent of the transfers. There were no maternal deaths. There were 8 fetal deaths during labor and 15 neonatal deaths; the combined intrapartum/neonatal mortality rate was 2 per 1,000 births. Twelve of the deaths were babies with lethal congenital anomalies; the mortality rates for babies without serious anomalies were 0.7 fetal deaths during labor + 0.27 neonatal deaths = 1.0 per 1,000 births (Anderson & Murphy, 1995).

Mortality Rates as the Primary Measure of Safety

This chapter is about the safety of out-of-hospital births in the United States. The bottom line for safety is mortality. This section is about mortality. Information on deaths associated with childbearing is expressed as rates. The mortality rates used in this discussion, and elsewhere in this book, are defined as follows:

- The *maternal mortality ratio* is the number of women who die as a result of pregnancy per 100,000 live births.
- The *infant mortality rate* is the number of infants who die before reaching one year of age per 1,000 live births. Infant mortality includes neonatal deaths, which occur during the first twenty-eight days of life, and postneonatal deaths—deaths of infants who are at least twenty-nine days old but have not reached their first birthday. The *neonatal mortality rate* is the number of neonatal deaths per 1,000 live births. The *postneonatal mortality rate* is the number of postneonatal deaths per 1,000 live births. Most neonatal deaths are caused by problems associated with the pregnancy and birth. Postneonatal deaths are more likely to be caused by other influences, including the quality of infant nutrition and child

care and environmental safety. Babies who are born dead are not included in either the numerator or the denominator of the infant, neonatal, and postneonatal mortality rates.

- Intrapartum deaths are fetal deaths that occur during labor and delivery. The *intrapartum mortality rate* is the number of fetal deaths during labor per 1,000 births. Intrapartum deaths are also referred to as "stillbirths." The denominator for this rate includes all of the births, not only those in which the baby is alive when it is born.
- This book uses "total mortality" as a shorter term that includes fetal deaths during labor (intrapartum deaths) and infant deaths during the first twenty-eight days of life (neonatal deaths). The *total mortality rate* is the number of intrapartum and neonatal deaths per 1,000 births (total births, not just live births).
- Many books, and some of the research reports on which this summary is based, use "perinatal mortality" or the "perinatal mortality rate" to include intrapartum and neonatal deaths. However, perinatal deaths also include late fetal deaths that occur before the onset of labor, as well as fetal deaths during labor and infant deaths during the first twenty-eight days of life. Reporting of fetal deaths at all phases of pregnancy is very incomplete; thus the *perinatal mortality rate* (the number of perinatal deaths per 1,000 total births) is not very reliable. In addition, because this chapter is about the safety of labor and delivery in nonhospital birth sites, fetal deaths that occur before the onset of labor are not at issue. The term is rarely used in this book.

Maternal Mortality

None of the studies summarized in this chapter reported any maternal deaths, which are relatively rare in the United States. Maternal deaths have resulted from home births and births in free-standing birth centers; the inci-

dence is unknown, but is probably very low. In-hospital deaths caused by anesthesia and other complications of cesarean sections are a much more significant source of maternal mortality in the United States.

Intrapartum and Neonatal Mortality

Intrapartum and neonatal mortality rates from studies of the safety of out-of-hospital births in North America are summarized in Table 13. This section explains the organization of Table 13 and provides some information on the studies.

An attempt was made to include findings from all published studies of out-of-hospital births attended by midwives in the United States and Canada. This effort was assisted by access to information from a thorough search for home birth studies being conducted by investigators at the University of Texas Health Science Center at San Antonio (Fullerton, 1996). Findings from some studies are not included in the table because they were redundant with other studies and thus would not add to our understanding of the relatively safety of out-of-hospital births. Because the several studies by Dr. Lewis Mehl (now Mehl-Madrona) were based on an accumulating data set, data from only the final, largest data sets are presented: data on 3,545 home births attended by forty-six direct-entry midwives in eight states from 1970 through 1985, and data on 4,107 home births attended by family physicians in two states from 1969 through 1981 (Mehl-Madrona, 1996/1997). The NBCS is the only birth center study included in Table 13, and, except for information on out-of-hospital births attended by CNMs in the study of all births in Washington State in 1981–1990 (data shown in Table 11), and data from the entire U.S. in 1989 (data shown in Table 12), the ACNM Home Birth Committee study is the only study of CNM home births included in Table 13. Both of the studies shown in the second part of Table 13 reported on more than eleven thousand births and included the majority of practitioners in its category.

Table 13

Mortality Rates from Studies of Planned Out-of-Hospital Births Attended by Midwives, Selected Studies of Other Planned Out-of-Hospital Births, and Low-Risk Births Attended by Physicians in Hospitals for Comparison Purposes, Studies Conducted in North America, 1969–1994*

Location	Years	Number of Births	Birth Attendants	Intrapartum Mortality Rate†	Neonatal Mortality Rate**	Total Mortality Rate†
Data on All Out-of-Hospital Births Attended by Specified Categories of Midwives in a Particular Geographic Area						
North Carolina[1]	1974–76	768	DEMs	NA	4.0 (0.0)	??
Arizona[2]	1978–81	1,449	Licensed DEMs	1.4	1.4 (0.0)	2.8 (1.4)
Missouri[3]	1978–84	725	Unrecognized DEMs	NA	8.3	??
		1,770	MDs, DEMs, and CNMs	NA	2.8	??
Washington[4]	1981–90	6,944	Licensed DEMs	NA	1.7	??
		4,054	CNMs	NA	1.7	??
Toronto, Ontario[5]	1983–88	1,001	DEMs	0.0	(2.0)	(2.0)
Vermont[6]	1989–94	678	DEMs	NA	0.0	??
National Studies That Tried to Include All Practices in a Certain Category						
Eighty-four birth centers[7]	1985–87	11,826	81% CNMs + MDs + DEMs	0.4 (0.3)	0.8 (0.3)	1.3 (0.7)
Term births		9,871	81% CNMs + MDs + DEMs	0.2 (0.2)	0.7 (0.3)	0.9 (0.5)
Postterm		1,306	81% CNMs + MDs + DEMs	1.5 (1.5)	2.3 (0.8)	3.8 (2.3)
Ninety home birth practices[8]	1987–91	11,081	CNMs	0.7 (0.7)	1.4 (0.3)	2.0 (0.9)
Studies of Selected Out-of-Hospital Birth Practices: Births Attended by Direct-Entry Midwives and/or Family Physicians						
Eight states[9]	1970–85	3,545	46 DEMs	5.4	5.9	9.9
Vermont[10]	1981–85	253	DEMs	7.9 (7.9)	7.9 (4.0)	15.8 (11.9)
California[11]	1985–91	461	DEMs	0.0	0.0	0.0
Sonoma Co., California[12]	1976–82	453	1 OB + 1 DEM	2.2	2.2	4.4

Study	Years	N	Attendant	†Fetal deaths during labor	**Intrapartum & neonatal mortality	‡Infant deaths
The Farm, Tennessee[13]	1971–89	1,707	DEMs, MDs, Amish midwives	NA	NA	8.8 (5.4)***
California and Wisconsin[9]	1969–81	4,107	Family physicians	1.7	4.1	5.8
Urban Ontario[14]	1976–86	280	One family physician	0.0	7.1 (3.6)	7.1 (3.6)

Low-Risk Births Attended by Physicians in Hospitals

Study	Years	N	Attendant	†Fetal deaths during labor	**Intrapartum & neonatal mortality	‡Infant deaths
One academic hospital[15]	1969–75	12,055	Obstetricians	NA	(0.5–1.1)	??
One community hospital[16]	1974–75	4,144	Physicians	1.0	3.4	4.3
Fifteen hospitals[17]	1977–79	10,521	Physicians	NA	1.7	??
National sample[18]	1980	2,935	Physicians	NA	2.5	??
All in Washington[4]	1981–90	23,596	Physicians	NA	1.0	??
One academic hospital[19]	1982–85	14,618	Obstetricians	0.0	1.0	1.0
Twelve hospitals[20]	1982–85					
Term births		8,135	Physicians	0.0	2.1 (1.9)	2.1 (1.9)
Postterm		3,457	Physicians	0.0	2.6 (2.1)	2.6 (2.1)

* This table can only be properly interpreted in conjunction with an understanding of the accompanying written text. Using the table in isolation is likely to result in misinterpretation. There were significant differences between the studies shown on this table related to the socioeconomic status of the women and screening criteria.

Key: NA = Data not available; DEM = direct-entry midwives. Numbers in parentheses are mortality rates excluding fetuses and infants with lethal congenital anomalies.

†Fetal deaths during labor per 1,000 births.

**Intrapartum mortality and neonatal mortality per 1,000 births.

‡Infant deaths during the first 28 days of life per 1,000 live births.

***Rate based on all women who initiated prenatal care at the Farm, including some twins and breech deliveries, many women of low socioeconomic status, and thirty-one women who were referred to hospital care prior to the onset of labor. See discussion on pages 368 and 369.

References: [1]Burnett et al., 1980; [2]Sullivan & Beeman et al., 1983; [3]Schramm et al., 1987; [4]Janssen et al., 1994; [5]Tyson, 1991; [6]Vermont Vital Statistics System, 1996; [7]Rooks et al., 1989; [8]Anderson & Murphy, 1995; [9]unpublished mortality rates from the data set used in Mehl-Madrona & Madrona, 1997; [10]Carney, 1990; [11]Booker, 1991; [12]Koehler et al., 1984; [13]Durand, 1992; [14]Schneider & Soderstrom, 1987; [15]Neutra et al., 1978; [16]Amato, 1977; [17]Adams, 1983; [18]See discussion, page 371; [19]Leveno et al., 1986; [20]Eden et al., 1987.

The NBCS reported findings from 52 percent of all birth centers in operation from mid-1985 through 1987. The ACNM home birth study included from 61 to 72 percent of all home births attended by CNMs from 1989 through 1991. Although other studies of both kind of births have been published, their findings are similar to findings in the much larger, more inclusive studies.

Table 13 presents information on the intrapartum and neonatal mortality rates found during fifteen studies of out-of-hospital births attended by midwives or physicians in North America between 1969 and 1991 and similar information from seven studies of low-risk women who gave birth in U.S. hospitals between 1969 and 1990.* The studies are presented in four categories. Within each group, the studies are presented in a general chronological order and by the kind of care provider.

- Data from the six previously described area-wide studies or data sets are presented at the top of the table. The data from North Carolina, Arizona, Missouri, Washington, and Toronto were presented in published papers. The data from Vermont was provided by staff of the Vermont Vital Statistics System at the request of the author of this book. A small, unpublished prospective study from Vermont (included in the third set of studies in Table 13) had found very high levels of both intrapartum and neonatal mortality during the early 1980s. More recent data was requested to determine whether current direct-entry practice in Vermont was generating a high level of mortality. No neonatal deaths were reported in Vermont during this later period (1989–1994). No data are available to determine whether any *intrapartum* deaths were associated with home births attended by direct-entry midwives in Vermont during that period. These data also cannot account for deaths that occur in a hospital after the mother is transferred in from an out-of-hospital birth. These limitations apply to all except two of the six data sets in this group. Only the studies from Arizona and Toronto can provide information on fetal deaths during labor, as well as neonatal deaths.

- The next group includes the NBCS and the ACNM Home Birth Committee study. Both were large national studies that tried to include all members of their class.

- The third group includes seven studies that were based on data from one or more specific out-of-hospital birth practices or services.
  —The first three lines of data are based on home births attended by direct-entry midwives.
  —The next line presents data from a practice in which a midwife and physician attended home births together.
  —The next line presents data from the Farm, in Tennessee. It is presented separately because the situation at the Farm is unique in many ways: Although direct-entry midwives attend most births that take place at the Farm, the data set includes births attended by physicians who work with the midwives. Some women who have had no prenatal care go to the Farm for the first time when they are in labor. Local physicians have asked the Farm midwives to serve a nearby Old Order Amish community, in which many of the births are to very high-parity women. Farm midwives and physicians also provide emergency backup for Amish midwives, who attend some births in that community. Some Amish families refuse to go to a hospital, even when there is a serious complication. All of the Amish births

---

*Several other studies of out-of-hospital births during this period have been published. Their findings are not shown in Table 13 because the detailed information needed for the table was not provided in the published report of the study.

were included in the study. The Farm midwives attend births involving some kinds of complications; a local physician taught them how to manage breech presentations and twins and provides backup during complicated births. The study followed all women who initiated prenatal care at the Farm, including some who were referred to hospitals before the onset of labor. The Farm study includes data on every pregnant woman attended by the Farm midwives during the first eighteen years after the community was started, beginning with the very first births, when the "midwives" had little (virtually no) experience (Gaskin, 1996). And, in addition to attending home births, the Farm operates a birth center and owned an ambulance (until a regular ambulance service became available in that community). Thus these data reflect a wide spectrum of births, birth sites, and birth attendants; include some very high-risk births; and cover a long period of time. The mortality rate would probably be lower if the study had been limited to births during the last ten years. Ina May Gaskin, who leads the Farm midwifery services, has become well-known for her expertise.

—The next two lines in this group present data from two studies of home births attended by family physicians— mortality rates from Dr. Mehl-Madrona's data on 4,107 home births attended by family physicians in California and Wisconsin, and data from a study of 280 planned home births attended within one FP practice in Ontario.

• Findings from seven studies of low-risk deliveries in hospitals are summarized at the bottom of the table. Data from six of these studies were used to provide context for findings from the NBCS (Rooks *et al.*, 1992c). The seventh low-risk in-

hospital birth group came from the study conducted in Washington State from 1981 through 1990 (Jannsen *et al.*, 1994). Data from these studies provide a frame of reference for the mortality rates found during studies of out-of-hospital births. These studies are described in greater detail in the following section on Comparison Groups.

The Farm study gave the total mortality rate, but did not break it down into intrapartum versus neonatal deaths. All of the other studies represented in Table 13 reported neonatal deaths, if any. Except for studies based solely on birth and death certificate data (four of the six area-wide studies), all of the other out-of-hospital birth studies also reported intrapartum deaths, if any, thus allowing calculation of the total mortality rate (intrapartum plus neonatal deaths per one thousand births). "NA," meaning that the information is not available, is filled in as the intrapartum mortality rate for those studies that did not report it; in that situation, question marks are inserted in the space for the total mortality rate, which is unknown.

A large proportion of the deaths associated with low-risk births are due to congenital anomalies. If the studies distinguished between deaths due to congenital anomalies and all other deaths, the mortality rates excluding deaths from lethal anomalies are presented in parentheses.

A few studies included fetal deaths that occurred prior to labor in their results. The rates presented in Table 13 are based only on intrapartum mortality and neonatal mortality; thus some of the rates are different from those presented in the referenced reports.

Comparison Groups

Most of the published papers provided some kind of comparison for the mortality found during the study, if only to note that the home birth mortality rate was lower than the rate for all births in the state or local community. Some of the studies presented more complicated comparisons, as discussed next.

The study of home births in Missouri compared the number of neonatal deaths associated with home births attended by physicians, CNMs, and qualified direct-entry midwives with the number of deaths one would expect if their clients experienced the same mortality rate as *all* women who had hospital births attended by physicians in Missouri during the same time period, that is, not just women having low-risk births. The actual number of intrapartum and neonatal deaths was 5; the expected number, based on the rate for in-hospital births was 3.92. The two numbers were not significantly different (Schramm *et al.*, 1987).

The study from Washington State compared the neonatal mortality rate associated with out-of-hospital births attended by licensed direct-entry midwives with rates for births attended by CNMs and rates for low-risk in-hospital births attended by physicians; differences between the rates were not statistically significant (Janssen *et al.*, 1994).

The Farm study compared outcomes for women who initiated prenatal care at the Farm with outcomes in a data set developed by excluding women who would have been ineligible for care at the Farm from a national sample based on all fetal death and birth certificates filed in the United States in 1980.* Because women with twins, breech presentations, and some other kinds of complications are not automatically excluded

from care at the Farm, women with those complications were not excluded from the comparison group. In addition, LBW births and fetal deaths had been deliberately oversampled in the national survey used as a basis for the comparison group. The Farm study used data analysis methods to compensate for the oversampling. Nevertheless, the cesarean delivery rate for the comparison group was more than 60 percent higher than the rate for the nation as a whole during the year of the survey—26.6 percent, compared with 16.5 percent for the entire United States in 1980. It is not clear why the cesarean rate for the comparison group was so high. The perinatal mortality rate for women in the comparison group was not significantly different from that associated with births at the Farm, for which the cesarean delivery rate was only 1.5 percent (Durand, 1992).

The studies of low-risk births attended by physicians in hospitals (i.e., the data presented at the bottom of Table 13), provide a general frame of reference for making judgments about the mortality rates reported in the studies of out-of-hospital births. Each of the comparison studies created a low-risk pregnancy data set by excluding women with certain characteristics or outcomes from a larger database. Mothers of LBW infants and women with multiple gestations, nonvertex presentations, repeat cesarean sections, or significant medical or prenatal complications were excluded from most if not all of the comparison studies.

---

*The comparison group for the Farm study was derived by deleting women who had no prenatal care, out-of-hospital births, nonphysician birth attendants, prepregnancy diabetes or hypertension, anemia (hematocrit lower than 28), Rh negative blood with positive antibody screen, or weight greater than 135 kilograms from the data set resulting from the 1980 U.S. National Natality/National Fetal Mortality Survey (NNS/NFMS). The survey was based on a probability sample of all births that occurred in the United States during 1980 for which a birth or fetal death certificate had been filed.

- The first study (12,055 births at an academic hospital, 1969–1975) stratified 15,846 live births at the Beth Israel Hospital in Boston into five risk categories (Neutra *et al.*, 1978). A score derived by summing weights assigned to individual risk factors was used to assign women to a specific risk category. Three-fourths of the women were in the lowest risk group.
- The second study (4,144 births in a community hospital, 1974–1975) sepa-

rated maternity patients at a hospital in Cincinnati into high-risk and low-risk groups. In addition to the other exclusions, women with meconium-stained amniotic fluid, postterm pregnancies, oxytocin stimulation, or prolonged rupture of the membranes were excluded from the low-risk group, which included 57 percent of the women in the study (Amato, 1977).

- The third study (10,521 births at 15 hospitals, 1977–1979) screened data on nearly 19,000 live births in fifteen hospitals in southeastern Minnesota to identify 10,521 low-risk pregnancies. Mothers of LBW infants and parous women whose babies were in breech position were retained in the low-risk group. Women carrying twins, women who had repeat cesarean sections, women with significant medical or prenatal complications, and women who were younger than nineteen or older than thirty-four were excluded. Only about 55 percent of the women in the original data set remained after those exclusions (Adams, 1983).

- Births in the "national sample" were derived from data in the 1980 National Natality Survey (a probability sample of 9,941 live births that occurred in the United States during 1980), which was culled to omit, in addition to the usual "high-risk" exclusions, women who smoked more than ten cigarettes per day, women who consumed more than three alcoholic drinks per week, women who had fewer than four prenatal visits, and women who were unmarried, black, or less than eighteen years old. Only 30 percent of the original sample were retained in the low-risk group, which was purposefully designed to approximate the women in the National Birth Center Study.

- The next line of data was taken from the study that linked birth and death certificates from Washington State for 1981 through 1990 (see Table 11). The process by which the low-risk in-hospital physician care group was created was described earlier.

- The next study (14,618 births at an academic hospital, 1982–1985) started with data on 17,759 live births at Parkland Memorial Hospital in Dallas. In addition to all of the usual exclusions, the low-risk group created by these researchers also excluded women whose labor had been induced by oxytocin and women whose labors were complicated by problems such as meconium in the amniotic fluid or an abnormal fetal heart rate. After all the exclusions, only 42 percent of the original group of women remained in the low-risk group (Leveno *et al.*, 1986).

- The last study on the table (8,135 term births and 3,457 postterm births at twelve hospitals, 1982–1985) screened 60,456 births at hospitals included in a Midwestern perinatal referral network to identify 11,592 "uncomplicated" term and postterm pregnancies in women between the ages of sixteen and thirty-nine. The low-risk group that remained after the screening included only 19 percent of the women in the original data set (Eden *et al.*, 1987).

Although these seven studies include births during a period of twenty-two years, there is no apparent time trend. Most of the improvement in neonatal mortality during that period was due to increased survival of LBW infants, who were excluded from six of the seven comparison studies. Although there was no time trend, there was considerable variability in the mortality rates reported by these hospitals. The data from the national sample and the study based on all births in Washington State may provide the best comparison of neonatal mortality, since both studies included the wide variety of hospitals in which births actually occur. Unfortunately, neither study—both based on birth and death certificates—could provide information on the incidence of intrapartum deaths. In fact, only three of the seven comparison studies provided information on intrapartum mortality. In addition, only the two studies based on birth and death certificates were able to truly measure neonatal deaths. The other studies, based on hospital data only, would have missed any neonatal deaths that occurred after the infant's initial discharge from the hospital. Although it is rare for a newborn who has been discharged from the hospital in which it was born to die during the first twenty-eight days of its life, one of the fifteen neonatal deaths in the NBCS was an apparent case of sudden infant death syndrome (SIDS) involving a baby who was healthy at birth and in good condition when discharged from the birth center. The fact that such deaths are included in the rates reported by some studies but not others further complicates the use of these data as a standard for judging rates found during studies of out-of-hospital births.

Interpretation of the Mortality Rates Summarized on Table 13

Table 13 was constructed to facilitate comparison of the mortality rates found in studies of out-of-hospital births attended by midwives or physicians under varying circumstances, and to compare those mortality rates with mortality found during studies of low-risk women who deliver their babies in hospitals. The total mortality rates found during the seven studies of low-risk hospital births ranged from 1.0 to 4.3 deaths per 1,000 births. Four of the studies lack data on intrapartum mortality (and thus lack data on total mortality), and exclusion of women who experienced meconium stained amniotic fluid or abnormal fetal heart rate patterns makes the study of 14,618 births in an academic hospital from 1982 through 1985 of questionable value for the purpose of this chapter. Even without information on stillbirths, the neonatal mortality rate for very low-risk women in the 1980 National Natality

Survey was 2.5 per 1,000 births; thus the total mortality rate for this nationwide representative sample of very low-risk births was at least 2.5, if not higher. The low neonatal mortality rate from the study of births in Washington State (1 death per 1,000 live births) is significant because it is based on the largest number of births over the longest time period, including births in 1990, and because it is representative of low-risk in-hospital births for an entire state. The highest total mortality rate (4.3 per 1,000 births) was from a single community hospital during 1974 through 1975. The best comparison group for our purpose may be the last study on the table, which included births from twelve hospitals in a perinatal network, and presumably included all levels of hospitals; total mortality was 2.1 deaths per 1,000 term births and 2.6 per 1,000 postterm births.

Based on this array of studies, one might conclude that out-of-hospital birth services and practices that take care of low-risk women and experience mortality of more than 3 or 4 deaths per 1,000 births provide care that is less safe than care in a typical U.S. hospital. The rest of this section compares the mortality rates reported in the fifteen studies summarized in Table 13 against this standard, taking into consideration the strengths and limitations of each study and the circumstances of the out-of-hospital birth practices that generated the data. Of the fifteen studies of out-of-hospital births summarized in Table 13, only ten presented data on both intrapartum and neonatal mortality or, in the case of the study from the Farm in Tennessee, provided data on total mortality. Only two of those nine include all births attended by a specified category of care providers—direct-entry midwives in both studies—in a specified geographic area over a specified period of time. Four of the studies that provided data on both intrapartum and neonatal mortality were small, based on fewer than 500 births. In addition, several of the data sets are quite old, based primarily on births during the 1970s. This information is far from adequate to satisfy all questions about the safety of out-of-hospital births in the United States. The data are, however, sufficient to reach some tentative conclusions.

The most significant data sets are the studies from Arizona and Toronto; the National Birth Center Study; the ACNM home birth study; and the two large cumulative data sets on home births attended by direct-entry midwives and family physicians between 1969 and 1985. The total mortality rates found during the first four studies on this list were low—between 1.3 and 2.8 deaths per 1,000 births. Considering only the six data sets on this list, the studies that found rates higher than the standard defined by the studies of low-risk hospital births were heavily weighted by data from the 1970s, when the home birth movement was new and most people who attended home births—physicians, as well as truly *lay* midwives—were inexperienced.

In addition, the higher rates came from practices that attended out-of-hospital births for women with high-risk pregnancies. A recent analysis of data based on one thousand matched pairs of women from the two large data sets accumulated by Dr. Mehl-Madrona since the early 1970s demonstrates the effect of breech, twin, and postterm deliveries on the mortality rates associated with out-of-hospital births.* It also explains why the mortality rate was higher for the births attended by midwives than for the births attended by physicians (Mehl-Madrona & Madrona, 1997). Many of the midwives who contributed data to this data set did not discourage women with these high-risk conditions from attempting a home birth. Although some family physicians also ac-

cepted women with these complicating factors, most of the physicians followed a policy that called for referring women with these conditions to hospitals for delivery. When all women with any of these three high-risk factors (breech presentation, twins, or post-term pregnancies) were excluded from the matched-pair data set, the total mortality rate for both groups fell to two to three deaths per 1,000 births—levels that are well within the standard set by hospitals. In addition, once the high-risk births were omitted, the mortality rates were low regardless of whether the births were attended by midwives or physicians. The issue of attending high-risk births in an out-of-hospital setting is further discussed in the section on "High-Risk Pregnancies" later in this chapter.

There was great variation in the experience and preparation of the midwives who attended the births included in these studies. Taken together, the studies reviewed in this chapter point to the importance of training and experience, and of having some means to assess and ensure the competence of individual midwives, whether through regulation by state authorities or a certification program operated by a midwifery organization.

The very first study published by Dr. Mehl-Madrona reported on 287 births attended by midwives associated with the Santa Cruz Birth Center during the early 1970s; there were no deaths† (Mehl *et al.*, 1975). Although the study reported on births from a very early phase of the development of direct-entry midwifery in this country, the midwives who started the birth center were heavily involved in training and very concerned about quality. As noted in Chapter 4, they closed the birth center in 1976 because it had begun to attract a wider

---

*The matched pairs in this study were taken from the large data sets accumulated by Dr. Mehl-Madrona. Findings from the recent matched-pair study are not shown in Table 13, but the two large data sets from which the matched pairs were drawn are included in the table. The mortality rates from these two large data sets—one for direct-entry midwives and one for family practitioners—had not been published prior to their publication in this book.

†Data from this study are not shown in Table 13 because these births are among the 3,545 home births attended by direct-entry midwives in eight states, 1970–1985, which are represented in Table 13.

group of midwives. The original group realized that the birth center did not have the structure necessary for quality control and felt that they should not continue to operate the center under those circumstances (Bowland, 1993).

Another study from California (461 births, 1985–1991, shown in Table 13) also reported no deaths. Only 4 percent of the births in that study occurred before the California Association of Midwives (CAM) had developed its certification process. All of the other births in the study were attended by midwives who had met the criteria required for certification by CAM (Booker, 1991).

Studies in Vermont and Missouri found high mortality rates associated with care provided by direct-entry midwives who were not involved in any kind of certification process and good outcomes for midwives who were. The small prospective study of births attended by direct-entry midwives in Vermont from 1981 through 1985 found high rates of both intrapartum and neonatal mortality, with total mortality of almost 16 deaths per 1,000 births. The Missouri study was based on births during approximately the same period (1978–1984). Although it could not provide information on intrapartum deaths, the level of neonatal mortality associated with care provided by midwives who were not affiliated with the Missouri Midwives Association (8.3 deaths per 1,000) was virtually the same as the neonatal mortality rate in the study from Vermont (7.9 per 1,000). If neonatal deaths represented only half of all deaths associated with the births in Missouri, as they did in Vermont, the total mortality rate for births attended by unaffiliated midwives in Missouri might also have been approximately 16 deaths per 1,000 births.

The Vermont study was completed before direct-entry midwives in Vermont had developed a certification process. The unaffiliated midwives in Missouri were not members of the Missouri Midwives Association and had not demonstrated that they met the standards of that organization. Some were

identified as "religious midwives."[*] During the same time period, there were no neonatal deaths among 396 births attended by midwives who were members of the Missouri Midwives Association.[†] The Vermont Vital Statistics System reported that no neonatal deaths had been associated with home births attended by direct-entry midwives in Vermont during a later period.

Outcomes improved with increased experience and in-service training of the midwives in Arizona. Of twenty-six midwives licensed to practice in Arizona at the time of the study, twenty-two had passed the qualifying examination and four who had not taken the examination were "grandfathered" in because they had been practicing under an old "granny midwife" law. One of the only two preventable deaths found during the study involved a breech birth attended by a midwife who was licensed under the grandfather clause. She attended this birth in the mother's home, even though Arizona's licensing rules require midwives to refer breech deliveries to physicians (Sullivan & Beeman, 1983).

The neonatal mortality rate for out-of-hospital births attended by licensed direct-entry midwives in Washington State was the same as the rate for out-of-hospital births attended by CNMs. Three years of formal midwifery education is a requirement for licensure of a direct-entry midwife in Washington (Janssen *et al.*, 1994).

Low mortality in the study from Toronto was associated with care provided by midwives who abided by the rules and protocols of the local midwifery association (Tyson, 1991).

The lowest total mortality rates in studies with at least 1,000 births were associated with care provided by licensed direct-entry midwives in Arizona; unlicensed direct-entry

---

[*]See discussion of "Christian Midwives" in Chapter 9.

[†]Data on their births were combined with those of physicians and CNMs attending home births in Missouri between 1978–1984. Data on those births are presented in Table 13.

midwife members of the Ontario Midwives Association; care provided, mainly by CNMs, in well-established birth centers; and home births attended by CNMs. Outcomes found during each of these studies are similar to outcomes for low-risk births in hospitals.

Differences in the Proportion of Deaths That Occur During Labor

Only three of the seven studies of low-risk hospital births reported on intrapartum as well as neonatal mortality. Two of the three found no fetal deaths during labor; the third found a low rate of stillbirths. These findings suggest that neonatal deaths may constitute nearly all of the mortality associated with low-risk hospital births. In contrast to this, deaths found during out-of-hospital birth studies are divided between intrapartum and neonatal deaths; this was the case in all but two of the studies in Table 13 that reported both components of total mortality. Intrapartum deaths accounted for 29 percent of all deaths in the data on 4,107 births attended by family physicians and about one-third of the deaths in the two studies in which most or all of the care was provided by CNMs (both studies in the second grouping in Table 13). Six studies of direct-entry midwifery care outcomes reported both intrapartum and neonatal mortality. No deaths were reported in the study of 461 home births in California (1985–1991), and no intrapartum deaths were found during the study of 1,001 home births in Toronto (1983–1988). In each of the other four studies, half or nearly half of the deaths occurred before the baby was born.

One possible explanation for the virtual lack of intrapartum mortality in the studies of in-hospital births and its presence in most of the studies of out-of-hospital births is that the ability to conduct a rapid cesarean section during childbirth in many or most hospitals may save the lives of some babies who would have died during labor in an out-of-hospital setting. But there is another possibility: Several out-of-hospital birth studies

that reported stillbirths nevertheless reported low overall mortality rates; the total mortality rates from those studies were no higher than the neonatal mortality rates reported by several of the studies of low-risk births in hospitals. This suggests that the ability to achieve a rapid cesarean delivery of infants who are in distress during labor in a hospital may result in the live births of some moribund infants. This would shift some inevitable deaths from the intrapartum period to the neonatal period. In that case, the cesarean section would have been to no avail.

Postterm Births Result in Higher Mortality

Pregnancies that continued, undelivered, beyond 42 completed weeks based on the best estimate of the date of conception are considered *postterm* or *postdates*. The use of the term *postdates* instead of *postterm* acknowledges that the date of conception is an estimate. As many as 70 percent of pregnancies that are thought to be postterm are probably not really biologically prolonged; the error is based on the difficulty of determining the actual date of conception. Several adverse pregnancy outcomes are significantly increased in actual postterm pregnancies (Cunningham *et al.*, 1993). Two of the studies shown in Table 13 provided separate information on mortality rates associated with *term* deliveries (those that are neither *preterm*, i.e., occurring at less than 37 completed weeks of gestation, or *postterm*, occurring at more than 42 weeks). The NBCS provided this information on 9,871 term and 1,306 postterm births in free-standing birth centers. A study conducted at twelve hospitals that are part of a perinatal referral network in the midwest provided this information on 8,135 term and 3,457 postterm births. The findings from these two studies, both quite large, are instructive:

- In both studies, in-hospital births and out-of-hospital births, the total mortality rate for postterm births was higher than the rate for term births.

- The increased mortality associated with postterm status was much greater for the births that occurred in birth centers than for the births that occurred in hospitals. *The postterm mortality rate was more than four times higher than the rate for term pregnancies among women who initiated their care in birth centers, but was only 25 percent higher among women who initiated their care in hospitals.*

Low Morbidity Associated with Home Births

One consistent finding of Dr. Mehl-Madrona's matched control group studies is much lower rates of complications during labor and lower rates of both maternal and newborn morbidity associated with home births. For example, in a study that matched 1,040 home births attended by family physicians (67 percent) and midwives (31 percent direct-entry midwives, 2 percent CNMs) with births attended by physicians in two hospitals in Madison, Wisconsin, the in-hospital births were much more likely to be complicated by fetal distress (a sixfold increase), maternal hypertension (a fivefold increase), meconium in the amniotic fluid (three and a half times as many cases), shoulder dystocia (eight times higher), and postpartum hemorrhage (three times higher). Apgar scores for babies born in the hospital tended to be lower, and they were thirty times more likely to sustain physical injuries during the birth and almost four times more likely to require resuscitation. The in-hospital birth newborns were also four times more likely than those born at home (or in the hospital following a transfer from a home birth) to acquire an infection during the neonatal period. Low use of obstetric interventions during home births seemed to explain the difference in the incidence of morbidity (Mehl, 1977).

Transfers During and After Labor, and Cesarean Deliveries

Table 14 shows the percent of hospital transfers and cesarean deliveries found during some of the studies shown in Table 13. The transfer rate includes women transferred during labor and instances in which either the mother or the baby was transported to a hospital shortly after the birth. Three of the low-risk in-hospital birth studies included at the bottom of Table 13 provided information on cesarean deliveries; cesarean rates found during those studies are shown at the bottom of Table 14. Total mortality rates shown in Table 13 are repeated in Table 14. Most of the out-of-hospital birth studies with the best outcomes reported transfer rates of 16 or 17 percent. The lowest transfer rates were associated with home births attended by physicians.

Low-risk women who give birth in hospitals are much more likely to have a cesarean section than those who attempt to give birth at home or in a birth center. This difference is almost certainly due in large part to the use of continuous internal fetal monitoring and epidural anesthesia during childbirth in American hospitals. (See discussion in Chapter 10.)

Attending High-Risk Births at Home

Alaska is the only state that specifically authorizes midwives to deliver twins or babies in breech position; some state laws prohibit it explicitly. Midwifery is conceptualized as appropriate care for low-risk births, and twins, breech, and postterm deliveries are associated with increased risk. Some of the women who became midwives during the 1970s learned to deliver babies in breech position from Grand Midwives or rural doctors, or learned from experience. Vaginal breech delivery is abetted by a relaxed mother who has confidence in her birth attendant, and calmness and patience on the part of the midwife

Table 14

Transfer, Cesarean Delivery, and Total Mortality Rates from Studies of Out-of-Hospital Births Attended by Midwives, Selected Studies of Other Out-of-Hospital Births, and Low-Risk Births Attended by Physicians in Hospitals, Studies Conducted in North America, 1969–1991*

Location	Years	Number of Births	Birth Attendants	Transfer Rate (%)	Cesarean Delivery Rate (%)	Total Mortality/ 1,000 Births
Data on All Home Births Attended by Direct-Entry Midwives in a Specified Geographic Area: Studies With Follow-Up of Transfers						
Arizona[1]	1978–81	1,449	Licensed DEMs	23.0	NA	2.8 (1.4)
Toronto, Ontario[2]	1983–88	1,001	DEMs	16.5	3.5	(2.0)
National Studies That Tried to Include All Practices in a Certain Category: Studies With Follow-Up of Transfers						
Eighty-four birth centers[3]	1985–87	11,826	81% CNMs + MDs + DEMs	15.8	4.4	1.3 (0.7)
90 home birth practices[4]	1987–91	11,081	CNMs	10.0	3.0	2.0 (0.9)
Studies of Selected Out-of-Hospital Birth Practices: Births Attended by Direct-Entry Midwives and/or Family Physicians						
Eight states[5]	1970–85	3,545	45 DEMs	4.6	1.4	9.9
California[6]	1985–91	461	DEMs	15.8	5.6	0.0
Sonoma Co., California[7]	1976–82	453	1 OB + 1 DEM MDs,	6.4	2.9	4.4
The Farm, Tennessee[8]	1971–89	1,707	DEMs, MDs, Amish midwives	11.8	1.5	8.8 (5.4)†
California and Wisconsin[5]	1969–81	4,107	Family physicians	2.3	0.9	5.8
Low-Risk Births Attended by Physicians in Hospitals						
Fifteen hospitals[9]	1977–79	10,521	Physicians		5.5	
National sample[10]	1980	2,935	Physicians		8.4	
Twelve hospitals[11]	1982–85					
Term births		8,135	Physicians		8.3	2.1 (1.9)
Postterm		3,457	Physicians		17.6	2.6 (2.1)

*This table can only be properly interpreted in conjunction with an understanding of the accompanying written text. Using the table in isolation is likely to result in misinterpretation. There were significant differences between the studies shown on this table related to the socioeconomic status of the women and screening criteria.

Key: NA = data not available; DEM = direct-entry midwife. Numbers in parenthesis are mortality rates excluding fetuses and infants with lethal congenital anomalies.

† Rate based on all women who initiated prenatal care at the Farm, including some twins and breech deliveries, many women of low socioeconomic status, and 31 women who were referred to hospital care prior to the onset of labor. (See discussion on pages 368 and 369.)

References: [1]Sullivan & Beeman, 1983; [2]Tyson, 1991; [3]Rooks *et al.*, 1989; [4]Anderson & Murphy, 1995; [5]unpublished data from the data set used in Mehl-Madrona & Madrona, 1997; [6]Booker, 1991; [7]Koehler *et al.*, 1984; [8]Durand, 1992; [9]Adams, 1983; [10]See discussion, page 371, [11]Eden *et al.*, 1987.

or physician—a hands-off policy, allowing the delivery to proceed without intervention up to a certain point. Some midwives probably did the right thing out of ignorance at first, and learned that vaginal breech deliveries can be successful at a time when cesarean section for breech presentations was *de rigueur* in hospitals (it still is in many hospitals). A paper published in 1992 synthesized findings from thirteen studies of breech deliveries that had been published since 1979 (Weiner, 1992). When babies with lethal congenital anomalies were omitted from the data, the mortality rate for deliveries of babies in breech position was virtually the same whether accomplished vaginally or by a cesarean section. A cesarean section does not significantly improve outcomes for babies in breech presentation, but imposes a much greater risk of morbidity on the mother (Collea *et al.* 1980; Cunningham *et al.*, 1993).

Ina May Gaskin, of the Farm community in Tennessee, has developed a video and other methods for teaching the techniques for vaginal delivery of selected women whose babies present in breech position. Breech presentation is often associated with other problems, especially congenital anomalies or preterm delivery, so it is important to select which cases might be appropriate for a vaginal delivery in an out-of-hospital setting. Fifty-seven of the 1,827 women who had birth care at the Farm between 1970 and 1993 had babies in breech position (Gaskin, 1993). This amounts to 3.1 percent of all births at the Farm during this period, which is the normal incidence (Cunningham *et al.*, 1993). Seventeen of the 57 were transported to a hospital for delivery, 6 were home births attended by a physician, and the midwives delivered the remaining 36. Four babies died, 3 from lethal anomalies and 1 from complications of prematurity; the mother had been taken to a hospital as soon as labor started. There were no deaths of viable ba-

bies born at term. Some women travel to the Farm specifically to have a vaginal breech birth (Gaskin, 1993).

Some midwives resist describing breech presentation as an abnormality, considering it a variation of normal. One of the studies by Dr. Mehl-Madrona that is not shown in Table 13 reported data from two midwife practices and three family physician/RN practices operating in northern California during the mid-1970s (Mehl *et al.*, 1977). Data were provided on 1,146 births; 21 of them (1.8 percent) were breech presentations. The paper noted that one of the women whose baby was in breech presentation was delivered by cesarean section after being transferred to a hospital. The report did not indicate whether any of the other women with babies in breech presentation were transferred, and breech presentation was not listed as a complication. This suggests that breech presentations were treated as variations of normal and delivered at home. Six sets of twins were delivered at home successfully. Another study (the report of an obstetrician/direct-entry midwife practice in Sonoma County, California, included in Table 13) did not mention how many of the births were breech, but noted that the only fetal death during labor was a fetus in breech presentation. One of the deaths in the study from Arizona was a baby in breech presentation. The study from Washington State also found that some of the licensed midwives were delivering high-risk women at home, including those carrying twins or babies in breech position. The neonatal mortality rates for births attended by both CNMs and licensed direct-entry midwives declined when high-risk births were removed from the analysis (see Table 11).

Laws to regulate direct-entry midwives have been debated in various states. Some direct-entry midwives have argued that breech and twin deliveries should be allowed, becuse they believe that their outcomes for breech deliveries are at least as good as the mother can anticipate if she delivers in a hospital (Morningstar, 1994; Trepiccione, 1994). There is recognition, however, that assisting with a breech birth requires special training and experience and is beyond the skills of most midwives. Some direct-entry midwives advocate and apparently practice disobedience of laws that prohibit midwives from attending breech births at home. In addition to their concerns for women they have taken care of throughout pregnancy, they are concerned that the art of assisting in vaginal breech deliveries will die out if midwives are prohibited from this practice (Tully, 1993).

A recent study by Dr. Mehl-Madrona is pertinent to this issue, even though the data are relatively old. Because of his home birth experience and research, he is sometimes asked to serve as an expert witness in lawsuits involving bad outcomes of home births. Most of the suits in which he has testified arose from births involving complications such as breech presentation, twins, or postdate deliveries. He conducted this analysis of his accumulated data on out-of-hospital births (described earlier) out of curiosity and a sense of responsibility for the home birth movement his own studies have helped to support: The study compared outcomes for one thousand matched pairs of women who had home births between 1969 and 1985. Each matched pair included one woman whose birth was attended by a direct-entry midwife and one whose birth was attended by a family physician; they were matched to be identical in maternal age group, socioeconomic status, parity, race, and medical risk using a standardized risk-scoring system, modified to not consider breech presentation, twins, or postdates as risk factors, since he wanted to investigate their effect on outcomes (Mehl-Madrona & Madrona, 1997). Total perinatal mortality among the midwife-attended births included three fetal deaths before labor, six fe-

tal deaths during labor, and five neonatal deaths. The total perinatal mortality rate was fourteen deaths per one thousand births. Mortality among the births attended by family physicians included one fetal death prior to the onset of labor, two fetal deaths during labor, and two neonatal deaths. The perinatal mortality rate was five per one thousand births. The difference (fourteen per one thousand versus five per one thousand) was statistically significant ($p = 0.04$).

The researchers then examined the data to identify the number of babies with lethal congenital anomalies and the number of pregnancies involving twins, breech presentations, and postterm pregnancies. There was no significant difference between the two groups in the incidence of congenital anomalies, but most of the family physicians did not accept women with postdate pregnancies, breech presentations, or twin gestations for home births, and the midwives had significantly more births involving each of those high-risk conditions. The researchers then conducted a series of reanalyses of the data. When babies with congenital anomalies were deleted from the data set, the total perinatal mortality rates were reduced to twelve per one thousand for the midwives and two per one thousand for the physicians. The difference is statistically significant ($p < .05$). When babies with congenital anomalies and deliveries involving twins, breech presentations, or postdate deliveries were deleted from the data set, the total perinatal mortality rates were reduced to three per one thousand and two per one thousand. The difference is not statistically significant (Mehl-Madrona & Madrona, 1997). The midwives' outcomes were as good as the physicians' when they stuck to normal births. But because they did not stick to normal births, their actual mortality rates were higher.

The data from the Farm show that it is possible to organize a home birth service that can deal with breech deliveries safely. Dr. Mehl-Madrona's study—based on data reflecting care provided by a broad spectrum of direct-entry midwifery care ten or more years ago—shows that attending high-risk births at home may lead to an increased rate of deaths. All three of the conditions he identified as increasing the mortality rate in midwife-attended home births are also associated with increased mortality when the deliveries occur in hospitals. In the case of breech deliveries, the increased mortality remains, even if the babies are delivered by cesarean section. We do not have a study to compare the outcomes for these high-risk births when attended by a midwife at home versus typical care in hospitals.

The ACNM guidelines for home birth are clear regarding conditions that make a woman inappropriate for a home birth, including preterm deliveries, breech deliveries, and twins. Ninety-six percent of the CNMs who participated in the ACNM home birth study indicated that they would not attempt home births for women with twins or babies in breech presentation (Anderson & Murphy, 1995). Sixty-one percent considered gestation exceeding forty-two weeks a contraindication for home birth. All of the CNMs who would consider a home birth for a woman with any of these conditions had been attending home births for at least five years. Although some women carrying twins or babies in breech or other nonoptimal positions ("malpresentations") were among the 11,081 women included in the ACNM Home Birth Committee study, all of them were referred to physician care prenatally or were transported to a hospital as soon as the condition was diagnosed during labor. None of them gave birth at home. Two intra-partum deaths were associated with post-term deliveries (Anderson & Murphy, 1995).

There is a clear difference of opinion on this issue between nurse-midwives and direct-entry midwives. Part of the problem is a lack of research to assess the relative safety of managing some complications in homes versus hospitals. Part of the problem is philosophical, having to do with the definition of midwifery and parameters of "normal," and differences in the ethical framework created by the ACNM and MANA—one giving more emphasis to safety and one emphasizing women's rights to make their own informed choices about where they will give birth.

Summary

Studies that do not distinguish between planned and unplanned out-of-hospital births find higher rates of neonatal mortality among births that occur in nonhospital locations as compared to births in hospitals. Studies that examine outcomes of planned out-of-hospital births find lower mortality rates than for all in-hospital births—which include high- as well as low-risk women. There are powerful differences in risk (the underlying likelihood of experiencing a complication leading to fetal or neonatal death) between women who have planned out-of-hospital births and women who have births in hospitals. Because of these differences, it is very difficult to determine whether the pregnancy outcomes for women who have planned home births or use free-standing birth centers are as good, nearly as good, or better than the outcomes the same women would have experienced if they had gone to hospitals.

Some of the ways in which these groups of women differ involve characteristics that seem to have an effect on pregnancy outcomes—age, race, marital status, parity, socioeconomic status, medical and obstetric history, and behaviors such as smoking. Although it is possible to match a sample of home birth mothers with other pregnant women based on some of these characteristics, these relatively easy-to-measure characteristics may not be the real causes of the difference in risk. Instead these characteristics may be associated with other, less well recognized factors that are much harder to measure, such as stress and how the women feel about being pregnant. Hospital care for childbirth is widely available to women in this country; it takes positive action for a woman to give birth in a nonhospital setting.

This unusual decision and proactive planning required to have a home birth self-select a group of women who are highly committed to having a healthy pregnancy and baby and are willing to assume responsibility to make it happen. It is assumed that the attitudes and determination exhibited by women who give birth in out-of-hospital settings have a positive effect on their pregnancies. However, as described in the section on birth centers, a study conducted at a birth center associated with a hospital in Miami found that women who were *assigned* to the birth center when the hospital was crowded experienced the same good outcomes as women who were given an option and chose birth center care.

In addition to any differences in the underlying level of risk of women who choose to have an out-of-hospital birth, the screening and referral practices of midwives and physicians who provide care to these women adds to the disparity in risk between women who have out-of-hospital births and women who have births in hospitals. Out-of-hospital birth practitioners constantly assess their clients for complications and high-risk conditions; most of them adhere to strict eligibility criteria and refer women with serious complications to a hospital-based practitioner for care during birth. In addition, 10 to 15 percent of the women who begin labor under the care of a midwife at home or in a birth center are transferred to a hospital because of a complication. Prenatal screening and referrals and transfers during labor all function to remove the women who are most likely to have poor pregnancy outcomes from the out-of-hospital birth population and to concentrate high-risk women in hospitals. As a result of all of these forms of selection, it is difficult to make meaningful comparisons between the mortality rates associated with home births and births in hospitals. Trying to compare neonatal mortality rates is particularly problematic, because neonatal mortality accounts for almost all of the deaths associated with hospital childbirth but only half to two-thirds of the mortality arising from out-of-hospital births. Comparing neonatal mortality rates from out-of-hospital births with those from in-hospital births will always make the outcomes of out-of-hospital births look relatively better than they are.

We know from studies of home births in other countries, especially the Netherlands, that home births can be safe. However, conclusions based on out-of-hospital births conducted under one set of circumstances may not be valid under a different set of circumstances. Studies of out-of-hospital births should not be seen as tests of a universally defined service; rather they are evaluations of the effectiveness of both the prenatal screening and referral practices and the labor and delivery care provided by specific birth centers or home birth practices or by all members of a certain category of out-of-hospital birth attendants in a particular geographic area during a particular period of time. The outcomes vary depending on many factors. Studies that report on all births in a specified geographic area reflect the range of quality that exists in actual practice.

Small individual studies are not powerful enough to provide reliable information about the occurrence of rare events, i.e., mortality associated with low-risk births in any setting. A collection of small retrospective studies or a large study that aggregates data from many out-of-hospital birth practices may give a false impression due to bias affecting which services analyze and publish their data and which practitioners participate in a retrospective study; most people are disinclined to advertise unfavorable results. Assuming that it is impossible to conduct large randomized trials of out-of-hospital births in the United States, the most reliable conclusions will be based on prospective studies that include a large number of births and all or most of the practitioners in a certain category, collect data on intrapartum as well as neonatal mortality, include outcomes for women and babies who are transferred to hospitals because of complications, and take measures to ensure the accuracy and completeness of the data. Based on these criteria, the three most reliable studies reported to date are the study of births attended by direct-entry midwives in Arizona and Toronto, the NBCS, and the ACNM home birth study.

The studies from Arizona and Toronto reported on all births attended by midwives during a six-year period, and both studies were large enough to result in reasonably reliable findings. The total mortality rate was low in both studies—1.4 deaths per 1,000 births in Arizona and 2 per 1,000 in Toronto, excluding babies with lethal congenital anomalies. Although neither group of midwives had formal training, midwives in both studies adhered to strict regulations. In Arizona the regulations were enforced by the state. Most of the midwives who attended the births included in the Toronto study were members of a midwifery association that implemented a program of voluntary self-regulation. One of the few preventable deaths in Arizona was due to a midwife breaking the rules to attend a breech delivery at home. The National Birth Center Study included most birth centers that were in operation during the data-collection period, 1985 through mid-1987. Prospectively collected data tracked the progress and outcomes of almost all of the 11,814 women who were admitted to birth centers in labor, with very complete follow-up of those transferred to hospitals. There were 1.3 intrapartum and neonatal deaths per 1,000 births, only 0.7 excluding babies with lethal anomalies. The ACNM home birth study reported outcomes for the majority of home births attended by CNMs between 1987 and 1991. There were 2.1 deaths per 1,000 births (less than 1 if we exclude babies with lethal anomalies).

Appropriate comparison studies of low-risk deliveries managed by physicians in hospitals report total mortality rates between about 1 and 4 per 1,000 births. The mortality rate for home births attended by midwives in

the Netherlands is about 1 per 1,000 births (Treffers, 1993). Mortality rates found during the Arizona and Toronto studies, the NBCS, and the ACNM home birth study are similar to the good outcomes achieved in the comparison studies. Studies that have found higher mortality rates reported outcomes of home births attended by lay midwives and family physicians when the home birth movement was young and most people who attended home births were inexperienced. In addition, the studies that reported higher rates tracked practices and services that were willing to attend out-of-hospital births for women with high-risk pregnancies. There have been very few studies of births attended by direct-entry midwives. Most of those that are available are old and do not reflect changes in the training and practice of those midwives who are trying to increase standards and professionalize.

The following are some other general observations about the outcomes of out-of-hospital births based on the available studies:

- Low birth weight caused by preterm births accounts for a very large proportion of all neonatal deaths in the United States. Most midwives refer women who go into labor before term to physicians. As a result of that referral pattern, as well as the low-risk characteristics of home birth mothers, and perhaps the nutritional focus of care provided by midwives, relatively few LBW babies are born in out-of-hospital settings. The dearth of low-weight babies results in low neonatal mortality relative to the rate for the nation as a whole. In addition, as many as one-third to one-half of all deaths associated with out-of-hospital births are fetal deaths during labor. In contrast, nearly all deaths associated with low-risk births in hospitals are neonatal deaths. Because of both of these reasons, *it is never appropriate to compare neonatal mortality rates for out-of-hospital births to general neonatal mortality rates.*

- It is possible to identify a low-risk population of women for out-of-hospital births; however, it is not possible to identify a group of women who have no risk at all. Ten to 15 percent of the women who begin their labor care in an out-of-hospital setting, or their babies, are transported to hospitals during labor or shortly after the delivery. About three-fourths of the transfers are made during labor and one-fourth after the birth. Most of the transfers during labor are due to slow progress and are not emergencies. However, even in a well-screened group of healthy women, about 8 percent may experience a serious complication and 2 to 3 percent may need emergency transfers to a hospital. Women who have never had a baby before are more likely to be transferred, but they are not more likely to experience a serious complication or emergency (based on the NBCS).
- Transfer rates are lower for out-of-hospital births attended by physicians as compared with midwives. But there is no evidence that the outcomes of out-of-hospital births are better if the birth is attended by a physician.
- Higher transfer rates may be associated with lower rates of total mortality.
- Services that exclude women whose babies are in breech presentation, women carrying twins, and women with postterm pregnancies have the lowest mortality rates. Very few CNMs are willing to attend births involving twins or breech presentation in nonhospital settings, and none of the studies that reported relatively high mortality rates were based on care provided by CNMs. Some direct-entry midwives do attend these births, even though only one state sanctions this practice. We do not know whether women excluded from home births for these reasons have better outcomes in hospitals than they would have had at home.
- Women who give birth at home or in a free-standing birth center seem to have a much lower incidence of complications and morbidity, including meconium-stained amniotic fluid, fetal distress, shoulder dystocia, and birth injury to the baby. The greater use of interventions in hospitals probably accounts for at least some of the higher incidence of complications.
- Out-of-hospital birth reduces unnecessary cesarean sections, cutting the cesarean section rate to half or less compared with low-risk hospital births.
- There was great variation in the preparation of the direct-entry midwives who attended the births included in these studies. Better outcomes are associated with more training, longer experience, and having some means to assess and ensure the competence of individual midwives.
- All studies that ask women whether they were satisfied with their care during childbirth find that most women who give birth at home or in a birth center are highly satisfied with their experience. Many women choose these options because they are dissatisfied with previous births in hospitals.

It is not possible to make any generalized statement about the safety of out-of-hospital births attended by midwives in the United States. Home births are safe in Holland because they have designed and developed a system in which all of the necessary components are in place. The Dutch system is described in Chapter 13. Although the United States does not have this kind of system, the available evidence indicates that births attended by either midwives or physicians in homes and birth centers in this country can be as safe as in-hospital births when the following conditions are in place:

- The midwives must be competent, that is, have the necessary knowledge, skills, and judgment. At the individual level, this requires thorough education and training, substantial experience, and a degree of humility. At the system level, it requires excellent education and training programs, methods to test the competence of individual midwives, and authority to prevent incompetent midwives from practicing. The system needs to provide opportunities for midwives to acquire adequate experience while attending births with another completely qualified midwife or physician. All midwives should participate in on going processes of continuing education, self-assessment, and peer review.

- There must be good prenatal care, with careful screening to detect and address complications and identify high-risk conditions, and the development of good communication and trust between the midwife and the pregnant woman and others who will be present during the birth.

- There should be more than one knowledgeable person at the birth—either two midwives or a midwife and a trained, experienced assistant.

- There should be clear, universally accepted criteria regarding referral of high-risk women for hospital births. These criteria should be known within the population of women who might seek home births, as well as within the midwifery community.

- There should be no disincentives to transporting women and newborns to the hospital. Transports should be viewed and accepted as an expected part of a program of out-of-hospital births. They should not be seen as failures by the mother and her family, or the midwife.

- There must be access to rapid means to transport women and newborns to hospital care. Emergency medical technicians need appropriate training to support out-of-hospital births.

- There must be competent and reliable obstetrical backup at a nearby hospital.

This crucial component requires an effective working relationship between the out-of-hospital midwife and the doctors and nurses at the hospital. The hospital personnel must trust the judgment of the out-of-hospital birth midwife, and an out-of-hospital birth midwife must be able to rely on the hospital personnel to respond appropriately when she calls to say that she is bringing a woman or newborn into the hospital. This means that the midwife must have authority, either personal authority based on competence, self-confidence, and reputation, or authority based on her role.

Some babies and women die for lack of immediate access to interventions that are available only in the hospital. But the opposite is also true: Some babies and women die as a result of overuse of interventions that are applied too frequently in hospitals. Currently, out-of-hospital births are an option exercised by a very small minority of women. Most of them are well informed and make this choice through a thoughtful, responsible decision-making process. If that choice exposes them to any risk greater than they would experience during a hospital birth, the difference is small. At the same time, that choice protects them and their babies from unnecessary medical interventions. The freedom to make this choice is very important to some women and their families. In most places, midwives are the only birth practitioners who have both the competence and the commitment to ensure the viability of out-of-hospital births as an option for American women. In addition to the women who are choosing out-of-hospital births currently, some additional women would prefer to give birth at home or in a birth center if all of the conditions just listed could be ensured and if out-of-hospital birth options were covered by major mainstream health care financing plans.

Chapter 12
Effects of Midwifery Care on Costs and Other Special Contributions

This chapter deals with two separate but related contributions of midwifery to maternity care in the United States—reduction in health care costs and providing attractive, effective care to socioeconomically high-risk women. With nearly four million births per year, pregnancy and childbirth make enormous demands on the nation's health care system. A large proportion of births are to young women who are poor or relatively poor and do not have private health care insurance. All responsible parties believe that it is cost effective for society to provide health care to pregnant women and to young children. Both the short- and long-term financial and social costs of failing to do so are grave. Yet the cost of providing the care is very high, and some of the women who are most likely to have problems during pregnancy are not reached by the health care system or do not participate in the available care in a way that

makes a difference. The high overall cost of care is an important factor in limiting access to care for some American women. The United States provides the world's most expensive maternity care but has worse pregnancy outcomes than almost every other industrialized country. The difficulty of reaching socially distressed women with maternity care that engages them in a way that can make a difference is one of the circumstances that contributes to this conundrum.

Over the years the public policy emphasis has ebbed and flowed between concerns about access to care, concerns about the quality and effectiveness of maternity care, and concerns about cost. Concern about the cost of providing care dominated during the first half of the 1990s. Concern about these problems has been the underlying motivation for long-standing government and philanthropic support of nurse-midwifery.

The Effect of Midwifery on Health Care Costs

Although there are many reasons to think that midwifery care is especially cost effective, few studies have attempted to measure the actual economic impact. This section summarizes the reasons why a cost savings is often assumed and the findings from those few studies. Many people assume that midwifery care is less expensive because midwives earn less than physicians. Although most midwives do earn less than most physicians, the fee for basic maternity care provided by a midwife may be the same or nearly the same as the fee for care provided by physicians who practice in the same geographic area as the midwife. Because midwives provide care to fewer women during a given period of time, they cannot earn a living while charging significantly less than a physician charges to provide a maternity care "package" (all routine care) to a low-risk pregnant woman. Midwives spend more time with each client during prenatal, postpartum, and other office or clinic visits, and stay with their patients throughout labor and delivery. Much of the cost savings from use of midwifery care comes from achieving excellent outcomes with fewer procedures that add to the cost of the basic maternity care package.

Cost Savings from Nurse-Midwifery Care with In-Hospital Births

The first study of the economic impact of nurse-midwifery care examined the effects of a hospital-based nurse-midwifery service established to serve low- to moderate-income women in four rural Georgia counties in 1972 (Reid & Morris, 1979). Before the program began, these women delivered their babies at the hospital, but many arrived for delivery having had little or no prenatal care. As the program developed, the infant mortality rates for the four counties decreased, with marked declines in the incidence of low birth weight (LBW) preterm births and infants exhibiting signs of pathology. Data were collected to provide estimates of expenditures for perinatal care, including hospital costs and charges for physician services, but not for additional charges for care related to complications or for care provided to newborns. Estimated costs of perinatal care decreased by almost 30 percent per birth in the four-county area during the first three years of the program (the period studied). Most of the savings came from shorter postpartum hospitalizations and use of less, expensive personnel. The per patient costs were less even though the average number of pre-natal visits per woman was much higher. In addition, while the birth rate decreased by only 6 percent in three nearby counties, the number of births in the four target counties fell by 28 percent. Effective provision of family planning services contributed to the reduction in over-all costs, which was even greater than calculated, because the study did not measure the costs of providing care to newborns, who were both fewer in number and much healthier after the nurse-midwifery service started.

A study conducted in Salt Lake City during 1979 and 1980 found that the mean hospital bill for forty-eight women whose births were attended by nurse-midwives was $114 less than the average bill for forty-five women whose babies were delivered by physicians (Cherry & Foster, 1982). Women with serious complications or cesarean sections were excluded from both groups. To the extent possible, the physician clients were matched to nurse-midwifery clients on delivery date, parity, age, use of forceps, medication used during the delivery, infant birth weight, Apgar scores, complications, and whether the birth took place in a birthing room or a delivery room. It was not possible to find matches for all of the women on use of anesthesia and use of a birthing room versus a delivery room. However, anesthesiology services were not included on the hospital bill, and the hospital did not have a reduced fee for use of the birth room. Thus the findings did not reflect savings due to reduced use of anesthesia and reduced use of a quasi-surgical delivery room. The study design also excluded the possibility of reflecting differences in costs associated with varying utilization of cesarean sections. The differences in charges that were recorded arose from shorter mean length of stay and somewhat less use of many supplies and services, including fewer intravenous infusions (IVs).

Another study compared charges for all maternal and newborn care provided to 29 clients of the nurse-midwifery service at the University of Michigan Women's Hospital and 29 clients of physicians at the same hospital. The MD clients met the nurse-midwifery service's low-risk criteria and were matched to the CNM clients on delivery date, maternal age, and infant birth weight. Women who had cesarean sections were excluded. Both groups of women had essentially normal pregnancies and similar care, except that the MD clients had much higher utilization of technical procedures. Cost data included all billings from the first prenatal visit through two months postpartum for the mothers and until two weeks after birth for the babies. The basic professional fee charged by the nurse-midwifery service is the same as the basic fee for care provided by obstetricians. However, the average total charge for care provided to the obstetricians' clients was $548 higher than the total for the CNMs' clients, with significantly higher charges for electronic fetal monitoring (EFM), anesthesia, and use of delivery rooms. MD clients also had higher bills for services rendered by anesthesiologists and pediatricians. CNM clients had higher charges for postpartum clinic visits, which are billed on a per-visit basis (Krumlauf *et al.*, 1988).

This study was later expanded to include 471 women cared for by CNMs and 710 women with equivalent risk status who were cared for by obstetricians. The expanded study utilized additional information in an attempt to explore alternative explanations for differences in care, as well as costs, between the two groups of women. Although the women in both groups were low risk at entrance into care, the women who obtained their care from physicians experienced slightly more medical problems during pregnancy and birth; in addition, they were significantly more likely to indicate during prenatal care that they wanted to have procedures such as EFM and epidural anesthesia during labor and delivery. These differences largely accounted for the higher use of high-cost elements of care and thus for the higher hospital and professional fees charged to the women who obtained their care from physicians (Oakley *et al.*, 1996).

A study of the effectiveness of certified nurse-midwives in a large health maintenance organization in southern California included an analysis of costs (Bell & Mills, 1989). The study compared staff costs per office visit, per delivery, and per pregnancy at eight Kaiser Permanente medical centers that had the same wage scales. The obstetrics and gynecology department at the Kaiser Medical Center in Anaheim was staffed with eleven obstetricians, five nurse practitioners (NPs), and five CNMs. The CNMs assisted the obstetricians in the care of complicated pregnancies and high-risk deliveries, shared the prenatal care of women with uncomplicated pregnancies with the NPs, and managed the uncomplicated births. None of the other seven medical centers used CNMs. The Anaheim Medical Center had the lowest per delivery and per pregnancy personnel costs of all eight Kaiser medical centers in that part of California. The obstetrics and gynecology department reduced its payroll costs by approximately 13 percent by using nurse-midwives during 1982. (See Chapter 8 for more information on this nurse-midwifery service.)

The most recent study compared obstetric care provided to low-risk pregnant women by a random sample of obstetricians ($N = 54$), family physicians ($N = 59$), and certified nurse-midwives (*N* = 43) providing care to women in urban areas of Washington State in 1989 (Rosenblatt *et al.*, 1997). Forty-seven percent of the pregnant women who initiated care with these doctors and midwives between September 1988 and August 1989 met the study's low-risk criteria. Eleven women who met the criteria were randomly selected into the study from the practice of each of the participating clinicians. The CNMs were less likely than either kind of physician to use continuous EFM or to induce or augment labor with oxytocin, and their patients were less likely to have epidural anesthesia. The cesarean section rate for their patients was 8.8 percent, compared with 13.6 percent for the obstetricians' patients and 15.1 percent for the family practitioners' patients. Little difference was observed between the practice patterns of the obstetricians and the family physicians. The 1989 fee schedule used by Blue Cross of Washington was used to approximate the cost of the obstetric care rendered to each woman in the study. Based on this method of estimating costs, the obstetricians' more active approach to managing labor and delivery was associated with 12.2 percent greater use of resources than the more selective use of procedures practiced by nurse-midwives. Most of the difference was due to greater use of anesthesia and longer hospitalizations for women having cesarean sections.

Cost Savings from Use of Birth Centers and Home Births

The National Association of Childbearing Centers conducts periodic surveys to determine the average cost of complete care in a free-standing birth center and the average hospital and professional fee charges for an uncomplicated vaginal birth in hospitals located in the same communities as the birth centers. Fifty-three birth centers participated in the 1993 study. The average cost for complete care at those birth centers, which were located throughout the country, was $3,268. The average cost for maternity care provided by physicians and hospitals in the same communities was $6,034 for care including a two-day post-partum hospital stay, $4,763 for care including a twenty-four-hour postpartum hospital stay, and $5,436 for use of an in-hospital birth room with relatively brief hospitalization. Women using a free-standing birth center (or their health insurance companies) saved 46 percent compared to hospital care with a two-day stay, 31 percent compared to hospital care with a twenty-four-hour stay, and 40 percent compared to use of an in-hospital birth room with a variable but brief postpartum stay (National Association of Childbearing Centers, 1995). Although the costs of both birth-center and hospital care have increased since the first survey was conducted in 1984, the percentage of savings associated with use of a birth center has remained constant.

The total cost is greater for women who are transferred to a hospital during a birth center birth. An analysis of the effect of transfers on the cost of providing birth-center care to a population of women was conducted using costs at a specific birth center and a specific hospital (Stone & Walker, 1995). Women transferred to the hospital had to pay the complete fee for a hospital birth. It was assumed that 10 percent of the births would involve serious complications, which is higher than the rate found during the National Birth Center Study (7.9 percent). It was further assumed that every woman who had a serious complication would be transported to a hospital in an advanced life-support ambulance for a fee of $250. Only 47 percent of serious complications experienced by women and infants during the National Birth Center Study resulted in transfers. (Some complications occurred during or so close to the time of birth that it was not possible to transfer the patient until after the crisis has passed; then, if the complication had been managed successfully, there was often no need for a transfer.) Only 2.4 percent of women in the National

Birth Center Study had emergency transfers, and ambulances were used for only 65 percent of the emergency transfers (Rooks, *et al.*, 1992c). The outcomes were excellent with this low level of emergency transport, indicating that the assumptions on which this cost-effectiveness analysis were based greatly overestimated the need for use of ambulances. Despite these overestimates of costs, the analysis determined that a birth center is the most cost-effective childbirth setting for low-risk women and would remain so even if the need for transfers were much greater than it really is.

Home births are much less expensive than births in hospitals. A study conducted in Washington State found that the total cost of a home birth attended by a midwife might be as much as 70 percent less than the combined cost of a hospital birth with care provided by a physician (Washington Department of Licensing, 1987). Information gathered during the early 1990s found that home births attended by a licensed direct-entry midwife in Florida cost from $700 to $1,600, compared with $4,500 for a normal hospital birth (Suarez, 1993).

Providing Care to Underserved, Hard-to-Serve Women

One of the greatest benefits of nurse-midwifery to American society continues to be its long-standing involvement and interest in providing care to women who have lacked access to effective care because of poverty, rural isolation, or barriers related to culture or language. In many cases these barriers exist despite sustained efforts to make care more accessible. As explained in Chapter 5, most women find their way to a hospital when they are in labor. The larger problem is lack of early and consistent prenatal care for women who are at high risk of low birth weight and other poor pregnancy outcomes due to poor nutrition and hygiene, inadequate housing, smoking and use of drugs, sexual or physical abuse, untreated health

problems, infections, and lack of resources, information, experience, self-confidence, and social support. These women need prenatal care that gives them hope and engages them in a partnership of supported self-care during pregnancy. They also greatly need to have a positive, rather than a frightening, undignified experience during labor and delivery, and to come out of that experience feeling proud of themselves and their ability to bring forth life and be a mother. These are the women who most need to be encouraged to reach down and touch their baby's head as it is being born and to experience fully the wonderful first hour of intimate contact between a mother and her newborn. They need encouragement and help to breast-feed their babies and empathetic support and ready access to advice for dealing with the problems that beset any new mother, along with sensitive counseling and assistance for initiating family planning.

In 1986, both the Institute of Medicine (IOM) and the American Nurses' Association started processes to develop information and recommendations for improving utilization of prenatal care. The IOM Committee to Study Outreach for Prenatal Care published its report in 1987. The report recommended that prenatal care for socioeconomically disadvantaged women be provided in a personal, caring environment in which patients are treated with respect, telephone consultations are easily available, and there is continuity-of-care in the relationship between the primary care provider and the patient. Small or decentralized services were recommended to avoid the feeling of a large, impersonal bureaucracy. Care providers were advised to respond to women's concerns, recognize patients' needs for acceptance and emotional support, and understand and try to overcome barriers related to culture. The report noted CNMs' special contribution to providing care to low-income women, adolescents, members of minority groups, and women who live in inner cities and rural areas, and recommended that means be found to overcome legal restrictions and "obstetrical customs" that limit their practice (IOM, 1987).

The American Nurses' Association convened four regional conferences that focused on barriers to prenatal care. The conference report described three categories of nonfinancial barriers: barriers related to the health care system, barriers arising from women's interactions with society, and barriers related to health care providers. The section on health care provider barriers described "negative personal characteristics" (being rude, insensitive, judgmental, hostile, condescending, patronizing, or racist); inadequate teaching, communication, and counseling skills; failure to keep current; poor communication between professionals providing services to the same woman; discrimination against certain kinds of women; inadequate education about the psychosocial and cultural aspects of providing care to pregnant women; inconsistent application of standards of care; turf battles between different kinds of professionals; and inadequate knowledge and use of community resources. Greater use of nurse-midwives and nurse practitioners was identified as one of the many strategies for reducing the barriers (Curry, 1987).

Chapter 7 used data from several sources to describe the women whose babies are delivered by midwives. Nurse-midwives play a special role in the care of Native American women, and, as reflected in the IOM report on outreach for prenatal care, CNMs' general clientele have a higher-than-average concentration of social, economic, and behavioral risk factors associated with poor pregnancy outcomes.

Research on "Underserved," "Hard-to-Serve" Women

Many statistical analyses have been conducted to identify maternal characteristics associated with late or no pre-natal care and low birth weight and other poor pregnancy outcomes. Little research has been done to describe and explain the circumstances of women who do not use prenatal care even when it is seemingly available. This section summarizes information from a study of women who had little or no prenatal care before delivering babies at Denver General Hospital from 1989 through 1991, and the women's reasons for not seeking prenatal care (Meikle *et al.*, 1995). Babies born at this hospital were seven times more likely to be very low birth weight if their mothers had no prenatal care. By the time this study was started, it had become clear that expanding eligibility for Medicaid does not guarantee that low-income women will use prenatal care at all, or that they will enter a program of prenatal care during the first few months of pregnancy (Piper *et al.*, 1990). This study was conducted to determine why. More than 600 low-income women who had delivered at the hospital having had fewer than five prenatal visits throughout their entire pregnancy or no visits until the last three months of their pregnancy were interviewed on the day after their delivery. Forty-eight percent of them were Hispanic; 26 percent were black. More than one-fourth were teenagers; two-thirds had not completed high school. Eighty percent were not married, and nearly 70 percent had at least one other child. Eighty-seven percent of the pregnancies were unintended. Sixty percent of the women planned to raise their new babies by themselves, although most (65 percent) had a monthly household income of no more than $500 (Meikle *et al.*, 1995).

Asked why they had not started prenatal care earlier, almost half of the women cited a belief or attitude as the most important reason; one-fourth cited financial problems as most important. Financial reasons were more important to white women; attitudinal reasons were more important to black and Hispanic women. Attitudinal reasons fell into two major categories: (1) not wanting to be pregnant (being afraid to find out that she was pregnant, considering an abortion, not wanting to think about being pregnant, and not wanting anyone to know that she was pregnant) and (2) thinking that prenatal care was not important or needed (because she was getting advice from friends, was not having any problems, or thought she knew how to take care of herself). Less frequently mentioned reasons included system problems such as difficulty getting an appointment, having had a bad previous experience with doctors or nurses, not knowing where to go for care, and difficulty getting a baby-sitter or transportation. Many of the women also cited personal reasons such as frequent moves, homelessness, being on drugs, and being in jail. Nearly one-third of the women had a history of physical or sexual abuse. Some had experienced several serious problems while pregnant or just before they conceived, including separation or divorce, worsening financial concerns, drug addiction, alcoholism, or the deaths of close friends or family members. Many reported constant arguing at home; more than 40 percent said they were depressed, sad, or blue during the last six months of pregnancy. One-fourth of the women felt that they "can't do anything right" or are "helpless in dealing with life problems" (Meikle *et al.*, 1995).

Summary

Consideration of cost effectiveness must include both costs and effectiveness. In assessing midwives' contributions to the cost effectiveness of the reproductive care provided to women in the United States, the high long-term social and financial costs of failing to provide care that succeeds in engaging the healthful hopes of the women who are most socially distressed and disparate from their care providers must be considered in the equation. Although nurse-midwives could increase their short-term "productivity" by having brief prenatal visits, thus seeing more patients in an hour (as some are being pressured to do), short-term savings are likely to be offset, if not overtaken, by diminished effectiveness. Quality

maternity care should not be conceptualized as only a cost, but also as an investment in better pregnancy outcomes and a healthier, more positive start for families.

Midwifery care may reduce the total cost of maternal and infant health care in many ways. Although the financial benefits of the effects of midwifery care have been measured in only a few instances, and then not completely, it is reasonable to assume that many aspects of midwifery care are associated with reduced costs.

Nurse-midwives have focused on reaching underserved and hard-to-serve women with care that these women are willing to participate in consistently and effectively. Involving these women in effective care results in better pregnancy outcomes; reduced morbidity for the mother and baby; more breast-feeding; a more positive start for young families; and mothers who are more knowledgeable and confident in caring for their babies, more likely to bring their babies for routine health care, including immunizations, and more likely to use contraception in order to delay another pregnancy.

There is some evidence that nurse-midwifery care may help to reduce the incidence of low birth weight among socioeconomically high-risk women; the strongest evidence exists for an effect on preventing very low birth weight among infants born to socioeconomically high-risk black women. The financial and social benefits of preventing these outcomes are enormous.

Large cost savings could be achieved by moving more low-risk births out of hospitals into the less expensive settings of birth centers and homes. Costs could be reduced by 30 to 70 percent.

Nurse-midwives were the pioneers of early hospital discharge for well-prepared, healthy mothers and babies. Early discharge was picked up by hospital administrators and third-party payers as a way to save money and has become a controversial issue in which physicians argue that early discharge is unsafe and will hurt mothers and babies and cost more money in the long run. Nurse-midwives have avoided these problems by providing the education and support needed to make it easier and safer for women to return to their homes relatively quickly after giving birth in hospitals.

Nurse-midwives save money by managing many hospital births in the same bed and room in which the woman labored, instead of moving her to a surgical-style delivery room. Nurse-midwives also reduce costs by using labor and delivery procedures more selectively, less routinely, and less frequently than they are used by most physicians.

Midwives provide support for successful breast-feeding. This saves hospitals some money, and saves mothers and families much more money; formula for an infant costs more than $300 per year (Oski, 1993). Reduced infant illness associated with longer breast-feeding also saves money, in part through reduced need for pediatrician visits and hospitalization during the first year of life.

Midwives are contributing to a slow reduction in the incidence of cesarean deliveries. Cesarean section rates are much lower for women whose births are attended by midwives. The difference is most dramatic for women who have home births or births in free-standing birth centers, but the impact is more far reaching for births in hospitals. Midwives have a particularly good record regarding VBACs, that is, increasing the proportion of successful vaginal births among women who have had prior cesarean deliveries.

Some of the reduction in cesarean section rates associated with midwifery care is attributable to the low-risk status of the women midwives take care of and to their clients' preferences regarding the use or avoidance of certain procedures during labor, including epidural anesthesia, which is associated with a two- to threefold increase in cesarean deliveries. Although many Amer-ican women really want an epidural, the lack of midwifery care leaves many women with no source of consistent, effective support during labor and no access to alternative methods to relieve and cope with the stress and pain of labor. Women who understand the risks associated with epidural anesthesia may have the confidence to forgo it only if they can count on having the intensive, personal skilled support of midwifery care.

A study that assigned women to midwifery or medical care on a random basis found that obstetric residents could achieve a cesarean section rate as low as the midwives' rate when they took care of similar women. But this occurred in a public hospital with a Hispanic clientele and obstetric leaders who were committed to avoiding unnecessary cesareans.* This study showed that it is possible for physicians to achieve a very low cesarean section rate, but this is the exception, not the rule. Midwives routinely achieve good pregnancy outcomes with few cesarean sections. In addition to the impact of their care on the women they serve, midwives contribute to preventing unnecessary cesareans by demonstrating an alternative approach to managing many aspects of labor and delivery to others. Nurse-midwives who work in close contact with physicians influence their colleagues, just as the physicians influence the midwives. The study just described was conducted in a teaching hospital that had had a vigorous nurse-midwifery service for more than fifteen years. Slowly but surely midwifery is affecting the professional and public paradigm regarding the nature of appropriate care for pregnant women. This influence extends beyond the minority of women who have personal experience with midwifery care.

---

*See Chapter 10 for more information on factors that influence the cesarean delivery rate and the study conducted at the Los Angeles County/University of Southern California Women's Hospital.

Chapter 13
Midwifery in Europe, Canada, Australia, New Zealand, and Japan

This chapter provides information on the International Confederation of Midwives and an overview of midwifery and maternity care in countries that are similar to the United States culturally or in terms of economic and general social development and medical standards. The infant mortality rate is higher in the United States than in every country included in this review.

Canada is the only country discussed in this chapter in which midwives do not play a clear, widely accepted role in the care of all or most pregnant women. The role of midwives in those countries varies widely—a full, independent midwifery role in some countries and a circumscribed, dependent role in others. Nevertheless, the countries of North America are distinct among those in this peer group because midwifery is not assumed to be an inherent part of all or virtually all maternal health care services in either Canada or the United States. This is

changing in a few places in Canada, and nurse-midwives play a critical role in some components of the health care system in the United States. Still, midwives in North America fill niches or struggle to create, hold, or expand a place for midwifery practice in systems in which midwifery is an alternative, but not the standard. We can learn much from observing the circumstances where midwifery is the standard of care.

Most midwives look to the Netherlands as providing the best example of the performance of a well-established, autonomous midwifery profession. Several factors originating within its history and culture have made the Netherlands uniquely resistant to modern obstetrics' demand for universal hospitalization and technical surveillance during childbirth. Thus, although the proportion of home births has declined somewhat in the Netherlands, cultural factors, excellent medical leadership, excellent outcomes of home births attended by midwives, and the cost-effective policies of the national health care insurance system have supported a vigorous home birth tradition in the Netherlands. With approximately a third of its births at home over an extended period, the Netherlands has had a consistently low rate of infant mortality. Its infant mortality rate for 1992 was 6.3 per thousand, the tenth lowest rate in the world. The U.S. infant mortality rate for 1992 was 8.5 per thousand, and we ranked 22th in the world (NCHS, 1996b).

After admiring the steadfast excellence of midwifery in the Netherlands, the next most striking impression from this review is that midwifery is blossoming in the English-speaking countries of our peer group. The dissatisfaction with impersonal, pathology-oriented obstetric care that led to the development of lay midwifery in the United States during the 1960s and 1970s was experienced throughout the Western world. Criticism and demand for change in individual countries were strengthened by international communication and interaction facilitated by activities of the World Health Organization (WHO) and the International Confederation of Midwives (ICM), and by the growing strength of the consumer and women's movements, heightened international interest in perinatal research, and the flow of ideas and information generated by books and journals. Demand for alternative kinds of maternity care arose simultaneously in many countries. Seeds of change sown during the 1970s now seem to be coming to fruition, creating an exciting international array of new developments in midwifery. Although there are important similarities from one country to another, historical differences have led to unique aspects of midwifery in each country.

Virtually every country has experienced increasing medicalization of childbirth since the early 1970s, with efforts to centralize births in large tertiary hospitals and closure of many small maternity units. Midwives de-

cried the loss of normal childbirth but seemed unable to stem the tide; their discouragement was reflected by declining enrollment of midwifery students in England and the United States during the early 1980s, as midwifery seemed to be losing its special role and a wider variety of careers became available to women. General practice physicians also experienced a diminishing role in the care of pregnant women in many countries (e.g., the Netherlands, Great Britain, and the United States), and the number of obstetricians expanded. Midwifery has made a comeback in some countries on the strength of consumer demand. The reduction of the family physician's role in maternity care may be more permanent.

Government-initiated reviews of maternity care in Britain and Australia sought the views of the women who use the services. The voices of women resounding through the reports of those reviews called attention to satisfaction and dissatisfaction as vital measures of the quality of the care provided to pregnant women. Many women were not satisfied with the care they were receiving. They wanted midwives, and they wanted an opportunity to develop a trusting relationship with an individual midwife, and real midwifery, not midwives subjugated to the obstetricians' paradigm of pathologic childbirth. The same dissatisfactions and desires were expressed by women in New Zealand and several Canadian provinces, where change came from the enactment of new laws. But whether initiated by influential reports or legislation, rapid and remarkable change began in all four countries as a result of democratic governments asking not just doctors, but women, to tell them what was wrong and what was needed to improve the care and experience of women having babies.

In some countries, groups consisting of both midwives and consumers organized to demand better maternity care for the women of that country. The strong partnership between midwives and women in New Zealand is described later in this chapter.

But New Zealand was not unique. Politically active groups of midwives and consumers arose in several countries. Examples of such organizations in countries that are not focused on in this chapter include Femme, Sage-Femme in France, Foreldre og Fodsel in Denmark, and Nascita Attiva in Italy (Wagner, 1996a). Midwifery has been empowered by consumers in these countries, renewed in spirit, embracing the changes women want and committed to developing midwifery models that will make it practical to provide continuity of care within a national health care system. New models of care are being conceptualized, tried, tested, and examined.

Most of the midwives in most of the countries discussed in this chapter are employed by their governments, usually working shifts and providing care during only one part of the maternity cycle. Providing continuity of care is one of many challenges that accompanies the recent changes. Regardless of increased legal independence in some countries, midwives need to collaborate with physicians. Although the clinical issues remain the same, midwives in some countries are having to learn to negotiate with physicians from a new role and position. Newly "independent" midwives in New Zealand are experiencing some of the practice barriers that U.S. nurse-midwives have been dealing with for years, such as restrictions imposed by hospitals as a condition to the "privilege" of admitting women for care. Hospital privileges are not needed by New Zealand midwives who work shifts in government hospitals. Midwives everywhere—even in the Netherlands—need to learn to deal with new technologies, such as ultrasound (Tymstra, 1993). New expectations for continuity of care and midwife shortages in several countries (e.g., the Netherlands and Japan) are producing burnout. Shortages in some countries are exacerbated by midwives leaving the profession for various reasons, including low pay. Midwives in Britain, Canada, and Australia are trying to find ways to achieve the new, larger objectives of midwifery care without producing burn-out.

The history of midwifery in several of these countries reveals a struggle with nursing over control of the profession. Direct-entry midwifery education died out in the United Kingdom, Australia, New Zealand, and Japan, as midwifery became subsumed under nursing. This trend is being reversed in some of those countries, where midwives are reasserting their independence from nursing, as well as medicine. New direct-entry midwifery education programs have been started in the United Kingdom and New Zealand; both are countries in which direct-entry midwifery had existed earlier. A recent survey conducted by the World Health Organization found that 46 percent—slightly less than half—of all midwives in industrialized countries are nurses (Peters, 1995). But they are thought of and referred to as "midwives," not "nurse-midwives;" no distinction between nurse-midwives and direct-entry midwives is made in the countries that have both.

Although the standard length of direct-entry education is three years, midwifery education programs are getting longer in some countries. The standard is now four years in the Netherlands. There is also a small trend toward moving midwifery education into institutions of higher learning. In countries in which the midwifery role is strong, large numbers of young women apply for the limited number of places in midwifery schools, and entrance is very competitive. The social class level of midwifery students in Great Britain has risen with the more prominent role of midwives in the British health care system (Allison, 1994). Midwives in many countries are becoming more involved and experienced in research. Small numbers of men are joining the profession in some countries.

Home births declined everywhere during most of this century, even in the Netherlands. Home births have begun to increase in Denmark, England, Germany, New

Zealand, and Japan—all due to recent changes made to accommodate the expressed desires of women. The proportion of home births in the Netherlands stopped declining in the mid-1980s and now seems to be relatively stable at about one-third of the country's births. There is increasing interest in free-standing birth centers in some countries, especially Germany and Australia, where many birth centers have been developed since the beginning of the 1990s.

Purpose of This Chapter

The subject of this book is midwifery and childbirth in America—in the United States. The purpose of this chapter is to provide an international context for understanding midwifery and maternity care in the United States. It is a restricted purpose, and the information presented has limitations. Much of the information came from published papers and reports. Although the chapter benefited greatly from the review and critique of individuals who know much more than I about the situations in specific countries, it is not based on the same level of complex historical and current knowledge and understanding that is behind the other chapters. And it is uneven. For instance, I was able to obtain information and discuss issues affecting midwifery in Canada with several different people, with different perspectives. I did not have access to a wide range of perspectives about midwifery in any of the other countries. I have also come to believe that there is some bias in the reports about midwifery in other countries that are published in the United States. Even though each article and document may be completely accurate, the telling of any story has a bias—what is included in the story, and what is left out. "Publication bias" affects which stories are told at all, particularly which news articles about midwifery in other countries are picked up and which research reports are published or summarized in journals that are widely read in the United States.

Ulla Waldenström, a Swedish midwife who teaches midwifery at a university in Australia, reviewed my draft of the section on Australia. Although she was interested in the history and did not disagree with the facts presented, she felt that the composite picture was too rosy and not truly representative of the actual situation. She spoke of the high use of epidurals and the high rate of cesarean sections in Australia; the identity crisis the midwifery profession is facing due to new expectations caused by changes in obstetric practices, women's expectations, and midwifery education; and the limitations of the traditional midwifery role and traditional midwifery education at a time when information is expanding rapidly and midwives, as well as physicians, are expected to base their practice on research. This book deals with these issues in relation to midwifery in the United States. Although the same issues affect midwives throughout the world, I do not have enough understanding of the events, history, and context of midwifery in other countries to go beyond a relatively superficial kind of reporting.

Despite these limitations, this chapter is important to an understanding of midwifery and childbirth in America. Midwifery has been stunted here. It is important to understand that our situation is aberrant, to realize how different it is in other countries, and to be aware of some of the remarkable recent trends and other events.

The International Confederation of Midwives

The first international midwives' meeting was held in Berlin in 1900; it drew more than one thousand midwives from nine European countries. Training was the main subject of discussion. The International Midwives Union was founded in 1919; it focused on midwifery in Europe. The International Midwives Union held five international meetings, the first in Belgium in 1919, the last in 1938. India sent representatives to the meeting held in 1934—the first official participation by non-European midwives. In 1954 the International Midwives Union adopted a new constitution with a wider international focus and reorganized itself as the International Confederation of Midwives. ICM's mission is to improve the standard of care provided to mothers, babies, and families throughout the world; to support and advise midwifery associations; to advance provision of maternity care; and to develop the role of the midwife as a professional practitioner in her own right (ICM, 1996). ICM is trying to find ways to make it more feasible for midwifery organizations in developing countries to afford ICM membership and for midwives from developing countries to attend ICM congresses and play a more active role in the organization.

The ICM established a permanent secretariat and convened its first meeting, in London, in 1954; it was attended by midwives from more than fifty countries throughout the world (Raisler, 1994). The ICM has held congresses every three years since then. The first ICM congress outside of Europe was held in Santiago, Chili, in 1969 (Woodville, 1971). Two ICM congresses have been held in North America. The American College of Nurse-Midwives hosted the 1972 ICM Congress in Washington, D.C. The Midwives Association of British Columbia hosted the 1993 ICM Congress in Vancouver. The most recent ICM Congress was held in Oslo, Norway, in May 1996. The 1999 congress will be held in the Philippines. The triennial congresses provide an invaluable opportunity for midwives from different cultures to share information and learn from one another. This exchange has played a powerful role in changes affecting midwifery in many countries during the past decade.

Headquartered in London, the ICM was for a long time heavily subsidized and housed by the Royal College of Midwives, which is, by far, its largest member. National midwifery organizations pay membership fees. The U.S. Agency for International Development (USAID) provided financial support for the 1972 Congress and additional funding from 1972 through 1979 for activities directed at educating midwives in family planning and training traditional birth attendants. USAID support made it possible for ICM to rent its own office space and hire its first staff (Raisler, 1994). ICM continues to receive grants from national and international development assistance organizations for work intended to improve maternal and infant health care in developing countries.

A new constitution adopted in 1981 introduced a process for regional representation; this has allowed non-European members to play a more active role (Raisler, 1994). Representatives of member organizations comprise the ICM Council, which meets immediately before each triennial congress. The organization is run by a three-person board of management and by its major officers, whose terms begin at the end of one triennial congress and extend through the next one. The president is the leader of the midwifery association that will host the next congress.

The United Nations (UN) recognized ICM as an official nongovernmental organization (NGO) in 1957. This gives ICM the right to be represented at meetings of WHO and other UN agencies. During the 1960s a study group comprised of representatives of the ICM and the International Federation of Obstetricians and Gynecologists produced a book on *Maternity Care in the World*, which described maternal and child health services in 210 countries (Raisler, 1994). ICM has participated in a variety of WHO and UNICEF activities, including the "Safe Motherhood Initiative" to combat maternal mortality in developing countries. ICM publishes policy papers on issues related to midwifery, such as legislation, education, research, and professional accountability (Raisler, 1994).

Twenty-five hundred midwives from seventy-one countries attended the 1996 ICM

Congress. The midwifery organizations of fifty-three countries were represented by official delegations that participated in the business meetings. The 1996 Council adopted a "Global Vision for Women" and specific goals for serving midwives throughout the world during the period from 1996 through 2002. The United States was represented by both the American College of Nurse-Midwives and the International Section of the Midwives Alliance of North America. Seven countries are represented by more than one national midwifery organization.

Midwifery in Europe

There are several fundamental differences between maternity care in western Europe and North America. Midwifery is an integral part of maternal health care in Europe—the standard for the care of healthy women in most countries. Every Western European country has a large group of practicing midwives. Every woman in Europe is guaranteed maternity care by her government. The rates of both infant mortality and cesarean deliveries are lower in most western European countries than in the United States, and every country in western Europe spends less of its gross national product on health care (Wagner, 1988).

Most European countries have had laws to regulate midwifery, publicly supported schools to educate midwives, and professional associations to represent midwives since the beginning of the twentieth century (Devitt, 1979; University of Washington, 1980). All European countries have some form of government-financed health care. Most midwives work for government health services, providing prenatal and postpartum care in clinics or working in hospital labor and delivery suites. Because of the way these jobs are structured, relatively few midwives provide continuity of care to their clients. A woman who receives prenatal and postpartum care from a midwife who works in a

clinic in the woman's community will probably receive care from a different midwife, whom she has not met before, during labor and delivery in a hospital (Miller, 1987). Midwives in some countries make home visits to pregnant women, or, more commonly, to mothers and their babies shortly after the birth. Although most countries includes home visits as an integral part of their maternity care program, public health nurses, rather than midwives, are responsible for postpartum home visits in some countries (Miller, 1987).

There is great variation in the role of midwives in the many countries of Europe. Midwives practice as autonomous practitioners in the Netherlands, but play a secondary role to physicians in some countries. Midwives in some countries provide complete care to virtually all women with normal pregnancies, from conception until the end of the postpartum period, and provide family planning and other services at the end of the childbearing cycle. In other countries, most midwives provide care only during labor. Each country has its own pattern for combining the services of midwives, general practitioners, obstetricians, and nurses in the care of pregnant and postpartum women. The role of each is defined by law, to some extent, but also by the policies and practices of the national health care and health insurance systems. For example, although midwives provide prenatal care to all women in Denmark (five to eight visits), all Danes are registered with a general practitioner (GP), and most women also make three visits to their GP during pregnancy and return to their GP for their six-week postpartum examination (Miller, 1987; Hoúd, 1997). In this case, the postpartum examination, which is viewed as the last component of the care associated with pregnancy in the United States (and is done by the woman's pregnancy care provider), is used to mark the woman's reentry into her usual, that is, not pregnant, health care, which is provided by her GP. Midwifery is exceptionally strong in the Netherlands for many reasons, including long-standing policies and practices of the national health insurance system.

The role of midwives in Europe has also been affected by the worldwide trend toward an increasing focus on the pathologic potential of pregnancy. As a result of this conceptual change, higher and higher proportions of women are being defined as high risk and obstetricians have become more involved in the care of women with uncomplicated pregnancies. With this has come increasing or even routine use of technical procedures, especially during labor and delivery. These changes have resulted in decreased use of GPs and decreased authority for midwives in some countries, turning some of them into obstetrician assistants. Another consequence has been reduction in the availability of small maternity services, with concentration of a growing proportion of births in the high-volume obstetric units of tertiary hospitals. This results in dissociation between prenatal care, which is often provided relatively close to where women live, and childbirth care, which is provided by hospital-based midwives and obstetricians. The cumulative effect of all of these trends was dissatisfaction among many midwives and childbearing women and the development of an international movement promoting alternatives to the care provided through the government health services. This dissatisfaction prompted an investigation that resulted in an influential report published by the Office for the European Region of the WHO in 1985. The report documented these trends and described midwife-centered alternative forms of maternity care being developed in North America and eight countries in the European Region of WHO.

The number of "independent midwives" (those working outside of the government systems) has increased to some degree. However, many health care systems will not pay for services provided outside of the government system, and there are few role models for independent health care practice in many countries. Working outside of the system, without retirement and other fringe benefits, is too financially insecure for many midwives. Actually, the term, *independent midwife* is applied to two kinds of midwives, those who work in the community (i.e., not in hospitals or clinics) but are part of the government system, and midwives who work privately (i.e., are not part of the government system at all).

Midwives in some European countries are experimenting with different ways to increase their ability to provide continuity of care within the national health care system, for example, by forming small teams of midwives who provide complete care to a limited number of clients. This system is widely used by Dutch home birth midwives and in the United Kingdom (U.K.). Finding ways to implement continuity of care is a work in progress, and efforts are being made to measure the effects of providing this kind of care. A paper reporting the results of a randomized, controlled trial of "midwife-managed care" versus "shared care" was published in *The Lancet* (a leading British medical journal) in 1996 (Turnbull *et al.*, 1996). The study was conducted at a hospital in Scotland. Each woman who was assigned to "midwife-managed care" received all or most of her care from a particular midwife, from her first prenatal visit through childbirth and the postpartum period; when her midwife was not available, the woman received care from a midwife who was a colleague of the woman's usual midwife. Women in the control group received care from a variety of physicians and midwives and did not see the same midwife throughout their pregnancies. The women who received continuity of care from midwives were less likely to have had their labor induced with pitocin, had fewer episiotomies, and were significantly more satisfied with their care.

Home deliveries declined markedly throughout Europe during the last forty years, even in the Netherlands, which remains the renowned exception to the rule of nearly universal hospitalization. Home births accounted for 31 percent of births in the Netherlands in 1991. Although home births had fallen to only 1 percent of births in England and Wales by 1984, an important report issued by a parliamentary committee in 1992 challenged the assumption that hospitals are the safest place for all women to give birth. That report led to additional investigation of the quality of maternity care provided by the National Health Service and a virtual about-face in U.K. policies regarding maternity care. The United Kingdom has embarked on a remarkable effort to "change childbirth" by making it more responsive to women's needs and preferences, moving away from frequent use of obstetrical interventions and creating new models of community-based maternity care in which every pregnant woman has the opportunity to choose a midwife to provide her care throughout her pregnancy. Recommendations of the 1993 *Changing Childbirth* report have been widely accepted; a concrete five-year implementation plan with measurable objectives for assessing progress in achieving the recommendations has become the new national policy. One result is an increase in home births (Allison, 1994).

Free-standing birth centers or "birth houses" have been opened in Austria, Denmark, Germany, and Switzerland, and birth centers located in hospitals have been developed in Sweden, Denmark, and Norway (Waldenström & Nilsson, 1993; Stallings, 1995; Friedrich, 1996; Hoúd, 1997). Birth center care usually features continuity of care, with each woman receiving all of her care from the same small team of midwives from her first prenatal visit, during the births, and through the postpartum period. A randomized trial was conducted to measure women's satisfaction with care provided at an in-hospital birth center in Sweden and to compare it with the degree of satisfaction expressed by women who received standard obstetric care (Waldenström & Nilsson, 1993). The women who had been assigned to the birth center expressed greater satisfaction with each phase of their care (prenatal, childbirth, and postpartum), and were especially satisfied with the psychological aspects of their experience.

Physicians in some countries still promote themselves as the best source of primary care for pregnant women, and midwifery is being marginalized in some countries. But there is a strong countermovement. During the 1980s obstetricians convinced the government to close down all midwifery schools in Spain. Midwives joined with women's groups in protesting this change, and all of the schools have since reopened. Also during the 1980s the German Obstetrical Society asked the national government to eliminate the law (which had been on the books for centuries) that requires a midwife to be present at every birth. Midwives and women's groups joined together to protest the proposed change; the law remains (Wagner, 1996a). As described later in this chapter, midwifery has experienced a renaissance in the United Kingdom.

Midwifery Education and the European Economic Area Midwives Directives

Every Western European country requires students to complete "gymnasium" before entering a midwifery education program. Although gymnasium is academic, the training provided in most European midwifery schools is similar to that provided in a trade school. There is, however, a small trend toward making the training longer and placing midwifery education in universities.

Nursing education is required for entrance into midwifery education in some countries (e.g., Norway, Scotland, Sweden). In other countries students enter midwifery education directly (e.g., Denmark, France, the Netherlands). Some countries maintain both educational routes to professional midwifery (e.g., Belgium, the United Kingdom, Germany). Direct-entry midwifery education is developing rapidly in England.

The European Economic Area (EEA) includes fifteen countries that are full members of the European Union and three that are not full members of the Union but are members of the European Free Trade Association.* Countries that belong to the EEA are required to bring their national laws into accord with EEA directives within a specified period of time. One purpose is mutual recognition of the major health professions in order to make it easier for qualified professionals to move between EEA countries. The EEA produced the E.U. *Midwives Directives* in 1983. Midwives credentialed in countries whose laws comply with the directives are eligible for midwifery licensure in all other EEA countries. Because of differences in the status and training of midwives in the member states, it took ten years to develop the directives. Although the process was lengthy, the negotiations were productive. The *Midwives Directives* are unique among all E.U. professional directives because they include a definition of the scope of practice of a midwife and an outline of the activities a midwife must be able to perform (Winship, 1996). The E.U. *Midwives Directives* authorize member nations to educate either nurse-midwives or direct-entry midwives; however, every EEA country must recognize and allow both kinds of midwives to practice. Both types must be treated as equivalent in the country's midwifery practice law.

Between 1989 and 1994 the European Midwives Liaison Committee (representatives of the midwives' associations from each E.U. country) conducted a study to determine the extent to which actual midwifery practice in each E.U. country conforms to the scope of practice specified in the E.U. *Midwives Directives* (European Midwives Liaison Committee, 1996). This has important

*The following countries are members of the European Economic Union: Austria, Belgium, Denmark, Finland, France, Germany, Greece, Holland, Ireland, Italy, Luxembourg, Portugal, Spain, Sweden, and the United Kingdom. The three other countries included in the European Economic Area are Iceland, Liechtenstein, and Norway (Winship, 1996).

ramifications because the midwifery education programs in *every* E.U. country must be able to prepare midwives who are competent to practice in *any* E.U. country.

The *Midwives Directives* require a formal midwifery education program that is at least three years in length—two years for students who are already qualified in nursing (Official Journal of the European Communities, 1980). Some countries had to increase the length of their programs to comply with the directives (Forestier, 1983). In addition, the Netherlands has increased the length of its midwifery course to four years. England has developed both three-year diploma (nondegree) and four-year degree programs for preparation of direct-entry midwives. Several countries have moved some midwifery education into universities, in part because of the desire to increase midwives' sophistication and skills in producing and using the results of research (e.g., Iceland). Nevertheless, most midwives currently practicing in Europe were trained in three-year, nonuniversity programs (Wagner, 1996a). Midwifery education is free in most countries, and students receive a government salary or stipend. A few universities in a few countries offer one-year post-basic courses for midwives who want additional preparation for roles as educators or administrators (Hoúd, 1997).

In 1984, the EEA established a committee to advise the European Commission on the training of midwives. Three experts from each member country sit on the committee. Although most members of the committee are midwives, some countries have appointed obstetricians or civil servants who are neither midwives nor obstetricians to represent them on the committee (Winship, 1996).

Having a Baby in Europe–A WHO Report from the Early 1980s

Criticism of the maternity care provided through government health services spread in Europe during the 1970s. Delegates attending the 1979 annual meeting of the European Region of WHO asked that a committee be established to investigate the care being provided to pregnant women in their countries. The resulting Perinatal Study Group collected information, in part through a survey that was completed by 23 of the 33 countries in the region, which includes Russia, the Eastern European countries of the former Soviet Union, Turkey and Morocco, as well as the countries of Western Europe (WHO Regional Office for Europe, 1985).

Midwives were practicing in 19 of the 23 countries. There were more than three times as many midwives as obstetricians. Eighteen countries provided estimates of the proportion of births attended by midwives, obstetricians, and others. A midwife was the primary attendant at all or nearly all normal births in half of those countries; obstetricians attended all or most normal births in all of the other urban countries and two of the other rural countries. An obstetrician and a midwife attended every birth, normal or complicated, in one country. Obstetricians and midwives shared the normal deliveries in two countries; obstetricians and traditional birth attendants shared them in a rural country. Midwives also played a role in some or all complicated births in one-third of the urban countries and three-fourths of the rural countries. General practitioners did not play a major role in childbirth in any of these countries. Obstetricians were playing an increasing role in normal births in several countries. In some countries midwives were attending normal births in government hospitals, while obstetricians attended normal births in private hospitals.

Most women received prenatal care from a different person (whether a midwife or a physician) than the person who took care of her during labor and delivery. Because most hospital staff worked eight-hour shifts, few women even had continuity of care throughout labor and delivery (WHO Regional Office for Europe, 1985).

Home births accounted for less than 5 percent of the births in all but two countries.

The Netherlands and Denmark were the only countries in which every woman with a normal pregnancy could choose where she would like to give birth. All other countries had explicit or implicit hospital-birth-only policies, although there were some midwife-assisted home births in rural parts of several large countries. In countries with "monopolistic governments" (i.e., communist or totalitarian), few women could choose which hospital to use for childbirth; it was predetermined, based on where they lived. In "pluralistic" (i.e., democratic) countries, women might be able to choose between a smaller community hospital and a larger district hospital. But maternity homes and obstetric units in small hospitals were disappearing in many countries. Births were becoming centralized in a few very high-volume hospitals in several countries (WHO Regional Office for Europe, 1985; Hoúd, 1997).

Women had little choice about use of procedures or the presence of other people during labor and delivery. Women in ten countries had no choice regarding use or nonuse of analgesia and anesthesia. Use of obstetric interventions was increasing. The cesarean section rate ranged from 4 percent to 12 percent (WHO Regional Office for Europe, 1985).

Rooming-in was increasing but not fully in place in most countries, although six countries had established national policies to encourage rooming-in. In wealthier countries, this policy was established to facilitate breast-feeding and good mother–infant attachment; in less developed countries, rooming-in was practiced because of lack of space in government hospitals. Although a few monopolistic countries had rooming-in "experiments" in selected hospitals, there was no rooming-in at all in several countries.

A midwife or public health nurse made at least one home visit during the first days or weeks after the mothers and babies had left the hospital in 20 countries. Midwives made the home visits in most countries that had routine home visiting; specially trained nurses made the visits in most countries in which only special risk cases were visited (WHO Regional Office for Europe, 1985).

The Alternative Maternity Care Movement

At some point the Perinatal Study Group realized that it had been looking at only the official maternity services and thought they could learn something by looking at the alternative services that had been created in response to dissatisfaction with the officially provided care. A midwife (Susanne Hoúd) and a sociologist (Ann Oakley) were teamed to study this phenomenon in the European region. They visited ten countries in which alternative care systems were being developed, including Canada and the United States, as well as Denmark, France, the Federal Republic of Germany, the Netherlands, Sweden, the USSR, the United Kingdom and Yugoslavia. Canada and the United States were included because of the importance of alternative services in North America and their connection to the alternative service movement in Europe (WHO Regional Office for Europe, 1985).

"Alternative services" were defined as those outside the usual or "official" pattern of perinatal care. The two researchers identified eight alternatives that existed in at least some settings in most of the countries they visited. Expanding the choices available to women was considered a critical element in defining an alternative service:

- Attempting to provide continuity of care, that is, to make it possible for women to have a continuous relationship with one care provider during prenatal care and labor and delivery.
- Developing home-like "birth rooms" in hospitals. These rooms provide privacy and enable the woman to labor and deliver in the same room and avoid use of a surgical-type delivery room.
- Allowing women to assume various positions while giving birth.

- Using birth chairs or birth stools.
- Permitting the presence of friends and relatives at birth.
- Eliminating preparatory baths, enemas, and shaves as a routine part of childbirth care.
- Trying to reduce use of interventions during labor and birth, including use of oxytocin to induce and augment labor, use of continuous electronic fetal monitoring (EFM), use of forceps and vacuum during vaginal births, and cesarean deliveries.
- Conducting Leboyer-style births, with dimmed lights and gentle treatment of the newborn.

Actual implementation of these alternatives varied among and within countries. Alternative services were found to exist within both the official insurance- or government-financed health care system and the private health care system. Some existed entirely outside of the health care system, such as lay midwives in the United States.

Midwives were the "key" figure in the alternative perinatal services that the research team identified as being most alternative. The report noted a general worldwide decline in the status and power of midwives and determined that the objective of most alternative services was restoration of the skills and services that midwives have traditionally offered to women—emphasis on the normalcy of childbearing, continuity of care, and sensitivity to the psychosocial as well as the clinical aspects of pregnancy and childbirth.* Even in western European countries with a comparatively strong midwifery tradition, the researchers noted a tendency for

---

*The wording of the report's description of the situation in the United States and Canada is an interesting reflection on the great gap in the role of midwives in these countries as compared with Europe: "In some areas of North America, midwifery is actually illegal and there is no official provision for midwifery training. . . ."

midwives working in hospital obstetric units to either become assistants to the physicians or to be replaced by nurses. Midwifery was not expanding in any of the countries; there was no country in which midwifery training or job opportunities were increasing (WHO Regional Office for Europe, 1985).

The report noted "a widespread opinion among proponents and users of alternative perinatal services that direct entry to midwifery training (whether provided officially or unofficially) is preferable to a combined nursing and midwifery training. The midwife who enters her profession without a nursing background is considered more likely to view pregnant women as people rather than patients and to see childbearing as a social as well as a medical phenomenon. Direct-entry systems are also thought to be more likely to encourage older women with personal experience of childbirth to enter midwifery" (WHO Regional Office for Europe, 1985).

Maternity care consumer groups had developed in all eight of the nonsocialist countries surveyed. The main complaints driving these groups were (1) not enough choice as to place of birth, (2) inadequate conditions for women giving birth in hospitals, and (3) the overuse of technology. These dissatisfactions and the existence of alternative maternity services were observed to have had some impact on the official or mainstream health care systems; some alternatives had been incorporated into the care provided in hospitals (WHO Regional Office for Europe, 1985).

The following are some of the conclusions made by Houd and Oakley on the basis of their study:

- The critique of mainstream maternity care and the development of alternatives in so many countries was seen to form an international movement with a core of common aims and strategies.

- The provision of alternative maternity care was becoming quite profitable due to the demand among middle-class consumers. This development does nothing to enhance the degree of choice, freedom, and control available to women who must depend on publicly financed health care.

- Although midwives and others involved in the alternative maternity care movement are highly skeptical of routine obstetric interventions, "this is rarely matched by an attitude of caution about the safety and effectiveness of alternative methods." The report stressed the importance of evaluation for promoting the acceptance of alternative methods.

- Alternative maternity care services "give great prominence to the role of the female midwife and to the way in which her autonomy as the manager of normal childbearing had been diluted over the years."

- There is "a tendency among some providers of alternative services to consider that those women most at risk according to conventional medical criteria are those who most need alternative forms of care."

- There is a demand for sharing of both information and decision making, "in other words, an absence of the hierarchy separating user and provider that is built into the official health care system of most developed countries today."

The three major recommendations in *Having a Baby in Europe* were (1) to unite the medical and the social approaches in order to improve perinatal care, (2) to apply careful scientific evaluation to all aspects of perinatal care, and (3) to increase the role of women in defining their health needs, planning their services, evaluating their services, and making choices about how they as individuals will use these services. The conclusion section of the report also included this statement:

> The potential of care for pregnant women goes far beyond what exists at present. It appears that several rather major shifts in the care system will be necessary to begin to realize this potential: a shift from care provided at the secondary or tertiary level to care provided at the primary care level; a shift from relying mainly on specialist physicians to relying mainly on midwives; a shift from focusing on abnormality to focusing on normality; and a shift from focusing on clinical medical issues to combining the medical and social approach. Such shifts will take time but can be done in steps. (WHO Regional Office for Europe, 1985).

Midwifery Practice During the Early 1990s

The European Midwives Liaison Committee studied midwifery practice in twelve European countries between 1992 and 1994*: Data were collected from (1) the "competent authority" for midwifery in each country (the person with the greatest responsibility and authority for midwifery education and practice within the legal structure of the country), (2) midwives in charge of individual midwifery services, and (3) a random sample of practicing midwives. The study showed great variation. What is seen as normal midwifery in some countries is not part of midwifery practice in some other countries. The study also revealed that midwives are involved in some activities that are not permitted under their national laws

---

*Belgium, Denmark, France, Germany, Greece, Italy, Ireland, Luxembourg, the Netherlands, Portugal, Spain, and the United Kingdom. Some European countries were not included, for instance, Austria, Finland, and Sweden. None of the Eastern European countries were included. In addition, complete data were not available for Italy, Portugal, and Spain.

or regulations. For example, midwives in Greece are not allowed to take action to release shoulder dystocia—when the baby's shoulder becomes stuck after the head has emerged during birth, a situation that is a true emergency. Two-thirds of Greek midwives who attend births indicated that they act in the face of this emergency, regardless of the rules (European Midwives Liaison Committee, 1996).

The study examined the extent to which midwives in each country provide specific elements of reproductive health care (European Midwives Liaison Committee, 1996).

- Midwives in all of these countries provide family planning information and advice to individual women during pregnancy and the postpartum period. In most countries they also provide this information to groups of nonpregnant, pregnant, and postpartum adult women. Midwives in at least six countries provide family planning information to groups of public school students. Although some midwives in almost every country insert intrauterine contraceptive devices (IUDs) and provide other methods of contraception (such as fitting diaphragms and prescribing oral contraceptives), midwives do not play a significant role in the actual provision of contraception in any of these countries.
- Five of the twelve countries do not provide explicit authority for midwives to diagnose pregnancy, and midwives in Germany, Luxembourg, Portugal and Spain are relatively unlikely to do so. On the other hand, diagnosis of pregnancy is an integral part of the care provided through most midwifery services in France, Greece, and Ireland. In many countries, most women see a physician first and are not referred to a midwife until after their pregnancy has been confirmed.

- Midwives in all of these countries are authorized to provide prenatal care to normal pregnant women, and from 80 to 100 percent of midwives in Denmark, Greece, the Netherlands, Ireland, and the U.K. do so. This is not the case in Belgium, Germany, Luxembourg, and Spain, in which physicians provide most of the prenatal care. Paradoxically, midwives in Belgium and Spain are less likely to provide prenatal care to women with normal pregnancies than to play a role in the prenatal care of women who have known complications or high-risk conditions. In fact, midwives in most E.U. countries play significant roles in the prenatal care of women with complications. The only exceptions are Germany and Spain (in which few midwives are involved in prenatal care at all) and the Netherlands (in which midwives play the main role in all phases of the care of normal pregnant women, but have a very small, secondary role in the care of women with complications).

- Some midwives in each of these countries perform ultrasonograms for the purpose of identifying high-risk pregnancies. Performing ultrasound examinations is considered part of the routine prenatal care expected of midwives in Denmark, France, and the U.K.

- Midwives in every country except Portugal and, to an extent, Luxembourg, provide a program of instruction regarding self-care during pregnancy, preparation for childbirth, and preparation for parenting.

- Midwives in every country are authorized to conduct normal vaginal births on their own responsibility. Midwives attend virtually all normal births in Denmark and France, 90 percent of normal births in Germany, between 70 and 80 percent of normal births in Ireland and the U.K., about 43 percent in the Netherlands, 10 percent in Greece, and very small proportions in Belgium and Luxembourg. The majority of Dutch midwives and about 40 percent of French midwives manage labor entirely on their own authority. In all other countries, less than 15 percent of midwives practice independently. However, most of those who do not work independently work under the policies of the maternity unit in which they practice. Except for Belgium, relatively small proportions work directly under the supervision of another person; when they do, the supervisor is usually a physician.

- Although midwives are allowed to attend home births in all of these countries, the Netherlands is the only country with a significant proportion of home births (about one-third of all births). Home births account for 1 to 2 percent of births in Belgium, Denmark, Germany, and the U.K., and less than 1 percent in the other countries.

- Midwives in all of these countries except the Netherlands are more likely to use electronic fetal monitoring than to use a fetoscope to monitor the fetal heart rate.* Full implementation of continuous EFM requires applying an electrode to the scalp of the unborn fetus (usually by screwing it into the scalp) and inserting a pressure gauge into the intrauterine space by pushing it around the fetal head. Although midwives in most of these countries apply the fetal scalp electrode, except for those in France, they are unlikely to insert the intrauterine pressure catheter.

- The majority of midwives practicing in Denmark, France, Greece, and the U.K. prescribe and administer some kind of calming or pain-killing medications to

---

*No information was collected on use of portable doppler equipment to monitor the fetal heart rate intermittently. This equipment, which is easier to use than a fetoscope but does not provide continuous monitoring and does not attach the woman to a machine, is preferred by many midwives in the United States.

at least some of the women they take care of during labor and delivery. The use of such drugs is very rare among midwives in the Netherlands, Ireland, and Portugal. Somewhere between 25 and 50 percent of midwives in the other countries use these kinds of drugs. Midwives in at least five European countries employ analgesics (for pain relief) on their own authority, that is, without the approval of a physician. (This information was only available for nine of the twelve countries, so the actual number of countries that provide this authority may be higher.)

- Midwives in France and Luxembourg have legal authority to prescribe and administer oxytocin during the first and second stages of labor (before the baby is born), and the majority of midwives in both countries do so on occasion. Midwives in Spain do not have that authority, but most do so anyway on occasion. The majority of midwives in all other countries except the Netherlands administer oxytocin to women during labor when it has been prescribed by a physician.

- Although midwives in every country cut episiotomies and midwives in most countries repair them, very few midwives in Belgium, Germany, Italy and Luxembourg repair episiotomies and perineal tears. Midwives in Belgium and Germany are not allowed to suture episiotomies and repair tears, although some do. Midwives in Italy and Luxembourg are allowed to, but most do not. Although 97 percent of midwives in Portugal cut episiotomies, only about half of them repair episiotomies and only 41 percent repair tears.

- Midwives in every country are allowed to deliver babies in breech presentation in case of an emergency. In actual practice, Denmark, France, and the Netherlands are the only countries in which more than half of the midwifery services

allow midwives to attend breech deliveries under normal circumstances.

- Approximately 10 percent of midwives in Denmark use vacuum extraction as part of their normal practice, and half of them use it in an emergency. Between 10 and 17 percent of midwives in France, Germany, Italy, and Spain use vacuum as an emergency measure. At least a few midwives in every country use it during an emergency. This is also true for use of forceps, although their use is not considered part of normal midwifery care in any of these countries. Small proportions (between 1 and 6 percent) use forceps in an emergency. None of these countries specifically authorize midwives to use either operative approach to assisting a vaginal birth on a routine basis. Denmark specifically allows midwives to use vacuum during an emergency.

- Oxytocin is used during the third stage of labor (after the baby is born but before the placenta has been expelled) to prevent or control hemorrhage. Prophylactic use of oxytocin is recommended during the third stage of labor for women who have higher-than-average risk of postpartum hemorrhage and women who might be endangered by even an average amount of blood loss (WHO, 1996). In addition, use of oxytocin may be critical in the face of actual postpartum hemorrhage. Nevertheless, five of the countries included in this study do not authorize midwives to administer oxytocin after the birth of the baby. The majority of midwives in all of those countries except Portugal ignore the lack of official authority and administer oxytocin during the third stage of labor when needed, without consulting a physician.

- Midwifery practice in Europe includes emergency resuscitation of the newborn and examination of the newborn for full development, birth injuries, and visible malformations.

- Most midwives in eight of the twelve countries provide care to mothers during their postpartum hospitalization. Midwives are somewhat less likely to assume responsibility for the babies than for the mothers during the post-birth hospitalization; midwives in only five of the twelve countries provide care to healthy newborns in the hospital.
- At least half of the midwives practicing in Germany, the Netherlands, Spain, and the U.K. provide care to postpartum mothers and their babies after they return home. (In the case of the Netherlands, the midwives continue to provide home care to mothers who never left their homes.)

Midwifery in Selected Countries

Midwifery in the Netherlands and Britain is of special interest; each is described in a separate section of this chapter. Selected aspects of midwifery in several other European countries are described here. Similar information is not provided for each country. Aspects of practice and education that are unique or of special interest are emphasized. These summaries are based on written documents published during the first half of the 1990s and input from senior midwives from some countries, who reviewed early drafts. Along with information on midwifery in the Netherlands and Britain, these summaries provide a general idea of the variation and similarities of midwifery education and practice in Europe during this period.

Austria: The law requires a midwife to be present at every birth, and most of them work in the labor and delivery units of large hospitals. Midwives who work in smaller hospitals are more likely to provide complete maternity care. There are also several kinds of private midwifery practices. Although many private midwives provide only prenatal and postpartum care, some hospitals allow privately paid midwives to attend births in the hospital. In addition, some midwives attend home births (about 2 percent of all births in

Austria), and there are about thirty free-standing birth centers, some led by midwives and some by physicians. However, most Austrians are accustomed to obtaining health care through government services, and most midwives prefer to work within the system, which provides financial security and other benefits of government employment. Nevertheless, many women want continuity of care, and some midwives are experimenting with ways to provide it. At one physician-directed birth center in Vienna, small midwife teams provide complete care to women from the twenty-eighth week of pregnancy through the postpartum period (Friedrich, 1996).

Denmark: Pregnant women go to their GP for an initial screening examination and if they become ill, and see an obstetrician only if they are referred by either their GP or their midwife. Otherwise, they receive prenatal care from midwives in midwifery centers that are close to the women's homes. Most women who are referred to an obstetrician for a consultation return to the midwife, after which the obstetrician and midwife may share the woman's care. Although only 2 percent of births are in homes, most midwives attend births in homes as well as hospitals. The proportion of home births is rising, and there are four in-hospital birth centers in Copenhagen. Water births are quite common (Houd, 1997). GPs may not attend deliveries in hospitals. Women receive childbirth care from midwives unless they are under "shared care" because of complications. No matter what complications arise during a birth, there will always be a midwife, in addition to the doctors. Most women do not see a physician at any time during a hospital birth. Midwives deliver twins and breech presentations; obstetricians perform cesareans and take care of women with serious complications. Midwives visit the women in the postpartum hospital wards, although nurses provide the actual care. Women bring their babies and return to the midwifery centers for later postpartum/postnatal care. Women return to their GP for their six-week postpartum examination (Flanagan, 1990; McKay, 1993; Wagner, 1996a; Hoúd, 1997).

Most Danish obstetricians respect midwives as separate professionals with an essential role. Obstetricians in Denmark do not give midwives "orders." They discuss the case together and then each carries out their role in implementing their decisions (Wagner, 1996a). The country's two midwifery schools (direct-entry) receive up to one thousand applications for eighty new-student positions per year (Hoúd, 1997).

Germany: Encouraged by rising popular support, during the 1980s German midwives began to challenge the increasing medical domination of childbirth in Germany. A 1985 law authorizes independent midwifery practice and requires a midwife to be present at every birth (Scheuermann, 1995). Physicians provide most of the prenatal care. About one-third of all German midwives work in hospitals; one-third are in independent practice, and one-third hold part-time jobs. Although there is some unemployment (due to the falling birth rate, changes in the health care system, and a large influx of midwives from East to West Germany after reunification), there is significant unmet demand for independent midwifery services (Friedrich, 1996).

Most births occur in hospitals, where they are attended by both a physician and a midwife; there are no obstetric nurses. If an episiotomy is cut, a physician usually sutures it, although midwives are qualified to do so. Women stay in the hospital for six days and are visited by a midwife after returning home. Although most births follow the high-tech style of Western obstetrics, some hospitals are developing a homeopathic approach. At least fifteen free-standing birth centers have been established. A few midwives attend home births (Scheuermann, 1995).

There are 57 midwifery colleges (Friedrich, 1996). Each is affiliated with a major university or city hospital and receives four hundred to one thousand applicants for only ten to fifteen spaces for new students each year (Scheuermann, 1995). Although the training is mainly directed toward working in a hospital, each student spends two to four weeks with an independent midwife (Friedrich, 1996). Some midwifery schools require nursing as a prerequisite, others don't.

Sweden: Midwives provide 80 percent of prenatal care and more than 80 percent of the family planning services in Sweden (Lindmark & Nyberg, 1997). Prenatal care and classes and postpartum care and contraception are provided in "mothercare centers," which are close to the women's homes and are adjacent to child health clinics. Each woman has eight to twelve prenatal visits with a midwife and sees a physician once or twice during pregnancy. Although most women see the same midwife throughout prenatal care, they will have a different midwife when they go to the hospital. Midwives who work in mothercare centers are completely separate from those who work in hospitals (Wagner, 1996).

Midwives attend all normal births in public hospitals. In private hospitals they manage the labor but not the delivery. It is arranged this way because the payment goes to whoever delivers the baby and this is the form of payment for private physicians, whereas the midwives are paid a salary by the hospital (Lindmark & Nyberg, 1997). Midwives also attend many complicated births, the latter under an obstetrician's supervision. Although midwives have independent responsibility for managing uncomplicated pregnancies, midwives and obstetrician-gynecologists work together very closely. Midwives attend breech deliveries, if the obstetrician is busy, use vacuum and forceps, and extract the placenta manually, if needed. There are about seven midwives for every gynecologist (Lindmark & Nyberg, 1997). EFM is common; 25 percent of women have epidurals, and one-fourth to one-half of labors are augmented with oxytocin (Lindmark & Nyberg, 1997; Waldenström & Nilsson, 1993). However, Swedish obstetrical practice has been influenced by Dr. Michel Odent (see Chapter 6). "Low-tech" methods, such as laboring in a pool of water, are also common. Midwives are respected practitioners, who receive much credit for Sweden's low perinatal mortality rate—the fifth lowest in the world in 1992 (NCHS, 1996b). Home births are even less frequent than in the United States—about one birth in two hundred. A midwife-run birth center has been developed in one hospital (Waldenström & Nilsson, 1993). Swedish midwives are also employed in "youth clinics," that provide education about sex and relationships, counseling for prevention of sexually transmitted diseases (STDs), contraceptive counseling, abortion counseling, examinations for STDs, and support in dealing with psychological and social problems (Lindmark & Nyberg, 1997).

All students must complete a three-year nursing program and have at least six months of experience as a graduate nurse before applying to midwifery programs, which are eighteen months in length. Although both programs (nursing and midwifery) are taught in universities, they are not thought to be sufficiently academic to lead to a degree. Students are, however, expected to participate in research (Waldenström, 1993). Students must attend at least 100 women during labor, including at least fifty for which they provide care during the entire labor and delivery (Lindmark & Nyberg, 1997).

The Netherlands: Autonomous Midwives and Many Home Births

Midwives throughout the world look to the Netherlands as the epitome of the full role of midwifery in the care of a nation's mothers. Dutch midwives practice autonomously and have high professional status. Along with general practitioners, whose role is declining, midwives are responsible for all aspects of the care of women having normal pregnancies and births in the Netherlands. In addition, the Netherlands is the only modern country in which a large proportion of births occurs at home. The strong role of midwives

in the Netherlands has continued unbroken for many centuries.* In recent decades, midwifery has benefited from the unwavering support of Dr. J. G. Kloosterman, one of the country's leading and most influential obstetricians.† In addition, midwifery and home births are consistent with a cultural consensus that birth is a private, family matter and a natural process that should not be interfered with. These factors, and the strong domestic focus of Dutch life, have made the Netherlands relatively resistant to modern obstetrics' push for universal hospitalization and routine technological surveillance during childbirth (Hiddinga, 1993).

Legal Status and Protection of Midwives' Role

The role of midwives in the Netherlands has been secure since the medical practice act es-

---

*One of the main distinguishing characteristics of Holland has been a long-standing separation between state and church. During the Dutch Republic (1579–1795), midwives were relieved of their religious duties (baptism and reporting signs of heresy or immorality), which had been a major responsibility since the Middle Ages. This allowed midwifery to be established as a medical occupation under the control of the state. At that point, the criteria for recruiting midwives changed from piety to good reputation plus the ability to read and write and experience attending deliveries. Early secularization of midwifery was an important step toward professionalization, setting Dutch midwifery apart from midwifery in other parts of Europe. Several authors have also noted that the relationship between midwives and physicians during the seventeenth and eighteenth centuries was characterized by greater cooperation and recognition of mutual dependency in the Netherlands, as compared with other European countries (Abraham-Van der Mark, 1993a).

†Dr. Kloosterman, a former professor of obstetrics and gynecology at the University of Amsterdam, was director of the Midwives Academy in Holland from 1947 to 1957. Dr. Kloosterman's long support for midwifery is based on cultural values and his concern that "modern western obstetrics is perverting the physiology of human parturition" as obstetricians on the lookout for pathology interfere in ways that cause pathology (Kloosterman, 1985). In the 1970s, Dr. Kloosterman became editor of the obstetric textbook used in medical schools throughout the Netherlands (Hiddinga, 1993). As a result, his views were very influential.

tablished the role and authority of both general practitioners and midwives in 1865 (Hingstman, 1994). Although the law has been revised several times over the years, the legal status of midwives remains the same; midwives are independent practitioners limited to the supervision of normal pregnancy and childbirth. In fact, with the passage of time, the authority of midwives has expanded to include prescription of certain kinds of medicine, external version of a fetus in breech presentation, and cutting and repairing episiotomies and suturing lacerations. These additions to their role were necessary to allow them to remain independent. When the law that regulates midwives was revised in 1979, the word for "midwife" (vroedvrouw) was replaced by the word that means "obstetrician" (verloskundige). Thus midwives are called by the word that means "expert in obstetrics," while obstetricians are referred to as "gynecologists" (Hiddinga, 1993).

Legislation to protect midwives from competition by physicians has been in place since 1925. Although originally motivated by concern about the higher fees charged by GPs, in 1953 the secretary of health emphasized that the policy is not based on cost, but quality; midwives have more training in obstetrics than GPs and "can assist at birth with patience—still the most important condition for normal obstetrics" (Abraham-Van der Mark, 1993a).

Every Dutch citizen is covered by health insurance. Approximately two-thirds obtain their coverage through the national health insurance system; those with incomes above a certain level have private health care insurance. A pregnant woman covered by the national insurance system must use a midwife unless none is available in her area or she has a complication that requires an obstetrician. If a midwife is not available, she may go to a GP. Midwives and GPs have the same scope of practice in regards to pregnancy; both provide prenatal care in community-based primary care sites and attend births in homes and short-stay "normal" birth units in

hospitals. Women with private insurance can use either a GP or a midwife but must pay the difference between a midwife's and the GP's fee (Hingstman, 1994). There has been a shortage of midwives, who were the only attendant at 43 percent of all births in the Netherlands in 1992 (de Veer & Meijer, 1996; European Midwives Liaison Committee, 1997). The proportion of births attended by GPs fell from 46 percent in 1960, to 11 percent in 1989, and 8 percent in 1995 (Hiddinga, 1993; Treffers, 1993; Hoope-Bender, 1997). Few GPs continue to practice obstetrics (Abraham-Van der Mark, 1993b). Although a midwife may attend the birth of a woman whom she has referred to a physician, midwives do not attend the births of most high-risk women and are not usually present at a birth attended by an obstetrician. The national health insurance system will not pay for care provided by an obstetrician unless it occurs in a teaching hospital or is required because of a condition included on an authorized list (Van Teijlingen & McCaffrey, 1987).

Place of Birth and Cesarean Deliveries
Short-stay normal-birth units were introduced in 1965. They are an increasingly popular option for women who perceive hospital births as safer than home births but want to return home as soon as possible (Van Daalen, 1993). Currently about 63 percent of births attended by midwives are in homes and 37 percent are in hospitals (de Veer & Meijer, 1996). Home births fell from 74 percent in 1958, to 35 percent in 1979, and 31 percent in 1995, in part because of the acceptance of short-stay hospitalizations, and because of expansions in the list of indications for an in-hospital specialist delivery. Reduction in family size also played a role, because women are somewhat less likely to have their first birth at home (Abraham-Van der Mark, 1993b). Although the proportion of home births has been relatively stable at about one-third of all births since 1978, the government is subsidizing the midwifery or-

ganization's efforts to prevent any further fall in the utilization of home births (Hoope-Bender, 1997).

Although the indications for consulting an obstetrician are the same whether the woman labors at home or in the hospital, referrals are more frequent for women who begin labor in a hospital (Treffers, 1993). The cesarean delivery rate associated with births that begin at home is very low—only 0.4 percent in one study (van Alten *et al.*, 1989). The overall cesarean section rate for the country is 7 percent (Treffers, 1993).

A National System for Sorting Women by Risk Status

Although the high proportion of home births is the most conspicuous element of maternity care in the Netherlands, Dr. Pieter Treffers, a Dutch obstetrician, considers home deliveries only a detail; in his view, early identification of obstetric pathology and a clear, universal system for sorting women into different care groups based on risk is the fundamental characteristic of the system. Primary care provided by midwives and GPs is the first level of the three-level system. The secondary level is care provided by obstetricians, who accept referrals and transfers from midwives and GPs based on the presence of a complication or a condition that increases the risk associated with the pregnancy. The third level is care provided in the perinatal centers associated with the country's eight university hospitals; obstetricians working at the secondary level refer women with the most serious kinds of complications to specialists at the tertiary centers. Midwives and GPs decide whether women can deliver at home (or in a short-stay in-hospital birth center) or need to be sent to an obstetrician; however, these decisions are based on nationally established guidelines (Treffers, 1993). About 38 percent of women who begin maternity care at the primary level (midwife or GP) are referred to an obstetrician at some point during their care. Obstetricians are required to refer a woman who has been treated for a prenatal problem back to her midwife or general practice physician once the problem has been resolved (de Veer & Meijer, 1996).

Use of a list of indications for treatment by an obstetrician was started by Dr. Kloosterman in 1973. Concern about increasing medicalization of birth led to revision and clarification of the list and rules in 1987. In contrast with the old list, the new list includes some conditions that require the midwife or GP to send the women for a "consultation" visit with an obstetrician, but do not require referral. After the consultation, the obstetrician and midwife or GP discuss the case and usually come to a shared decision on who will be responsible for further care of the woman. But sometimes they disagree; a recent nationwide survey found considerable differences of opinion among midwives, GPs, and obstetricians on risk selection issues (Meijer *et al.*, 1996). When they disagree, it is the midwife's or GP's responsibility to decide whether the woman is low-risk and can remain in primary care, or is high-risk and must be referred to an obstetrician (Abraham-Van der Mark, 1993a). This change in the rules was rejected by the majority of obstetricians, who believe that they are more competent to detect and judge risks associated with pathology (Meijer *et al.*, 1996). Some obstetricians refuse to refer patients back to midwives and GPs under these circumstances, and the obstetricians' professional organization made a formal complaint to the board of the national health insurance system. The decision in favor of the midwives was maintained, in part but not exclusively, because of cost considerations (Abraham-Van der Mark, 1993a). Nevertheless, cooperation among midwives, GPs, and obstetricians is usually good at the local level (Treffers, 1993).

The list of indications for a hospital birth (other than use of a short-stay normal-birth unit) includes both medical and social indications. Social indications include living in poor housing, use of hard drugs, psychiatric problems, and plans to give the baby up for adoption (Abraham-Van der Mark, 1993b).

Home Nursing Assistance for Postpartum Mothers

A maternity home care nursing assistant makes one or two prenatal visits in the home (McKay, 1993), helps during the home birth, and provides full-day in-home care of the mother and newborn for up to eight days after the birth. Home care is also provided after short-stay hospital births, but not after a regular hospital birth, which includes a period of postpartum hospitalization. The home care assistant performs necessary household chores, helps the mother with breast-feeding and child care, provides information and instruction, and tries to make the mother feel more comfortable, knowledgeable, and confident in caring for her baby (Abraham-Van der Mark, 1993b; Van Teijlingen, 1990). Maternity home care assistants complete a three-year course, must pass an examination, and are supervised by the woman's midwife or GP (Van Teijlingen, 1990; Magill-Cuerden, 1977; Treffers, 1993). The purpose is to provide support during the transition from one family constellation to the next; the training is based on that function (Hoope-Bender, 1997). Although envied, the Dutch home health care system has been threatened and, in large cities, cut back by reduction in government funds (Abraham-Van der Mark, 1993b). About 75 percent of postpartum women receive the service (Hingstman, 1994). However, it is considered an essential part of the system; some believe the country could not continue to have a high proportion of home births without this support (Van Teijlingen, 1990). Although the Netherlands has the world's tenth lowest overall infant mortality rate, it is fourth lowest in postneonatal deaths, which often results from suboptimal parenting or hazards in the home environment. Home care during the postpartum period may contribute to the country's very low rate of postneonatal mortality.

Safe Home Births

Although infant mortality rates for most European countries declined during the last half of the 1950s and during the 1960s, the decrease was slower in the Netherlands than in Scandinavian countries that adopted high rates of hospitalized childbirth. Slipping from first place in this international ranking led to a prolonged debate about whether the Netherlands should give up home births and follow the universal-hospitalization practices of other European countries. Studies examining the data in several ways led to the conclusion that the slower decline in the Netherlands' perinatal mortality rate could not be explained by its high proportion of home births (Scherjon, 1986; Treffers & Laan, 1986; Damstra-Wijemga, 1984). Although the debate focused on perinatal mortality, the value of the home birth experience for women and their families also received attention. Doctors supporting home births warned that further medicalization of childbirth might increase infant mortality because of iatrogenic problems associated with obstetric interventions and the inevitability of infections spread through hospitalization (Abraham-Van der Mark, 1993b).

A Limited Scope of Practice

Midwifery has been strictly regulated since enactment of the 1865 law that established it as an independent profession. The 1865 law prohibited use of instruments, medicine, and other procedures, and imposed strict rules that midwives cannot be involved in the care of women with complications (Abraham-Van der Mark, 1993a). Dutch women who have home births expect and receive virtually no medications during labor. The birth of a baby is viewed as a natural process that should not be interfered with and as a normal part of human life.

Education

Dutch midwifery schools must produce midwives who can function autonomously; the educational standards have become more rigorous over the years, and recruitment is competitive. Every year about 1,000 individuals apply for approximately 120 openings at the country's three colleges for midwives. Men have been eligible since the 1970s, and 3 percent of practicing midwives are male. The midwifery program was increased from three to four years in 1994. Students enter after at least five years of secondary education (Oudshoorn, 1993). All Dutch midwifery schools were directed by obstetricians until 1991, when a midwife was appointed as director of one of the three schools (Abraham-Van der Mark, 1993a). Now all three schools are directed by midwives (Hoope-Bender, 1997). Midwifery education is completely separate from nursing. Dr. Kloos-terman in particular believes that a nursing background is detrimental to midwives because midwives must be able to think independently and challenge doctors, whereas nurses must learn to be subservient to doctors (Mehl-Madrona & Madrona, 1997; Hoope-Bender, 1997).

Practice Arrangements and Conditions

In 1990, only 15 percent of all Dutch midwives were employed by hospitals; 71 percent were in independent practice. About a third of those in private practice worked alone; others worked with a partner or in small groups. Although the number of midwives increases every year (Hingstman, 1994), there is a shortage relative to need; as a result, each midwife attends an average of 150 deliveries per year. Some are leaving the profession under the strain of this work load. Midwives are expected to be available to their clients nearly continuously. The pay is not high, and many feel it is impossible to combine marriage and a family with midwifery. As a result of these pressures, Dutch midwives are moving away from their tradition of solo practice, with many forming group practices, which make it possible to have a husband, children, and other interests (Abraham-Van der Mark, 1993a, Hoope-Bender, 1997). Midwives employed in teaching hospitals help teach the medical students, who must pass an examination given by a midwife before they are allowed to work on the labor ward (Friedrich, 1996).

Great Britain: Demands for a New Approach to Maternity Care

Midwives have played a major role in maternity care in Britain since passage of the Midwives Act in 1902. Most attended home births as independent practitioners until the mid-1930s, when Parliament passed a law requiring the establishment of government-financed maternity services. Nearly all health care in England was brought under the government when the National Health Service (NHS) was established a decade later. Most British midwives have been employed by the NHS since then.

Over the years, British maternity care has been strongly influenced by government-commissioned "expert" reports. The 1970 Peel report was the first of several recommending that, for safety's sake, all births should be in hospitals. A startling reversal of that recommendation occurred in 1992.

The first tabulation of British births by place of birth, done in 1927, found that 85 percent of all births took place at home. By 1964 the proportion of home births had fallen to 28 percent; by 1974, it had fallen to only 4 percent (Chamberlain, 1988). Despite this sharp decline, many women continued to prefer home births. A study based on a random sample of 2,400 women who had given birth in England and Wales in 1975 found that 92 percent of those who delivered at home but had a previous in-hospital birth preferred the home delivery (O'Brien, 1978). Nevertheless, home births had dropped to only 1 percent by 1984 (Chamberlain, 1988). A 1984 report by the Maternity Services Advisory Committee approved of the change, stating that, "As unforeseen complications can occur in any birth, every mother should be encouraged to have her baby in a maternity unit where emergency facilities are available (Expert Maternity Group, 1993).

The "no-birth-can-be-treated-as-normal-until-it's-over" attitude that decimated home births in the United Kingdom (as in the United States) and the seemingly inexorable encroachment of technological management of labor and delivery made many midwives feel that the battle for normal childbirth had been lost. Although midwives continued to be the senior person present at three-fourths of births in England and Wales, their ability to exercise judgment that affected patient care became significantly narrowed after the transition of birth into hospitals (Weitz, 1987). The presence of midwives at birth did not decline, but their role and status did (Renfrew, 1997).

The concern about medicalization of childbirth, fragmentation and diminished quality of care provided to pregnant women, and loss of the true midwifery role led to the development of a powerful consumer movement during the 1970s and 1980s, and the creation of several vocal, effective consumer organizations, including the National Childbirth Trust and the Association for Improvement in the Maternity Services (Renfrew, 1997).

There was also discontent among some midwives, especially younger midwives at some schools. In 1976 ten midwifery students and one practicing midwife started the Association of Radical Midwives as a loosely organized support, study, and political action group for midwives who believed that medical definition and control of childbearing had eroded midwives' role and skills and was harming mothers and babies. The association focused on reducing medical intervention in childbirth, developing more direct-entry midwifery training programs, and promoting natural childbirth, home births, and staffing patterns that provide continuity of care (Weitz, 1987).

By 1987 the Royal College of Midwives, (the huge, long-standing professional organization for midwives in Britain) joined the cause with their own set of proposals for restoring the midwife's role. Both groups proposed that midwives should be organized into small teams that would provide continuity of care for a defined caseload of women throughout pregnancy and the postpartum period. Both organizations also criticized the then-current policy whereby general practitioners served as "gatekeepers" to all other health services; they proposed that pregnant women should be able to engage a midwife directly. An editorial in *The Lancet*, a prestigious British medical journal, supported these proposals, pointing out that socially disadvantaged women, who are most in need of early prenatal care, are least likely to have a relationship with a GP, and that forcing them to go to a doctor first creates a barrier and disincentive. A study had found that 30 percent of people living in some parts of inner London were not registered with a GP (Anonymous editorial, 1987).

In 1991 a committee made up of eleven members of Parliament began a year-long, in-depth investigation of the quality of the maternity care being provided by the National Health Service (NHS). All concerned parties, whether users or providers of maternity care, were invited to submit their views in writing, and more than 450 written submissions were received. The committee also heard oral testimony from representatives of professional and consumer organizations, visited maternity hospitals and clinics in the Netherlands and Sweden, as well as the United Kingdom, and had access to advice from two midwives, two obstetricians, a pediatrician and a general practitioner (Tew, 1992).

In 1992 the House of Commons Health Select Committee submitted its report on Britain's maternity services. Known as the Winterton report, it was a turning point in maternity care in Great Britain. Contradicting the 1984 Maternity Services Advisory Committee statement that "every mother should be encouraged to have her baby in a maternity unit where emergency facilities are available," the 1992 report concluded that "the policy of encouraging all women to give birth in hospitals cannot be justified on grounds of safety" and asserted that maternity care in Britian should no longer be based on a "medical model of care." Noting the absence of adequate research about interventions "such as epidurals, episiotomies, cesarean sections, electronic fetal monitoring, instrumental delivery and induction of labor," the Winterton report concluded that women should be able to choose "on the basis of existing information rather than having to undergo such interventions as routine." In fact, "women should be given unbiased information and an opportunity for choice" in all aspects of their care, "including the option, previously largely denied to them, of having their babies at home, or in small maternity units." The National Health Service has not "done nearly enough to respond in practical terms to the call by women to be involved as full partners in the decisions made about their care" (House of Commons Health Committee, 1992).

The report recommended that the country abandon its policy of closing small rural maternity units and that hospital delivery practices be changed in order to provide privacy, make delivery units look like a normal room rather than an operating theater, ensure that laboring women and their companions have access to refreshments, allow women to be "in control" of their labor, and make it possible for a woman to assume any comfortable position during labor and delivery. "In the area of postnatal care above all others, attention must be turned away from a medical model of care to a woman-centered approach which takes full account of their social needs." The report recommended that the Medical Research Council be given sufficient funds to support a full program of research on maternity care and urged that attention should also be given to increasing knowledge "of the true costs of the current pattern of delivery of maternity care" (House of Commons Health Committee, 1992). Several of the committee's conclusions and recommendations related to midwifery:

- "We conclude that there is a strong desire among women for the provision of continuity of care and carer throughout pregnancy, and . . . the majority of them regard midwives as the group best placed and equipped to provide this."
- Most maternity care should be community based and near the woman's home. Obstetric and other specialist care should be readily available by referral from midwives or general practitioners.
- Schemes should be established to enable women to get to know one or two health professionals during pregnancy who will be with them during labor and birth, whether at home or in the hospital, and who will continue to provide care to the mother and newborn after the birth.
- The Department of Health should fund "extensive pilot schemes in the establishment of midwife-managed maternity units within or adjacent to acute hospitals. We further recommend funding of an extensive program of establishing small team midwifery care using community-based clinics." The country should "move as rapidly as possible toward a situation in which midwives have their own caseload and take full responsibility for the women who are under their care" (House of Commons Health Committee, 1992).

"Changing Childbirth"—A Mandate to Improve Maternity Care

In response to this report, the government established an expert committee to review and make recommendations regarding NHS policies on maternity care, especially during childbirth. An Expert Maternity Group was established under the Parliamentary Under Secretary of State for Health, drawing members from women who use the NHS and professionals who provide maternity care. The expert group conducted extensive site visits and interviews to obtain first-hand information, held a conference on maternity care, and commissioned several studies about women's perceptions about the care available to pregnant women in England (Expert Maternity Group, 1993). The following information on the role of the midwife is taken directly from their report:

> From the evidence we received, we recognized that women have great confidence in the midwifery profession. . . . Importantly, the midwife is able to work across a variety of settings, and is able to be with the woman when and where needed, ensuring that she remains the focus of care. Legally midwives are able to practice independently. When a pregnancy is uncomplicated they are able to be responsible for providing and arranging all the maternity care that is needed for a woman and her baby. If abnormalities are suspected or occur, the midwife is obliged to refer to a doctor, and to continue to provide care working with the doctor. When a woman has a complicated pregnancy and books with an obstetrician, the midwife's role is to provide any additional support and advice that may be necessary.
>
> In the past, changes in the organization of maternity care have resulted in midwives working in a fragmented way, tending to specialize in particular aspects of care, rather than providing total care to a group of women. In an attempt to achieve greater continuity, over 40 percent of maternity services have recently introduced team midwifery . . . although midwives might have been apprehensive in advance of taking up their new responsibilities and patterns of practice, once they became accustomed to the new way of working they have found it more satisfying.

The Expert Maternity Group's report was entitled *Changing Childbirth*. It laid down principles of good maternity care, stated specific objectives and a plan of action for changing childbirth in the United Kingdom within a five-year period, and identified indicators for measuring success. The three principles of good maternity care stated in the report are as follows: (1) The woman must be the focus of maternity care. She should be able to feel that she is in control of what is happening to her and make decisions about her care, based on her needs and full discussion with the professionals involved. (2) Maternity services must be readily and easily accessible to all. They should be sensitive to the needs of the local population and based primarily in the community. (3) Women should be involved in the monitoring and planning of maternity services to ensure that they are responsive to the needs of a changing society. In addition, care should be effective, and resources should be used efficiently.

A "Patient's Charter" lays out the rights of patients within the system. The report challenged all components of the NHS to review their services and develop a strategic plan in order to achieve the *Changing Childbirth* objectives. Ten indicators were identified in order to measure their success. Although the plan is multifaceted, many of the objectives affect the role of midwives, or the way GPs and obstetricians relate to midwives. The following is a summary of those objectives and indicators for measuring success in achieving the objectives (Expert Maternity Group, 1993):

- Every woman should know one midwife who ensures continuity of her midwifery care—the "named" midwife. Wherever possible, the named midwife should be located in the community; she should feel comfortable practicing in both the community and the hospital.
- The woman should know the name of the person who has primary responsibility for planning and monitoring her care and she should have a voice in selecting her "lead professional". A woman with an uncomplicated pregnancy should, if she wishes, be able to have a midwife as her lead professional for the entire

pregnancy, including childbirth in a hospital. If she has medical problems or pregnancy complications, her lead professional may be a GP. In that case, there must be good communication between the woman's midwife and her physician. The lead professional for at least 30 percent of women should be a midwife.

- Seventy-five percent of women should be cared for in labor by a midwife whom they have come to know during pregnancy.
- Midwives should have direct access to some beds in all maternity units.
- At least 30 percent of women delivered in a maternity unit should be admitted under the management of a midwife.
- Women should receive clear, unbiased advice and be able to choose where they would like their baby to be born.
- All front-line ambulances should have a paramedic able to support a midwife during an emergency transfer of a woman from a home birth to a hospital.
- Concern was expressed that the number of GPs taking part in labor and delivery care is falling steadily. GPs who want to provide maternity care were encouraged to receive appropriate training. Midwives and GPs were advised to work in partnership in the best interest of the woman.
- The knowledge and skills of the obstetrician should be used primarily to provide advice, support, and expertise for the care of women with complicated pregnancies. However, women with uncomplicated pregnancies should be given an opportunity to meet a consultant obstetrician and may choose to book a consultant obstetrician as their lead professional, via their GP or midwife.

The report advocated "team midwifery" as a way to achieve continuity in the person providing care to a particular pregnant woman. The standards being sought are for the midwifery team to have no more than six midwives, for each team to provide total care to a defined caseload of women, for at least half of the women to have their baby delivered by a midwife who is known to the mother, and for there to be teamwork in all aspects of patient care. The report acknowledged that making continuity of care a reality will require substantial flexibility from midwives and their service administrators and advised that "as midwives accept more responsibility, their terms of employment, including remuneration, may need to be reviewed" (Expert Maternity Group, 1993).

In 1993 the Institute of Manpower Studies reported that one-fourth of the team midwifery services established during 1990 had been discontinued by the end of 1991, in many cases because of dissatisfaction on the part of the midwives (Dunlop, 1993). Nevertheless, midwives are trying to find ways to achieve the changing childbirth goals, and early research has found that continuity of care makes a difference. In 1996, *The Lancet* published results of a randomized clinical trial that compared outcomes of continuity of care provided by a known midwife with outcomes of care provided by a variety of midwives, GPs, and obstetricians. Results of this study, which used the "gold standard" method for discerning differences between two kinds of care and was conducted in Scotland are heartening: Low-risk women randomized to care by a "named midwife," who met the woman during her first prenatal visit and provided most of her subsequent care, had significantly fewer interventions during labor and delivery and were significantly more satisfied with their care than women randomized to standard care. Women who received continuity of care from a midwife were also less likely to develop hypertension or bleeding during the prenatal period, and were less likely to have labor induced with oxytocin. They had fewer vaginal examinations during the first stage of labor and were more likely to complete the birth without either an episiotomy or a perineal laceration (Turnbull *et al.*, 1996).

The *Changing Childbirth* recommendations have been adopted as official government policy. In 1994 the Royal College of Obstetricians and Gynaecologists, the Royal College of Midwives, the Royal College of General Practitioners, and other groups joined to express agreement with its main tenets (Kitzinger, 1995). Many women are now able to choose their place of birth and primary care provider. Home births have risen slightly (Renfrew, 1997). There are significant limitations, however. Most midwives currently practicing in the U.K. were trained in hospitals and have no home birth experience. To truly make home births available, many midwives would need assistance to develop the necessary skills. Better emergency back-up services would also need to be developed (Renfrew, 1997). Midwives constrained by a large caseload rarely offer home birth, because it would require them to be on call continuously without pay (Sandall, 1996). A requirement for two qualified individuals to be present at each home birth increases the logistical problems (Dunlop, 1993). It is clear that, although most British women probably feel safer in a hospital, the demand for home births (about 8 percent in a recent study) is greater than midwives are currently filling (Young, G., 1993). In addition midwives are leaving the profession because of low pay (an average of about $27,500 per year) and increased workloads (Lyall, 1995).

Midwifery Education and the Resurgence of Direct-Entry Midwifery

There has been great change in midwifery education, as in practice. Prior to changes made during the early 1990s, nurse-midwives completed three-year nursing programs, and then some worked as nurses before going into midwifery and some entered midwifery school immediately. The post-nursing midwifery program was eighteen months—a total of four and a half years of education in nursing and midwifery. Direct-entry programs could be completed in only two years and three months but tended to attract older women, many of whom had prior education in other fields. Compared with students entering nurse-midwifery programs, those entering direct-entry programs were more likely to be married with children, and most had some kind of health care experience. Although older when they entered midwifery, they tended to practice longer than nurse-midwives. But nurse-midwives predominated the profession, and the government seemed to lose interest in direct-entry education. One problem related to the qualifications to teach in a government-run school. Nurse-midwives had two certificates; direct-entry midwives had only one. All direct-entry programs were in schools that also had a nurse-midwifery program. Many nurses wanted to become midwives, and most of the faculty were nurse-midwives. During the last half of the 1970s and the early 1980s all but one direct-entry program closed. Although it accepted only ten students a year, there were three hundred applicants on the waiting list for the last school, which closed during the early 1980s (Allison, 1994).

The government was responsible for midwifery education. No tuition was charged to students, and those who entered as nurses were paid their regular nursing salary while in school. This also tilted the educational system toward nurse-midwifery.

A troubling shortage of midwives was attributed in part to a decline in applications to nurse-midwifery education programs during the 1980s (Haire, 1990). However, there was also a greater, long-standing problem of midwifery training wasted on graduates who obtained midwifery "qualification" in order to advance their status in the British civil service and did not ever practice midwifery, or practiced for only one or two years (Robinson, 1986). Perhaps all government bureaucracies link education with rank, salary, and opportunities for promotion. For nurses in the huge British National Health Service, midwifery training counted as a postgraduate qualification that could lead to career advancement, even if one had no particular interest in midwifery. The problem had been identified by

1923, when a midwifery certificate had already become an essential qualification for appointment as a matron at many hospitals (Robinson). Only about half of the midwives who qualified for the Midwives Roll (i.e., new graduates) between 1975 and 1981 ever practiced as midwives. Midwifery training was not wasted on direct-entry midwives, who entered midwifery because they wanted to be midwives, not because they were competing for better roles in the nursing hierarchy.

Turf battles between nursing and midwifery contributed to a resurgence of interest in direct-entry midwifery. The English National Board for Nursing, Midwifery and Health Visiting's practice of appointing "generic education officers" meant that midwifery schools and training courses could be approved by nursing educators who were not midwives. Midwives worried about losing control of midwifery education (Brain, 1990).

In 1989, the Department of Health provided funds to develop fourteen direct-entry midwifery education programs in sites throughout England. The plan met great enthusiasm. Direct-entry midwifery had become a movement during the period leading up to and following the two landmark reports, and it had the early support and full involvement of the Association of Radical Midwives. Leaders of this movement hoped to produce midwives capable of fully implementing the spirit as well as the mandate of the *Changing Childbirth* policies—midwives who are research based, health focused, and woman centered. Thirty-two direct-entry midwifery education programs were in operation by June 1993, and nearly eight hundred students had been enrolled. There are both three-year diploma programs and four-year degree programs; each program is linked to an institution of higher education. As of mid-1994, about 85 percent of the student positions were in diploma programs. The number of post-nursing programs declined as the number of direct-entry programs increased (Kent *et al.*, 1994). As of 1994, approximately 30 percent of midwifery students were in direct-entry programs (Allison, 1994).

Postnursing and direct-entry midwifery education have both moved out of hospital-based midwifery schools into midwifery departments in universities. Because of British midwives' large role in maternity care, there is no shortage of clinical experience for midwifery students. Moving midwifery education out of hospital-based schools has created the opposite problem: Hospitals can no longer count on students to carry part of the workload. Many midwifery services have lost both the students and the funds that paid the students, which have sometimes been shifted to other parts of the health service (Renfrew, 1997).

Emphasis on Evidence-Based Practice and Research: Even before British midwifery education moved into universities, British midwives had become very active in research, in part as a means to show the value of midwifery care in an attempt to reverse the then declining status of midwifery. British midwives have accepted the need to base their practice on evidence to a degree that is different from nursing in the U.K. and from midwifery in most other countries. There is an emphasis on randomized controlled clinical trials and consistent rigor in adhering to solid research methodology. British midwives have published a series of monographs reporting the results of their research, publish two journals devoted to midwifery research (*The Royal College of Midwives Current Awareness Bulletin* and the *Midwives' Information and Resource Service**), and an annual "Research and the Midwife" conference (Robinson & Thompson, 1989).

Canada

Midwifery was illegal or outside of the law in all but the remote northern parts of Canada

---

*The Midwives' Information and Resource Service is also known as "MIDIRS." It was described in Chapter 9.

throughout this century until the mid-1990s, when four provinces (of ten) enacted new midwifery laws. On January 1, 1994, Ontario became the first Canadian province to establish midwifery as a legally sanctioned health profession and began a process intended to integrate midwives into the government-funded health services. Direct-entry midwifery in Canada, as in the United States, evolved as a maturation of the lay-midwifery/home-birth movement that started during the 1970s. Direct-entry midwifery is the model applied in Ontario, and home birth experience is required. Registered midwives in Ontario attend births in homes and are eligible for hospital privileges; their services are covered by the government health insurance plan. Québec, Alberta, and British Columbia also enacted new midwifery laws between 1990 and 1995, the governments of Manitoba and Saskatchewan have announced their intention to do so, and midwifery legislation is under consideration in at least two other provinces. Midwives will be practicing under the new law in Alberta by late 1997. Midwives will be practicing under the new law in British Columbia by late 1997 or early 1998 (Kaufman, 1997a).

There is strong commitment to direct-entry midwifery. Most midwives who were practicing in Canada before the law changes and who were most involved in developing the new rules and regulations are apprentice-trained direct-entry midwives. It is seen as very important that midwifery is a *self-regulating* profession—free of legal control and educational domination by either medicine *or nursing*. The motivation to legalize midwifery grew out of a broader movement that values out-of-hospital settings as a way to protect and preserve the normalcy of childbirth. Direct-entry midwifery is strongly associated with home births, whereas nurse-midwifery is seen as a form of midwifery that has been attenuated by the influence of nursing and involvement in hospital births. Direct-entry midwives are thought to have a stronger com-

mitment to providing choice of birth place and continuity of care. None of the new laws requires nursing as a prerequisite to midwifery education. A nurse-midwifery education program and demonstration project that preexisted the new law in Alberta was discontinued—despite evidence of good outcomes, including a significant reduction in cesarean sections—because the university hospital in which it was based cannot provide the out-of-hospital birth experiences required by the new law. Foreign-trained nurse-midwives who lack recent out-of-hospital birth experience need to attend home births under supervision in order to acquire the necessary skills. But the demand for home births is limited in Canada, as in the United States. Tying midwifery to out-of-hospital births too tightly may make it difficult for midwifery to expand.

As of the end of 1996, there were two formally organized midwifery training programs in Canada: a program that is being implemented in three universities in Ontario, and a program in Povungnituk, in Northern Québec, where Inuit women are trained to serve as midwives for their own communities. So far, financial constraints have prevented the development of education programs to complement the new laws in Alberta and British Columbia. However, Alberta has issued a call for proposals to establish an education program based on the model being implemented in Ontario (Kaufman, 1997b). Québec's law authorizes midwifery in specified pilot projects as an experiment that is scheduled to end in 1998. Québec plans to establish a school after that date, assuming that new, more permanent legislation is enacted after evaluation of the current experiment (Daviss, 1996 & 1997).

Four years of postsecondary formal education in midwifery is the standard being built into the requirements of the regulating bodies. This is based on recognition of the need to erect high standards in order to build credibility for professional midwifery in a country where it has not existed for most of this century and in a country (and continent) in which university degrees are the common currency of professional education. However, every province that has grappled with the issues involved in midwifery legislation has tried to develop a way to recognize apprentice-trained midwives who were already practicing in the province through some means of individual assessment. Doing this in a way that is fair to all kinds of midwives while supporting the values that underlie the rules is a universal and continuing challenge.

History

The early history of midwifery in Canada was similar to that in the United States. Trained midwives were among the early colonists and immigrants. Midwives working in the colony of New France during the mid-1600s had been commissioned by the king of France, and there are records of requests to the British government to pay for the services provided by midwives in Nova Scotia (Knox, 1993). Midwives were a valued component of the developing health care system in eastern Canada and participated in the instruction of medical students at McGill University in Montreal during the mid-1800s (Burgin, 1994). However, there were few attempts to develop midwifery schools or the formal professional structures that had existed in the European countries from which the midwives came. The church oversaw the activities of midwives in some areas. Physicians tried to establish a system to bring midwives under medical supervision as early as 1790 in Québec (Knox, 1993). In addition to formally trained midwives, who tended to practice midwifery as a profession, women without formal training helped their neighbors during childbirth but did not see themselves as members of a profession (Knox, 1993).

Physicians found it difficult to make a living in the sparsely populated country. As they increased in number, they began to seek sole authority for childbirth, which could be the foundation for a successful practice (Knox, 1993). Although medical practice

acts were passed in every province during the late 19th century (O'Neil & Kaufert, 1990), none was able to prevent midwives from assisting women during births. But as the number of physicians increased, so did their efforts to dominate and monopolize health care (Knox, 1993). Midwifery was effectively outlawed in provinces where the legal definition of medical practice included the care of pregnant women. Although midwifery was not explicitly illegal in the other provinces, and some midwives continued to work, they did so without government sanction and licensing, and no training programs were developed. "Lay" or "granny" midwives continued to assist women in remote rural areas and some indigent women in the cities. Few midwives were actually tried for illegal practice, and the few who were tried were seldom, if ever, convicted (Knox, 1993).

Midwifery began to disappear during the early decades of the twentieth century, as childbirth moved into hospitals and women welcomed the advent of obstetric anesthesia. During 1910, the Victorian Order of Nurses became interested in starting a midwifery school like the one that was being developed at Bellevue Hospital in New York City* (O'Neil & Kaufert, 1990). The idea was defeated by opposition from other nursing groups, as well as physicians. Nurses had a new and important role in hospital-based obstetrics and endorsed the idea that physicians could provide safer care to pregnant women (Knox, 1993). Nursing's early support for medical domination of childbirth contributed to Canadian midwives' preference for a direct-entry form of midwifery.

With the exception of Newfoundland, in which midwives continued in practice into the 1960s, only the most isolated areas retained any kind of midwifery after 1950 (Knox, 1993). During the 1960s and 1970s, the Canadian government built nursing sta-

---

*Bellevue opened the first tax-supported midwifery school in the United States. See section on "Midwifery at the Turn of the Century" in Chapter 2.

tions in remote outposts in the Yukon, Labrador, the Northwest Territories, Newfoundland, and northern Québec, and recruited foreign-trained nurse-midwives, mainly British, to staff the stations. *Nurse*-midwives were needed, because they were required to provide emergency and primary medical care, in addition to midwifery. The medical societies viewed this as a poor alternative to medical obstetrics, and the presence of midwives in the far north had no effect in the southern areas, where most Canadians live (Burgin, 1994; O'Neil & Kaufert, 1990; Daviss, 1996, 1997).

Midwifery resurfaced as an issue within the context of the counterculture and women's movements of the 1970s, and the discontent of pregnant women who wanted fewer medical interventions and a more natural form of childbirth. Realization that Canada was the only industrialized member of the World Health Organization that did not have professional midwives widened interest in midwifery within the women's movement, contributing to a political environment primed for consideration of change (Soderstrom *et al.*, 1990). During the last half of the 1980s, Alberta, British Columbia, Ontario, and Québec initiated processes to study issues related to legalization of midwifery (Burgin, 1994).

A shortage of maternity care providers in some parts of Canada may have also contributed to the political receptivity to the idea of midwives. Nationwide, about half of the babies have been delivered by family physicians and about half by ob-gyns. The proportion of FPs doing obstetrics has been falling; by the mid-1990s, only one in five FPs was delivering babies. Low pay for obstetric care combined with the high cost of liability insurance, the irregular and often long hours, and lack of confidence in the adequacy of their obstetrics training are all contributing factors. The increasing proportion of women entering family practice in Canada is also a factor. Many young female FPs want to start their own families shortly after they finish their residencies

and begin to practice. Being pregnant or mothers themselves makes them less able to cope with the time demands of obstetrics. Yet family physicians who do not include obstetrics in their practice from the start are unlikely to add it later. Instead of including full obstetrics in their practice, many FPs in Canada have developed "shared care" relationships with obstetricians, in which the FP provides prenatal and postpartum care and the ob-gyn does the delivery (Levitt, 1997). Consumer demand has been a very important factor in creating a place for midwifery in Canada, and the desire for continuity of care has been a consistent theme of consumer support for midwives.

Ontario

Ontario is the most populous province of Canada, and probably the most influential. Because it was one of the provinces that did not define midwifery as the practice of medicine, midwifery was not explicitly illegal in Ontario, and a small number of lay midwives began to attend home births there during the 1970s. There were also some formally trained nurse-midwives in Ontario—mostly recent immigrants from the United Kingdom and certain developing countries. Special efforts had been made to encourage immigration of nurses from the Caribbean Islands to deal with the shortage of nurses created by growth in the number of hospitals during the 1970s (Nestel, 1997). Most of the British nurse-midwives had little out-of-hospital birth experience, and their nursing credentials enabled them to work as obstetric nurses in hospitals. They had nursing licenses to protect and were not eager to challenge the system by attending home births in relatively inhospitable environments. Although the Caribbean nurse-midwives were more likely to have attended home births, they were nonwhite immigrants seeking citizenship in a predominantly white country and did not want to endanger their status by participating in a controversial practice. As a result, the formally trained nurse-midwives were not practicing midwifery. With the exception of two or three American and British nurse-midwives who were providing some midwifery care on an experimental basis but were mainly teaching nursing, apprentice-trained lay midwives were the only midwives practicing in Ontario during the early 1980s (Nestel, 1997; Daviss, 1996 & 1997; Bourgeault, 1997).

The professionalization of midwifery in Ontario was stimulated by the provincial government, which began a comprehensive review of the laws regulating all health professions in the province in 1983—the Health Professions Legislation Review (HPLR). Staff responsible for the HPLR were aware of the presence of both kinds of midwives and asked members of both groups to indicate whether midwifery should become a regulated health profession. If so, they would need to describe the formal education and other standards to be built into the regulatory legislation (Bourgeault, 1997).

The lay midwives' realization that regulation would require standardization of midwifery practice and education resulted in a serious debate about the advantages versus the risks and costs of regulation. Ultimately they decided to seek integration into the health care system and joined with the nurse-midwives to form a coalition to develop a single, strong response to the HPLR inquiry. The Midwifery Coalition also included a group of consumers. The midwives in the coalition went on to form the Association of Ontario Midwives (AOM). The consumers from the Midwifery Coalition formed a consumer task force that went on with its own set of activities in support of midwifery (Kaufman, 1997b). Discussions and negotiations within the AOM and between the AOM and the HPLR began in 1983 and continued into 1985. The midwives asked for self-regulation, multiple educational routes into the profession, authority to attend births in both homes and hospitals, and government funding of midwifery services. Although some midwives and consumers wanted an apprenticeship approach to

midwifery education, the educational model conceptualized within the AOM became more and more formal during the negotiations. Eventually they recommended that the standard for midwifery education be a four-year degree program with an ongoing clinical internship—a direct-entry midwifery program to which nurses would be welcome but not necessarily given advanced status. They didn't think a university degree was necessarily superior educationally, but they thought it was necessary politically and for social and professional credibility, so they recommended it (Bourgeault, 1997; Daviss, 1996 & 1997).

Creation of the AOM was critical to the professionalization of midwifery in Ontario. The AOM functioned as a voluntary regulatory body for practicing midwives during the decade leading up to actual legal regulation and served as the instrument for articulating the values of the profession and building them into the plans for implementation. In 1984, the AOM initiated a process for voluntary self-regulation of midwifery practice by AOM members. AOM standards required two midwives to attend every birth and specified conditions that are contraindications to a home birth and risk factors that require consultation with a physician (Tyson, 1991). The AOM conducts peer review and had a procedure for handling complaints and discipline (Kaufman, 1991). A study published in 1991 indicated that 55 midwives were practicing in Ontario at that time and that 48 of them were AOM members (Tyson, 1991). If those numbers were accurate, more than 85 percent of practicing midwives were members of the AOM. However, in 1992 (only one year later) the provincial government admitted 70 midwives into a special program for which only midwives who were already practicing in the province were eligible.* The Friends of Midwives consumer group believes that there may have been as many as 160 midwives practicing in Ontario

---

*The pre-registration program is described later in this chapter.

prior to legislation (not counting the immigrant nurse-midwives, who were not practicing). The issue of how many midwives were practicing prior to enactment of the new legislation is contentious.

A 1985 coroner's inquest into the death of a newborn following a home birth stimulated a wider public discussion of midwifery. The jury concluded that the death could have been prevented. To avoid such deaths in the future, the jury recommended that midwifery become integrated into the provincial health care system as a legally regulated profession and that a formal midwifery education program be started in Ontario. The HPLR incorporated the jury's recommendations into its official report. In January 1986 the government of Ontario announced its intention to integrate midwifery into the health care system and established a task force to make recommendations to assist the government in implementing its intent.

The first question addressed by the task force was whether midwifery in Ontario should be based on nurse-midwifery education or direct-entry midwifery education. The AOM recommended a direct-entry education model that could accommodate nurses. Nursing and medical organizations pushed for the nurse-midwifery model. During 1986 and 1987 the task force studied midwifery practice, education, and regulation in Denmark, the Netherlands, the United Kingdom, and the United States. Of those countries, only the United States makes systematic distinctions in legal status, place of practice, and education between nurse- and direct-entry midwives. The task force found that the direct-entry programs in the United Kingdom were recruiting a new kind of applicant; in contrast to most nurse-midwifery students in the U.K., most applicants to the direct-entry programs were older, came from more remote communities, had some informal midwifery experience, felt that midwifery was "a calling," and were making a midlife career change. The

task force noted that the direct-entry education program emphasized adult learning methods, the teaching was decentralized, and there was an emphasis on the social sciences, health promotion, health education, and feminist concerns. Faculty of the direct-entry program expected most of their graduates to develop private practices; home births were emphasized (Eberts *et al.*, 1987).

During its investigation in the Netherlands, the task force learned that nurses are not given advanced standing in midwifery education programs in that country and that many Dutch midwives feel that socialization into the nursing profession is damaging to future midwives (Eberts *et al.*, 1987). The task force also saw the effects of the division between nurse-midwives and direct-entry midwives in the United States and determined that its recommendations would "ensure the development of a well-educated and unified profession whose members would have an identical scope of practice regardless of the route of entry into midwifery" (Kaufman, 1991).

The task force report was published in 1987. It proposed that a fully funded midwifery education program be established in an existing university. The program should be autonomous—not part of either a medical or a nursing school. Graduates should earn bachelor of science degrees *in midwifery*, which should be required for entry into practice. It should be possible to compress the four-year curriculum into three calendar years to enable individuals to complete the course faster and to provide continuity of care for better student learning. Although individuals with prior midwifery or nursing education and experience should be assessed for advanced standing, all students should complete the full cycle of clinical midwifery learning experiences. The scope of practice should be based on the international definition of a midwife.* The

---

*The international definition of a midwife is presented in Chapter 1.

end product should be a midwife who can provide primary care to well women; the education program should not prepare midwives for participation in the care of high-risk pregnant women. The majority of clinical preceptors should be practicing midwives. The program should be developed by a network of cooperating institutions to enhance access, distance learning, bilingual instruction, and outreach to the far northern communities. Currently practicing midwives who apply for licensure should be individually assessed and specific educational plans should be developed to fill gaps in their prior preparation and experience. Midwifery care should be covered by the regular provincial health care financing plan; midwives should earn regular salaries, and their services should be accessible through a variety of existing health care facilities (Eberts *et al.*, 1987).

The ability of Ontario midwives to self-govern their practice through their professional association helped to convince the government to include midwifery in the legislative framework for self-regulated professions; it also influenced the task force to recommend creation of an autonomous governing body for midwifery (Kaufman, 1991). The task force recommendations were incorporated into a large legislative package intended to update the regulation of twenty-six health professions in Ontario. In 1989 an interim governing council was appointed to help the Ministry of Health prepare for the new law by developing standards of practice, certification mechanisms, and regulatory processes. The interim council was later replaced by a transitional council and, ultimately, by the College of Midwives, which includes representation by members of the public, the Ministry of Health, the College of Nurses, the College of Physicians and Surgeons, and the Association of Ontario Midwives (College of Midwives of Ontario, 1994; Kaufman, 1991).

A retrospective study of all home births attended by midwives in Toronto from 1983 through the middle of 1988 was published in 1991 (Tyson, 1991). The study reported on 1,001 births attended by twenty-six midwives. Seventeen percent of the mothers and/or their babies were transferred to hospitals during labor or soon after the birth; the cesarean section rate was 3.5 percent. There were no maternal deaths, no intrapartum deaths, and only two neonatal deaths, resulting in a total mortality rate of 2 per 1,000. Ninety-nine percent of the mothers were breast-feeding their babies at 28 days postpartum. These were excellent outcomes, similar to findings from the National Birth Center Study, that had been published two years earlier, and similar to outcomes from low-risk births in hospitals (Rooks *et al.*, 1989).

The model of midwifery practice defined by the College of Midwives of Ontario is based on continuity of care, informed choice, and choice of birth place as fundamental tenets of midwifery. Midwives are expected to serve as the primary care providers for their clients throughout pregnancy and the first six weeks postpartum, to attend births in the setting chosen by each woman, and to accept full responsibility for their own clients. Continuity of care should be achieved through a relationship that "develops over time between a woman and a small group of no more than four midwives." Two midwives should be identified and act as the client's primary care midwives throughout the course of care. One or both of those midwives will be present for the birth except in unusual circumstances, when other midwives from the small group will attend the birth. Two fully qualified midwives should be present at every birth, regardless of the birth setting; both must be skilled in neonatal resuscitation and the control of maternal hemorrhage. Although all midwives should be competent to attend births in all settings, the College of Midwives encourages out-of-hospital births in order to promote normal childbirth (College of Midwives of Ontario, 1994).

The law implemented in Ontario in 1994 is based on the model of midwifery practice defined by the College of Midwives of Ontario. Criteria for registration as a midwife include: (1) successful completion of a special one-time Pre-Registration Program for Experienced Midwives or possession of a baccalaureate degree in midwifery from a recognized institution in Ontario (currently this means the program being implemented in three universities), and (2) carrying professional liability insurance (Kaufman, 1997b). Midwives apply for hospital privileges according to the rules and procedures that apply to physicians (College of Midwives of Ontario, 1994). They have independent authority to prescribe medications and order laboratory tests, are salaried, and their services are covered by the alternative payment program of the government's health care payment system. Although the law does not require midwives to have a formal association with a physician, they must adhere to mandatory guidelines regarding consultation and transfer of care (*Quickening*, 1993). Indigenous "aboriginal midwives" who attend aboriginal women are exempt from regulation under this legislation.

Two kinds of educational programs were implemented in preparation for the new Midwifery Act. In 1992, a one-time Pre-Registration Program for Experienced Midwives was started for the purpose of qualifying midwives who were already practicing in Ontario for licensure under the new law. Admission criteria required having attended at least sixty births during the prior six years, including at least thirty in Ontario. The program was conducted at an institute in Toronto during the fifteen months prior to legalization (Nestel, 1997). The faculty consisted of experienced European midwives. The program was designed to be flexible, anticipating that most students would continue practice while in the program (*Gazette*, May 1992). The program included: (1) a one-month didactic component, including a review and assessment of the individual's ex-

perience in home and hospital practice, a technical update, and administration of a written test of midwifery knowledge; (2) assessment of clinical skills; and (3) a period of placement in the provincial health-care system (*Quickening*, 1993). Seventy midwives were admitted to the program (Axelrod, 1994). The European midwifery tutors were, in general, impressed by the knowledge and skills of the apprentice-trained midwives in Ontario (Hoúd, 1997).

In September 1993 a baccalaureate midwifery program was started at McMaster University, with satellite programs at two other universities. Thirty-three students were selected from more than four hundred applicants. One campus accommodates part-time students, who may take as long as seven years to complete the program. One university offers some components of the curriculum in French. Many components are offered through distance education (Bourgeault, 1997). Anyone who has completed baccalaureate level courses that cover the same material as courses required in the midwifery program can challenge an individual course, and relevant experience, such as working in a sexual assault center or an abortion clinic or teaching childbirth education classes, is considered. No automatic advanced standing is given to nurses. The first class—a total of 18 students from the three universities—graduated in September 1996. When the program is operating at full capacity, it should produce 25 to 40 graduates per year (Kaufman, 1997b).

Neither the Pre-Registration Program nor the baccalaureate program address the circumstances of midwives who immigrated to Canada after completing formal midwifery training in other countries—for example, the United Kingdom, Eastern Europe, the West Indies, India, or the Phillippines (*Gazette*, May 1992; Nestel, 1997). Approximately 40 percent of the individuals expressing a desire to practice midwifery in Ontario since 1986 were classified as "visible minority" women. Almost none of the midwives who emigrated to Ontario from "Third World" countries are able to work in their profession (Nestel, 1997).

A special program intended to address this situation was started in the fall of 1994. Referred to as the Prior Learning Assessment process, it is a long process that includes an assessment and teaching, and it is still undergoing change (Kaufman, 1997b). Currently it involves (1) a midwifery-specific English-language test, (2) a portfolio assessment, (3) a multifaceted intensive assessment, and (4) discussion of professional issues related to midwifery in Ontario (Bourgeault, 1997). It took three years to get the process started, and it is slow and cumbersome. A great deal of paperwork is required to document completed course work and the number of births attended in both homes and hospitals. It is difficult to obtain records from hospitals in some countries, and no credit is given for courses that were not taught at a university-degree level, although a degree is not required. More than 120 foreign-educated midwives applied to the Prior Learning Assessment program during 1994. As of February 1997, only 7 had been registered, although many were still in various stages of the process. Some of the women who have not succeeded in being registered had practiced and taught midwifery for as many as fifteen years (Daviss, 1996 & 1997; Nestel, 1997).

As of January 1997, approximately 90 midwives had been licensed to practice in Ontario. Midwives work in practice groups of two or more, sometimes in community health centers. Their pay is based on the number of births they attend. Their services are fully funded by the province and are legally accessible to all women who are experiencing a normal, uncomplicated pregnancy and birth (MacDonald, 1997). Midwives attended approximately 2,300 births in Ontario during 1996—between 1 and 2 percent of all births in the province (Kaufman, 1997a).

Québec

Midwifery became an issue in Québec as part of a broad debate about the medicalization of pregnancy and the care of pregnant women. Articles and cartoons supporting midwifery were published in Québec journals and newspapers throughout the 1980s. In 1985, the Ministry of Health and Social Services announced its intention to legalize midwifery. With the exception of the medical associations, by 1987 there was wide support for legalization—from many women's organizations and several governmental offices in addition to the Ministry of Health and Social Services* (Vadeboncoeur, 1996). Polls taken during the early 1990s found that 93 percent of Québec consumers approved of midwifery practice in hospitals and 81 percent approved of midwives practicing in free-standing birth centers (Burgin, 1994).

Although the government of Québec announced its intent to legalize midwifery earlier than Ontario did (in 1986), progress was slower and less complete in Québec. The difference has been attributed to very strong opposition from the medical establishment and division between lay-midwives and nurse-midwives in Québec, and more organized and effective consumer support in Ontario, (Vadeboncoeur, 1996). Several coroner's inquests into deaths associated with home births dampened consumer support for home births, and they lobbied primarily for birth centers (Daviss, 1996 & 1997). In addition, the context provided by the Health Professions Legislation Review process both stimulated and structured the legalization process in Ontario (Vadeboncoeur, 1996).

Prior to 1990, physicians had allowed only one midwifery service to be established in Québec—at an Inuit birth center in Povungnituk, a strong remote community that wanted to stop evacuating its pregnant

---

*The Office des Professions du Québec, the Conseil des Affaíres Sociales (Vadeboncoeur, 1996).

women to hospitals in southern Québec. The community organized and sponsored the birth center, and physicians in the community supported the idea and helped implement the service (Daviss, 1997a). Home-birth midwives from southern Québec and Ontario were recruited to staff the birth center and train Inuit women in midwifery. It is not possible to perform a cesarean section at the birth center, and transport to a hospital where a cesarean can be performed took up to eight hours and was not available during much of the year because of weather. As a result, the midwifery teachers and students had to learn to cope with problems on their own. Although the students' training was limited to the care of women during pregnancy and birth, in less than a year women from villages throughout the area were going to the Inuit student midwives for advice on all kinds of "women problems," including domestic violence and alcoholism among their family members (Wagner, 1996a).

The government initially resisted the development of additional birth centers, preferring to address the need for maternity care in other parts of northern Québec by using airplanes to fly pregnant Inuit women to cities in southern Québec during the early part of the last month of their pregnancies. The women were housed in dormitories until they went into labor and were admitted to a hospital. The Inuit culture has a long tradition and respect for midwifery, and many Inuit women have a strong desire to give birth in their own community. They were strongly discouraged from attempting to do so, with warnings that they might die if they refused to go to southern Québec. The plight of these native Canadians increased public support for midwifery in Québec (Burgin, 1994).

In 1990, Québec adopted legislation that authorizes midwifery practice until 1998 in seven new pilot projects. The pilot projects opened in 1994. One closed in 1996 due to medical opposition and lack of midwifery staff, so there are now a total of seven projects, including the birth center in Povungnituk. The six new midwifery projects are viewed as an experiment, to be evaluated; further progress toward legalization of midwifery in Québec will be based on assessment of the outcomes of this experiment (Vadeboncoeur, 1996).

The 1990 legislation also created a committee charged with establishing training standards and assessing the competency of midwives who apply to work in the projects. It was estimated that sixty-four midwives would be needed to provide care to one hundred to three hundred women per year in each project. The plan called for retraining that number of midwives through a program that the provincial government would operate (Moreau, 1992). As in Ontario, there were two kinds of midwives in Québec at the beginning of the 1980s: (1) formally educated foreign-born midwives (mainly nurse-midwives), most of whom were not practicing midwifery, and (2) practicing midwives, most of whom were self-taught or had been trained by a more experienced self-taught midwife. Each group is represented by a separate organization (Vadeboncoeur, 1996). The midwives who applied for the government retraining program included native Québecers, who had been practicing as lay midwives and met the standards of the Practicing Midwives Alliance of Québec, and both direct-entry and nurse-midwives, who were immigrants and had received their training elsewhere (Hatem-Asmar, *et al.,* 1996). As of January 1996, only 16 midwives had completed the retraining process, and the government acceded to demands for a second program. As of March 1997, 49 midwives had completed the process and were legally authorized to practice midwifery in the pilot projects, and 39 of them were practicing (Vadeboncoeur, 1997). Although some practicing midwives have not been accepted into either program, they can continue to practice, because midwifery is not illegal. Uncredentialed midwives are not punished or barred from practice, but cannot work in the birth centers that are at the center of the government projects (Daviss, 1996).

Alberta

The history of midwifery in Alberta includes a short-lived, hospital-based nurse-midwifery education program at the University of Alberta; a consistent but low volume of home births attended by a small number of mostly apprentice-trained midwives; a pilot nurse-midwifery program in a tertiary hospital in Calgary; and a new law that was enacted in 1992 but had not been fully implemented by the end of 1996. Maternity care provided by a physician is free to pregnant women, but they must use their own funds to pay for midwifery care. Lack of third-party payment and hospital privileges has kept the number of births attended by midwives low. As in the United States, the proportion of planned out-of-hospital births is less than 1 percent.

Midwifery became recognized as a profession in Alberta on the basis of a 1992 amendment to the Health Disciplines Act; however, several additional steps were needed to establish midwifery as a legally regulated profession. Standards and regulations were approved in November 1994 and were slated to go into effect in August 1995. Although the regulations require four academic years of postsecondary midwifery education, the educational requirement can be waived for individuals who meet experience requirements* and pass a written examination. Enforcement of the regulations was suspended in order to give the government time to process the applications of the midwives who were already practicing in the province. Although no more than 30 midwives were actually practicing in Alberta at that time, the government received more than 100 applications. As of the end of 1996, approximately 60 individuals had submitted portfolios documenting their midwifery experience, and 40 people had taken the exam. Actual registration was due to commence in March or April of 1997 (James, 1997).

The new law will authorize midwives to attend births in homes, birth centers, and hospitals, provide for prescription privileges, and require that midwives provide continuity of care to their clients and carry malpractice insurance. Although women may engage a midwife directly (i.e., no referral will be needed), the provincial health plan pays for physician services only. With the exception of a pilot project in Calgary, no midwives were allowed to attend births in any hospital in Alberta as of the end of 1996 (James, 1997).

During the 1940s or 1950s, the University of Alberta began to teach an advanced practical obstetrics course to prepare graduate nurses to provide midwifery service in rural areas. As the health care system changed, the need declined; the course was terminated in early 1980s. In 1987 (five years before midwifery was recognized as a profession in the law) the University of Alberta established a nurse-midwifery demonstration project and initiated a nurse-midwifery education program that combined a certificate in midwifery with a master's degree in nursing (Burgin, 1994; Burkhardt, 1996). The program was designed before the regulations for the new law were written, and it could not provide all of the experiences required for registration under the new law. It was terminated in 1993. The regulations are based on direct-entry midwifery and require home birth experience. Nevertheless, the pilot nurse-midwifery program in Calgary has been very successful. A small randomized controlled trial was conducted to compare outcomes for women assigned to the nurse-midwifery service with those for low-risk women who received their

---

*The applicant must have attended at least 60 births, including at least 10 hospital births and 10 out-of-hospital births; must have served as the primary midwife for at least 40 of the 60 births, and must have provided continuity of care (prenatal, labor, delivery, and postpartum care) to at least 30 of the women.

care from physicians (Harvey *et al.*, 1996). The most important finding was a large, statistically significant difference in the rate of cesarean sections—4 percent for the nurse-midwives' clients, compared with 15.1 percent for the physicians' clients. Women who received their care from nurse-midwives were also significantly less likely to have episiotomies and several other kinds of obstetric interventions, their hospital stays were shorter, and their babies were less likely to require neonatal intensive care.* Nevertheless, this hospital-based nurse-midwifery model is not what the consumers who lobbied for midwifery in Alberta asked for (James, 1997).

The ability to waive the educational requirement of the law means that midwives who have received all of their training through apprenticeships will continue to be able to apply for registration in Alberta. This will allow experienced apprentice-trained midwives who move to Alberta in the future to become registered. However, the requirement for hospital as well as home birth experience and the relatively low volume of home births in Alberta could make it difficult for a person without prior experience to enter the profession through this route. The requirement for malpractice liability insurance also works against apprenticeships; a registered midwife who accepts an apprentice for training must have liability insurance that covers the apprentice. In the early 1980s, there were only six midwives working in two practices in the entire province—one practice in Calgary and one in Edmonton. As of the end of 1996, there were about thirty. Although there has been some increase in home births, the increase in midwives has been greater than the increase in home births. It is not clear that there is enough demand for midwifery services to justify developing an educational program, so long as the provincial health plan refuses to pay for midwifery care (James, 1997).

---

*This study is also discussed in Chapter 10.

British Columbia

In 1982 a nurse-midwifery demonstration project was started at Grace Hospital in Vancouver, British Columbia (Burgin, 1994). Grace Hospital is a major obstetric referral center for the entire province. Four nurse-midwives staffed a low-risk prenatal clinic located in the outpatient department of the hospital, under the supervision of obstetricians. Only 51 women had received prenatal care through the nurse-midwifery clinic by 1984. A study was conducted to compare the prenatal care provided by the midwives to 44 women who attended this clinic and the prenatal care provided by family physicians to 88 similar women in their offices with criteria reflecting standards of the local medical community. The results of the comparison were reported in a paper published in the *Canadian Medical Association Journal* in 1988. The prenatal care received by the nurse-midwives' patients was judged to be of higher quality than the care received by the family physicians' patients (Buhler *et al.*, 1988).

In June 1993 the British Columbia Minister of Health expressed support for legalizing midwifery and establishing a College of Midwives in B.C. A committee to advise the government on implementation of legalization was established shortly thereafter.

Midwifery was formally recognized as a health profession in British Columbia in 1995. It is regulated by the College of Midwives of British Columbia, which was established under the law. The provincial minister of health appoints members of the board of the college, three of whom represent the public. Midwives will have to be registered by the College of Midwives in order to practice within the provincial health care system. No midwives had been registered as of the end of 1996.

The College of Midwives submitted the final draft of its bylaws to the Ministry of Health in December 1996. The model of care developed by the College was adapted from those in place in Ontario and Alberta. Midwifery practice will be based in communities, and midwives will attend births in both home and hospital settings. No determination has been made regarding public funding of midwifery services. The College has organized an Interim Multidisciplinary Midwifery Registration Panel to design the registration process. Registration is expected to begin in late 1997; it cannot begin until the cabinet approves the bylaws of the College of Midwifery (Benoit, 1997). Women who want a midwife-assisted birth will be required to consult a physician during the first three months of pregnancy. The Ministry of Health also plans to conduct a demonstration project to determine how home births could be most safely and efficiently provided within the health care system. The home birth demonstration project is expected to be completed in 1998 (Benoit, 1997). The ministry is also considering establishing birth centers (Seattle Midwifery School Bulletin, 1995).

Provinces in Line for New Laws:
Manitoba and Saskatchewan
In 1995 Manitoba announced its intent to regulate midwifery and make it available to women through the provincial health insurance plan. It was recommended that midwifery be a self-regulating profession with multiple routes of entry. A Midwifery Implementation Council was created to develop a process to assess the education and experience of midwives already practicing in the province as a basis for registration. As in Québec, there are two separate midwifery organizations in Manitoba, one for nurse-midwives and one for apprentice-trained direct-entry midwives. Neither organization wants to require nursing as a prerequisite to midwifery education and practice in their province (Robinson, 1997).

The first accomplishment of the Midwifery Implementation Council was to bring a diverse group of midwives together to develop a "competency chart" that describes basic midwifery practice. The next challenge was to determine a fair and effective way to

assess the varied knowledge and skills of midwives who are seeking the right to practice in Manitoba. The Midwifery Implementation Council gave preliminary approval to adopting the NARM certification process as an important part of this assessment.* To begin the NARM process, a midwife must be able to document that she has served as the primary attendant during at least ten out-of-hospital births; there is no requirement to have attended a specific number of births in hospitals. Acceptance of the NARM process as the legal standard would have excluded the majority of midwives in Manitoba from licensure—nurse-midwives educated in other countries and some native Manitobans who endured dislocation and high financial costs to obtain nurse-midwifery education and certification outside of Manitoba. None of them have significant home birth experience. When the Midwifery Implementation Council understood this problem, it asked NARM to suspend the requirement for out-of-hospital birth experience for midwives seeking NARM certification as a requirement for licensure in Manitoba (Robinson, 1997).

In addition to fairness and equity, the Midwifery Implementation Council realized that it would be difficult to enact a new midwifery law for Manitoba if the proposed regulations would exclude most nurse-midwives. The number of direct-entry midwives is very small. To justify the expense of creating the bureaucratic machinery to support the new profession, it will be necessary to have realistic plans for building a profession capable of establishing midwifery as a choice for all childbearing women (Robinson, 1997).

Saskatchewan established a Midwifery Advisory Committee in 1994. The committee was created to provide the Minister of Health with information relevant to determining whether there is a need for midwifery in the province. The report was due at the end of 1996. Although only four mid-

---

*The NARM process is described in Chapter 9.

wives were practicing in Saskatchewan in early 1996 (Daviss, 1996), there is growing consumer support for midwifery. In 1997 the government of Saskatchewan announced its intent to professionalize midwifery and bring it into the provincial health system (Daviss, 1996 & 1997).

The Varying Reactions of Physicians

Canadian medical organizations have made a variety of responses to the new visibility and legality of midwives in their midst. In 1987, the Canadian Medical Association published the results of a survey which found that most Canadian women were satisfied with the care being provided by physicians (Sullivan, 1987). Many physicians argued that there was no need for midwifery services on a large scale and that flaws in the current system could be corrected without midwives (Blais *et al.*, 1994). Canadian physicians who had received part or all of their medical training in Great Britian tended to be more positive.

The Ontario Medical Association contributed to the process in their province by forming a committee that collaborated with the government, midwives, and consumers during the period preceding passage of the Midwifery Act (Vadeboncoeur, 1996). A 1986 survey of physicians delivering babies in Ottawa-Carleton, Ontario, found that nearly half agreed that midwives who meet certain standards should be licensed (Stewart & Beresford, 1988; Blais *et al.*, 1994).

Physicians in Québec reacted differently. A 1991 survey found nearly universal opposition to legal recognition of midwives among physicians practicing obstetrics in Québec, despite wide acknowledgment of shortcomings in the care provided to pregnant women and recognition of some advantages of legalized midwifery: One-fourth to one-third of the physicians doubted that pregnant women receive enough information about nutrition and agreed that the psychological aspects of pregnancy are often neglected; 40 percent agreed that more

progress must be made to humanize maternity care. Nearly half agreed that the cesarean section rate (nearly 20 percent at that time) was not medically justified, and one-fourth believed that midwives could "restore women's confidence in their capacity for natural childbirth" and that introducing midwifery would reduce the use of cesarean sections and episiotomies and allow obstetrician–gynecologists to focus their efforts on high-risk pregnancies. But 34 percent of family physicians thought that "in the long run, midwives will take the place of general practitioners who practice obstetrics," 22 percent of obstetrician–gynecologists thought that legal recognition of midwives would decrease their own clientele, more than three-fourths of both kinds of physicians thought that "giving birth without the aid of a physician is dangerous for the health of the mother and the baby," and most thought that midwives are not necessary in the current system of care (Blais *et al.*, 1994). Every step of the process in Québec has been opposed by every medical association in the province (Vadeboncoeur, 1996).

Observing the difference in reaction between physicians in these two provinces, a professor of family medicine at McGill University in Montreal, Québec, attributed the "calmness, maturity, and cooperativeness" of both family physicians and obstetricians in Ontario to the increasing withdrawal of both kinds of physicians in Ontario from "the maternity care arena." The obstetricians were aging and not being replaced, and only one-third of family physicians in Ontario were practicing obstetrics, as compared with two-thirds of family physicians for the entire country of Canada, and 80 percent in some provinces. Thus he explained the different reactions of physicians in Ontario and Québec, which are adjacent to each other and are similar in geography and population density and distribution, as different understandings of how midwifery would affect them personally. Attrition within obstetrics in Ontario was causing an increased workload. Obstetricians in Ontario understood that midwives were needed, and they were willing to relinquish their role as primary care providers for normal pregnant women and move into the role of consultant and specialist. Although obstetricians and family physicians were also dropping out of maternity care in Québec, the issue there became lodged within a broader concern about the need to prevent nonphysicians (including acupuncturists and homeopaths) from encroaching on the practice of medicine. This set up a strong stance against proposals to legalize midwifery (Klein, 1991).

Australia

Australia was colonized by the British in the early 1800s. Midwives arose from the community as needed, and some trained midwives arrived from England. As in the United States, midwifery is regulated by the laws of specific states. State by state, midwives lost control of their profession to nursing during the early 1900s. Eventually laws or rules were passed requiring all midwives to be nurses. In a sequence that by now should seem familiar, childbirth was moved into hospitals and became increasingly medicalized and the true midwifery role seemed to be lost until a corner was turned, based on women's dissatisfaction with the maternity care provided through the government-run services. Reviews and investigations of maternity care at both the national and state level conducted during the late 1980s quantified the dissatisfaction and provided a focal point for discussions of needed change. These investigations led to recommendations that midwives should play a larger role and that emphasis should be given to increasing the proportion of women who have an opportunity to develop a relationship with the midwife who will attend their births. Midwives are experimenting with ways to accomplish this objective. New birth centers have been opened; more midwives are providing prenatal care, as well as care during labor and delivery; and team

midwifery has been established in several mainstream hospitals. A randomized controlled trial of team midwifery found improved outcomes and reduced costs, as well as significant improvement in women's satisfaction with their pregnancy-related care.

History

The history of midwifery in Australia compresses many aspects of the development of midwifery in the Western world into a very short time frame; the first British settlement in Australia was not established until nearly the beginning of the nineteenth century. The rapid development of midwifery in Australia is in stark contrast to the very slow development of midwifery in North America, although both were vast, sparsely populated continents colonized predominantly by the British. British midwifery was much more developed by the time Australia was colonized, and British midwifery training and traditions were established in Australia relatively quickly. Yet, because the country itself is young, many developments in the midwifery profession are still relatively new. The development of midwifery in Australia also provides examples of some cycles that seem to be nearly universal, issues and themes that recur in many countries: the inevitable development of lay midwifery where unmet needs exist, the ability of midwives to cross social and cultural barriers to provide care to women during labor, and nursing's usurpation of midwifery's authority for self-regulation in many areas.

New South Wales, the first British colony in Australia, was settled by convicts and their keepers in 1788. Because some of the female convicts were pregnant and there were no experienced midwives among them, midwives developed by force of need. A female convict from one of the first boats began to practice as a midwife within a few days of her arrival. She was soon joined by "a kindly 'madam' and former shop-lifter who mended her ways to become a busy midwife." By 1820, an obstetric confinement unit had been built and the colonial governor created a paid position for a midwife, who could be either a convict or a free woman, but was paid less if a convict. A doctor was available, who could be called for complications. The nonconvict settler women gave birth at home, with the help of a relative, neighbor, or servant (Hayes & Bayliss, 1984).

Additional settlements were established between about 1800 and 1835, several as penal colonies. As in New South Wales, wherever there was a concentration of women, some form of lay midwifery had to develop. The first shipment of female convicts arrived in Tasmania in 1820. They were housed together and soon developed a lay midwifery service, which also took care of women in the nearby town. The physician could order a particular convict to be released so that she could be with a woman who was in labor in the community. In time, midwives trained in Britain joined the free community in Tasmania (Garrison *et al.*, 1984).

The first trained midwives began to arrive in what is now Melbourne, Victoria, within ten to fifteen years of its settlement in 1835 (Adair *et al.*, 1984). However, there may have been no formally trained midwives for many years after the first settlements were established in the Northern Territory and Western Australia during the 1920s (McDonald & Davis, 1984; Keenan *et al.*, 1984). Women helped one another during childbirth; some eventually became known as midwives based on skills honed on experience and, sometimes, guidance provided by physicians (Keenan *et al.*, 1984). Aboriginal women assisted at the births of the first women settlers in South Australia, which was settled (without convicts) in 1836. Eventually a few physicians and midwives arrived, and lying-in homes were built (Conboy, 1984).

The discovery of gold in New South Wales in 1851 led to a period of rapid growth of population and wealth. By 1860, wealthy families had developed the practice of hiring a "ladies' monthly nurse," who moved into their home one week before a baby was due and stayed for three weeks after the birth. Midwives for the common folk, known as "grannies," walked or drove a horse and buggy to attend home births and then stayed to cook for the family, care for the other children, maybe even milk the cow, while the mother rested. The pay for the grannies was minimal (Hayes & Bayliss, 1984).

Midwifery schools were developed in lying-in hospitals in Melbourne, Sydney, and South Australia during the second half of the 1800s. A hospital in Melbourne started a midwifery training program in 1862. By 1888, the Women's Hospital offered two midwifery courses, a one-year course (nine months of midwifery and three months of gynecology) and a six-month course that did not include gynecology. In 1893, a two-year midwifery course was started, and a one-year Diploma of Midwifery course was introduced for nurses (Adair *et al.*, 1984). The first midwifery school in Sydney was started in 1875. During the next two decades, lack of access to maternity care and poor outcomes for destitute women motivated the development of three additional schools in hospitals on the outskirts of Sydney (Hayes & Bayliss, 1984). The first lying-in hospital in South Australia opened during the 1890s and quickly started a midwifery training program for nurses (Conboy, 1984). By the end of the 1800s, some women from Western Australia and the Northern Territory were going to Sydney or Melbourne for nursing or midwifery training (Keenan *et al.*, 1984; O'Brien & Green, 1984).

Midwifery schools opened in other parts of the country during the early 1900s, and there were efforts to improve the quality of midwifery training, to require midwives to register, and to limit registration to midwives who had evidence of training. In 1901, Tasmania became the first Australian state to pass a midwifery law*. The first Tasmanian

---

*This was one year before enactment of the first midwifery act in England. Thus a British penal colony that was not established until the early 1800s regulated midwifery earlier than England itself.

midwifery training program did not open until six years later (Garrison *et al.*, 1984). The first formal midwifery training program in Western Australia was started in 1909; four years later Western Australia passed a law that required midwives to register and restricted registration to midwives with a training certificate or evidence of extensive experience (Keenan *et al.*, 1984).

Despite the presence of four midwifery schools, only 10 percent of midwives practicing in New South Wales in 1904 had evidence of formal training, and there was concern about the training standards of several of the schools. In addition, the birth rate was falling, and infant mortality seemed to be increasing. A commission assigned to investigate these circumstances recommended hospitalization for childbirth. Because of fear of infection, babies born in hospitals were separated from their mothers and kept in centralized nurseries. Visitors were restricted, and children were not allowed to visit their mothers in the hospital. As the teaching hospitals became increasingly crowded, some midwives opened small, private lying-in hospitals that were closer to women's homes, and the government established community-based "baby health centers," where new mothers were encouraged to breast-feed and taught how to take care of their babies (Hayes & Bayliss, 1984).

By the early 1900s some nurse-midwifery training programs had been started, although most midwifery schools did not require nursing. This changed during the next twenty-five years, as nursing organizations gained authority for midwifery education and practice. The following is the story of that transition in Victoria, including a struggle between the Australian Trained Nurses' Association and physicians at the major lying-in hospital in Melbourne for control of midwifery standards:

In 1895, the Melbourne District Nursing Society organized a home birth midwifery service in association with Women's Hospital. By 1901, only certified nurses could be employed in the Women's Hospital midwifery service, which had been recognized by the Australian Trained Nurses' Association as an approved training school for nurses. From then on, the curriculum of the school was determined in conjunction with the nurses' association, which also played a role in the administration of examinations (Adair *et al.*, 1984).

In 1903 the Victorian Trained Nurses' Association established a nurses registry, including a special registry for nurses trained in specialty areas, such as midwifery. In 1910 the Victorian Trained Nurses' Association decided to push for mandatory state registration of nurses (Adair *et al.*, 1984).

In 1912 Women's Hospital began to lobby for a separate midwives act. A separate law for midwifery would allow the hospital to develop midwifery training programs to meet its needs, without reference to the rules of the nurses' association (Adair *et al.*, 1984).

In 1915 two bills were introduced in the legislature, one for nursing and one for midwifery. The nursing bill did not pass, but a law to regulate the training, registration and practice of midwives was enacted. It established a three-member Midwives' Board with authority to determine the qualifications for registration to practice midwifery in Victoria. Two of the three Board members were physicians. The Board established a minimum age and made registration mandatory; a woman who called herself a "midwife" but was not registered was subject to penalty. An examination that had to be passed as a qualification for registration was initiated in 1917. Two midwifery training programs were approved by the Midwives' Board, including the one at Women's Hospital. All instruction had to be provided by a physician or a registered midwife (Adair *et al.*, 1984).

A Nurses Board was established in 1923. A Nurses Act passed in 1928 amended the

Midwives Act and gave all functions of the Midwives Board to the Nurses Board. There were no midwives on the Nurses Board. In 1929 the Nurses Board adopted regulations that required the matron (i.e., principal) of every midwifery school to be registered as both a nurse and a midwife. A rule adopted in 1941 required one member of the Nurses Board to be a midwife as well as a nurse. The Victorian Nursing Council succeeded the Nurses Board in 1958. In 1966 the Victorian Nursing Council eliminated direct-entry midwifery training by adopting a rule that required all students entering midwifery training programs to be registered general nurses. The post-nursing midwifery curriculum in Victoria was one year in length. By 1983, 11 hospitals in Victoria were operating post-nursing midwifery education programs; between them they graduated 600 midwives per year. (In contrast, only 238 nurse-midwives were certified in the entire United States in 1983.) The first college-based midwifery program in Victoria was started in 1983. The degree to be awarded was a Bachelor of Applied Science in Advanced Nursing (Adair *et al.*, 1984).

Similar transitions occurred in New South Wales, South Australia, and Western Australia. As in Victoria, nursing and medicine struggled for control of midwifery educational standards in South Australia. The coalescence of nursing and midwifery worked both ways. Community health nursing was a very important part of health care in sparsely populated areas. By 1920 all nursing positions in the Northern Territory required qualifications in both general nursing and midwifery. This kind of rule requires nurses who have no particular interest in midwifery to take midwifery training.

Home births continued to be important in Australia until after the second World War. When the war ended there was a surge in population and, with the new availability of antibiotics, blood transfusions, and trans-

portation, a rapid shift of births to hospitals in urban states, such as New South Wales. By 1950 almost all births in New South Wales occurred in hospitals. Over time, the small, private maternity hospitals closed (Hayes & Bayliss, 1984). Although childbirth began to move into hospitals in Western Australia after the end of World War II, midwives continued to attend home births in both rural and urban parts of Western Austria. Some midwives practiced in small maternity centers in rural areas, sometimes with and sometimes without a general medical practitioner (Keenan *et al.*, 1984).

During the 1960s and 1970s some women in Australia, as elsewhere, accused obstetricians of having transformed the care of women during pregnancy and childbirth by an overemphasis on pathology. Although most births continued to occur in hospitals, there was a strong interest in free-standing birth centers and a resurgence of interest in home births (Hayes & Bayliss, 1984). A 1984 report by the Tasmanian midwives noted that both midwives and consumers had become increasing dissatisfied with the maternity care being provided in Tasmania (Garrison *et al.*, 1984).

Recent Events and the Current Situation

During the late 1980s three of the most populous Australian states conducted comprehensive reviews of their maternity services. The report of the review conducted in New South Wales was published in 1989; reports of the reviews conducted in Western Australia and Victoria were published in 1990. All three reports recommended that midwives play a greater role in the care of women giving birth (Biro & Lumley, 1991). Two of the reviews also recommended increasing the number of birth centers (Rowley *et al.*, 1995).

A survey to measure the extent of satisfaction and dissatisfaction with maternity care was conducted as part of the information gathering for the Ministerial Review of Birthing Services in Victoria. A survey form was mailed to every woman who had given birth in Victoria during one particular week in 1989 (Brown & Lumley, 1994). The purpose was to determine whether the complaints and concerns expressed in written testimony and during public hearings conducted as part of the review were widely shared or were held by only a few elite women. Many relatively high socioeconomic status women had written or participated in the meetings, and some observers assumed that well-educated women with "unrealistic expectations" were the only ones who were strongly dissatisfied and critical of the childbirth care being provided in Victoria. Seventy-one percent of the women who had babies during the specified week responded to the survey. Women who were single, did not speak English, or were less than twenty-five years of age were least likely to respond; otherwise, the results were representative of all childbearing women in Victoria* (Brown & Lumley, 1994).

Two-thirds of the women were satisfied with the care they had received; 27 percent had mixed feelings; 6 percent were very dissatisfied. There was no association between socioeconomic status and the likelihood that a woman was unhappy about her care. The factors most strongly associated with dissatisfaction were lack of involvement in decision making, not having been given enough information, having had many interventions during labor and delivery, and perceiving the caregivers as not very helpful. Women having first babies were more likely to be dissatisfied if their baby was delivered by a

physician instead of a midwife, although the difference (44 percent dissatisfied versus 28 percent dissatisfied) was not statistically significant. Most of the dissatisfaction arose from care provided during labor and delivery; most women were relatively satisfied with their prenatal care (Brown & Lumley, 1994). Women who received all of their prenatal care from a single primary care provider (obstetrician, GP, or midwife) and those who received care from a small team of caregivers (such as the care provided to women who have home births, care in birth centers, and care shared between a midwife and the woman's general practitioner) were most satisfied with their care. Women who attended public hospital clinics were least satisfied (Lumley *et al.*, 1990). More than one-third of childbearing women receive their health care from the private sector; somewhat less than two-thirds use public facilities (Waldenström, 1996, 1997).

The National Health and Medical Research Council of Australia also issued recommendations for improving the care of pregnant women in Australia. All of these reports—three statewide reviews and a National Health and Medical Research Council report—identified lack of continuity of care as a specific source of dissatisfaction among women receiving care in Australia, concluded that women benefit from receiving care from a midwife with whom they have developed a relationship, and recommended greater use of midwifery teams as a way to enhance continuity of care.

These recommendations led to experimentation with "team midwifery" and other ways to achieve continuity of care and a randomized trial to assess the effect of continuity of care provided by a team of midwives on events during pregnancy, neonatal outcomes, maternal satisfaction, and costs. The randomized trial was conducted at a teaching hospital during 1991 and 1992 (Rowley *et al.*, 1995). More than 800 women were randomly assigned to team midwifery care or routine care (provided by a variety of mid-

---

*About 40 percent of women who give birth in Victoria receive care in public hospitals; 45 percent are patients of private obstetricians, 11 percent are patients of private family physicians, and a few use in-hospital birth centers or have home births (less than 1 percent). Midwives provide much of the care in hospital obstetric suites, although they were the main or only professional attendant at only 22 percent of the births of the women who participated in this study, $N = 790$ (Brown & Lumley, 1994).

wives and doctors) when they initiated care at the hospital's prenatal clinic. The women who received team midwifery care attended more prenatal classes, required less pain medication during labor, and were more likely than the women who received care from many midwives and physicians to give birth without any form of intervention. In addition, their babies had fewer low Apgar scores and needed less resuscitation, and the women expressed greater satisfaction with the information they had received, felt more able to discuss anxieties and participate in decision making, and were more likely to feel that their caregivers were interested in them as individual people. Team midwifery care was associated with nearly a 5 percent reduction in the overall costs of the care (Rowley *et al.*, 1995).

"Shared care," based on a formal cooperative arrangement between a maternity hospital and practitioners who work in the community, is another way to provide continuity of care. A shared care midwifery service operated by a small, inner-city primary health care agency and a maternity hospital in Melbourne received a national Best Practice award in 1995. The award highlights care that is measurably cost efficient, effective, high quality, and produces outcomes that are valued and desired by the community. Most of the women who use the shared maternity care program at the North Richmond Community Health Centre (NRCHC) are refugees from Vietnam or Timor, a politically troubled island of Indonesia. The women are not integrated into Australian society and tend to feel alienated by the public hospital system. The shared care model made it possible for the midwives to get to know these women within the context of their own homes and lives, giving the midwives a deeper understanding of their clients. It also enhanced collaboration and trust between midwives and physicians and between the hospital and community-based practitioners and led to the development of effective working relationships with people

in the schools, city government, and the welfare, housing, and emergency services agencies. Midwifery care has become part of the social support network of the women who use the NRCHC program (Carberry & Carey, 1996).

Home births have a long history in Australia, and there is some continuing demand for them, especially in South Australia and Western Australia. Several studies of home births attended by midwives or doctors and midwives were published during the late 1980s and early 1990s (Howe, 1988; Crotty *et al.*, 1990, Woodcock *et al.*, 1990). Nevertheless, planned home births comprised only 0.5 percent of Australian births between 1985 and 1990 (Bastian & Lancaster, 1992). Because small maternity homes were part of the country's history, the idea of free-standing birth centers did not require a conceptual leap of faith. Birth centers began to be developed during the late 1970s and proliferated during the 1990s, due to government funding provided through a new Alternative Birthing Services program (Whelan, 1994). More than fifteen new birth centers have been opened since 1990 (Waldenström, 1996 & 1997).

These alternative models of care affect only a minority of women. About 8,000 women were booked for birth center care in 1995; about half that number actually gave birth in a birth center. The new team midwifery models within traditional hospitals provide care to between 1,000 and 1,500 women per year. A minority of midwives are involved in providing these kinds of services, which are available to slightly less than 4 percent of the women who give birth in Australia in an average year (Waldenström, 1997). The majority of Australian midwives are government employees and work shifts in hospital labor and delivery units. Being a member of a small team of midwives who provide continuity-of-care to a caseload of women requires being "on call" much of the time and has a major impact on midwives' personal lives. Australian midwives are conducting research in order to better understand the experiences of midwives who are trying to implement new models of midwifery care within mainstream maternity services, such as working as members of small midwifery teams that practice in large hospitals (Brodie, 1996).

Many Australian midwives have no involvement in prenatal care. In some hospitals, especially in the private sector, midwives working in labor and delivery wards are dependent on doctors and thus function more like obstetrical nurses than midwives. In some places, midwives call a physician to conduct vaginal examinations during labor and do not suture tears and episiotomies. A recent survey found that 35 percent of the midwives who work in birth centers were not suturing tears—a very high figure, considering that birth centers are organized in a way that encourages midwives to practice independently (Waldenström, 1996 & 1997).

Nevertheless, there are many very positive circumstances for midwifery in Australia. Australian women are, in general, very satisfied with the services provided by midwives. In addition many Australian obstetricians are dissatisfied with their long, irregular hours, feel pressured by the threat of malpractice litigation, and are seeking new ways to practice, and many general practitioners are abandoning obstetrics. These conditions within the medical community may open new opportunities for midwives to develop collaborative associations with obstetricians (Waldenström, 1997).

Midwifery Education

An experienced Swedish midwife who is currently leading a midwifery education program at an Australian university has voiced concern about the amount of clinical training. The nurses boards in some Australian states have low experience requirements for midwives, in some cases requiring only five vaginal assessments of progress during labor and only fifteen to twenty deliveries. Arguments to increase clinical training standards have failed

due to limited access to patients, especially in settings where midwifery and medical students have to share the available clinical experience. In addition, some nurses who receive midwifery training do not go on to practice midwifery (Waldenström, 1997). This further dilutes the clinical learning experiences available to students who will actually assume a midwife's responsibility for care of women.

In 1989 the federal government of Australia took the position that all nursing education, including midwifery education, should move away from hospital-based training to institutions of higher education. The Australian College of Midwives agrees, and also believes that midwifery education should be conducted in tertiary medical centers. Some distance learning programs have been developed to extend the reach of university and tertiary-hospital-based midwifery education programs to students in remote areas (Glover, 1996).

New Zealand

New Zealand is a relatively sparsely populated country consisting primarily of two islands, which together include territory somewhat smaller than Great Britain or Japan, but with a population of less than four million (Stimpson, 1996). Its indigenous people are Maori. It was colonized by the British at about the same time as most of the Australian colonies, around 1820. Although a modern, Western country, New Zealand retains an important agrarian base and a large rural population. The health care system is a hybrid, with elements of a nationalized system coexisting with a vocal private sector (Rosenblatt, 1994). Although health care is guaranteed to everyone, current reforms are trying to move it toward further privatization (Young, D., 1993). New Zealand created a formal regionalized perinatal care system in 1975, with three levels of facilities and risk-based clinical guidelines for referring or transporting high-risk women from lower to higher-level facilities.

Until the recent changes described in this section, most midwives were employed by state-run hospitals (Rosenblatt, 1994). The typical sequence of care for a pregnant woman included prenatal care provided by her family doctor (a GP), with referral to an obstetrician if complications were detected, or prenatal care provided through a hospital clinic. Midwives provided care during labor; because the midwives worked shifts, a woman having a long labor might receive care from several midwives. The doctor was expected to appear in time to actually deliver the baby. Postpartum care in the hospital was provided by midwives, with an occasional visit by the doctor. Specially trained nurses made home visits to the mother, especially to check on the baby, after they returned home (Cole, 1996; Wagner, 1996). A few midwives attended home births (Guilliland, 1997).

History

During early colonial times, well-trained midwives assumed responsibility for their own practice (Stimpson, 1996). Although a law making midwifery an autonomous profession was enacted in 1904, physicians soon wanted a larger role in the care of pregnant women, and childbirth moved increasingly into hospitals. Midwifery devolved into a form of obstetric nursing, and "midwives lost their sense of responsibility and accountability as independent practitioners, lost their sense of professional identify as separate from nursing, and above all, lost their place in the community as respected guardians of birth" (Pairman, 1996). The loss of the midwifery role was solidified by passage of the Nurses Act of 1971, which gave ultimate authority for the care of all pregnant women to physicians and made it illegal for a midwife to provide any service to a woman who was not under the care of a physician. The midwife needed only to carry out the doctor's instructions, assist him "when he arrives to deliver the baby," and clean and comfort the mother and baby after the delivery (Stimp-

son, 1996). However, midwives continued to provide most of the care during labor, and the postpartum period, and were the real decision makers in the numerous smaller birthing units (Guilliland, 1997).

In 1983 a group of women formed "Save the Midwife" as a consumer lobbying group dedicated to reversing the loss of midwifery authority (Donley, 1990). Ultimately, midwives also realized the need for political activation and for a national midwifery organization that is separate from the New Zealand Nurses' Association (Donley, 1990).

A Recent Renaissance: In 1988 midwives and activist women began to work together to reestablish midwifery as an independent profession in the law and to create the New Zealand College of Midwives (Pairman, 1996). Both goals were achieved within two years. In 1989 the New Zealand College of Midwives was established and the Minister of Health (a woman) proposed that the Nurses Act be amended to allow independent midwifery practice (Donley, 1990; Stimpson, 1996). Despite strong medical opposition, the recently established New Zealand College of Midwives and its consumer partners carried the day. In 1990, the leader of the opposition said he was not willing to fight the women of the country and conceded. A 1990 amendment to the Nurses Act authorizes midwives to provide all care needed by normal pregnant women without medical supervision, including ordering diagnostic tests and prescribing all medications consistent with their role in pregnancy and birth (there is no stipulated list). The law recognizes women's desire for informed choice in maternity care and directs midwives to work in partnership with women. Pregnant women must be informed about their options regarding who will be their "lead maternity carer," prenatal and childbirth classes, and the place of birth. A woman may choose to receive care from a midwife, a GP, an obstetrician, or a combination of care providers, but one person must be identified as the "lead maternity carer" (Cole, 1996). The legislation was also intended to facilitate the establishment of direct-entry midwifery education programs (Young, D., 1993). The Minister of Health challenged the midwives to use their new autonomy to increase the choices and quality of care offered to child-bearing women (Stimpson, 1996).

The New Zealand College of Midwives (NZCOM) quickly became a unique voice in the international midwifery community. During the 1993 congress of the International Confederation of Midwives (ICM), the NZCOM introduced and took the lead in promoting its position that the midwifery profession is based on a partnership between women and midwives and that midwifery associations should encourage consumers to participate in the activities of the organization. This position was adopted by the ICM. The NZCOM is implementing that policy and has developed a model for midwifery practice that is based on the partnership concept: The partnership between a midwife and a pregnant woman is based on continuity of care, which allows time for the partners to get to know and trust each other. The partnership itself should be based on principles of individual negotiation; equality, shared responsibility, and empowerment; and informed choice and consent (Guilliland & Pairman, 1995). Members of NZCOM ask their clients to provide written evaluations of their care, which are considered during annual reviews conducted by a committee of the College (Young, 1993). Midwives and consumers participate in the annual reviews (Stimpson, 1996). "Partnership" has become part of the midwifery culture of New Zealand (Pairman, 1996).

While midwifery was acquiring a new law, a new professional organization, and a new philosophy, the entire health care system in New Zealand was undergoing radical deregulation intended to move away from the centralized national health care system model toward a more pluralistic "privatized" system. Although maternity care is still paid for by the government, the components of the system now have to compete for clients, and thus for funds. Small maternity hospitals are fighting to stay open (Young D., 1993).

Independent Midwifery Practice

The convergence of deep changes and invigoration within the midwifery profession and a general loosening of the health care system created an entrepreneurial environment in which midwives are developing new practices, new models of practice, new organizational arrangements, and new forms of collaboration with physicians. For example, one group of midwives and general practitioners is planning to establish a primary maternity consortium within which they will develop and implement a model of care intended to maximize the mother's and family's involvement and make the most appropriate use of midwives, general practitioners, and specialists. New free-standing maternity units are opening, in some cases through conversion of small rural hospitals. Some midwives and physicians are forming joint practices; other midwives are working in midwifery groups and teams that have easy access to obstetric consultants. Midwives are advertising their services, and women are being given choices regarding both the place of birth and the desired caregiver for each component of the maternity cycle. Continuity of care is the model, but it can be achieved in many ways (Young D., 1993). Although some midwives and doctors are "focusing on the value of their common ground rather than their differences" (Young D., 1993), some physicians have found it difficult to work in an equal partnership with midwives (Stimpson, 1996).

As in Australia and the United Kingdom, midwives in New Zealand are experimenting with their new responsibilities and the challenge to provide continuity of care. In the words of a New Zealand midwife who spoke at the 1996 ICM Congress, "Continuity in a practical sense means being available twenty-four hours a day, seven days a week.

This means that partners and children can no longer know when she can be with them or rely on her presence at business activities or school functions. Many midwives have exhibited signs of burnout after only six months of independent practice. . . . Independent midwifery is a total life change and a major exciting challenge." Self-employment is new to midwives in New Zealand, who are having to learn to manage their time and limit their caseload (Guilliland, 1997). The New Zealand College of Midwives recommends that independent midwives accept no more than forty to sixty clients per year if they are providing full continuity of care. As midwives gain experience as self-employed practitioners, they are choosing to practice in pairs (partnerships) within a group of four to six midwives, which enables them to have scheduled time off, to be covered in case of illness, and to be able to meet the needs of two clients who need care at the same time. The 1990 amendment to the Nurses Act requires that they be paid (by the state) at the same rate as a general practitioner (Gulbransen *et al.*, 1997).

Other problems also need to be worked out. All of them are issues American nurse-midwives have been working on for years. Most women who want care from a midwife want to give birth in hospitals. Midwives who are not employed by a hospital need "access" (i.e., privileges) to admit their clients to a hospital and provide care for them there. At first some hospitals refused to give access to midwives who had less than a certain number of years of experience or required midwives and GPs who attend births at the hospital to have a backup agreement with an obstetrician (Stimpson, 1996). Hospital access problems have since been largely resolved through guidelines established by a unit of the government (Guilliand, 1997). In addition, midwives and physicians lack experience in how to work together when the midwife is "independent." Collaboration in the care of women whose risk status changes and who need care from both an obstetri-

cian and a midwife is easier when both are salaried employees of the same institution, and that was the only experience of most midwives and obstetricians in New Zealand until recent years. It takes a while to work out the communication and trust required to create the necessary flow of care and authority when short-term medical consultation or intervention is needed for a client of a self-employed midwife.* Early problems caused by pharmacists who were unaccustomed to filling prescriptions written by anyone other than a physician have been resolved through guidelines produced jointly by the New Zealand College of Midwives and the Pharmacists' Society (Guilliland, 1997).

Independent practice is not for everyone. Some midwives work "under the umbrella" of a GP's practice, in some cases providing nearly all maternity care to women in his practice, in others providing only specific aspects of the care, for example, just prenatal care, just care during labor, or just postpartum care. In addition, many midwives continue to work shifts in hospitals. All hospitals have introduced team midwifery or a "Know Your Midwife" scheme, ranging from one-to-one care to teams with as many as twelve midwives (Guilliland, 1997). A woman meets every midwife on her team, usually two or three midwives, during prenatal care and can rely on having one of them take care of her during labor and delivery. Approximately 75 percent of women now know the midwife who attends them during labor (Guilliland, 1997).

Home births had increased to more than 2 percent of births in 1993 (Gulbransen, 1997), and 3 to 5 percent of births in Auckland (the largest city in the country). Midwives attended 36 percent of all births in

---

*See discussion of collaboration with physicians in Chapter 8, especially the difference between the role of physicians in a midwifery practice or service as compared with medical/midwifery partnerships and teams.

New Zealand in 1994—16 percent as the sole practitioner and 21 percent with a GP (Young D., 1993). All midwifery schools now offer direct-entry degree programs, nurse-midwifery programs are continuing, and the number of midwives is increasing (Stallings, 1995; Guilliland, 1997).

Japan

Japan has the lowest infant mortality rate of any country in the world. Japan's infant mortality rate in 1992 was 4.5 deaths per 1,000 live births. The United States had the 22nd lowest mortality rate—8.5 deaths/ 1,000 live births, which was nearly twice as high as the rate in Japan that year (National Center for Health Statistics, 1996).

Japan's excellent pregnancy outcomes are attributed to many factors. Everyone is covered by health-care insurance, and there are no qualitative differences in care based on type of insurance coverage. Public health organizations work with mothers' club members, who disseminate health information and encourage and assist pregnant women to enroll in prenatal care. This system is effective but does not reach into some parts of the largest cities, in which most people live in nuclear families and many women work. Most births occur to women within the optimal age range for childbearing, and there are few births to unmarried women. Abortion is available when contraception fails, and few births are unwanted. Most Japanese citizens are well educated and seek medical advice. All pregnant women receive a *Maternal and Child Health Handbook*, in which all information about the pregnancy is recorded. The book becomes the first health record of the child. The woman is given the book when she reports her pregnancy at the town hall and keeps it with her, bringing it to every prenatal visit, to the hospital when she goes to give birth, and to every episode of child health care until her child reaches the age of six and receives a different health record book on entry into school. During the mother's week-long postpartum hospitalization, a nurse or midwife makes sure that the mother and newborn establish effective breast-feeding. At least 70 percent of Japanese babies are still breast-feeding at two to three months of age, even though additional foods may have been introduced. Low-income families receive government subsidies (Leppert, 1993; Kondo, 1997).

History

A law enacted in 1899 established midwifery as a professional occupation. Midwives were authorized to practice independently. Prior to the United States' influence on Japan at the end of World War II, there had been a very long tradition of a large proportion of Japanese births taking place in homes. When the U.S. Army occupied Japan after the war, American army nurses (who had no experience with professional direct-entry midwifery) became concerned about home births being attended by midwives who had not been trained as nurses (Wagner, 1996; Kondo, 1997). Enactment of a new Public Health Nurse, Midwife, and Nurse Law (law number 203) in 1947 restricted new midwifery licenses to midwives with previous training as nurses (Fukuzawa, 1984). There has been no direct-entry midwifery education in Japan since 1951 (Stallings, 1995).

Childbirth in Japan underwent fundamental change during the first twenty-five years after the war. In 1950, more than 95 percent of births occurred in homes, and a midwife was the primary attendant for 90 percent of all births in the country. Economic changes and population growth during the 1950s and 1960s resulted in a substantial downsizing of homes—to the extent that there was not enough room for a comfortable birth in the average Japanese home. Responding to this change, some midwives developed birthing units in their own homes, and there was a significant shift of home births from mothers' homes to midwives' homes, which were classified as midwifery clinics. By 1965, only 16 percent of births occurred in homes, and about an equal proportion occurred in midwifery clinics. By 1975 only 1 percent of births were in homes, and only 10 percent were attended by midwives in the absence of a physician. By 1991 only one in a thousand births was at home and midwives were the "primary" attendant at less than 2 percent of all births. (Doctors are considered to be the primary attendant for all births at which both a midwife and a physician are present, even if, as is the usual case in both hospitals and clinics operated by physicians, the midwife assists the delivery while the physician watches. As a result, the data on the proportion of births attended by midwives in Japan is misleading.) Births in midwifery clinics fell from about 13 percent during the mid-1960s, to 7 percent in the mid-1970s, and 2 percent in 1985. In 1991, 56 percent of all Japanese births were in hospitals, 43 percent were in clinics operated by obstetricians, and 1 percent were in midwifery "clinics" (Fiedler, 1996).

Efforts to Reestablish Midwifery Birthing Homes

Most of the midwives who owned homes with enough space to accommodate a birthing unit are old and have stopped attending births. At the same time, younger midwives cannot afford to buy such large homes, and many lack experience with home births. Yet both midwives and consumers are interested in resurrecting the home birth tradition. In 1997 the Japanese Midwives' Association initiated a full-time one-year program to prepare experienced midwives to open and operate birthing homes. The program includes a technical update, including training in ultrasonography and precepted experience in a midwifery birthing home. The Midwifery Association plans to provide this training for nine or ten experienced midwives each year. Three midwives started the program in 1996 and completed it in 1997; nine started it in 1997 and will finish in 1998. The number of home births is beginning to increase (Kondo, 1997).

Current Practice

Although obstetricians provide prenatal care to most women, midwives play a major role in childbirth. Japanese culture accepts birth as a normal physiologic process that should be handled with little technological intervention. Labor and delivery are seen as a vulnerable period requiring medical consultation or supervision, but not routine medical intervention. Midwives attend women during labor and attend all normal deliveries in hospitals. Obstetricians are not usually present during labor, but must be present for the birth in case of a complication that requires intervention. If there is a need for administration of local anesthetic, cutting an episiotomy, or application of forceps, the midwife steps aside and the obstetrician performs the procedure. When his special tools and skills are no longer needed, he steps aside, allowing the midwife to complete the birth. The use of obstetric tools seems to distinguish when an obstetrician needs to play a direct physical role in the woman's care. Midwives may deliver twins and babies in breech presentation, with an obstetrician in the room. The obstetrician will probably not step in to provide direct care unless his tools are needed (Fiedler, 1996). Women's groups are protesting overuse of obstetric interventions, and obstetricians are becoming more cautious about using them (Kondo, 1997).

Because of the underlying attitude that birth is normal, and because of the influence of midwives, most Japanese women eat and drink during labor and walk from the labor room to the delivery room. They do not receive analgesia and anesthesia routinely (Fiedler, 1996). The cesarean delivery rate was 14 percent in 1993—up from 8 percent in 1984. (The cesarean section rate for the United States was 22 percent in 1993.) Midwives are generally not viewed as an authoritative source of information about pregnancy and birth. Japanese women tend to view them "as ancillary specialists who function as intermediaries, interpreting and explaining the obstetrician's diagnoses and recommendations . . . since most obstetricians are male and all midwives are female, midwives are viewed as good supplementary sources of information and emotional support because of their direct understanding of childbearing and female physiology" (Fiedler, 1996). Although relatively few midwives are in independent practice (slightly more than 12 percent in 1994), women do see *them* as experts, addressing them as "sensei," a term that implies respect for a person with special expertise (Fiedler, 1996; Kondo, 1997). Midwives teach childbirth classes and provide nutrition education and contraceptive counseling and services (Leppert, 1993).

Education, Employment, and Retention of Midwives

Nurses complete the compulsory nine years of basic schooling and three years of high school, followed by a three-year nursing education program at a junior college or a four-year nursing program at a college or university. Graduates of three-year junior college nursing programs may take midwifery as a separate one-year course; most enter the midwifery course immediately after completing their basic nursing program. For those who take nursing at a college or university, the basic nursing education is largely completed during the first three years of the programs, leaving most of the fourth year for electives. Thirty-one of the nation's 46 baccalaureate nursing programs offer a one-year midwifery course as a year-four elective. Whereas there may be 50 to 100 students in each basic nursing class, only five to ten students will be accepted into the midwifery elective. Many more apply, so the midwifery faculty can be selective.

Although the midwifery elective lasts for a full academic year, students also have to take some nursing courses during that time. The minimum number of credits allotted to the midwifery elective is eight, although some schools have increased the elective to eighteen credits by extending the program through the summer. Many midwifery faculty believe that, even with a summer extension, there is not enough time for adequate training in midwifery. For at least ten years the National Midwifery Education Council has recommended that midwifery be taught as a full-year (32 credits) postgraduate program, preferably at the master's level. Nurses who are not midwives outnumber the midwives and have a more powerful voice in determining the nursing curriculum; thus the recommendation of the Midwifery Education Council has not been accepted. Nevertheless, at least one school is planning to offer midwifery as a master's degree program, and one or two others hope to follow (Kondo, 1997).

More than 23,000 midwives were practicing in Japan in 1994. With approximately 1,180,000 births in 1994, there was slightly less than one midwife for every 50 births. Approximately 80 percent of the midwives worked in hospitals, 12.2 percent (almost 3,000 midwives) attended home births—mostly in midwifery "clinics" within the midwife's home (Kondo, 1997). Some work in physician-operated "clinics" (essentially small private hospitals). The number of midwives had been declining due to retirement of a large group of aging midwives (Fukuzawa, 1984; Leppert, 1993), but has recently begun to rebound. But midwives continue to be in short supply, a problem that is receiving attention. Burnout contributes to the problem (Matsuoka *et al.*, 1996).

Chapter 14
The Current Situation and Recommendations for the Future

Chapter 13 describes midwifery and maternity care in some of our "peer" countries—those whose level of wealth, development and medical sophistication make them an appropriate comparison group for the United States. An American midwife cannot read that chapter without becoming jealous. Why are things so much better, not just for midwives, but, more importantly, for pregnant women in those countries? And how can we move maternity care in this country into a situation that is more like theirs? If we were to design the best maternity care for women in the United States, we would plan a system far different from what we have. But it does no good to design a better system starting with a blank piece of paper. We are where we are for many reasons, including the history of the development of midwifery, obstetrics, and family practice in the United States, the structure of our government and

health care system, and characteristics of our culture.

The purpose of this final chapter is to provide an analysis of our current situation, including a recap of the relevant history, because that is the necessary starting point for making plans to improve things. I have reached some conclusions, and I make some recommendations, but relatively few. America is a perplexing backwater in both midwifery and maternity care in general. Panels of experts have discussed the problems that account for this over many years. This book notes the recommendations of some of those panels, beginning with the 1925 White House Conference on Child Health. The most recent were recommendations made by the Institute of Medicine and the National Commission to Prevent Infant Mortality during the 1980s. During the 1990s several other groups made recommendations that call for adopting a midwifery model of care as the means to improve maternity services in the United States. Although I have added a little, my main objective in writing this book was not to make recommendations but to provide a clear description and understanding of the current situation. The situation existing in the United States near the end of the twentieth century contains both constraints and opportunities for improving the care and outcomes for pregnant women in this country.

The role of midwifery is growing in the United States, but it continues to be a niche filler, an alternative, a way to close gaps in the availability of care. If midwifery is to play its full role, to make its full contribution to the health and well-being of American women and their babies and families, it needs to move out of the alternative, niche-filler column and be recognized and actualized as an essential part of the system that provides maternity care. This chapter argues that this should happen. But, unlike the countries discussed in chapter 13, the United States does not have a national health care system. No single agency or organization is responsible for making and implementing a national health care plan. We are not like Great Britain, where the recommendations in *Changing Childbirth* are being applied throughout the nation. The American health care "system" is not a system at all, but a network of separate components and systems. The kind of care available to pregnant women in the United State is not determined by some small set of health care policymakers but arises from the decisions and choices of hundreds of thousands of parties—state and local government bureaucrats, officials, and legislators; professional associations and other nongovernmental organizations; individual hospitals, health care plans, insurance companies, medical staff committees; doctors, nurses, midwives, and, ultimately, consumers. Chapter 14 is addressed to members of this large and diverse group of health care policymakers.

The historical events and developments and most of the research findings and other evidence that support the statements made in this chapter are presented and documented in the other chapters. References that document the sources of information presented in other chapters are not repeated. References are provided for information that is not presented elsewhere in this book.

Two Ways of Viewing Pregnancy and Birth

The division of the care of pregnant women into two separate fields—eventually the professions of midwifery and medical obstetrics—began in ancient times and has continued into the present. Each of these disciplines is based on a different understanding of the nature and significance of pregnancy and childbirth. *Midwifery* is essentially female, developing out of the social, informational, physical, and material support women have traditionally provided to one another in time of need. Midwives view pregnancy as a critical, very important, vulnerable, but normal part of women's lives. *Obstetrics* developed to deal with the pathologies of pregnancy. Each of these perspectives calls forth a different approach to the care needed by pregnant women: the medical model and the midwifery model.

- As a specialty of medicine, the main focus of obstetrics is the diagnosis and treatment of pregnancy complications and the management of diseases affecting pregnant women and the fetuses they carry. This focus is vital because, although most pregnancies are normal, serious complications and diseases are not uncommon and can be deadly. However, physicians have expanded the proportion of pregnancies considered abnormal or pathologic by using monitoring devices that overdiagnose complications, by basing diagnoses on overly narrow definitions of normal, and by treating variation from those definitions as pathologic. The desire to identify complications early has led to the use of a sequence of preemptive interventions (to prevent complications or to treat them before there is evidence that they exist) and a focus on "risk factors" (conditions that are not pathologic but are associated with an increased incidence of complications). In many instances, the distinction between risk factors and actual pathology has been lost, and women with high-risk factors are treated as though they have actual complications. Prenatal care focuses on screening for abnormalities. Childbirth is closely monitored and controlled.

- Midwives believe that pregnancy and birth are fundamentally healthy processes, which have many normal variations. Midwives are experts in protecting, supporting, and enhancing normal pregnancy and childbirth. A large part of the midwife's attention and concern focuses on her client as a person, a unique individual, in the context of her family and her life. The midwife is interested in the woman's expectations and experience of her pregnancy—her perceptions and beliefs; her knowledge, opinions, questions, and worries; her feelings, satisfactions and dissatisfactions, comforts and discomforts; her desires, decisions, and actions; and the effect of all of these on her pregnancy, her fetus, her labor, delivery, breastfeeding, postpartum recovery, and her development as a mother. Midwives see the pregnant woman as an active partner in her own care. A large part of the midwife's role is to give her clients the information and support they need to make their own decisions.

- Both of these perspectives are valid and important; the extent to which one or the other should be given priority varies with different women. Conceptually the two fields are complementary rather than competitive. Throughout the world, but in the United States more than any other country, the inherent complementarily turned to competition when medicine usurped the midwifery role by medicalizing normal childbirth. This has resulted in a long-standing, ongoing conceptual competition between the midwifery and medical models of care for pregnant women.

The medical model gained the upper hand in the United States during the early part of this century. It has maintained its preeminence because women fear death or damage to themselves or their infants and believe that doctors know more than midwives and have more effective treatments and thus can save them and their babies from danger, and because doctors and hospitals promise relief from the pain of giving birth. When the transition from homes and midwives to hospitals and physicians began and achieved critical momentum, most doctors did not have superior knowledge about childbirth and had few effective treatments. As we learned later, most women and their babies were safer if they gave birth at home. "Twilight sleep" enticed women into hospitals before the invention of antibacterial agents, blood transfusions, and drugs to treat toxemia—the medical miracle treatments that did save women's lives. Eventually these highly effective treatments became widely available; as a result maternal mortality fell sharply after about 1935, adding real weight to the importance of medical care for pregnant women. But the damage caused by obstetric anesthesia was also becoming evident, especially the short-term effects of anesthesia on newborns, who entered the world limp and unresponsive to their need to breathe. Thus the mass movement of birth into hospitals and wide use of obstetric anesthesia elicited a counterforce—the natural childbirth movement, which began during the 1930s. Although lay women were major players in the development and effectiveness of this movement, physicians who had seen the danger of anesthesia also played a critical role.

Since then the two paradigms have vied with each other, competing for the scientific upper hand and the acceptance and loyalty of women. In actual practice, there has been some merging of the models. Everyone acknowledges the importance of medical treatment for women with pregnancy complications; the standards of the American College of Nurse-Midwives require all certified nurse-midwives (CNMs) to practice in settings that provide access to medical care. Similarly, most people now acknowledge the importance of the social and emotional aspects of pregnancy and childbirth to some extent; hospitals and physicians who at first resisted women's requests to have their husband or another support person with them during labor now "allow" it, and the practice is widespread. Thus instead of two distinct, mutually exclusive ways of managing birth, there is a wide continuum, with some examples of more extreme or pure renditions of each paradigm at the ends of the continuum, but most practices falling toward the middle. If childbirth practitioners were placed on this continuum and plotted on a frequency curve, the curve might be bimodal*—relatively few examples of the pure expression of each paradigm, most practices incorporating elements of both, and two distinct peaks in the curve, one reflecting practices that adhere more to the midwifery model and one reflecting practices that adhere more to the medical model.

The relative height of the peaks reflecting the central tendency of each model would be different in every country. In Holland, a large proportion of the births would cluster around the peak that reflects application of the midwifery model; the peak representing the medical model would be smaller. The opposite would be true in the United States. In addition, such curves—if the data existed and had been plotted periodically—would be seen to change over time. The factors that cause these changes—events and developments that give more weight to one paradigm or the other—include the concerns that caused women to leave their homes and go to hospitals for childbirth in the first place, especially fear of danger and the desire to avoid pain.

Favorable and Unfavorable Trends

Some things *are* changing in the United States, but the change is slow and minimal, and much of it is in the wrong direction. Here is the good news:

- Midwives are attending more births—5.5 percent in 1994, compared with 1.7 percent in 1980. Although the proportion more than tripled, midwives attend only slightly more than one of every twenty births. But this is a significant change, and it is continuing.
- The cesarean section rate has fallen every year since 1988, down from almost 25 percent since then, to slightly less than 21 percent in 1995.
- The use of forceps is declining, from 5.5 percent in 1989 to 3.8 percent in 1994.
- Women are now more likely to avoid an episiotomy.

Despite these improvements, there are many unfavorable trends:

- Labor was induced in 14.7 percent of births in 1994—up from 9.0 percent in 1989. Inductions are increasing by more than one percentage point per year; if this rate of increase continues, the induction rate will be more than 22 percent by the year 2000. Another 15.2 percent of women received oxytocin to strengthen and speed their labor after it had started spontaneously. As many as 30 percent of American women may be

---

*The "mode" is the most frequent value in a set of data. A bimodal frequency curve has two modes.

receiving oxytocin as part of their treatment during labor.

- More than 80 percent of women who gave birth in 1994 were attached to electronic fetal monitoring (EFM) equipment, up from 68 percent only five years earlier.

- The use of epidurals is not measured at the national level, but it is high and not decreasing. In some hospitals, virtually every woman has an epidural.

- The reduction in cesareans and forceps is nearly balanced by an increase in the use of vacuum extraction. Although this is a less invasive and risky procedure, it is evident that large numbers of American women—more than 30 percent altogether—are unable to give birth to their babies on their own. The rate of normal spontaneous births remains below 70 percent.

The other path seems so clearly better. Why is the United States so stuck in the medical model? The research and other data that have supported the changes in the other countries—evidence of high costs, little or no benefits, and damage, especially to women, from treating all births as though they were likely to result in problems—are available to doctors in this country. In fact, much of the research was done here. Why is our system so intractable?

Brief Recap of the Medicalization of Childbirth in the United States

The history of how the obstetric paradigm became predominant in this country is laid out in the historical chapters of this book. Events during the second decade of the twentieth century were especially important in setting American obstetrics on this course:

- In 1910 the Carnegie Foundation for the Advancement of Teaching published Abraham Flexner's critical report on medical education in North America. After visiting every medical school in the United States and Canada, Flexner concluded that America was oversupplied with badly trained doctors and recommended that most medical schools then in operation should be closed, that only the best should remain open, and that all schools that remained in operation should be strengthened based on the model provided by Johns Hopkins. Flexner singled out obstetrics as making "the very worst showing" (Flexner, 1910).

- In 1911 the leading professor of obstetrics at Johns Hopkins conducted his own study, which confirmed Flexner's findings. The obstetric professors who responded to Dr. Williams' survey believed that most women were safer with midwives than with general physicians. Dr. Williams's 1912 article in the *Journal of the American Medical Association* recommended better pay for doctors who practice obstetrics, hospitalization for all deliveries, and gradual abolition of midwives in large cities; the midwives should be replaced by "obstetrical charities," which would serve as sites for training physicians (Williams, 1912).

- In 1912 the federal government established the Children's Bureau to provide accurate information on the health of children, among other responsibilities. One of its first acts was collection of data which revealed that the U.S. infant mortality rate was higher than rates for the major countries of Europe. Midwives were widely assumed to be responsible for our poor standing.

- Twilight sleep was introduced into the United States (from Germany) in 1914. Upper-class women formed "twilight sleep" societies. Obstetric anesthesia became a symbol of the progress possible through medicine.

- In 1915 the Association for the Study and Prevention of Infant Mortality published a paper in which Dr. Joseph DeLee, author of the most important obstetric textbook of that time, described childbirth as a pathologic process. "Obstetrics has a great pathologic dignity—it is a major science of the same rank as surgery . . . even natural deliveries damage both mothers and babies, often and much. If childbearing is destructive, it is pathogenic, and if it is pathogenic it is pathologic. . . . If the profession would realize that parturition viewed with modern eyes is no longer a normal function, but that it has imposing pathologic dignity, the midwife would be impossible even of mention" (DeLee, 1915).

- In 1920 Dr. DeLee proposed a sequence of medical interventions designed to save women from the "evils" that are "natural to labor": Specialist obstetricians should sedate women at the onset of labor, allow the cervix to dilate, give ether during the second stage, cut an episiotomy, deliver the baby with forceps, extract the placenta, give medicine to help the uterus contract, and repair the episiotomy. DeLee changed the focus from responding to problems as they arise to preventing problems through routine application of interventions to control the course of labor. His article was published in the first issue of the *American Journal of Obstetrics and Gynecology* (DeLee, 1920).

All of the interventions DeLee prescribed did become routine: All but 8 percent of the white women and 26 percent of the black women included in a large nationwide study conducted between 1959 and 1965 were anesthetized when they gave birth; most of the white women's babies (57 percent) were delivered with forceps (National Institute of Neurological Disease and Stroke, 1972). Seventy percent of women who delivered babies in 1977 had episiotomies.

Interventions developed after DeLee's time have also been incorporated into the routine care of pregnant women. Continuous electronic fetal monitoring was introduced in 1960. Two studies demonstrating that EFM produces little or no benefit when used during low-risk births were published during the late 1970s; one of them showed a clear association between routine use of EFM and increasing use of cesarean sections (Neutra *et al.*, 1978; Haverkamp *et al.*, 1979). The association between EFM and cesarean deliveries is now well established. In 1988 the head of obstetrics at Harvard Medical School described EFM as a "failed technology" but predicted that it would be hard for obstetricians to stop using it in the absence of a substitute, in part because of their fear of being sued (Ryan, 1988). One of four babies born in America that year was delivered by cesarean section. Use of EFM increases yearly. Epidural anesthesia was developed to replace the sedation recommended by DeLee. It affects virtually all aspects of labor and delivery and, like EFM, increases the rate of cesarean sections.

The Effects and Effectiveness of High-Tech Childbirth Care

Other features of childbirth care in the United States include its high cost and a high rate of cesarean sections; both are corollaries of a maternity care model that has incorporated into routine care many procedures that were originally developed for managing complicated labors. The loss of normal childbirth is another corollary of this kind of care. People who have never experienced or seen a normal birth may not comprehend this loss, but it is a profound loss—to individuals and to our culture. Childbirth is a sexual function—part of the intricately designed and orchestrated, deeply organic system for conceiving, bearing, bringing forth, and nurturing human offspring. Like sex itself, it operates and involves and affects us on many levels. Like making love, it is physical—physiologic, but it is also more. It works best in an environment of intimacy, privacy, and expressiveness. It is vulnerable; there can be problems, sometimes it needs help. But most often it doesn't; it is a powerful force, with its own intelligence—an involuntary bodily process. In the words of Dr. Michael Odent, the French physician whose work is discussed in chapter 6, "One cannot help an involuntary process. The point is not to disturb it" (Odent, 1994). When we numb women, making them unable to stand, walk, and move naturally, destroying the organic unity of the mind, body, and spirit and overriding the body's inbred timing and control of labor, we dilute the natural power of normal birth. That results in unintended consequences. And that is only one level of our loss.

The purposes of this expensive, disruptive care are to prevent any damage to the baby during its journey into the world and to make labor less painful and stressful for the mother. These are excellent goals; the efforts are well intended. But they have had many unintended negative consequences. None of the procedures is without some kind of risk. Most were introduced into widespread practice prior to any research demonstrating that they were safe and effective when widely applied. When careful studies were conducted, some procedures that are still widely used were found to be not useful or even dangerous when used routinely. Babies can be and have been injured, although, more commonly, it is the mother.

The Scientific Evidence

In 1979 the former director of a prestigious epidemiology research unit in England identified obstetrics as the specialty with the worst record of basing its practice on sound research. This scolding stimulated an international effort to review and summarize findings from the best studies of the effectiveness of methods used to care for pregnant women and their newborns, resulting in publication of *Effective Care in Pregnancy and Childbirth*, a 1,500-page book that recorded this information, and a much smaller book, *A Guide to Effective Care in Pregnancy and Childbirth*, which presents conclusions from that review in a manner that is accessible to clinicians. Infor-

mation from the 1995 edition of *A Guide to Effective Care in Pregnancy and Childbirth* is used throughout this book.

Obstetrics' reputation for not basing its practice on scientific evidence flows in part from the fact that most pregnancies are normal. Common sense approaches were often used without scientific testing, since they did not seem equivalent to actual medical treatments. The history of problems resulting from this approach is very long. Near the beginning of the current century physicians at Harvard and Johns Hopkins published two papers, both of which concluded that cases of childbirth fever (the leading cause of maternal death at that time) could be reduced by shaving the area around the woman's vagina (the perineum). Shaving was quickly adopted as a standard of good obstetric care. It did not matter that another cause was known for the problem shaving was supposed to reduce.* It made sense to doctors, who were accustomed to shaving skin before surgery, that delivery would be cleaner without hair. The first controlled trial to measure the efficacy of perineal shaving, published in 1922, found that washing the pubic area with soap and water was as effective as shaving. That conclusion was corroborated with another controlled trial, conducted during the 1960s. By that time, however, episiotomies had become routine, and shaving makes it easier to repair (stitch) the episiotomy. However, both controlled trials found that shaving does not reduce infections. In fact, there is a tendency in the other direction—more infection among the women who were shaved, due to minor abrasions cause by shaving. Although most hospitals have

_____

*Work dating from the mid-1800s had shown that most cases of childbirth fever were due to a lack of thorough handwashing. Despite this knowledge, childbirth fever remained an important cause of maternal death in the United States. The belief that "dirty" midwives were responsible for most cases of childbirth fever (totally unfounded, when studied) contributed to the campaign to eliminate midwives during the early 1900s.

dropped the practice, some women are still shaved before delivery. As of 1993, 16 percent of Canadian hospitals still had policies stipulating that all women should have at least a partial shave before delivery (Levitt *et al.*, 1995). Small hospitals were more likely to have this policy than large hospitals, and this study was conducted in Canada, not the United States. Nevertheless, not shaving is counterintuitive to many physicians and nurses, and the practice has taken a very long time to die. Most women dislike being shaved, and some experience discomfort as the hair grows back (Enkin *et al.*, 1995).

The effort to collect and synthesize information from randomized controlled trials of perinatal care, which resulted in the books on effectiveness of care during pregnancy and childbirth, expanded into a broader effort known as the Cochrane Collaboration (named for the British epidemiologist whose statement about the poor research base for obstetric practice stimulated the work on perinatal care). It has led to increased emphasis on the importance of "evidence-based practice" in all areas of medicine. Based on this work, we can no longer say that a great deal of American obstetric practice goes forth without adequate research. It is now more accurate to say that many interventions are used routinely or frequently *in spite of* research that has clearly shown that the procedure is being used inappropriately in this country.

The last chapter of *A Guide to Effective Care in Pregnancy and Childbirth* places all forms of care that were examined during this extensive research review into six categories, based on the evidence from well-controlled comparison studies. The six categories range from (category 1) forms of care that are clearly beneficial to (category 6) forms of care that are clearly ineffective or harmful. The intermediate categories include forms of care that are likely to be beneficial or not, based on less than conclusive evidence (categories 2 and 5) and, in the middle, forms of care with a trade-off between beneficial and adverse

effects (category 3) and forms of care for which the effectiveness is unknown (category 4). Table 15 lists all items from those six categories that are forms of care applied to women having normal pregnancies and births. Forms of care used to treat or manage specific problems are not included.

Only nine items are included on the list of forms of care that are clearly beneficial. Only one—folic acid supplementation—is a medical intervention. Only two are care that is required during labor and delivery: emotional and psychological support and maternal mobility and choice of position. Neither of them is truly available to most women who deliver their babies in most hospitals in the United States. Most of the others relate to providing nonmedical aspects of support to women during prenatal care, especially for socioeconomically disadvantaged women, or providing conditions to help women breastfeed successfully.

The list of items in category 6 (forms of care that are likely to be ineffective or harmful) is much longer and includes some kinds of care that many American women are still being subjected to: routine enemas and shaving during labor, keeping women on their backs with their feet elevated during the second stage of labor, using episiotomies frequently or routinely, taking care of babies in central nurseries and giving them fluids to supplement their mother's breast milk. A substantial number of American mothers are subjected to many of these practices; yet each of these procedures has been found to be ineffective when used routinely, and many of them are associated with an increased risk of complications.

EFM is included on this list if it is used without the ability to do fetal scalp blood sampling. Fetal scalp blood sampling requires making a small incision in the baby's scalp to obtain a sample of blood and testing the blood for chemical changes that reflect the degree of oxygenation. The technique for obtaining the blood is cumbersome, time consuming, and difficult and uncomfortable for

Table 15:

Elements of the Care Provided to Low-Risk Pregnant Women Classified by the Evidence Regarding Their Effectiveness*

Category 1: Forms of Care That Are Clearly Beneficial

Folic acid supplementation (or high folate diet) for all women contemplating pregnancy.

Programs to help women stop smoking.

Giving women their own medical records to keep during pregnancy to enhance their feeling of being in control.

Supplementation of diet as necessary.

Emotional and psychological support during labor and delivery.

Maternal mobility and choice of position during labor.

Consistent support for breast-feeding mothers, including personal support from a knowledgeable person.

Unrestricted breast-feeding.

Support for socially disadvantaged mothers to improve child care.

Category 2: Forms of Care That Are Likely to Be Beneficial

Access to care for all childbearing women.

Social support for childbearing women.

Financial support for childbearing women in need.

Legislation on paid leave and income maintenance during maternity or parental leave.

Midwifery care for women with no serious risk factors.

Continuity of care for childbearing women.

Antenatal classes for women and their partners who want them.

Advice to avoid excessive alcohol consumption during pregnancy.

Avoidance of heavy physical work during pregnancy.

Regular monitoring of blood pressure, urine, and fetal growth during pregnancy.

Screening pregnant women for blood group isoimmunization, syphilis and Chlamydia (a kind of vaginal infection).

Respecting women's choice regarding place of birth and companions during labor and delivery.

Presence of a companion on admission to a hospital.

Giving women as much information as they desire.

Woman's choice of position for the second stage of labor and for giving birth.

A variety of methods to relieve pain in labor, for example, maternal movement, position changes, touch, massage, music.

Trial of labor after previous cesarean sections (if the previous scar is in the lower part of the uterus).

Keeping babies warm immediately after birth.

Giving the newborn vitamin K to prevent hemorrhagic disease.

Encouraging early mother-infant contact.

Encouraging breast-feeding as soon as the mother and baby are ready.

Providing skilled help with the first breast-feeding session.

Correct positioning of the baby at breast.

Allowing mothers access to their own supply of symptom-relieving drugs in the hospital.

Consistent advice to new mothers.

(continued)

*Adapted from Tables 1 through 6 in Enkin M, Meirse MJNC, Renfrew M, Neilson J, *A Guide to Effective Care in Pregnancy and Childbirth, Second Edition*, Oxford University Press, New York, 1995.

Table 15:
Elements of the Care Provided to Low-Risk Pregnant Women Classified by the Evidence Regarding Their Effectiveness *(Continued)*

Category 2: Forms of Care That Are Likely to Be Beneficial (Continued)

Allowing women to choose how long to stay in the hospital.

Telephone access to advice and information after women go home from the hospital.

Psychological support for women depressed after childbirth.

Flexibility in breast-feeding practices.

Category 3: Forms of Care With a Trade-off Between Beneficial and Adverse Effects

Legislation restricting type of employment for childbearing women.

Use of a formal risk-screening system.

Routine use of ultrasound during early pregnancy.

Certain kinds of tests to screen for congenital anomalies.

Asking all women to count fetal movements as a way to assess fetal well-being.

Screening for toxoplasmosis (a kind of infection).

Using EFM with fetal scalp blood sampling[†] instead of other ways to monitor the fetal heart rate.

Narcotics to relieve pain in labor.

Inhalation analgesia to relieve pain in labor.

Epidural analgesia to relieve pain in labor.

Early artificial rupture of the membranes in spontaneous labor.

Giving all women oxytocin to aid detachment and delivery of the placenta.

Applying antibiotic ointments to the eyes of all newborns.

Category 4: Forms of Care With Unknown Effectiveness

Formal "preconceptional care" to help nonpregnant women prepare for pregnancy.

Social support for women with characteristics associated with increased risk of preterm labor and birth.

Supplementing the woman's diet with fish oil, calcium, magnesium, or zinc.

Avoiding foods that cause allergies in some people.

Changing salt intake during pregnancy.

Routine use of ultrasonograms to assess the placenta during prenatal care.

Routine ultrasonograms plus electronic fetal monitoring to assess fetal well-being during pregnancy.

Routine cervical assessment or home uterine activity monitoring to prevent preterm birth.

A short period of electronic fetal monitoring when the woman is admitted to the labor unit.

Routine artificial rupture of the membranes during early labor to look for meconium.

Pressing on the unborn baby's head or pinching its scalp with a clamp to see if this stimulation results in an increase in the fetal heart rate (a sign of healthy reactivity).

Routine examination of the amniotic fluid by shining a light through the membranes covering the cervical opening as a means to look for meconium during early labor.

Routine repeated blood pressure measurements during labor.

Putting pressure on the perineum during childbirth as a way to prevent tears.

Clamping the cord earlier instead of later.

Pulling gently on the cord until the placenta is delivered.

Pain relief methods such as immersion in water, acupuncture, acupressure, and hypnosis.

Early use of oxytocin to augment slow or prolonged labor; "active management of labor."

Applying antiseptics to the cord routinely.   *(continued)*

---

†Fetal scalp blood sampling involves testing blood drawn from the baby's scalp veins for the level of oxygenation.

Table 15:
Elements of the Care Provided to Low-Risk Pregnant Women Classified by the Evidence Regarding Their Effectiveness (*Continued*)

Category 5: Forms of Care That Are Unlikely to Be Beneficial

Involving doctors in the care of all women during pregnancy and childbirth.

Involving obstetricians in the care of all women during pregnancy and childbirth.

Not involving obstetricians in the care of women with serious risk factors.

Fragmentation of care during pregnancy and childbirth (i.e., many people involved in the care, no continuity).

Advice to restrict sexual activity during pregnancy.

Prohibiting all use of alcohol during pregnancy.

Imposing dietary restrictions during pregnancy.

Routine vitamin and iron supplementation in well-nourished populations (except folic acid).

High-protein dietary supplementation.

Routine use of ultrasound to estimate fetal size late in pregnancy.

Using edema (visible fluid retention) to screen for pre-eclampsia.

Use of several tests to screen for pre-eclampsia (for example, the "roll-over" test).

Screening for "gestational diabetes."

Blood glucose measurement and glucose challenge testing as part of routine prenatal care.

Urine tests to measure placental proteins or hormones.

Routine screening and treatment for certain kinds of vaginal infections in pregnant women without symptoms.

Not allowing women to eat and/or drink during labor.

Giving routine intravenous infusions of fluid during labor.

Using face masks during vaginal examinations.

Frequent vaginal examinations performed at regular intervals.

Several forms of pain relief during labor, for example, biofeedback, sedatives, and tranquillizers.

Telling women when and how to push, breathe, and bear down during the second phase of labor.

Arbitrary limitation of the duration of the second stage of labor—i.e., by attempting to deliver the baby faster.

Massaging the perineum during the second stage of labor.

Routine manual examination of the uterus after delivery to make sure that no fragments of the placenta remain.

Applying silver nitrate to the baby's eyes to prevent infection.

Suctioning all babies routinely.

Giving the baby a medicated bath to reduce infection.

Wearing hospital gowns in newborn nurseries.

Not allowing the newborn's siblings to visit for fear of infecting the baby.

Routine measurement of the mother's temperature, pulse, blood pressure, and uterine size during the postpartum hospitalization.

Not allowing women to use their own nonprescription, symptom-relieving drugs while in the hospital.

Administering nonprescription, symptom relieving drugs at set intervals.

Having breast-feeding mothers use nipple shields.

Switching the baby from one breast to the other before the baby terminates nursing at the first breast.

(continued)

Table 15:
Elements of the Care Provided to Low-Risk Pregnant Women Classified by the Evidence Regarding Their Effectiveness (Continued)

Category 6: Forms of Care That Are Likely to Be Ineffective or Harmful

Restricting women's diets in the hope of preventing pre-eclampsia.

Teaching pregnant women to do anything to prepare their breasts and nipples for breast-feeding.

EFM (with or without stimulating contractions) as a screening measure during prenatal care.

Routine use of enemas during labor.

Routine shaving of the pubic area prior to delivery.

Using EFM without access to fetal scalp blood sampling during labor.

Using rectal examinations to assess the progress of labor.

Requiring women to lie flat on their backs during the second stage of labor.

Putting women's feet up in stirrups for delivery.

Using episiotomies routinely or frequently.

Using ergometrine instead of oxytocin to stimulate uterine contractions after the baby is born but before the placenta has delivered.

Restricting contact between the mother and her newborn.

Taking care of babies in central nurseries.

Limiting the amount of time the baby can nurse.

Having mothers apply creams or ointments to their nipples.

Giving water or formula by bottle to breast-feeding babies (to supplement the mother's milk).

Giving mothers samples of baby formula to take home.

Encouraging breast-feeding women to drink even when they are not thirsty.

Use of oral contraceptive pills by women who are breastfeeding.

Weighing breast-fed babies before and after feeding to measure intake of breast milk.

---

the woman (Enkin *et al.*, 1995). Use of EFM without the ability to do fetal scalp blood sampling results in overdiagnosis of fetal distress, which results in unnecessary interventions, including cesarean sections. Use of EFM in hospitals that have the ability to do fetal scalp blood sampling is a form of care that brings both benefits and adverse effects (category 3). However, even when EFM is used with fetal scalp blood sampling, the results are no better than when a midwife listens to the fetal heart at regular intervals with an instrument that is placed on the woman's abdomen temporarily—as compared with internal EFM, which requires that equipment be pushed up into the uterus and screwed into or pinched onto the baby's head. Despite clear evidence that EFM is no better than noninvasive methods and that its use without fetal scalp blood sampling, which is painful and expensive, results in unnecessary cesarean sections, 80 percent of women who gave birth in the United States in 1994 had EFM.

In an effort to improve pregnancy outcomes, American obstetrics has wielded an armamentarium for controlling labor and delivery. The weapons have captured the wrong enemy. Problems during childbirth are not the cause of our high rate of infant mortality.* Preterm labor and retarded fetal growth—the causes of low birth weight and our high infant mortality rate—are unaffected by the high-tech childbirth care on which we spend most of our time, attention, and money. Greater, more intensive surveillance and control of labor is not what is needed to improve the health of America's mothers and babies. In addition,

---

*This statement should not be taken as a dismissal of the dangers of childbirth, which are real to both babies and mothers. The obstetric procedures that are used excessively in the United States and have been widely called into question represent a level of surveillance and intervention that exceeds the elements of necessary care.

it causes problems. Normal childbirth is not a wayward force; it does not need to be controlled.

Brief Recap of the Development of Midwifery in the United States

The history of midwifery in the United States is very different from the way it developed in other countries. Midwifery developed along with medicine in the British Isles and Europe, and both professions developed earlier there than here. Effective laws and government-supported schools integrated midwifery into the overall health care systems of most European countries relatively early. When medicine began to develop educationally and as a profession in the United States, there was no parallel elevation of midwifery, which was practiced exclusively by women. Except for recent immigrants, many of whom could not speak English, few American midwives had any formal midwifery training. Most did not start to deliver babies until they were middle aged, worked out of their homes, and did not think of themselves as members of a profession.

When America's high infant mortality rate was discovered, it was easy to blame the midwives. Yet, analysis of data in preparation for the 1925 White House Conference on Child Health and Protection led to the conclusion that "untrained midwives approach, and trained midwives surpass, the record of physicians in normal deliveries." The conference report ascribed this record to the physicians' overuse of "procedures which are calculated to hasten delivery, but which sometimes result harmfully to mother and child," while midwives wait patiently and let nature take its course. (White House Conference on Child Health and Protection, 1932).

Various approaches were proposed to reduce the nation's high rates of both maternal and infant mortality; most of the proposals had to do with midwives. Private practitioners and academic obstetricians wanted midwives to be eliminated as soon as possible and controlled by doctors in the meantime. Public health leaders, and some physicians in the South, doubted the feasibility of providing medical care to all pregnant women and proposed programs to train and supervise midwives, who would be expected to refer complicated cases to physicians. Federal legislation passed in 1921 provided funds to help states improve their own maternal and child health services. Midwifery training programs developed with funds from the Sheppard–Towner Maternity and Infancy Protection Act improved pregnancy outcomes in New York City, Newark, Philadelphia, and certain other cities. The American Medical Association lobbied against the Sheppard–Towner act, and Congress allowed it to expire in 1929. Similar scenarios were played out at the local level. Those who supported training of midwives lost the battle; those who wanted to eliminate midwives accomplished their purpose. Midwives attended one-half of all births in the United States during 1900. By 1935, the proportion had dropped to one-eighth. Women wanted anesthesia and presumed the advantages of modern medicine. As society accepted the medical paradigm of childbirth, midwifery was stigmatized as poor quality care that was used only by women who had no other choice. This assumption was never entirely true, but it fit and reinforced the dominant paradigm.

As midwifery declined, the incidence of infant deaths from birth injuries increased. Infant mortality due to birth injuries increased by 44 percent in the United States between 1918 and 1925; researchers attributed the increase to an "orgy" of obstetrical interference in birth (Devitt, 1979; Loudon, 1992).

Maternal mortality began a steep decline during the mid-1930s coincident with the availability of sulfa drugs, antibiotics, blood transfusions, and medicines to treat pregnancy-induced hypertension. Careful analysis of maternal mortality in many countries between 1800 and 1950 led to the conclusion that there are two kinds of obstetric care that result in high maternal risk: One kind of poor care is provided by untrained midwives who are ignorant of basic procedures, the other is provided by overzealous or poorly trained doctors who interfere in childbirth in dangerous ways. Sound practice by well-trained midwives was found to result in low maternal mortality rates even in populations that were socially and economically deprived.

Nurse-midwifery was introduced as a means to provide care to women who lacked access to physicians. For the first fifty years after its introduction in 1925, nurse-midwifery grew and developed in the maternity care gaps left by medicine: care of poor whites in rural Appalachia; care of poor blacks in Harlem and Alabama; care of poor Mexican-Americans in New Mexico. Nurse-midwives did only home births until the mid-1950s, when they were needed to help obstetricians cope with the post-war baby boom in some large, inner-city public hospitals. They were needed because the maternity units were overwhelmed by the large number of women, and they were needed to improve the quality of the care. Obstetric leaders speaking at a 1968 conference on midwifery described the "shameful and humiliating circumstances" experienced by poor, black women who sought care in "our great public hospital clinics" and "conditions and attitudes of callousness" at Harlem Hospital that "almost defy description." (Silver, 1968; Barnes, 1968). Obstetricians who had worked with nurse-midwives described the interest, competence, and dedication they brought to their work and the need to introduce those attitudes into charity-hospital obstetric services in order to "produce a more humanitarian quality of service" (Swartz, 1968). Yet all agreed that nurse-midwives should be restricted to caring for the poor: "Without careful and effective preventive measures, we may be faced with a new profession in private entrepreneurial practice, a development which must be avoided at all costs" (Silver, 1968).

Nurse-midwives did not complain, because most of them had become midwives for the purpose of improving the care and experience of pregnant women who were poor. Many early nurse-midwives were Catholic nuns, or the Protestant equivalent, or came from public health nursing. They knew the problems of poor mothers and babies, developed nurse-midwifery as a means to address those problems, and based it on the British model. Based on their backgrounds, their model, and their goal of serving women who had little money and many health problems, they needed an institutional base and the involvement and support of physicians. Nurse-midwives did not venture from care of the poor—because their hands were full with the needs of the women they were serving and because they could not do so and retain their institutional and medical support. Although highly respected by those who knew it, nurse-midwifery reinforced the concept of midwifery as an alternative for women who cannot afford a doctor.

Lay midwives were opposite from this in virtually every way. They arose from a free-spirited, antiauthoritarian, antibureaucratic movement—young, middle-class college students and graduates with the nerve and verve to buck the medical paradigm. They initially took care mainly of women like themselves. They did not need or want institutional support. Some acquired training and backup from individual physicians, but those who did not were willing to work without it. They were of great interest and very attractive to the women's movement and the press, and some were eloquent writers. They exploded the concept of midwifery as care only for the poor, and they were reviled by obstetric leaders. Their greatest supporters were their clients, with whom they developed a pure and compelling form of midwifery. They have made important contributions to midwifery in this country and have provided a model and inspiration for "radical" and "independent" midwives in other countries. Thus they have played an important role in the international renaissance of midwifery. Yet most have had no formal midwifery training, and they remain in noninstitutional, out-of-hospital practice. Out-of-hospital births peaked at 1.5 percent of all births in 1977 and have since fallen back to a very stable 1 percent.

The role of nurse-midwives has both broadened and increased. The lay midwives' example encouraged them into the private sector (shortly before it began to collapse into managed care), and CNMs now serve women in all strata of society. However, they continue to play a particularly important role in care of women who are poor and socially disadvantaged. They have also been attractive to health maintenance organizations. Nurse-midwives now attend one of every twenty births (1994) and provide a wide range of other kinds of women's health care. The number and percent of all U.S. births attended by CNMs increased each year between 1989 (the first year for which this information is available) and 1994 (the most recent year for which data are available).

There was a sharp increase in the demand for nurse-midwives during the 1980s, as health care costs sky rocketed and access to care for uninsured women increased. The major constraint to their role was the slow and limited production of midwives. Several prestigious health policy advisory groups called for greater use of midwives to help meet the needs of socioeconomically high-risk women, and actions were taken to increase the nation's capacity to educate midwives.

Access to midwifery care is increasing. Because of their impressive record, cost advantages, consumer demand, and the increased production of nurse-midwives, midwivery is being incorporated into more parts of the mainstream, regular health care system. Direct-entry midwives are gaining increasing access to third-party payment and medical backup in states with progressive laws, for example, Washington, which requires all health insurers and health maintenance organiza-

tions (HMOs) to provide access to all categories of health care providers who are licensed or certified by the state. Licensed direct-entry midwives are placed in a separate category from CNMs in Washington; as a result, all health insurers and HMOs, must include some licensed midwives in the panels of health care professionals available to their subscribers.*

Benefits of the Midwifery Model

During the "midwifery debate" (from about 1910 to 1935) several concerns were raised about what might happen if midwives were replaced by obstetricians. It was predicted that the high fees charged by physicians would make it financially impossible to replace midwives with maternity services provided through charity hospitals. There was concern that investing resources in obstetrics instead of midwifery would result in lack of access to care in rural areas, because obstetricians tend to move to cities. There was concern about harmful results from overuse of obstetric interventions.

Eventually all of these concerns became manifest as problems. The reemergence of midwifery, both nurse-midwifery and lay and direct-entry midwifery, has contributed to solving those problems, although its contribution has been limited by the relatively small number and role of midwives in this country.

- Both kinds of midwives take care of women who would otherwise lack access to care, including women who live in rural areas, women whose religious beliefs do not allow them to use mainstream physicians and health care facilities, and women with limited financial resources and no form of health care insurance.

---

*A federal district court decision released in May 1997 overturned this law on the basis that it preempts a federal law that governs benefit plans employers provide to workers.

- Nurse-midwives make a special contribution by providing more attractive, effective care to socially marginalized women who are dependent on publicly financed care, especially pregnant teenagers and women whose stressful, sometimes chaotic lives and unhealthful habits and practices may compromise their pregnancies. Nurse-midwifery care may contribute to better birth weights among babies born to some of these women.
- Midwifery care helps to reduce the cost of providing care to pregnant women, deriving savings for public institutions responsible for providing care to the poor, HMOs, and the families of women who pay for their own care.
- Midwifery care is associated with reduced use of cesarean sections and reduced maternal morbidity from complications of obstetric interventions (such as episiotomies).

Midwives have not had a regular place in the American health care system, but have filled gaps and created niches based on their ability to meet specific needs. In the process they built a significant record of providing safe, effective care, improving the quality of care provided to indigent women, and achieving high levels of patient/client satisfaction and appreciation. In addition, midwives have demonstrated a different approach to the care of pregnant women—a different paradigm, introducing new methods and ideas that have had an impact on other maternity care providers and thus have improved care throughout the system.

The personal, supportive, respectful care provided by midwives is very attractive to women. Studies that have examined satisfaction with maternity care consistently find that, although most women are generally satisfied with the care they receive, the level of satisfaction is significantly higher among women who receive their care from midwives. Women who have had one birth with a midwife nearly always go to a midwife for any future births; some women overcome many barriers to obtain midwifery care in communities where it is hard to come by; word of mouth is the basis for the success of midwives in private practice. Nevertheless, most American women who choose midwifery care do not opt for the purest model, that is, home births, instead they choose a midwife or midwifery service that attends births in a hospital, where there is medical backup in case of an emergency and the potential availability of analgesia and anesthesia. Studies that compare nurse-midwifery care provided in American hospitals with the care provided to low-risk women by physicians in the same hospitals consistently find much less use of drugs and invasive procedures by the CNMs—usually about one-third to one-half of the use of those drugs and procedures by obstetricians in the same hospital. But most nurse-midwives do use the drugs and procedures "as needed". They differ from the physicians in how frequently they believe these methods are needed.*

Dominance of the Medical Model

Although many beliefs and values support the midwifery paradigm, the concerns that support the medical model have been, in general, more powerful. Cultural factors, practical implications flowing from the structure of the health care system, and financial considerations also play important roles in determining what kind of care American women receive during pregnancy, labor, and delivery.

Cultural Considerations

Many women want to have a full, rich childbirth experience and are fascinated and moved by stories and pictures of women having peaceful, obviously deeply satisfying, completely natural births. Yet few American women believe they can do this themselves.

---

*See table 10 in Chapter 10.

One explanation is that we have lost the cultural knowledge of the normalcy of birth. When most women gave birth at home, few women arrived at their own first labor without having sat with another woman giving birth. This experience supported a cultural belief that birth is normal and that women can and do go through it in ways that are positive, strong, and joyful. This experience has been lost, replaced by the usual television and movie depiction of childbirth as a clamorous emergency in which someone other than the mother, usually a physician, comes through as a hero. The cesarean section rate has been between 20 and 25 percent since 1983. One of every four or five American women who gave birth during the past dozen years did so by means of major abdominal surgery. The cesarean section rate is highest among well-educated, higher-income white women—the trendsetters of society. Expert opinion to the contrary, most of them are sure that *their* cesarean section was essential and saved their babies' lives. Few women facing birth today do not have a relative or friend who has had an emergency cesarean delivery. With no experience of normal childbirth and common, widespread evidence of the frailty and failures of childbirth, it is not surprising that women lack self-confidence.

Chapter 5 cites the findings of several researchers who have tried to understand why American women seem so willing to give control of their births to doctors and medical technology. Robbie Davis-Floyd, an anthropologist, puts the onus on our culture, which she characterizes as a *technocracy*, a society organized around an ideology of technological progress (Davis-Floyd, 1994). An important part of the United States' charisma is its association with technological progress. The desire to be modern and scientific primed American women to accept the medical paradigm of pregnancy and childbirth in the first place, early in this century. We have only recently become a little skeptical of the automatic pairing of the words "technological"

and "advances." "Scientific knowledge" is assumed to be more valid and important than other kinds of knowing, understanding, and wisdom. Technological methods are assumed to be more effective. Although other industrialized countries share these values, most new technologies come here first and fastest. The United States is accustomed to being at the cutting edge of developing and using technology to improve human life and solve problems. Medically controlled childbirth is consistent with our optimistic view of the potential of technology.

Davis-Floyd raised another issue when she described women she had interviewed who see pregnancy as something to be overcome, resent its potential to disrupt their lives, and do not want to "drop down" into their female biology (Davis-Floyd, 1994). The midwifery model encourages women to "get into" being pregnant, to enjoy it, be proud of it, and learn and grow from the experience. Although her heart is clearly with this model, Davis-Floyd interviewed women who want the "mind–body separation" epidurals provide and may "prefer the orderliness and controllability of cesarean over the uncontrollable and chaotic biological process of birth" (Davis-Floyd, 1994). Surely there is a continuum with—at the extremes, some women who revel in the sexuality of pregnancy and childbirth, and some who would prefer to be unconscious.

Ignorance and Confusion About Midwifery

But if this range of preferences exists among women in America, it must exist in every country. So why are we so different? A big part of it is simple ignorance about midwifery. Widespread ignorance and confusion about midwifery are the legacy of the history of midwifery in this country. Midwifery had a widely acknowledged, unquestioned place in Europe and Great Britain over a long period during which it was defamed and nearly extinguished in the United States. Nurse-midwifery made a comeback from that history through care of women who were poor and lacked access to physicians. If Americans know anything about our health care system, it is that we do not provide the best only to the poor. (Because of the use of charity hospitals for teaching physicians, the care offered to some poor people is superior in some ways to average private care. Nevertheless, there is a deep assumption that any model of care developed specifically to serve the poor could not be first class.) The other common perception of a midwife is of an uneducated "lay" midwife who attends home births.

The facts deny these assumptions: Both kinds of midwives now serve a wide spectrum of women; poor, disadvantaged women *and* well-educated professional women are both more likely than other women to receive care from a midwife. Ninety-five percent of births attended by midwives in the United States are attended by CNMs, 70 percent of whom have master's degrees, many from the country's leading universities. Standards for the education and certification of direct-entry midwives have been developed. Ninety percent of births attended by midwives occur in hospitals. A large proportion of Americans have no realistic idea of the education and role of midwives in the United States. That ignorance was the major reason the Carnegie Foundation initiated the writing of this book.

There are two tiers of books on pregnancy and pregnancy care at Powell's Books, in Portland, Oregon. New and used books are filed together; there are more than 450 separate titles on this subject. Two were written by CNMs, nine by direct-entry midwives. Many of the others do not mention midwives at all; of those that do, only a few are at all accurate in their depiction of midwifery. If midwives are included in pictures, it is often a picture from the Frontier Nursing Service, circa 1930, or a picture of a midwife attending a home birth. Home births are exquisite and wonderfully picturesque, but they are not the whole story of midwifery in this country.

Differences between nurse-midwives and direct-entry midwives add to the confusion.

Canada is the only other country that has had recent experience with midwives who practice without licensure or formally recognized midwifery training. Having two very different kinds of midwives and midwifery practice causes enormous confusion. It is not legal for direct-entry midwives to practice in some states. Some practice anyway, and some states have had a string of well-publicized arrests of midwives. A mile away, CNMs may be practicing in the state's most prestigious academic medical center. If they are taking care of women who are poor, their presence may be unknown to most people. Some states license two kinds of midwives, each with different educational and practice standards and different scopes of practice. New York is the only state that is attempting to apply the same standards to both nurse-midwives and direct-entry midwives. All other states that regulate both kinds of midwives do so under different laws. The standards for nurse-midwives and licensed direct-entry midwives are widely disparate in most states. For example, it is illegal for a CNM to practice as a nurse-midwife in Oregon unless she has a master's degree in nursing. There are no educational requirements for licensure as a direct-entry midwife in Oregon; a test must be passed, but there are no required years of training, no need to complete a recognized course, no necessary degrees. And being licensed is not necessary. One can practice, advertise, and be listed as a midwife in the *Yellow Pages* without a license. This is a recipe for confusion.

Nevertheless, midwifery is no longer new and known by very few women, and it is no longer only for the poor and the hippies. Women throughout society have experienced midwifery care—more and more women, a critical mass of women and their families.

Most physicians have had many more years of education than most midwives. Very little of that education focused on the needs and care of women having normal pregnancies. It is hard—counterintuitive—for people to understand that their additional education does not mean superior knowledge in the care of pregnant women who are not sick. The bodies of knowledge that underlie midwifery and obstetrics overlap, but they are unique bodies of knowledge. Most people assume that obstetrics encompasses midwifery, so that an obstetrician has all of the knowledge of a midwife and more. That is not the case.

Fear of Danger

The subject of ignorance and assumptions brings us to the fear of danger as a major bulwark of the medical model. The fear of danger rests on assumptions based on both truth and ignorance: Obstetricians are the experts on the complications and diseases of pregnancy and childbirth; their knowledge and skills assure the best possible outcome when pregnancy is complicated by pathology. Although most pregnancies are normal, a small proportion seem normal until a complication appears without warning; then, if you are with a midwife and not a doctor, it may be too late to obtain the necessary medical care in time. These statements have the great misleading power of truth when it is only part of the story. Other essential parts of the truth summarized here, are laid out in chapters 10 and 11:

- Midwives understand their role and the need for obstetric and pediatric expertise and care when there are serious complications. Midwifery education and training include a strong focus on the limitations of the midwife's scope of practice, early identification of complications, bringing medical expertise into the care of women and newborns who are at high-risk of serious complications in time for them to obtain the full benefit of medical care, and short-term management of unpredictable medical emergencies.
- Extensive research, conducted in this country and others, has found excellent outcomes of pregnancies when a midwife had primary responsibility for the woman's care. There is no longer any

valid scientific question about the safety of the care provided by professional midwives when the births occur in hospitals in which medical assistance is readily available.

- Although there has been much controversy about the safety of births attended by midwives (or physicians) in out-of-hospital locations, there is substantial evidence that births in homes and free-standing birth centers can be as safe as hospital births when a system of quality assurance is in place. One-third of all births in the Netherlands are home births attended by midwives. The Netherlands has long had one of the lowest rates of infant mortality in the world. A careful study of nearly twelve thousand births initiated in free-standing birth centers in the United States found a very low incidence of poor outcomes—mortality rates as low as those associated with low-risk births in America's leading academic hospitals (lower than mortality resulting from low-risk births in many American hospitals). Some babies and women die for lack of immediate access to interventions that are available only in a hospital. However, the opposite is also true: Some babies and women die because of overuse of interventions that are applied too frequently in hospitals.
- The education and training of obstetricians focuses on pathology, with little emphasis on the knowledge and skills required to protect and support the normalcy of childbirth. The tendency of many obstetricians to treat most or all pregnant women as though they were likely to develop a serious complication introduces iatrogenic risks associated with the overuse of procedures that cause complications themselves or as a result of interference in the normal progress of labor.

The more we study labor and birth, the more we realize the intricacy of the natural processes and the dangers and side effects of all efforts to change and control it. The authority of the medical approach to pregnancy and childbirth has been dealt a deep blow by the constantly mounting evidence of unproductive costs, lack of benefits, and harm associated with overuse of obstetric interventions. Based on their comprehensive review and synthesis of findings from studies conducted throughout the world, the authors of *A Guide to Effective Care in Pregnancy and Childbirth* caution that "It is inherently unwise, and perhaps unsafe, for women with normal pregnancies to be cared for by obstetric specialists even if the required personnel are available" (Enkin *et al.*, 1995).

Obstetrician–Gynecologists as Primary-Care Physicians

The United States has differed from our "peer countries" in having a laissez-faire health care system with no superimposed logic or strategy. Individuals have been free to shop for health care in the same way that they shop for other commodities, with the government providing a "safety net" (with holes in it) for people who can not afford market prices. Market forces and professional opinion are the dynamics that were supposed to regulate the system. As a result of this approach, we have too many specialists and not enough primary-care physicians. Many people have never had a regular physician who has gotten to know them and their problems over a period of time, and many people have not had the benefit of primary care that emphasizes health promotion and disease prevention as well as the management of common health problems. As a result, people end up needing expensive emergency care for acute health problems that should have been prevented.

Managed-care is supposed to deliver us from these short-comings of the laissez-faire system. Managed care is based on the concept that every person should have an ongoing relationship with a primary-care provider, usually a physician, who will provide most of his or her care and refer the individual to a specialist as needed. A few people might have a specialist as their primary physician. For instance, a person with a serious chronic liver disease might have a continuing relationship with a gastroenterologist. However, except for people with serious chronic medical conditions, people who receive care from specialists are expected to maintain a relationship with a primary-care provider. A person who is referred to a specialist for diagnosis and treatment of a nonchronic condition should be referred back to the primary-care physician when the specialist's services are no longer needed. This is the way it works in Europe and the United Kingdom. Under this scenario, women of reproductive age have an ongoing patient relationship with a general practitioner. When they become pregnant, the general physician may take care of them (in a few countries) or they may be referred to a midwife (in most countries) or an obstetrician (in very few countries, e.g., Germany, where obstetricians provide most of the prenatal care). At the end of the maternity cycle (four to six weeks after the birth), they return to the general physician.

Primary care has gained center stage because of managed care. Primary-care providers are supposed to provide most of the care to most of the people enrolled in managed care organizations and are the "gatekeepers" to the care of specialists. Which groups of health professionals are classified as primary-care providers has become a very big deal. There is wide agreement that general practitioners (physicians with no specialty training—a dying breed), family physicians, internists, and pediatricians are primary-care physicians. Pediatricians and internists who are qualified in subspecialties, for example, a pediatric oncologist or a gastroenterologist, are classified as specialists. Nurse-midwives, physician assistants, and nurse-practitioners also function as primary-care providers in some systems. There is an ongoing argument about whether obstetrician–gynecologists (ob-gyns) are primary-care physicians or specialists. Or whether, like pediatricians and internists, some are primary-care physicians and some are specialists. And whether individual ob-gyns can function in both roles. If obstetricians are primary-care physicians, they are the only ones in that category who are fully qualified as surgeons.

Chapter 5 includes a brief description of a 1991 conference on how ob-gyns can best meet society's needs during the twenty-first century. The conference was convened by the Josiah Macy, Jr., Foundation, which has had a long-term interest in improving women's health and health care. Thirty of the forty three conference participants were ob-gyns. The others included scientists from various research institutes, representatives of several women's health organizations, the former chairman of the nation's leading academic department of family medicine, a lawyer, the executive director of the organization responsible for accrediting health care organizations, and the president of the American College of Nurse-Midwives. The conference focused on the usual problems (inadequate access to care for poor women, women of color, and undocumented aliens; inadequate quality of the care provided to many poor women and women of color; overuse of technology), but also focused on the role of nurse-midwives, whether or not ob-gyns should function as primary-care providers, opportunities created by the increasing numbers of women ob-gyns, ethics, and quality assurance (Milliken, 1993).

Dr. Warren Pearse, then the executive director of the American College of Obstetricians and Gynecologists (ACOG), presented information on the current and expected future need for women's health care services and the numbers and capacity for training ob-gyns, CNMs, and family physicians to meet those needs. At the time of the conference (1991) the nation was experiencing a "maternity care crisis." Dr. Pearse's data showed that many obstetricians were retiring early and others had stopped delivering babies; the

number of physicians entering family practice was low, and the proportion of family physicians providing maternity care was declining; there were relatively few nurse-midwives, and the annual production of new nurse-midwives was low and stagnant. Meeting the projected needs for care would require the participation of all of these categories of care providers—*and* a 10 percent increase in the number of positions in obstetrics and gynecology residency training programs. However, he believed that major changes in the numbers and mix of professionals providing women's health care were unlikely and argued that the system needed "fine tuning," not a revolution. He recommended that all three kinds of personnel should be trained together, should practice in collaborative relationships wherever possible, and that ob-gyns should be the "gatekeepers" of the system (Pearse, 1993).

Dr. Joyce Thompson, then president of the American College of Nurse-Midwives, said that ACOG's projections on the future numbers of nurse-midwives were too low and disagreed with Dr. Pearse's conclusion that fine-tuning is all that is needed. She said that a revolution is needed to improve the care provided to women and presented a model of women's health care that gives women control of their own health by educating them in self-care and health promotion. The education and training of nurses prepares them to provide this kind of care. Physicians are educated to provide *medical* care and treat illnesses, whereas nurses and nurse-midwives are educated to provide *health* care. Each should focus on what they have been prepared to do. She said it is not practical to use specialist physicians to provide primary care for women, most of whom are not ill, and predicted that fewer physicians and more nurse-midwives will be needed in the future (Milliken, 1993).

Most of the conferees agreed that a significant amount of the training of ob-gyns is oriented toward surgery and that they were not being trained as primary-care providers.

In the end, the conference recommended that ob-gyns be regarded as specialists, but the recommendation left an opening for their role in primary care: "Although primary care is not implicit in this professional definition, in given practice settings the obstetrician/gynecologist may choose to take responsibility for a woman's primary care." However, because "expensively trained specialists are not best used to provide primary care, the specialty should not formally incorporate primary care into its training" (Milliken, 1993). ACOG disagrees. As early as 1979, ACOG began to make policy statements that define ob-gyns as primary-care physicians (Hale, 1994; ACOG, 1994). Since then, the College has required ob-gyn residency training programs to include more emphasis and clinical experience in primary care, including the care of postmenopausal ("aging") women. Nevertheless, a 1994 analysis of the training required by primary-care physicians concluded that ob-gyns are less prepared in primary care than pediatricians, internists, and family physicians (Rivo *et al.*, 1994).

Actually, there are several aspects to the issue—whether ob-gyns *are* primary-care providers and whether they *should be* primary-care providers *for women having normal pregnancies, for nonpregnant women of reproductive age*, and *for women who are beyond childbearing age*. There is a clear answer to two parts of that question: Obstetricians *are* an important source of primary care for both pregnant and nonpregnant women of reproductive age in the United States. A study conducted during 1993 found that 16 percent of women were using an ob-gyn as their only regular physician and 33 percent had ongoing patient relationships with both an ob-gyn and either a family practitioner or an internist (Commonwealth Fund, 1996). Nearly half of the women were seeing ob-gyns on a regular basis. Obstetrician-gynecologists may not be adequately trained for this role, but they are improving their training programs.

Nevertheless, ob-gyns tend to limit their care to obstetric and gynecologic problems; family physicians and general internists provide the majority of outpatient care to women of reproductive age (Rosenblatt *et al.*, 1995). Family physicians provided 32 percent of all nonreferred outpatient care to women between the ages of 17 and 44 in 1989–1990. Ob-gyns provided 29 percent of this care, mainly in the form of prenatal visits and visits related to menstrual disorders and genital tract infections. However, they also provided slightly more than half of the visits that included a general medical exam. Women in this age group saw general internists for 9 percent of their outpatient visits, and saw a variety of specialists other than obstetrician-gynecologists for 30 of their outpatient visits, primarily visits to psychiatrists, orthopedic surgeons, urologists, dermatologists, and otolaryngologists.

Whether obstetrician–gynecologists *should* function as primary-care physicians is a separate question, and the answer is not clear. Much of the health care needed by women between the ages of about fifteen and fifty-five is in the reproductive-health arena—care related to preventing or facilitating conception, pregnancy, genital infections, screening for cancer of the reproductive organs (including the breasts), diagnosing and treating other pathologies of the genital tract (vagina, uterus, and ovaries), counseling for sexual dysfunctions, and providing hormone replacement to perimenopausal women. However, these are not the only health problems experienced by women of reproductive age. Of all women between the ages of fifteen and forty-four who lived in Boston and died during the 1980s, less than 3 percent died because of pregnancies or genital cancers (Katz *et al.*, 1995). Breast cancer, leukemia, motor vehicle accidents, other accidents, heart disease, homicide, suicide, liver disease, pneumonia and influenza, cerebrovascular disease, and AIDS each, individually, caused more deaths than were caused by problems arising from the genital organs other than the breasts. (Although AIDS and breast cancer arise from the reproductive organs—not exclusively, in the case of AIDS—the prevention, diagnosis, and treatment of neither condition is within the special purview of ob-gyns.)

Of course, focusing on deaths is not an accurate way to measure women's total needs for health care. The important point to be made from these data is that women of reproductive age have many kinds of health problems. Seventeen percent of the deaths were due to accidents or homicide. But 30 percent of the deaths were attributable, at least in part, to smoking; 32 percent were attributable, at least in part, to alcohol (Katz *et al.*, 1995). Suicide accounted for 6 percent of the deaths, AIDS accounted for more than 3 percent. Many of the deaths were at least theoretically preventable through the intervention of health care providers—*if they had a real knowledge of the women and an effective, supportive relationship*. We cannot expect the health care system to solve all the problems of our society. Yet one of the reasons for the focus on primary health care is the belief that a health care provider who develops a long-term relationship with his or her clients, gets to know them as individual human beings, and focuses on health education and preventive interventions will provide care that leads to better health and lower health care costs. Primary health care providers are supposed to attend to the emotional and behavioral conditions that contribute to these kinds of deaths.

If most women are to have only one primary-care physician (not two, although that is the case for about one-third of women currently), it is hard to say whether the primary-care physician should be an ob-gyn or an internist or family physician. If family physicians and internists are going to function as the primary-care physicians for reproductive-age women, should the women be sent to obstetrician–gynecologists or midwives for family planning care, or can that be handled by a family practitioner or internist? (Thirty percent of American women between the ages of fifteen and forty-four use a method of contra-

ception that requires prescription or administration by a health professional.) On the other hand, if ob-gyns are going to function as primary-care providers for nonpregnant women, they will either have to refer many women for treatment of common health problems or they will have to learn to treat those problems themselves. The Oregon Medical Association's guidelines, for instance, require all primary-care physicians to be competent to provide immunizations, blood pressure screening, diet and exercise counseling, injury and accident prevention, and education about alcohol, tobacco, and drug use. They should be able to evaluate common complaints (e.g., chest pains, headaches); to diagnose and manage routine chronic and acute problems (e.g., diabetes, respiratory infections); to coordinate care with other health care providers (including hospice care); and to perform common outpatient procedures (e.g., suturing cuts, removing ear wax.) If ob-gyns are to perform this role, their training will have to change (Husk, 1996).

In the short-run, who *should* be the primary-care physicians for nonpregnant women of reproductive age may be only an academic point. Ob-gyns currently occupy a lot of this territory; any changes will not happen quickly. But how this issue is resolved has long-term implications for midwifery. *Women who have an ongoing relationship with an ob-gyn when they are not pregnant do not switch to a midwife when they conceive.* The fact that almost half of all American women have an ongoing patient relationship with an ob-gyn creates a very different situation for midwifery than the situation that exists in our peer countries.

Another part of the question about whether ob-gyns are or should be primary-care providers for women has to do with women who are having normal pregnancies. In countries where midwives provide most of the care to most pregnant women, midwives are the primary-care providers for healthy women who are having normal pregnancies. Obstetrician–gynecologists function as specialists in both gynecology and obstetrics.

In contrast, ob-gyns function as both primary-care physicians *and specialists* in the care of pregnant women in the United States. Could that difference be part of the reason for the overmedicalization of pregnancy care in this country, for the overly intense focus on pathology? *Maybe overuse of high-tech care is a consequence of expecting physicians trained as pathology-oriented specialists to provide primary care.* Maybe there is an inherent conflict between the roles, making it difficult to be a proficient and artful practitioner of both roles simultaneously. In the maternity care system in the Netherlands, a woman is either in primary care or specialty care; she cannot be in both at the same time. Primary-care providers, whether midwives or general practitioners, follow clear criteria in deciding to refer or transfer a pregnant woman to an obstetric specialist. When the need for specialist care is over, the obstetrician refers the woman back to primary care. The transitions are very clear; there is no sliding back and forth. And many interventions are prohibited to the primary maternity care providers. If a woman needs those interventions, she is referred to a specialist. When one individual—an American obstetrician-gynecologist—is both the primary-care provider and the specialist, how easy it is for the distinction between "normal" and "complicated" to blur.

Does this blurring—the lack of clear distinction between normal and complicated and the ease of moving from one level of care to another—help to explain the overuse of interventions during normal pregnancies in the United States? I think that it does. The National Birth Center Study has been referred to many times in this book—a large, national, prospective study of care provided in eighty-four freestanding birth centers. Labor and delivery interventions were used very rarely. If a woman experienced significant complications or needed interventions that were inappropriate in an out-of-hospital birth setting (e.g., oxytocin or an epidural),

she was transferred to a hospital.* Subsequently a study was done to compare findings from the National Birth Center Study with information about the care provided by midwives and physicians committed to low-intervention care when they were taking care of low-risk women giving birth in hospitals. Some of the midwives and physicians who provided care to the women in the comparison study also participated in the National Birth Center Study. The purpose was to determine the effect of the birth site itself on the care provided. In both studies, the care providers believed in avoiding unnecessary use of labor and delivery interventions; both studies focused on low-risk women who were having normal births. There were significant differences between the care provided to the two groups of women in the use of nearly every kind of labor and delivery procedure. In every case the women who gave birth in hospitals received more interventions.

There may have been other reasons for the differences; the women in the comparison study did not choose to give birth in a birth center, so the two groups were different, regardless of their degree of measurable risk. However, the differences in use of almost every kind of procedure were considerable, and midwives and physicians who have discussed these findings think that they make sense. It is much easier to decide to use an intervention that is readily available and does not require a referral or any other kind of formalized decision-making process. It follows that it is easier, and therefore more likely, for a specialist who is functioning as a primary-care physician to employ his specialist skills more frequently than would occur if the same patients were under the care of a primary-care provider, whether a midwife or physician, who had to bring a specialist into

---

*The study methodology is described in Chapter 5. The major findings are described in Chapter 11.

the situation before the intervention could occur.

Maintaining clear distinctions between primary and specialist care is an important part of the logic of the concept of managed care. Allowing ob-gyns to function in both roles simultaneously undermines the logic. However, ob-gyns have to serve as primary-care providers because there are still too few family physicians and internists to provide primary care to nonpregnant women (although the number of family physicians being trained has grown rapidly in recent years)* and because there are too few midwives to take care of all women who are having normal pregnancies. So the primary-care/specialist-care breakdown has to blur in this area for awhile. In the long run, if the managed care approach works and becomes the major organizing principle for health care in this country, —in the long run, it would make more sense to train more midwives, family physicians, and internists, and fewer ob-gyns. An efficient system would provide all women with easy access to a single ambulatory care provider who can handle most illnesses, attend to psychosocial and health maintenance issues, and deal with each as an individual, as part of a family, and as part of the larger society. The traditional primary care specialties are the physician groups that are most likely to be able to fill this role (Rosenblatt *et al.*, 1995).

Pain as a Pivotal Issue

Pain—including fear of pain and the need for relief from pain—is the other major reason for the persisting dominance of the medical model. Women left midwives in the early part of this century in order to obtain twilight sleep and, later, general anesthesia, which were available only from physicians. During the 1930s Grantly Dick-Read, an

English obstetrician, published a book entitled *Childbirth Without Fear: The Principles and Practices of Natural Childbirth*. In it he argued that a significant part of the pain of labor and delivery results from muscle tension that is induced by fear and that healthy, self-confident women who appreciate birth as a normal process can experience childbirth without fear and thus with much less pain. Dick-Read's book and methods elicited strong opposition from British obstetricians, who accused him of abusing women by forcing them to suffer the pain of childbirth. His book was not published in the United States until 1944. When it was, it stimulated the beginning of the natural childbirth movement and the first natural childbirth education classes for pregnant women. The natural childbirth movement introduced the idea that giving birth can be a positive experience. Childbirth preparation classes—taught largely by nurses or women in the community, not as part of medical treatment and care—introduced an alternative concept of the appropriate role of pregnant women and doctors during birth; the woman's full role requires active use of not only her body, but also her mind and her spirit. Natural childbirth and obstetric anesthesia became the central themes and symbols in a resurrection of the contest between the midwifery and medical models for the care of pregnant women.

General anesthesia, amnesics, and heavy use of systemic painkillers were finally abandoned due to evidence of both short- and long-term ill effects on babies. Although the adverse short-term effects had been observed during the 1930s and 1940s, data demonstrating long-term effects of central nervous system depressants on infants did not become available until the late 1970s. In 1979 the Federal Drug Administration (FDA) convened a special meeting to discuss results of a large national study that found lingering behavioral and motor deficits in children whose mothers had received anesthesia or large doses of analgesics, including De-

---

*See the sections titled "Family Practice Physicians" and "Primary care Providers as Gatekeepers" in Chapter 5.

merol, which was in wide use in the country at that time. Anesthetics that were inhaled were the worst offenders, causing gross-motor-skill deficits (retarded ability to sit, stand, crawl, and walk) that did not seem to dissipate with time (*Medical World News,* 1979). Press and television coverage of the FDA meeting increased interest in natural childbirth and boosted the home-birth/midwife movement, increasing scientific support for the midwifery model of pregnancy care.

In 1982 an obstetric journal published an article that used findings from several studies to argue that (1) the bad reputation of obstetric analgesia had resulted from use of excessively high doses and other forms of gross abuse during earlier periods, (2) that proper use of analgesia and anesthesia leads to favorable outcomes, (3) that "the most frequent cause of fetal asphyxia in humans is likely to be maternal psychological or medical stress," which causes constriction of the arteries that carry blood to the placenta, and (4) that sedatives, analgesics, and general anesthetics "probably represent the single most important tool we have available (other than psychological support) to interrupt this basically destructive maternal physiological process" and thus prevent fetal damage from lack of oxygen (Myers & Williams, 1982). This article brought attention to the medical benefits of pain relief during labor and delivery. Although use of both natural and synthetic narcotics (such as Demerol) continues, high doses are usually avoided. General anesthesia is now used only for cesarean sections, and is not the preferred method of anesthesia for them. These methods were replaced by regional anesthetics—caudals, spinals, and then epidurals, the latter of which have become a mainstay of American obstetrics.

The Effectiveness, Untoward Effects, and Cost of Epidurals

Epidurals provide the most effective pain relief and do not affect the woman's level of consciousness. They are very popular among pregnant women themselves, and among ob-

stetricians, anesthesiologists, and labor-and-delivery-room nurses. But epidurals have serious drawbacks, including less effective contractions and an increased likelihood that the baby's head will not rotate into the optimal position for delivery. As a result, women who have epidurals experience higher rates of both cesarean sections and operative vaginal deliveries (use of forceps or vacuum to extract the baby). The cesarean section rate appears to be a full ten percentage points higher among women who have epidurals, with most of the increase due to cesareans performed because of dystocia (slow, nonprogressive labor); there may also be some increase in cesareans performed for fetal distress. The effect on cesareans can be reduced or eliminated by not starting the epidural until relatively late in the process of an individual woman's labor. But many women experience significant pain during the early phases of labor; postponing the epidural reduces its overall effectiveness in preventing pain. In addition, epidurals do not always work and do not work very well in some women. Having an epidural does not guarantee a pain-free birth.

The debate about the pros and cons of epidural anesthesia carries special weight because of the profound effect of epidural anesthesia on all aspects of labor and delivery. Epidurals have become the linchpin of the medical model: Continuous EFM and intravenous infusions are required and the use of oxytocin augmentation and some kind of operative delivery (vacuum, forceps, or cesarean) is much more likely. The woman is relatively inactive, will probably stay in bed, and can distance herself from the process to some degree. Everything tends to be quieter and more controlled. Some mothers and fathers watch television. Nursing care focuses on procedures, equipment, and information displayed on a television-like monitor; the woman does not need constant personal interaction and support. Not having an epidural is a necessary condition for a truly natural birth and results in a dramatically different experience—for the woman, her support person, and whoever takes care of her during labor. An unanesthetized woman is unlikely to stay in bed, will probably get in and out of bed several times, sit, walk, take a bath or shower, and assume a variety of positions. She needs almost constant personal attention, some of which can be provided by the person she has chosen to be with her during this experience. But she also needs much more attention from the nurse or midwife—touching, talking, holding, massaging, physical support, eye-to-eye contact, and constant emotional and social support. Labor with a woman who is in touch with her body is intense and may be unruly, immodest, and loud.

Women who have had epidurals are cut off not only from pain, but also from other sensations and neurological feedback that stimulate and orchestrate many voluntary and involuntary behaviors that contribute to the effectiveness of labor. Women who are not anesthetized experience a spontaneous desire to "bear down"—to use the musculature of their entire torso to supplement the force of their uterine contractions. During the 1980s CNM researchers at the University of Illinois used systematic observations and multiple biological measurements to study the effect of the bearing-down reflex during the expulsive phase of labor in women who were not anesthetized (Roberts *et al.*, 1987). When a contraction increased the intrauterine pressure to a certain point, the pressure seemed to trigger the bearing-down effort, but the intrauterine pressure at which this happened changed in relationship to the degree of cervical dilation and the position of the fetus. As the contractions became more intense, the number, duration, and amplitude of the women's bearing-down efforts increased. Although the women had not been instructed in how to push or breathe, most of them automatically adapted their breathing patterns in ways that tended to maintain oxygenation of their blood during contractions.

A leading obstetric textbook states that epidurals induced before labor is well established "may be followed by desultory labor" and that the cause of this phenomenon is not clear (Cunningham *et al.*, 1993). Surely part of the problem lies in the interruption of the neurological integrity that makes an unanesthetized woman respond to her labor spontaneously in the most efficient way. The inability to walk, squat, and assume a variety of other postures is also important. Maternal mobility and choice of position during labor are among the forms of care for which there is clear evidence of benefit (see Table 15). Because of this, obstetricians and anesthesiologists are trying to reduce the untoward effects of epidural anesthesia by improving the technique, including use of a lighter dose, called a "walking epidural." So far the use of the word "walking" in a "walking epidural" is extremely optimistic. Some women can stand and walk a few feet around their beds, with assistance. However, women with epidurals are attached to their beds and bedside equipment with several kinds of cords and tubes; even if the methodology were improved, actual walking would be limited.

Other effects of epidurals include increased body temperature of the mother, fetus, and newborn, perhaps due to the mother's reduced ability to dissipate the body heat generated by the intense activity of labor. Fever increases the metabolic rate and thus the need for oxygen. Because fever is often the first clinical sign of infection, fever during labor cannot be assumed to be benign. Because epidurals tend to increase the length of labor, they may also contribute to the incidence of fever caused by infection, which is more frequent when labor is prolonged. Because of the importance of diagnosing and treating infections, maternal fever may stimulate a number of diagnostic and therapeutic interventions during and after labor and delivery. Problems during the initial placement of the epidural may result in severe, sometimes incapacitating headaches. Several studies have found mild effects of epidural anesthesia on newborn behavior, although the data are not conclusive (Thorp & Breedlove, 1996). *A Guide to Effective Care in Pregnancy and Childbirth* indicates the authors' concern about the lack of adequate research to determine whether epidural anesthesia has effects on infants or long-term effects on mothers (Enkin *et al.*, 1995).

Financial costs should also be considered. Routine use of epidurals has enormous cost implications—$500 to $2,500 for the procedure itself, as well as costs related to increased use of forceps and vacuum, infectious morbidity, and the need to rule out infection in women and newborns who have fevers (Thorp & Breedlove, 1996).

The first randomized, controlled trial to observe the effects of epidural anesthesia was published in 1993 (Thorp *et al.*, 1993). The investigators stopped the study early, after they analyzed data from the first group of subjects and saw the very high rate of cesarean sections among the women randomized into the group getting epidurals. They determined that it would not be ethical to continue the study and reported their findings in an article that was published in the *American Journal of Obstetrics and Gynecology*. The journal received more letters to the editor about that study than it had received in response to any other paper it had ever published (Thorp & Breedlove, 1996).

The Nature of Pain During Childbirth
Although the pain of labor and delivery has a physical basis, the experience of the pain is subjective. How it is experienced differs from one society to another and is affected by women's expectations, what they have learned from other women, their self-confidence when they enter labor, the environment in which they labor, and the care and support they receive. One-third of women in the Netherlands choose home births knowing they will receive intensive midwifery support but will not have access to narcotics or anesthesia. Dutch midwives encourage women to discuss their expectations and fears about pain and urge those who seem overly fearful to go to a hospital.

Some American women can also tolerate the pain of labor. Of nearly 12,000 women admitted to American birth centers for labor and delivery, only 13 percent received any kind of central nervous system depressant (sedative, tranquilizer, or analgesic), and less than 3 percent experienced pain that was not adequately relieved. Two-thirds of the women who experienced unrelieved pain were transferred to hospitals; the others gave birth before they could be transferred, so the pain was, at least, short lived. Despite the lack of pain medication, the vast majority of the women were very satisfied with the care they received; they said they would use the birth center again themselves and would recommend it to their friends. Nevertheless, surveys and studies based on interviews find that most American women anticipate the pain of labor to be "awful"[*] and have little confidence in their inherent capacity to give birth.

Based on a worldwide review of studies on the management of labor pain, *A Guide to Effective Care in Pregnancy and Childbirth* concludes that "Satisfaction with one's childbirth experience is not necessarily dependent on the absence of pain. Many women are willing to experience some pain in childbirth, but they do not want it to overwhelm them" (Enkin *et al.*, 1995). Women who receive constant support during labor are significantly more satisfied with their care and are less likely to report that labor was worse than they had expected (Simkin, 1996).

Childbirth Education as an Alternative
Fear and anxiety potentiate pain and affect how we perceive and react to it. Childbirth

---

[*]One hundred and three college students gave their expectations of the pain of labor an average score of 4.4 on a scale in which 1 = no pain at all and 5 = intolerable pain. See Chapter 5.

education was developed for the purpose of preparing women with knowledge and skills intended to reduce their anxiety and give them tools to cope with the pain of labor. Most studies of childbirth education courses have found that their effectiveness is limited. Some studies have found that women who participated in a series of classes used somewhat less pain medication on average, reported less intense labor pain, were less likely to have their babies delivered by forceps, and had a more positive attitude about their birth experience. But labor is still painful, and there may be no reduction in the use of epidural anesthesia (Simkin, 1986a).

Support During Labor as an Alternative

The 1982 article that brought attention to the medical benefits of relieving the pain of labor (the article by Myers & Williams, discussed earlier in this section) identified "psychological support" as the only other important available tool for avoiding the maternal physiologic response to pain. The article did not follow through with a discussion of support during labor as an alternative to anesthesia. *A Guide to Effective Care in Pregnancy and Childbirth* provides a description of what is meant by "support" during labor and delivery. It includes physical comfort measures, emotional support, and a promise that the woman will not be left alone. It may include maintaining eye contact, walking with the woman, holding her hand, making sure she understands the purpose and result of every examination, keeping her informed about her progress, praising her efforts, giving her encouragement (Enkin *et al.*, 1995).

Hospitals and physicians have, with very few exceptions, not considered support during labor as a realistic alternative to the use of drugs. The idea of providing substantial support to women throughout labor and delivery has been given serious consideration only within the context of support provided by midwives (alternative care for women who want a special birth experience) or support provided by the woman's husband or other personal companion. Although some of the necessary support can be provided by the woman's own companion, there are many problems with assuming that the baby's father or another companion is able to provide all of the necessary support. Such individual's are inexperienced and are not trained in nonpharmacologic methods of pain relief. The baby's father is emotionally involved in the birth, is sharing the experience, and may need support himself. If there are tensions in the relationship between the woman and her companion, it may be difficult for the companion to provide effective support. Support provided by a knowledgeable, experienced person is needed (Enkin *et al.*, 1995).

In the past few years supporting women during labor has received attention as a way to reduce cesarean sections. Studies have shown that women who receive support from a trained, experienced person throughout labor have fewer cesareans (see Chapter 5). These studies were reported in the most prestigious medical journals and could not be dismissed because they were randomized, controlled trials and because of a wide consensus that the United States needs to reduce its cesarean section rate, in part because of the high financial cost. It is remarkable that the idea of providing support to women during labor has received more interest packaged as an intervention that can produce a medically advantageous outcome (reduced cesareans) than it receives in its more humble role as part of the humane care of pregnant women. The cross-cultural, age-old practice of providing social and emotional support to women during childbirth disappeared during the period when nearly all women had their babies under twilight sleep or general anesthesia. In the United States it has never recovered its place as an essential part of decent maternity care.

One reason for the lack of commitment to providing effective support to women during labor is that we do not have enough midwives to provide that kind of care. Although we have nurses, many people assume that hospitals cannot afford to hire enough nurses to provide one-on-one care to women during labor. In fact, the ratio of labor-and-delivery-room nurses to women in labor is nearly one to one in many hospitals. But the nurse's first obligation is to implement the physician's labor-management plan, and the nurses are very busy: setting up, monitoring and adjusting IVs, oxytocin infusions, and EFM equipment; assisting physicians while they perform other procedures; catheterizing anesthetized women who cannot control their bladders; telling women who cannot feel their contractions when to "push!"; moving semiparalyzed women from their labor beds to stretchers and then delivery tables, putting their feet in stirrups, and setting up the surgical equipment for episiotomies, and maybe forceps or vacuum extraction. Centralized monitoring, which allows a nurse to observe the EFM patterns of several patients while in a separate room (not with any of the women), may be one of the worst effects of EFM!

Midwife Approach to Pain Control
In addition to providing support, midwives are more likely to try pain relief methods that do not interfere with labor or introduce risk to either the mother or the fetus before they use methods that have known adverse effects. It is important to avoid causing additional pain by not using painful procedures unnecessarily. Having an intravenous infusion can be painful, vaginal examinations are uncomfortable, and having a pressure gauge pushed around the baby's head and into the uterus (a tight fit at best) can be painful. IVs and internal EFM can be avoided by giving women fluids to drink and using other equipment to listen to the fetal heart. Vaginal examinations can be kept to a minimum.

Walking, sitting, taking baths or showers, and changing position frequently help women relieve muscle pain, provide distraction from other discomforts, and facilitate the progress of labor. Midwives not only "allow" but encourage and assist women to be mobile during labor, and try to avoid procedures that require the use of tubes and cords that tie women to their beds. Use of specific positions and massage techniques can help to relieve specific kinds of pain: For example, having a woman assume a position in which her weight is supported by her hands and knees may relieve pain caused by the pressure the baby's head exerts against the bones of her lower back. An upright posture is associated with less pain during the second stage of labor. Applying steady counterpressure to a certain place on the lower back during contractions reduces back pain for some women (Enkin *et al.*, 1995). Many women get some relief from heat or cold applied through hot water bottles or ice packs. Sitting in a warm bath helps women relax; some report a significant reduction in pain. A cup of warm tea, soothing music, and dimmed lights can calm and comfort a woman who is experiencing pain. Touching, stroking, patting, massaging, and holding provide pleasurable sensations that draw the woman's attention away from her discomforts and communicate that she is cared for.

Midwives' use of pharmacologic methods of pain relief vary with their philosophy, the philosophy and wishes of their clients, and their access to these methods. American midwives are not unlike the Dutch midwives (noted earlier), who interview women regarding their expectations and fears about pain and their desire for specific methods of pain control. Women who are likely to need narcotics or an epidural are advised to go to a hospital. Likewise, American midwives who attend births in homes and birth centers cater to women who want a normal birth and are prepared to tolerate and cope with pain with the midwife's help.

CNMs who attend births in hospitals can administer sedatives and narcotics to their clients and can request initiation of epidurals (which are administered by an anesthesiologist or anesthetist). Table 10 in chapter 10 provides data on specific labor and delivery procedures used during the care of clients of six large, hospital-based nurse-midwifery services. The data were collected between 1981 and 1993. Two of the studies provided information on use of narcotic analgesia; four provided information on use of epidural anesthesia. Each of these studies had a control group consisting of low-risk women who were giving birth under the care of physicians. In five of the studies, the CNM clients and physician clients received care in the same hospital during the same period of time. In every study that examined it, the proportion of women receiving narcotics or epidurals was significantly higher among the women who received their care from physicians. Use of epidurals was more than twice as high among the obstetricians' clients in three studies. In one study, 11 percent of the nurse-midwives' clients had epidurals, compared with 53 percent of the physicians' clients.

Meeting the Special Needs of Socioeconomically High-Risk Women

The growth of managed health care and its impact on the health care system are discussed in Chapter 5. The move to managed care has affected nearly all parts of the health care system. In December 1995 a commission created by the Pew Charitable Trusts released its report on challenges facing the health professions as the United States moves into the twenty-first century. Most of the challenges result from circumstances created by the shift to managed care. The commission predicted that 80 to 90 percent of all Americans who have any kind of health care insurance will be enrolled in a managed care system within a decade.

We are still in a time of transition, so only the short-term results are known. However, large effects of the change are already clearly evident. Two important changes are an enormous shift of health care resources away from not-for-profit organizations into companies that are managed for profit and movement of large numbers of people who are eligible for Medicaid out of public sector health care into for-profit managed care plans. These changes are having a deleterious effect on public health agencies, public hospitals, and medical education programs that use public hospitals to provide clinical experience for medical students and physicians in medical-specialty training programs (residencies). They are also having an enormous impact on the care provided to pregnant women who are indigent, especially women on Medicaid, and on the network of services and special programs that had been developed to take care of them.

Professionals Who Focus on the Needs of Indigent Pregnant Women

Creation of the Children's Bureau in 1912 established a governmental interest in ensuring access to effective health care for pregnant women who are poor. This interest reflects both the decency of society and its self-interest. Enactment of the federal Medicaid law in 1965 escalated government's involvement. Since then a private/public coalition has developed both to provide this care and to study and im-prove it. Constituents of this coalition include the maternal and child health units of health departments at all levels of government, the maternal and child health departments of schools of public health, professional organizations (including the American College of Obstetricians and Gynecologists and the American College of Nurse-Midwives), researchers working in the large urban hospitals that provide care to many of the nation's poorest pregnant women and their babies, foundations, and organizations involved in the development and advocacy of public health policy. This functional but informal coalition brings together practitioners, researchers, and leaders from many disciplines —midwifery, obstetrics, family medicine, pediatrics, nursing, nutrition, social work, and the behavioral sciences—allowing people concerned with the health outcomes of the pregnancies of the nation's highest risk mothers to collaborate, learn from one another, and build on one another's work.

Nurse-Midwives' Contributions

Nurse-midwives work in a variety of roles in all parts of this system, and nurse-midwifery care is a highly valued part of the services provided through the system. Although limited in number, nurse-midwives provide a significant amount of care to women in some of the nation's busiest inner-city public hospitals. Nurse-midwives were brought into the obstetric departments of leading medical schools during the 1950s and 1960s in part to improve the quality of care being provided to women in those hospitals. Large hospitals with many obstetric patients needed large nurse-midwifery services; many started their own educational programs in order to prepare enough midwives. As a result, many nurse-midwifery education programs are based in the obstetric departments of large public hospitals or in universities affiliated with those hospitals.

Practicing, teaching, and conducting research in this milieu, nurse-midwives have focused on the many, complex problems of women who are both pregnant and poor, because poverty itself is the strongest correlate of problems during pregnancy. They have focused particularly on providing effective care to pregnant adolescents, working with women who are recent immigrants to this country, understanding the meaning of pregnancy and pregnancy rituals and care for women from different cultures, supporting pregnant women who are infected with the human immunodeficiency virus (HIV), and dealing with the problems of domestic violence and drug addiction as they affect both pregnant and nonpregnant women. Midwifery care, which is personal, respectful, supportive, and reaches beyond the medical aspects of a woman's condition and situation, has proven to be especially effective in meeting the needs of women who are dealing with many problems, whose lives are stressful, sometimes chaotic, some of whom have habits and lifestyles that can compromise their pregnancies. Nurse-midwifery care is associated with higher birth weights and may help to prevent low birth weight among babies born to some of these women. Within the relationship that can develop between a midwife and a pregnant woman over the many months of pregnancy, women who have had few successes in their lives can be helped to deal with problems successfully and can experience their pregnancies and births in a way that empowers them as individuals and as mothers.

High Proportion of Births to Socially Disadvantaged Women

The number of pregnant women with socioeconomic problems is large and may expand as a proportion of all pregnancies in the United States. More than one-third of pregnant women in America are on Medicaid; nearly a third are not married. There is also, and will be in the future, a growing need to provide effective care to pregnant women who are recent immigrants to the United States, many of whom do not speak English well, if at all, and are not familiar with our customs.

Short-Term Savings or Long-Term Cost Effectiveness?

State Medicaid managed care programs are allowing many medically indigent women to obtain care from private physicians and private hospitals. This is the first time that many of these women have been offered any choice in health care; many want to use the same doctors and facilities that are used by women who are not poor.

This change has moved many women away from special programs that were designed to meet their complicated needs. It has also moved them away from the people who have focused on these problems and from the institutions that have done most of the research. Moving them into a new kind of care constitutes an experiment. Because poor women have the highest incidence of poor pregnancy outcomes, the experiment is being conducted on our most vulnerable mothers and babies. Large parts of the experiment are being conducted without collecting the data necessary to evaluate the results. Nevertheless, we do have some data: Chapter 5 presented findings from several studies in several states, all of which raise concerns that routine care provided in private sector medical offices may not be sufficient for socioeconomically distressed American women. Two studies—one conducted in Kentucky and North Carolina and one conducted in Chicago—found an increased incidence of low birth weight when medically indigent women obtained their care from private physicians. In the study carried out in Kentucky and North Carolina, the association between private care and low birth weight was especially strong for very low birth weight births (babies born weighing less than three and a half pounds). These are the worst cases—the most important to prevent. In the study carried out in Chicago, the low birth weight rate was more than twice as high among Medicaid-eligible women who obtained their care from private physicians as compared to the rate for women who used the public clinics. Unpublished data from Florida, Oregon, and South Carolina corroborate the findings from the published studies.

Brief, impersonal prenatal visits that focus on only the physical aspects of pregnancy are not adequate to intervene in the problems and stresses that result in higher rates of low birth weight for socioeconomically disadvantaged women. Screening for pathology is essential but not sufficient.

However, not all the news is bad, and the bad news may not be permanent. Some people are being brought into regular health care for the first time in their lives. And some of the current problems may not be related to managed care per se, but may flow from the turmoil and other side effects of

the rapidity of the changes and the newness of some systems.

Many of the bad effects seem to result from a cost-saving mind-set that has gone beyond reducing unnecessary costs to reducing costs as much as possible in the interest of short-term profit. While there was a small reduction (1 percent) in the cost of health insurance between 1993 and 1994, there was an enormous growth in profits. Many hospitals and other parts of the system that were previously operated on a not-for-profit basis have been taken over by profit-oriented corporations. And there are indications that the reduction in health care inflation may have already ended. If so, the long-term ill effects will overwhelm the benefits.

The secret to success will be basing health care decisions not on short-term cost savings, but on long-term cost effectiveness. Long-standing HMOs have made an art form of examining long-term cost effectiveness. As a result, they have been leaders in health education and offering programs to help subscribers change unhealthful behaviors. HMOs were also leaders in providing nurse-midwifery services to women in private sector health care. Their motivation was cost effectiveness.

Recommendations Made by Other Groups

The situation described in this book is known to many people; it has generated many well-founded recommendations for change. This section summarizes recommendations made by several committees and organizations regarding the need for midwives or a midwifery approach to the care of pregnant women in order to improve access to maternal health care, the quality of maternal health care, and the outcomes of maternal health care in this country.

Recommendations from Prestigious National Institutes and Commissions

Over the years several high-level panels have studied the causes of poor pregnancy outcomes in the United States and made rec- ommendations to improve things. Such in- vestigations invariably focus on the problems of access to maternity care and the quality and effectiveness of that care, with emphasis on the particular problems and needs of so- cioeconomically disadvantaged women. The reports that result from these investigations invariably comment on the special contribu- tions nurse-midwives have made to improv- ing access and the quality of this care and call for increasing the numbers and use of nurse-midwives and reducing barriers to nurse-midwifery practice.*

The Institute of Medicine's 1985 report on *Preventing Low Birthweight* cited studies that found a reduced incidence of low birth weight associated with nurse-midwifery care of pregnant women who were at higher- than-average risk because of social and eco- nomic factors. Other studies had found that nurse-midwives spend more time with pa- tients during prenatal visits and always de- vote some of that time to patient teaching, and that CNMs' clients returned for a higher proportion of their prenatal appointments and were more likely than physicians' pa- tients to carry out instructions for self-care. The committee recommended that the na- tion rely more heavily on nurse-midwives to provide care to "hard-to-reach" high-risk women and that state laws be amended to support nurse-midwifery practice.

The Institute of Medicine's 1987 report on prenatal care noted that CNMs serve "dis- proportionate numbers of women who are poor, adolescent, members of minority groups, and residents of inner cities or rural areas" and that legal restrictions and "obstet- rical customs" limit their practice. The re- port characterized the country's maternity care system as "fundamentally flawed, frag- mented, and overly complex and urged the development of a new system that would

make appropriate use of both physicians and CNMs, supported hospital privileges for nurse-midwives, and called for improved col- laboration between physicians and CNMs.

In 1988 the National Commission to Pre- vent Infant Mortality called on state universi- ties to establish and expand nurse-midwifery education programs. The National Perinatal Information Center's 1992 report, *Perinatal Health: Strategies for the 21st Century*, called for nurse-midwives to play a major role in im- proving access to perinatal health care and recommended that CNMs be represented at all levels of policy and decision making in the perinatal health care system.

Recommendations from National Women's Health Organizations

The first years of the Clinton administration were energized by widespread expectation that federal legislation would result in some kind of a national health care program. In preparation for that reform, four long-stand- ing national women's health organizations worked together to develop a set of recom- mendations for "Childbearing Policy Within a National Health Program" (Women's Insti- tute for Childbearing Policy, 1994). The four organizations were (1) the Boston Women's Health Book Collective (authors of *Our Bod- ies, Ourselves* and related books), (2) the Na- tional Black Women's Health Project, (3) the National Women's Health Network, and (4) the Women's Institute for Childbearing Policy. The document was published in 1994.

It began with a summary: "Basic indica- tors of health show that present childbear- ing policies and practices have failed to meet the needs of women and children in funda- mental ways. A host of systemic problems lies behind these poor results. Of critical impor- tance is our inadequate attention to the con- ditions of everyday life, which are the primary determinants of health. In addition, our provision of clinical services involves se- rious and persistent problems of access, quality and cost." The statement calls for an

---

*See section on "Recommendations Regarding CNMs" in Chapter 5.

approach that emphasizes the everyday living conditions that influence health and provision of "primary care clinical services that are oriented towards prevention." It noted that midwives offer optimal primary care for childbearing women and newborns and identified free-standing birth centers as "a small-scale, health-oriented, accessible and highly appropriate setting for Primary Maternity Care." It urged a national health program to "recognize the midwife as the appropriate caregiver for most childbearing women," to support widespread implementation of a midwifery approach to care, to encourage the development and use of birth centers, and to support the choice of home birth. It included proposals for a systematic transition to a primary maternity care system, including expanding opportunities to educate midwives, implementing effective regulatory and reimbursement mechanisms, and supporting the strong research program needed to expand opportunities for women to receive care and give birth in "health- and birth-oriented nonmedical settings" (Women's Institute for Childbearing Policy, 1994).

Recommendations from a Consumer Advocacy Organization

In 1995 an independent consumer-advocacy group published "Encouraging the Use of Nurse-Midwives: A Report for Policymakers." It recommended expanding nurse-midwifery education with a goal of gradually adjusting the ratio of CNMs to obstetricians so that nurse-midwives can become the primary provider of care to low-risk pregnant women. The report and recommendations were based on a Public Citizen Health Research Group survey of the majority of nurse-midwives practicing during 1990 through 1992. A major finding of the study was low cesarean delivery rates (Gabay & Wolfe, 1995). Public Citizen is the consumer advocacy organization headed by Ralph Nader.

The Mother-Friendly Childbirth Initiative

The World Health Organization, UNICEF, and other international organizations concerned with the health and well-being of children are supporting a worldwide campaign to eliminate hospital practices that interfere with breast-feeding and replace them with practices that promote and support breast-feeding. It is called the Baby-Friendly Initiative; a major tool for accomplishing the goal of the initiative is a brief list of ten steps that need to be taken to create a baby-friendly hospital.

In 1996 a coalition of American maternity care organizations followed suit with a set of principles and ten steps required to create childbirth services that are friendly to mothers (Coalition for Improving Maternity Services, 1996). The coalition combines the expertise and energy of twenty-three organizations, including both national midwifery organizations, most major childbirth education organizations, the professional organization for nurses who specialize in women's health or obstetric and neonatal nursing, Doulas of North America, all major breast-feeding organizations, and other groups organized for the purpose of improving maternity services in the United States. Medical groups had opportunities to participate but did not.

The following is a summary of the ten steps for developing a mother-friendly hospital, birth center, or home birth service. Every aspect of the ten-step program is supported by research. A mother-friendly childbirth service should:

1. Offer all mothers unrestricted access to the birth companions of their choice, access to continuous emotional and physical support from a skilled woman (such as a doula) throughout labor and delivery, and professional midwifery care.

2. Provide accurate descriptive and statistical information about its practices, its use of interventions during labor and delivery, and the outcomes of its care.

3. Provide "culturally competent care"— care that is sensitive and responsive to the specific beliefs, values, and cus-

toms of the mother's ethnicity and religion.

4. Allow women to walk, move freely, and assume positions of their choice during labor and birth (except when restriction is necessary because of a complication) and discourage use of the lithotomy position (supine with her legs up).

5. Have clearly defined policies and procedures for collaboration and consultation between primary care providers and care providers at the referral level, and for linking the mother and baby to community resources for prenatal and postpartum follow-up and breast-feeding support.

6. Not routinely employ practices that are unsupported by scientific evidence, such as shaving, enemas, intravenous infusions, withholding nourishment, early artificial rupture of the membranes, and continuous EFM. Cesarean sections and use of oxytocin to induce or augment labor should be limited. (Percentages that should not be exceeded were given for each.)

7. Educate staff in nonpharmacologic methods of pain relief; not promote use of analgesic or anesthetic drugs not required to correct a complication.

8. Encourage all mothers and families, including those with sick or premature newborns or infants with congenital problems, to touch, hold, breast-feed, and care for their babies to the extent compatible with the babies' condition.

9. Discourage circumcision of male newborns for other than religious purposes.

10. Strive to achieve the WHO/UNICEF "Ten Steps of the Baby-Friendly Hospital Initiative" to promote successful breast-feeding: a written breast-feeding policy that is communicated to all health care staff; providing training to give staff the skills needed to implement the policy; informing pregnant women about the benefits of breast-feeding; helping mothers initiate breast-feeding shortly after giving birth; showing mothers how to breast-feed and how to maintain lactation during separation from their infants; not giving food or fluids other than breast milk to newborns except when required because of a medical problem; 24-hour-a-day rooming-in; encouraging breast-feeding whenever the infant seems to be hungry, not giving pacifiers to breast-feeding infants; and fostering the establishment of breast-feeding support groups and referring postpartum mothers to them.

Recommendations to Broaden the Objectives and Focus of Maternity Care

Now that maternal mortality is not a major threat in this country, the care of pregnant women has focused primarily on the fetus and the baby. Pregnancy is the incredible process by which a fertilized egg grows and develops into a new human being. A baby is such a fantastic outcome that society focuses almost exclusively on the baby as the sole product of this enterprise. But the baby is not the sole product. The other product of every pregnancy, especially every *first* pregnancy, is a mother (Heilmann, 1996). How well we grow and develop our mothers may be as important as how well we grow and develop our babies. The health of most babies is, ultimately, very dependent on their mothers. The baby is not the only product of a pregnancy; a healthy baby should not be the only goal.

More than 40 percent of American births are to women having their first baby. During her first pregnancy a woman is preparing for a radical change in her life. A pregnant women knows that she is facing enormous change and may be more open and ready for change than she has ever been before. She will go from being a daughter to a mother; for many women that means changing from a child to an adult. This process requires a restructuring of her self-concept and of her relationships with her own parents, her husband or other father of her child, probably her siblings, and the external world of friends, school, or work. America needs its babies to be born healthy. We also need pregnant women to go through this transition with all of the information, support, and encouragement they need to become strong, effective, self-confident mothers. Childbirth can be a profound experience. It can leave a woman with a new sense of her own competence and the power and importance of her role as mother. It can also leave her feeling violated and incompetent. The physiology of the mother and newborn prepare them to fall deeply in love when they reunite after their separation at birth. The quality of every aspect of this experience is important.

Problems related to pregnancy are only the tip of the iceberg of morbidities affecting our children, including neglect and abuse. One in three victims of physical abuse is a baby who has not yet reached the age of one. Contrary to public perceptions, much of the violence is perpetrated by women, including mothers.

The quality of a young child's environment and social experiences can have lasting effects on how the child develops. Research published during the last ten years has provided scientific support for long-standing observations that children who live in stimulating environments and are raised by caring adults learn more efficiently than other children. The brain develops much more rapidly during the first year of life than we understood before, but this development is vulnerable. The quality of the parenting and environment that affect a child during its first three years has long-lasting effects, determining how well the child will get along with other people, whether he will resolve disputes peacefully or through use of vio-

lence, how well she will learn to use words, whether he will be self-confident and able to explore the world without fear (Barnard, 1994; McCreary, 1996).

Many of our children live in very high-risk situations. Nearly one-third of the women who had babies in 1994 were not married—1.3 million babies with unmarried mothers. Among black births, 70 percent of the mothers were not married (Ventura *et al.*, 1996). Having reached that proportion, unmarried motherhood has become a norm. Of 12 million children under three years of age, one in four lives in poverty, one in four lives in a single-parent family (Barnard, 1994; McCreary, 1996).

What the health care system can do to help distressed mothers is limited. It cannot solve the underlying social and economic problems. However, it is not without resources. All but 1 percent of women who gave birth in the United States during 1994 had some prenatal care; 80 percent of all pregnant women and 68 percent of black pregnant women began prenatal care during the first three months of pregnancy. They had, on average, more than twelve prenatal visits (Ventura *et al.*, 1996). That is a lot of contact between pregnant women and the health care system during an extraordinary period in the lives of the young women—a lot of contact during a period that is rich with opportunity. Pregnancy is a time when people make important life decisions. Some women get married during this period, or decide to stay in unhappy marriages. Many people move—away from the family, back in with the family, or to a bigger place. Some quit school. Some people feel frightened; some feel trapped. There is a lot of physical abuse of pregnant women.

In addition, there is excitement and hope. I once attended an interesting continuing education session about drug-addicted or HIV-infected women who became pregnant and were offered abortions but decided to have their babies. Some of the women in the studies being reported had given birth to two or three babies under these conditions, even though they were rarely able to keep and take care of the babies after they were born. The people on the panel, who had worked closely with the women, believed that one reason the women could not give up their pregnancies was that, to them, being pregnant meant that there was hope—a baby meant a clean page, a fresh start, a chance to be a good mother, a chance to do it right. The page isn't always really clean; the hope isn't always realistic. But hope is a strong motivator; the desire to change creates readiness for learning. Pregnant women know their lives are going to change and that they are going to have to learn to do things they have never done before. Every woman wants her baby to be all right; in fact, she wants her baby to be healthy, strong, and smart! Every woman wants to know what to expect during labor and delivery and to be able to get through it with dignity. Every woman wants to be a good mother. For some women pregnancy, especially birth itself, may be a kind of epiphany—a deeply enriching spiritual experience. But even for the most distressed women, there is some spiritual element—a calling forth of resources aroused by the woman's intimate relationship with the baby in her body and by her sense of hope.

Prenatal care—more than twelve visits on average—occurs during this period of extraordinary physical, emotional, social, and often other change in a woman's life, when there is an unusual, perhaps unique readiness to learn and eagerness to rise to the occasion. But what kind of care do many women get, especially the women with the gravest problems and least resources? The woman or girl leaves her community to go to a clinic or doctor's office. She sits in a waiting room, urinates in a cup, stands on a scale, pulls up her sleeve to have her blood pressure measured, pulls down her pants for someone to palpate and measure her belly, answers a few questions from an authority figure who is scanning for pathology. She may be sent to a social worker

or nutritionist—special appointments with another person. The other special visits will be for routine (but usually unnecessary) ultrasounds, which she will love because she will get to "see" her baby and maybe find out if it is going to be a girl or a boy. But the primary focus is on her body—the possibility of pathology. The endpoint of the endeavor is the birth.

Chapter 5 describes the nation's long concern about low birth weight. Low birth weight is the problem behind our relatively high rate of infant mortality. In 1985 the Institute of Medicine published the report of a committee of experts who had spent two years studying how to prevent low birth weight. The major recommendation was for the nation to ensure that all pregnant women, especially those at highest risk, receive high-quality prenatal care. Chapter 10 summarizes research to assess the effectiveness of prenatal care as a means to reduce low birth weight. Many difficulties are associated with this kind of study, including selection bias and confounding. Another important problem is the inability to know what we are talking about when we discuss prenatal care. It is not like a shot of penicillin. Penicillin has been standardized; when you give a certain dose, you know exactly what you are giving. As long as the diagnosis is correct and it is the right drug for a particular germ, it does not matter too much how it is given. The right technique is important, but the therapeutic action is not dependent on the relationship between the patient and the person who administers the dose. None of this is true with prenatal care, for which the content, the context, and the relationship may all be critically important. This section focuses on recommendations to make prenatal care more effective, including recommendations made by a panel of experts and my own recommendations.

Public Health Service Recommendations on the Content of Prenatal Care

In 1986 the Public Health Service convened a panel of experts and asked them to examine and make recommendations about the content of prenatal care. A report on their findings, conclusions and recommendations was published in 1989 (Department of Health and Human Services, 1989). The expert panel recommended that prenatal care start before the woman conceives and that the focus of prenatal care should be expanded to include not only the pregnant woman, fetus, and infant, but also the family, not only during the pregnancy but throughout the infant's entire first year of life. The report spoke of the need for the pregnant woman and her support persons to be active participants in her prenatal care and asked for new emphasis on the psychosocial dimensions of prenatal care.

A Focus on the Mother

The Public Health Service report has been out for a decade. Although efforts have been made, the care provided to most pregnant women in America did not improve significantly, if at all, and the cost-cutting focus of the new managed care organizations has worsened the quality of care provided to many women.* The following recommendations and observations are mine:

- Prenatal care should be based on overt acknowledgment that most of the means to protect and maximize the health of an unborn baby lie solely within the power of the pregnant woman. It is she who will ultimately decide whether to smoke, drink, or use drugs. What she eats; whether and how she works, exercises, and rests; her hygiene; her exposure to sexually transmitted infections, violence, and psychosocial stress—all may affect the well-being of her baby and are largely beyond the control of the person providing her care.

---

*See the section on "Effects of Managed Care on Indigent Pregnant Women" in Chapter 5.

- Prenatal care cannot be maximally effective unless the pregnant woman and care provider join into a genuine partnership. That requires open communication, and that requires respect and trust. Open communication is especially important for women who have serious lifestyle or social problems, who are often reluctant to confide in authority figures. There are immense barriers between poor women and their care providers—barriers of social class and culture, often race or ethnicity, language or dialect, and in the case of male physicians, gender. Poor people are used to disdain and disrespect; the antidotes are authentic concern and respect. Smaller, less bureaucratic services in which clients become known as individuals and do not have to relate to large numbers of people make it easier to develop trust.
- Prenatal care should be part of a continuum of care that precedes and continues beyond the pregnancy, including family planning and access to abortions. We should not focus on birth as the endpoint of the care. Pregnancy should be seen as a time of preparing for not only the birth but the baby, and the necessary but exciting changes that will be required in the woman's life and in the lives of the father of her baby and all members of her family. We need to create strong linkages between those who provide maternal health care and those who provide services to promote better parenting and family conditions.
- We put too much emphasis on pathology. Think of the pregnancy as a beautiful apple that has been given to the woman; the whole time she is eating it, we are examining it for a worm. We need to detect and treat pathology, but we should expect normalcy, and help her expect it too. And we should be careful about "risk assessments." Some risk-scoring methods identify more than half of

the women as "high risk." What does that designation mean to pregnant women? Maybe we should do a "strengths and assets assessment" too—focus on her abilities, support system, and effective problem-solving strategies.

- Providing prenatal care through many dispersed clinics while centralizing deliveries in a single large hospital creates a schism between prenatal and childbirth care. Pregnant women see prenatal care as preparation for the coming birth and value it more when it is provided by the people who will be with them when they have their babies. Prenatal clinics that are dissociated from intrapartum care lose power in the eyes of their patients; pregnant women who do not value prenatal care will not obtain maximum benefit from it. They may not even bother to use it. I would like to see more small units that provide complete maternity care and are based in the community.

Watching Our Words

A 1992 article by an Australian woman who has studied maternity care but is not a doctor or midwife commented on the negativity of the language of obstetrics. "As a non-medical consumer," she wrote, "I am constantly amazed at the list of things women are told they have 'failed' at: they can 'fail' to dilate, to progress, to home birth, to breast feed— and their babies can 'fail' to thrive. Bits and pieces of them can 'fail' as well: contractions can be 'inadequate', as can their pelvis. Their cervix can be 'incompetent' (or merely 'unfavourable'). In the language of obstetrics and gynaecology, it is even possible for mucus to be 'hostile'!"* (Bastian, 1992). The terminology of failure and inadequacy "may

---

*"Hostile" cervical mucus is cervical mucus that is not conducive to conception. The object of the "hostility" is sperm. The term is used in assessments of the cause of infertility.

adversely affect a woman's confidence and self-esteem. Feeling ineffectual and impotent will not be help-ful to a woman in coping with the stresses of labour and motherhood. Nor should women be left with a view of their bodies as faulty machines, or their personal responses and 'performance' as inadequate." The title of the article was "Confined, Managed and Delivered: The Language of Obstetrics." The author contrasts these obstetric terms with "women labouring, being cared for, and giving birth." The obstetric terms connote restriction and passivity on the part of the woman, action and control on the part of the physician. Women with a previous cesarean section who want to deliver vaginally are "allowed" a "trial" of labor.

Although these criticisms were addressed to midwives as well as obstetricians, midwives in the United States and other countries are trying to turn this around, to put the focus on the woman as an individual, to recognize her as the most important person in the maternity care partnership, to emphasize the positive potential of pregnancy and childbirth, and to enhance women's confidence in their own ability to grow, to give birth, and to be a competent mother of a healthy child. Midwives no longer speak of "delivering babies" but say that they "attend births." The change is subtle, but it moves the action from the midwife to the mother.

Other Recommendations

All of the following recommendations flow from the situation described in this chapter and the other information contained in this book.

Women's Right to Access Both Maternity Care Models

Many women want medical model obstetrical care. With rare exceptions, those who do can exercise their choice. But some women do not want that kind of care. During the late 1980s and early 1990s the governments of

Great Britain and several Australian states conducted studies to determine what kind of care women wanted during pregnancy and childbirth. They found that most women wanted midwives; indeed, they wanted an opportunity to develop a relationship with an individual midwife and real midwifery, not midwives subjugated to the medical paradigm. Of course, British and Australian women have had experience with midwives, and most American women have not. But the United Kingdom, the United States, Canada, Australia, and New Zealand share a world of information and communication. The dissatisfactions that led to efforts to improve maternity care by fuller use of midwives in all of those countries, including a remarkable commitment to change childbirth throughout the United Kingdom, are experienced by women here. Many American women want a normal, fully experienced, self-empowering birth. Many who want that cannot implement their choice. The physical improvements that have been made in the maternity units of many American hospitals are important. Many women have access to private labor rooms. Most women are allowed to have a person of their choice with them throughout the birth experience. Some women labor and deliver in the same bed. More hospitals are providing time for women to hold their babies immediately after childbirth. Yet access to midwifery care is very limited.

The United States has relatively few midwives. That is related in part to national priorities for funding the training of various kinds of health professionals. In addition, significant barriers make it hard or impossible for some midwives to practice and make it hard or impossible for some women who want midwifery care to have it. Lack of access to midwifery care is becoming a greater concern as larger and larger proportions of Americans are enrolled in managed care organizations. A fundamental characteristic of managed health care is that subscribers must obtain all of their care from a limited group of care providers. Our health care system is undergoing significant change; many if not most of us may have to accept some restrictions in our health care choices. But expecting women to choose between a limited number of physicians or a limited number of midwives is one thing. Expecting women who want a midwife to accept a physician (or vice versa) is a restriction of choice that is of a different order.

The laws of Austria and Germany require a midwife to be present at every birth. The plan for improving maternity care in Britain calls for every pregnant woman to have a "named midwife," whom she can count on for advice, support, and care throughout her pregnancy. A law passed in New Zealand in 1990 recognizes women's desire for informed choice in maternity care; every pregnant woman can choose whether to have a midwife, a general physician, or an obstetrician as the primary person providing her care, and she must be informed about her choices.

Midwifery care has a solid record of safety and effectiveness. It is less expensive than care provided by physicians. A woman who chooses midwifery care will receive prenatal care with a heavy emphasis on education and support for prevention of complications, promotion of optimal health during pregnancy, and preparation for childbirth, breast-feeding, and the transition to motherhood. She will be more likely to go through labor without an epidural, less likely to have many other procedures during labor, and more likely to give birth without needing forceps, vacuum extraction, or a cesarean section. She will be less likely to have an episiotomy or an extensive perineal laceration. She will receive any help needed to breast-feed her baby effectively and for as long as possible. Given the examples of other countries; given the safety, effectiveness, and benefits of midwifery care; and given the importance of the qualitative aspects of the childbearing experience to many women and families, it is wrong to deny any American woman the option of choosing to have a midwife as her primary-care provider if her pregnancy is normal.

Both options—both pregnancy care paradigms should be available to all women. Every woman should have access to a midwife *if she wants one.* And every woman should have access to an obstetrician, if she prefers an obstetrician for primary maternity care or if she needs one because of pathology or a complication. It would be good to get rid of separate care for poor women—to give all women access to the same hospitals and physicians and midwives regardless of their financial status.

I do not advocate a rigid system based on risk assessment (as in Holland) for many reasons. Most American women are accustomed to using obstetricians, and all American women should have a choice. Some women want medical care during pregnancy and would not be comfortable or satisfied with a midwife. Women who want an epidural, EFM, et cetera, should be able to have the kind of care they want. But they should make an *informed* choice. Wherever a logical, risk-based system is imposed, that is, a system in which obstetricians only take care of women with complications (like the system in Holland), referrals need to work in both directions. Women who are referred to specialist care because of a complication should be referred back to primary care when the need for a specialist has passed. And we need to avoid confusing "risk" with "pathology." Just because a woman has characteristics or conditions that are associated with a higher-than-average incidence of bad outcomes does not mean that her pregnancy is not normal or that she will experience a complication.

Women's Right to Pain Control

Labor pain was long considered God's punishment of women for the sins and weakness of Eve. But women have always wanted relief from the pain. Pain control is an issue involving women's rights, as well as concerns about safety. Suffragettes, including many women doctors, organized the National Twi-light Sleep Association in 1915 to bring the message of pain relief to ordinary women (Har-per, 1994). Dick-Read was accused of abusing women by promoting natural childbirth.

Excessive pain is cruel to the mother and can cause a physiologic reaction that slows labor and threatens the well-being of the fetus. It is a deep responsibility of anyone who provides care to women during labor to attend to their pain, to minimize components of care that increase pain, to reduce the women's experience of pain as much as possible, to help them deal with it, to not allow them to be overwhelmed by pain. Use of methods to relieve pain play a vital role in the care of women during childbirth, regardless of who provides that care and the childbirth paradigm that is being followed. As with other aspects of the ongoing dialectic between the midwifery and medical approaches to childbirth, especially the use of technical interventions during births that are presumed to be normal, the issue is not that some interventions are bad and should never be used. The argument revolves around the circumstances in which it is appropriate to use specific interventions. Regarding pain control, the argument centers around the circumstances in which it is appropriate to use the most effective but most risky methods and the need to provide alternative measures to reduce and relieve pain, including the continuous support that any unanesthetized woman needs to cope with labor pain.

Actualization of women's rights as human beings must include giving them access to accurate information and realistic choices. All women should come to labor knowing about available methods of pain control, should have access to a variety of safe and effective methods, and should be able to exercise choice regarding what methods are used for them. Currently most pregnant women in this country do not have full and complete information about the effectiveness, limitations, side effects, and potential complications of epidurals. Nor do they have an adequate understanding of the nature of childbirth and the experiences of women who give birth without anesthesia but have the constant support of a midwife or doula. Nor can most American women realistically believe that they will receive intensive support and alternative methods of pain control if they choose to forego an epidural. In some hospitals, anesthesiologists enter the rooms in which women are laboring, often without a nurse to support them, and offer the women an epidural as a way out of pain. Making that offer at that time, under those conditions, may make it hard for a woman to resist. There is a place for epidural anesthesia—a need for it, as for all of the obstetric procedures that are identified in this book as being used too commonly. The issue is whether it is medically wise, cost effective, and ethical to offer the most risky method while withholding an important alternative.

The obstetricians who conducted the first randomized trial of epidural anesthesia stopped the trial because it is not ethical to assign women to a treatment that substantially increases the likelihood that they will require major abdominal surgery. Likewise, it is not ethical to fail to fully inform women of the many effects of epidural anesthesia on labor, including substantial increases in the need for cesarean sections and use of forceps or vacuum extraction to deliver babies. Nor is it ethical to offer women epidural anesthesia while not offering to provide them with the constant support of a skilled midwife, nurse, or doula.

Opportunities to Reduce the Long-Term Cost of Health Care

Enormous costs accrue from failure to prevent unintended pregnancies and births and preterm labor and low birth weight. Excessive numbers of cesarean sections cost more than $1.3 billion per year. Although no one has estimated the costs required to treat infants for problems caused by infections that spread through newborn nurseries, lack of

breast-feeding, poor bonding between the mother and her infant, and inadequate mothering during the baby's first year of life, we know that the costs are high. In addition, these are among our most important health problems and the cause of our high infant mortality rate. Reducing these problems— the source of so much unnecessary cost and damage—should be the major goal of changes to increase the cost effectiveness of the care provided to pregnant women. Accountant-driven administrators who focus on reducing the cost of the care should keep these goals in mind. It is folly to focus on reducing costs if the cost reductions compromise our ability to achieve these goals. The instability of the system during the past few years has made it hard for administrators to focus on long-term cost effectiveness. But even when people change from one system to another fairly rapidly, cost effectiveness, as well as every other value, demands that we organize maternal health care around reducing these problems. A health care service organized to reduce the long-term cost of providing care to pregnant women and young children would try to achieve the following:

- Educate adolescents about sex, sexuality, pregnancy, and sexually transmitted diseases.
- Provide sexuality and family planning counseling and contraceptive methods to sexually active women (and girls) who do not want to become pregnant. Provide ongoing clinical and personal support to women who are using a method of contraception. Provide abortion services as needed.
- Provide the best possible prenatal care, focusing on aspects of care that reduce the risk of low birth weight, including prompt identification and treatment of infections and helping women deal with smoking, nutrition, drug use, and stress. This kind of care takes time. Truly cost-effective care of high-risk women cannot

be achieved through brief, perfunctory prenatal visits. Women who miss appointments need follow-up, sometimes including home visits.

- Avoid unnecessary use of labor and delivery interventions that increase costs, complications, cesarean sections, and post-delivery morbidity.
- Promote mother–baby bonding and breast-feeding to reduce infant and child morbidity. Promote rooming-in as the standard of care to prevent newborn infections and promote breast-feeding and mother–baby bonding.
- Provide care that informs, strengthens, encourages, and supports the pregnant woman and mother.

Trying to save money by providing less than the most effective care is short sighted, even if you are only focusing on money. If you are focusing on the well-being of children, families, and society, saving money by providing less effective maternity care is indefensible. It is peculiar that health service administrators allow the wasteful use of expensive high-tech labor and delivery care while putting pressure on midwives to spend less time than they deem necessary with some women during prenatal care.

Training of Physicians, Midwives, Nurses, and Doulas

Much has changed since the 1991 Macy Foundation conference on the future of obstetrics and gynecology. Increased Medicaid payments for obstetric care and the musical-chairs effect of managed care have provided the incentives necessary for ob-gyns to provide care to women who are poor. The concern has shifted away from lack of access to care, at least for women who are on Medicaid, although lack of access to care continues to be a problem for women in rural areas. However, the number of both family physicians and nurse-midwives is increasing more quickly than was predicted in 1991. Nurse-midwives took the shortage of mater-

nity care providers during the late 1980s very seriously, set a goal of producing 10,000 nurse-midwives by the year 2001, and greatly increased their ability to educate nurse-midwives efficiently. Although these changes are in the right direction, the United States is not now in a position to make midwifery care available to all women, to offer skilled labor support to every woman during childbirth, or to provide the most effective kind of culturally sensitive, family- and woman-centered care to all of the country's socioeconomically high-risk prospective mothers. We have many obstetricians, many labor-and-delivery-room nurses, too few family physicians, relatively few midwives, and almost no doulas. Implementation of any of the changes recommended in this chapter has implications for the training of all of these categories of health care workers.

The American College of Obstetricians and Gynecologists has taken the position that ob-gyns are primary-care providers. But the logic of the recommendations made during the Macy Foundation conference remains: Ob-gyns are surgically trained specialists. In a logical, cost-effective system, their role as primary-care providers should diminish. Fewer should be trained. This recommendation is consistent with the analysis made by the Pew Health Professions Commission, which found that there are more medical specialists than needed and too few nurse practitioners, nurse-midwives, and physician assistants.

More midwives are needed. Many nurses want to become midwives, and the profession has developed more efficient training programs. Now the biggest constraint to preparing more nurse-midwives is financial support for nurse-midwifery education. Federal funds to support nurse-midwifery education are inadequate and very vulnerable at a time when there is a major bipartisan effort to cut the federal budget. State budgets are in the same situation. The 1995 report by the Pew Health Professions Commission called for funding medical education by creating a public–private payment pool tied to health care insurance premiums. The American Association of Medical Colleges and the American Medical Association support that idea. The Institute of Medicine has issued a report that calls for all public and private health care payers to help finance the training of health professionals. Health care services are the beneficiaries of the training of health professionals and should support their education. However, this is not likely to occur without federal legislation (Monroe, 1996). Funding for the education of nurse-midwives should be included in any laws that are proposed and any plans that are made to create a new, more stable mechanism for the training of physicians.

Funding of direct-entry midwifery education should be studied and acted on, although it is more problematic than the funding of nurse-midwifery education. In part, this is because the legal status, education, and role of direct-entry midwives varies greatly from state to state. Some states already provide some financial support for direct-entry midwifery education. This should be considered in other states where direct-entry midwives are licensed and help to increase access to maternity care. But funding of direct-entry midwifery education should not be linked to funding for nurse-midwifery education.

Physicians will always play an important role in the care of pregnant women in the United States, both as primary-care providers and as the specialists who collaborate with the primary-care providers. Nurse-midwives currently play important roles in teaching medical students about the care required by women who are having normal pregnancies. Their role in basic medical education should be expanded, and they should play a larger role in the training of family physicians and obstetrician–gynecologists. Chapter 10 included information about a study of differences in the obstetric care provided to low-risk women in Washington State by ob-gyns, family physicians, and nurse-midwives. The study was conducted by members of the Department of Family Medicine at the University of Washington School of Medicine. The paper reporting that study ended with a discussion of the policy implications of the findings from that and other studies: "Taken in its totality, this body of knowledge suggests that the approach to low-risk obstetrics as used in the real world by midwives has significant advantages for patients" (Rosenblatt *et al.*, 1997). The authors suggested that the application of this knowledge should be extended "by expanding the proportion of deliveries attended by midwives or by transferring some of the skills and philosophy that undergird midwifery to the physicians who practice obstetrics." Both need to be done.

In addition, it is important that physicians understand the role of midwifery. Physicians have enormous power and influence throughout the health care system. Family physicians, midwives, nurses, and obstetricians must be able to work together; they do it much better if they learn about each other's role and how to work together while each is learning his or her own role, that is, while they are in school. Physicians training to become family physicians, obstetrician-gynecologists, or pediatricians should learn about midwifery in general and should have opportunities to collaborate with midwives at some time during their residencies. The message about midwives that is being given to young family physicians at this point is particularly confusing. The American Academy of Family Physicians (AAFP) has maintained an anti-midwife position since 1980, when it issued a formal statement that opposed licensure for nurse-midwives, asserting that "the use of nurse-midwives is not in the best interests of quality patient care," and implied that midwifery should be abolished (see Chapter 5). In the light of massive evidence to the contrary, including the study and recommendation cited earlier (from the family medicine department that has been rated as the best in the nation), the AAFP should retract its outdated position and replace it with a statement on how family physicians and midwives can collaborate more effectively to meet the needs of the women and families they serve.

Labor-and-delivery-room nurses need to be better prepared and motivated to provide effective support and assistance to women during labor, including use of nonpharmacologic methods of pain relief. Nurse-midwives and nurse-midwifery education programs and direct-entry midwives and direct-entry midwifery education programs are potential resources for improving this aspect of the training of nurses—in undergraduate nursing education as well as in-service and continuing education. The Seattle Midwifery School, for example, currently operates a four-day labor-support course for childbearing women and couples, midwives, physicians, and nurses.

America needs doulas. Many more doulas are needed. Experience in childbirth education is a prerequisite for admission to a doula training program. Likewise, experience as a doula is valuable for individuals interested in becoming direct-entry midwives. Thus training and service as a doula may be a rung on a career ladder that leads to midwifery. Doulas of North America offers a certification program for doulas and information on workshops for the training of doulas. The Seattle Midwifery School operates doula training programs and a program for training childbirth educators as doula trainers.

In the paper he presented during the 1991 Macy Foundation conference on the future of obstetrics and gynecology, the executive director of ACOG proposed a recommendation that would have called for the preparation of a systematic report on the personnel needed to provide women's health care (Pearse, 1993). He suggested that such a report should be made every three years, and that it should be the responsibility of ACOG's Liaison Committee for Obstetrics and Gynecology. Although the conference did not make this recommendation, there *is* a need for periodic analysis of the human resources needed to provide health care to women, especially women of reproductive age. However, responsibility for conducting such studies should not reside in any organization that is affiliated with or dominated by ACOG, the ACNM, or the AAFP.

Recommendations Regarding Birth Centers and Home Births

ACOG has maintained a rigid position in opposition to the use of free-standing birth centers. ACOG's position states that the use of birth centers is discouraged until data are available to prove that care in birth centers is as safe as care in hospitals. There had been no adequate study of the safety of care in free-standing birth centers when ACOG developed this position. The organization's position on the subject has remained almost unchanged despite publication of the results of the National Birth Center Study in 1989. Although it was not a randomized, controlled trial, it provided sub-stantial evidence that well-managed birth cen-ters offer a safe alternative to hospital care for selected women. In 1982 a committee convened by the Institute of Medicine concluded that it would probably be impossible to conduct a large randomized trial of out-of-hospital births in the United States and urged investigators to use other research designs to provide information about the relative safety of birth in various birth sites (Institute of Medicine, 1982). The Institute of Medicine committee also noted that there is no conclusive evidence that births in hospitals are safer.

A lot can be learned from a noncontrolled study. In this case, the study was extremely large and included the majority of all birth centers in operation throughout the United States during the period of data collection. It was a prospective study and adhered to the highest research standards; the validity and reliability of the data were established; and there was very good follow-up of the women and infants who had been transferred to hospitals during or soon after labor and delivery. Lack of follow-up is the Achilles heel of many studies of out-of-hospital births.

The outcomes were compared with outcomes from five large studies of low-risk births in hospitals. In some of the comparison studies the "low-risk" group excluded women who exhibited no evidence of complications when they were admitted to the hospital labor-and-delivery suite if they experienced complications such as meconium and fetal distress during labor. Thus the women in most of the comparison studies were highly selected—much lower risk than the women in the birth center study. Yet outcomes from the birth center study were similar to the outcomes for these studies—several of which were based on care provided in the nation's leading academic medical centers. Outcomes from the birth center study were better than outcomes from studies that included a wider range of hospitals.

ACOG recently took the position of encouraging randomized trials of the safety of birth centers, while maintaining its opposition to the use of birth centers until the results of such trials are available. This action makes it appear as though the organization's opposition to birth centers is based on having a high standard for requiring scientific evidence as a basis for changes in practice. Given the strength of the evidence that birth center care can be safe, the lack of evidence for the safety and efficacy of many procedures that are in frequent use in obstetric departments throughout the nation, and the improbability of finding adequate numbers of women who would enter a study in which their birth site was determined randomly, ACOG's continued opposition pending evidence from a randomized trial is unreasonable. ACOG and the American Academy of Pediatrics (AAP) should reconsider their position on the use of free-standing birth centers. (The AAP and ACOG are joint authors of *Guidelines for Perinatal Care*, a periodically revised publication that presents the joint policies of both organizations on matters related to the care of pregnant women and newborns.)

Managed care organizations should become informed about birth centers. The Na-

tional Association of Childbearing Centers can provide extensive data about the safety and outcomes of birth center care, the financial savings associated with birth centers, national accreditation, state licensing regulations, and quality assurance. Workshops designed to explain the process of assessing the feasibility of starting a birth center are available.

The persistently low rate of planned out-of-hospital births raises questions about the viability and importance of both birth centers and home births. If very few women want to give birth in these settings, why should any action be taken to make them safer (e.g., by making it easier for direct-entry midwives to obtain medical backup) or to make them more accessible (e.g., by including them in more third-party health care financing plans)? Although there has been relatively little research on American women's preferences for childbirth care, most studies have found that the proportion of women who would like to give birth at home or in a free-standing birth center is significantly larger than the proportion who actually do so. The percent of home births attended by direct-entry midwives is much higher than the national rate in some communities, and a 1995 survey of members of the largest HMO in Washington state found that 8 percent of reproductive-age women were interested in the idea of a midwife-attended home birth and might choose that option if the cooperative would provide the same benefits for a home birth that it provides for a birth in one of the HMO hospitals.

Based on findings from that survey, home births attended by licensed direct-entry midwives (LMs) became available to members of the Group Health Cooperative of Washington in 1996. Each unit of the cooperative has agreed to contract with some LMs in its geographic area. To be eligible for a contract, a midwife must be licensed by the state and have professional liability insurance (available through a joint underwriting agreement).

She must participate in a quality assurance program to qualify for the insurance. The obstetrics departments of local Group Health hospitals provide the medical backup. All of these components—licensure based on education and examination, coverage by third-party payers, professional liability insurance, participation in a quality assurance program, and medical backup—need to be in place for any latent demand for home births to materialize. Until they are in place, we do not know what proportion of American women might want to use this kind of service. It is impossible to estimate the potential demand for a new service until the service is available and people know about it. Although the number of women using home birth services at this time is small, most women who have home births are ardent about this choice.

There are many possibilities for improving home births that are part of a well-organized health care system. The Group Health Cooperative of Washington's experience with LM attended home births should be carefully documented and studied from several perspectives, including pregnancy outcomes; patient satisfaction; costs; interdisciplinary working relationships between LMs and the doctors and nurses who work for Group Health; effects, if any, on marketing of Group Health within Washington's competitive health care environment; and any other impacts on the cooperative. Results from this analysis should be published in order to make the information available within the health care community.

The Possibility of Achieving These Recommendations

Several groups have called for midwifery to become the predominant paradigm for the care of pregnant women in the United States. My own recommendations call for midwifery care to be available to all women, for all women to be offered continuous personal support by a skilled person through-

out labor and delivery, and for the objectives of maternity care to be expanded, regardless of who provides the care. This section looks at major opportunities, as well as barriers to making these changes.

Potential Positive Effects of Managed Health Care

Managed care is the bull in the china shop right now. The move to managed care has resulted in termination of many special programs that used nurse-midwives to provide care to pregnant women with special needs, for example, programs for pregnant women who are members of migrant agricultural communities in some parts of the West. Many of these programs were developed during the late 1980s and early 1990s in response to a sense of crisis about lack of care for some groups of high-risk women and to high-level recommendations that the nation make better use of nurse-midwives to meet those needs. Some physicians who supported the development of nurse-midwifery services as a way to provide care to indigent women now see midwives as financial competitors and have withdrawn their support. A nurse-midwifery service cannot continue without medical collaboration. The effect on nurse-midwives has been severe because they play a large role in the care of indigent women. However, there has also been an effect on midwives in private practice. The dynamics of managed care work to aggregate health care resources into large systems that can contract for the care of large groups of people. The day of the solo practitioner or small partnership may be a thing of the past, for both midwives and physicians. Yet there is public demand for people to retain some degree of choice within these systems.

The move to managed care was motivated by the desire to improve access to care and reduce unnecessary costs. The hope for reducing costs relies in part on mechanisms to prevent the use of unnecessary care—to make health care more cost-effective. We can only hope that at the end of the period of turmoil, when the system settles down, those objectives will become predominant. Improving access to care and reducing unnecessary use of costly labor and delivery procedures would benefit America's mothers and babies. Midwifery fits into the picture perfectly. Many procedures that used to be done in hospitals have been moved into less expensive ambulatory-care settings located close to residential communities. Birth centers fit this model and produce extraordinary cost savings while reducing the rate of cesarean sections and providing care that is extremely satisfying to women and families. Managed care organizations will wake up to this some day. Managed care organizations are supposed to compete with one another at the local level; if they do they will become sensitive to factors that attract subscribers. Midwives are a draw for many women; lack of access to midwifery care is a negative. We should expect managed care organizations to become increasingly interested in measures of patient satisfaction. Midwifery care leads to very high levels of patient satisfaction.

In addition, the movement of poor women into private medical practices is creating a need for midwives in some of those practices. In 1995, the *American Journal of Obstetrics and Gynecology* published a paper that compared outcomes for low-income uninsured and underinsured women whose care was provided by nurse-midwives with outcomes for private patients whose care was provided by a group of ob-gyns. The ob-gyns who provided care to the private patients supervised and provided medical collaboration for the nurse-midwifery service. The private obstetricians were impressed that the outcomes for the medically indigent women were equal to those of their private patients, and the cesarean section rate for the indigent women was only half of the private-patient rate (Blanchette, 1995). The physicians attributed these excellent outcomes to "the effectiveness of midwives with good obstetric backup to manage complicated patients and

effect the compliance and behavior modification necessary to match the fetal outcomes of the private patients." Many private physicians in North Carolina have hired nurse-midwives in order to both take advantage of and cope with the large number of Medicaid-eligible women now seeking private care (Matyac, 1996).

Managed care systems place heavy reliance on primary care and need good teamwork to facilitate coordination of services between the primary and referral levels. Nurse-midwives have always worked with physicians in this model. Nurse-midwives have had a long, successful experience with HMOs. Nurse-midwifery care provided in these settings results in lower costs and high levels of patient satisfaction (Bell & Mills, 1989).

The move to managed care may provide an opportunity to redesign maternity care. Ideally, primary maternity care provided by midwives and primary care physicians and specialist care provided by obstetricians should be integrated into logically designed health care systems that emphasize primary care while providing access to specialist care to every woman in the system.

Barriers to Change

There are many barriers to moving maternity care in the United States toward the models provided by our "peer countries," in which virtually every pregnant woman has access to both midwifery and obstetrics. The most important barriers were discussed in the section on the dominance of the medical model. Additional barriers flow from the power of the status quo, the structure of our health care system, and the distribution of authority within the system.

The midwifery profession in the United States is relatively small, can only grow at a certain rate, and has not had a central role in maternity care in this country. In contrast, we have many experienced labor-and-delivery-room nurses and many ob-gyns. Although it seems circular to mention these factors as barriers, they are. If we were talking about politics, we would say that the medical paradigm has the advantage of incumbency.

If you go into any maternity unit in England, you will find midwifery. Its absence would be as strange as having a hospital without a kitchen; midwifery has an essential role. During the 1980s, its role weakened; now it is blossoming and advancing. But there was never a question about continuation of the role. Midwives in the United States do not have that security. A great deal of the energy of American midwives has always been directed toward creating, protecting and expanding a place for midwifery in a system in which it is not understood and is not thought to be essential. American midwifery has been enormously creative despite this burden, but there have been significant costs. Midwives in New Zealand used a period of significant change in their health care system to create new ways to provide continuity of care. During the same period, upheaval in the U.S. health care system required American midwives to focus on the struggle to survive. Although the move to managed care has been stressful for everyone in health care, there is no doubt that medicine will be part of every iteration of the evolving system. There *is* doubt about continuation of midwifery in the reconstructed, downsized versions of some local health care systems that have relied on CNMs for years. Midwifery is still seen as an alternative, an option, not a core component.

Every other developed country provides access to essential health care to all of its citizens, either through a national health insurance program or a national health care service. The lack of a national health service has allowed for pluralism in the U.S. health care system. That pluralism has made it possible to create and test new and different health care models, which may explain why free-standing birth centers, now becoming popular in other countries, were developed here first. But it is extremely difficult to mandate any kind of rapid change throughout the American health care "system," which is not really a system. The British National Health System has to respond to recommendations in a parliamentary report. There is no similar way to gain leverage on the American health care system. Health care policies in the United States are regulated by the laws of the federal government and the fifty states (plus the District of Columbia), and policies made by a large number of nongovernmental organizations and institutions. All levels of decision making are guided by judgments that are made by professionals, mainly physicians, who are expected to base their policy decisions on objective evidence (i.e., research) and act on behalf of society. American obstetricians have been selective in which research they respond to.

Seeking Complementarity

These recommendations and this book are not intended to disparage obstetrics or obstetricians. Obstetrician–gynecologists conducted most of the research that created the knowledge that sup-ports the changes that many groups are calling for. Individual obstetricians have always been among the leading wedge of people who have understood the damage and loss in-curred by treating normal pregnancy as though it were an illness. Obstetric leaders have been on the boards of the critical organizations and have supported and helped midwives. The changes that need to be supported and prepared for are not about midwives versus obstetricians. They are about what American women and babies and families and society need to support and facilitate and enhance normal childbearing and the transitions and important experiences that occur during pregnancy and during and after the experience of giving birth. The knowledge and skills of obstetricians are essential and must be available to all pregnant women—essential, but not sufficient.

America's competitive health care system has accentuated the competitive aspect of the medical/midwifery relationship. We need, instead, to accentuate their complementarity. We need to package the benefits of midwifery with those of medicine. No American mother should have to sacrifice one to have the other. The ideal approach is for professional midwives, family physicians, obstetrician–gynecologists and other health professionals to collaborate in reproductive health care teams that offer women and their families access to all of the services they need.

References

Abernathy TJ, Lentjes DM. Planned and Unplanned Home Births and Hospital Births in Calgary, Alberta, 1984–1987. *Pub Health Reports*. 1989;104(4):373–377.

AbouZahr C, Royston E. *Maternal Mortality: A Global Factbook*. World Health Organization, Geneva, 1991.

Abraham-Van der Mark E. Dutch midwifery, past and present: An overview. In Abraham-Van der Mark E. (Ed.), *Successful Home Birth and Midwifery: The Dutch Model*. Bergin & Garvey, London, 1993a, pp. 141–160.

Abraham-Van der Mark E. Introduction to the Dutch system of home birth and midwifery. In Abraham-Van der Mark E. (Ed.), *Successful Home Birth and Midwifery: The Dutch Model*. Bergin & Garvey, London, 1993b, pp. 1–17.

Acheson LS, Harris SE, Zyzanski SH. *Patient selection and outcomes for out-of-hospital births in one family practice. J Fam Prac* 1990;31: 128–36.

Ackerman D. The power of touch. *Parade Magazine*, March 25, 1990, pp. 4–5.

ACNM Certification Council, Inc. The National Certification Examination in Nurse-Midwifery: History of the modified-essay form. Author, Landover, MD, 1996.

ACNM Education Committee. Core competencies in nurse-midwifery: Expected outcomes of nurse-midwifery education. *J Nurse Midwifery* 1979;24(1):32–36.

Adair H, Harvey R, Jordan S, Lawson B, Harris P. Victoria. In McDonald W, Davis JA (Eds.), *History of Midwifery Practice in Australia and the Western Pacific Regions*. Western Australian Branch of the National Midwives Association of Australia, Perth, 1984, pp. 31–44. (Book prepared for the 20th Congress of the International Confederation of Midwives.)

Adams C. *Nurse-Midwifery in the United States: 1982*. ACNM, Washington, DC, 1984.

Adams C. *American Nurse-Midwifery: 1987*. ACNM, Washington, DC, 1989.

Adams JL. The use of obstetrical procedures in the care of low-risk women. *Women & Health* 1983;8:25-34.

Alan Guttmacher Institute. *11 Million Teenagers: What Can Be Done About the Epidemic of Adolescent Pregnancies in the United States?* Planned Parenthood Federation of America, New York, 1976.

Allen DI, Kamradt JM. Relationship of infant mortality to the availability of obstetrical care in Indiana. *J Fam Pract* 1991;33:609–613.

Alliance for Health Reform. News release: Alliance launches project promoting primary care. Author, Washington, DC, December 21, 1992.

Allison, J. Personal communication, May 1994. (Julia Allison was General Secretary of the Royal College of Midwives, London, England.)

Altemus M, Deuster PA, Galliven E, Carter CS, Gold PW. Suppression of hypothalamic-pituitary-adrenal axis responses to stress in lactating women. *J Clin Endocrin Metab* 1995;80: 2954–2959.

Amato JC. Fetal monitoring in a community hospital: A statistical analysis. *Obstet Gynecol* 1977; 50:269–274.

American Academy of Family Physicians. Professional liability study. Author, Kansas City, MO, 1986.

American Academy of Family Physicians. 1993–1994 compendium of AAFP positions on selected health issues. Author, Kansas City, MO, 1993.

American Academy of Family Physicians. AAFP facts about family practice, 1980–1991, and data resulting from annual surveys of family practice residency programs. Author, Kansas City, MO, 1994.

American Academy of Pediatrics and American College of Obstetricians and Gynecologists. *Guidelines for Perinatal Care*. Authors, Chicago and Washington, DC, 1983.

American Academy of Physician Assistants. General census data on physician assistants, 1993. Author, Alexandria, VA, 1993.

American College of Nurse-Midwives. Statement on home birth. Author, Washington, DC, 1971.

American College of Nurse-Midwives. Statement on home birth. Author, Washington, DC, 1976.

American College of Nurse-Midwives. Statement on practice settings. Author, Washington, DC, 1980.

American College of Nurse-Midwives. Certified nurse-midwives as primary care providers. Author, Washington, DC, October 31, 1992a.

American College of Nurse-Midwives. Expansion of nurse-midwifery practice and skills beyond basic core competencies. Author, Washington, DC, July 27, 1992b.

American College of Nurse-Midwives. Guidelines for the incorporation of new procedures into nurse-midwifery practice. Author, Washington, DC, November 1, 1992c.

American College of Nurse-Midwives. Standards for the practice of nurse-midwifery. Author, Washington, DC, 1993.

American College of Nurse-Midwives, American College of Obstetricians and Gynecologists, and Nurses Association of the American College of Obstetricians and Gynecologists. Joint statement on maternity care. Authors, Washington, DC, 1971.

American College of Obstetricians and Gynecologists. News release: Health department data shows danger of home births. Author, Chicago, January 4, 1978.

American College of Obstetricians and Gynecologists. Guidelines for vaginal delivery after a cesarean childbirth. Statement of the ACOG Committee on Obstetrics: Maternal and Fetal Medicine. Author, Washington, DC, 1982.

American College of Obstetricians and Gynecologists. Professional liability and its effects: Report of a 1987 survey of ACOG's membership. Opinion Research Corporation, Washington, DC, 1988.

American College of Obstetricians and Gynecologists. News report. *Birth* 1993;20(1):48. (Report based on data from an ACOG study.)

American College of Obstetricians and Gynecologists. The obstetrician-gynecologist: Primary care physician. Author, Washington, DC, 1994.

American College of Obstetricians and Gynecologists. Guidelines for implementing collaborative practice. Author, Washington, DC, 1995.

American College of Obstetricians and Gynecologists and American College of Nurse-Midwives. Joint statement of practice relationships between obstetricians and certified nurse-midwives. Authors, Washington, DC, November 1, 1982.

Anderson, R, Greener D. A descriptive analysis of home births attended by CNMs in two nurse-midwifery services. *J Nurse Midwifery* 1991; 36:95–103.

Anderson RE, Murphy PA. Outcomes of 11,788 planned home births attended by certified nurse-midwives: A retrospective descriptive study. *J Nurse Midwifery* 1995;40:483–492.

Andrews CM, O'Neil LM. Use of pelvic tilt exercise for ligament pain relief. *J Nurse Midwifery* 1994;39:370–374.

Andrulis DP, Acuff KL, Weiss KB, Anderson RJ. Public hospitals and health care reform:

Choices and Challenges. *Am J Public Health* 1996;86:162–165.

Angier N. Illuminating how bodies are built for sociability. *The New York Times,* April 30, 1996, pp. B5, B8.

Anisfeld E, Lipper E. Early contact, social support, and mother-infant bonding. *Pediatrics* 1983;72:79–83.

Anonymous editorial. Midwives of the future. *The Lancet* 1987;1(8534):664.

Arms S. *Immaculate Deception.* Houghton-Mifflin, Boston, 1975.

Armstrong P, Feldman S. *A Midwife's Story.* Ivy Books, New York, 1986.

Armstrong P, Feldman S. *A Wise Birth.* William Morrow and Company, New York, 1990.

Arthure H. The midwife—in Simpson's time and ours. *Br J Obstet Gynecol* 1973;80:1–9.

Avery GB. Editorial: Out of the vortex—neonatologists' treatment decisions for newborns at risk of HIV. *Am J Public Health* 1995; 85:1434–11450.

Avery MD, DelGiudice GT. High-tech skills in low-tech hands: Issues of advanced practice and collaborative management. *J Nurse Midwifery* March/April 1993;38 (Suppl):9S–17S.

Axelrod J. Personal communication, 1994. (Joan Axelrod is Conseillère en Services Ambulatoires, Unité due Financement Substitutif, Ministère de la Santé, Ontario.)

Bailey PP. The role of the Federal Trade Commission. In Rooks J, Haas JE (Eds.), *Nurse-Midwifery in America.* ACNM Foundation, Washington, DC, 1986, pp. 76–78.

Baldwin LM, Hutchinson HL, Rosenblatt RA. Professional relationships between midwives and physicians: Collaboration or conflict? *Am J Public Health* 1992;82:262–264.

Baldwin LM, Raine R, Jenkins LD, Hart LG, Rosenblatt R. Do providers adhere to ACOG standards? The case of prenatal care. *Obstet Gynecol* 1994;84:549–556.

Baldwin R. *Special Delivery.* IBP Books, Ann Arbor, MI, 1986.

Banta HD, Thacker SB. *Costs and Benefits of Electronic Fetal Monitoring: A Review of the Literature.* National Center for Health Services Research, U.S. Department of Health, Education and Welfare, Washington, DC, 1979. DHEW Publication 79-3245.

Barasch DS. The mainstreaming of alternative medicine. *The New York Times Magazine,* Part 2, October 4, 1992.

Barickman C, Bidgood-Wilson M, Ackley S. Nurse-midwifery today: A legislative update, Part II. *J Nurse Midwifery* 1992;37:175–209.

Barnard K. The quiet crisis. *Outlook,* Fall 1994; 7(3). (Published by the Center on Human Development and Disability, University of Washington, Seattle.)

Barnes AC. Training programs for the nurse-midwife in the United States. In *The Midwife in the United States: Report of a Macy Conference.* Josiah Macy, Jr. Foundation, New York, 1968, pp. 41–44.

Barnes CR. Primary concepts embodied in the "Philosophy of the American College of Nurse-Midwives." Paper submitted for a course at the Community-based Nurse-midwifery Education Program, Frontier School of Midwifery and Family Nursing, Hyden, Kentucky, October 1994.

Bartman BA, Weiss KB. Women's primary care in the United States: A Study of practice variation among physician specialties. *J Women Health* 1993;2:261–268.

Bastian H. Confined, managed and delivered: The language of obstetrics: *Brit J Obstet Gynaecol* 1992;99:9203.

Bastian H, Lancaster PAL. Home births in Australia 1988–1990. Sydney: *AIHW National Perinatal Statistic Unit and Homebirth Australia,* 1992.

Bastick T. *Intuition: How We Think and Act.* Wiley, New York, 1982.

Bayes M. The Midwife in the United Kingdom and a Report on "Maternity Care in the World." In *The Midwife in the United States: Report of a Macy Conference.* Josiah Macy, Jr. Foundation, New York, 1968, pp. 117–127.

Beal J. Nurse-midwifery intrapartum management. *J Nurse Midwifery* 1984;29:13–19.

Beauchamp N. Study groups and apprenticeship: One model of midwifery education. *Midwifery Today,* Spring 1992;21:32.

Beck LM. The nurse-midwife. *Clin Obstet Gynecol* 1972;15(2):357–369.

Becker E, Long M, Stamler V, Sallomi P. *Midwifery and the Law.* Peggy O'Mara; Santa Fe, NM, 1990.

Beebe JE. The passing of a friend—The realization of a vision: Mary Irene Crawford, C.N.M., Ed. D., in Memoriam. *J Nurse Midwifery* 1979; 24(5):37–38.

Beebe J. Initiation and maintenance of clinical learning sites in nurse-midwifery. *J Nurse Midwifery* 1980;25(1):29–32.

Beeman R. Personal communication, January 4, 1994. (Ruth Beeman is a retired nurse–midwife educator.)

Behrmann B. Witch hunt. *The Ithaca Times,* June 20–26, 1996, pp. 6, 10–12.

Belenky MF, Clinchy BM, Goldberger NR, Tarule JM. *Women's Ways of Knowing: The Development of Self, Voice and Mind.* Basic Books, New York, 1986.

Bell KE, Mills JI. Certified nurse-midwives' effectiveness in the health maintenance organization obstetric team. *Obstet Gynecol* 1989;74: 112–116.

Benner P. *From Novice to Expert: Excellence and Power in Clinical Nursing Practice.* Addison-Wesley, Menlo Park, CA, 1984.

Bennetts AB, Lubic RW. The free-standing birth centre. *The Lancet* 1982;1:378–380.

Benoit C. Personal communication, 1997. (Cecilia Benoit is associate professor in the Department of Sociology at the University of Victoria, Victoria, British Columbia.)

Benoit C, Wrede S, MacLean-Alley B. The midwifery knowledge debate in three countries: Life-world versus scientific ways of knowing. Paper presented during the Annual Joint Meeting of the Society for Applied Anthropology, the Society for Medical Anthropology, the Council on Nursing and Anthropology, and the Political Ecology Society, Seattle, Washington, March 6, 1997.

Benson RC, Berendes H, Weiss W. Fetal compromise during elective cesarean section II: A report from the Collaborative Project. *Am J Obstet Gynecol* 1969;105:579–586.

Bidgood-Wilson M. The legislative status of nurse-midwivery: Trends and future implications. *J Nurse Midwifery* 1992;37:159–160.

Bidgood-Wilson M, Barickman C, Ackley S. Nurse-midwifery today: A legislative update, Part I. *J Nurse Midwifery* 1992;37:96–140.

Biggs L. Caught between a rock and a hard place: Reflections of a social scientist involved in the development of midwifery policy. Paper prepared for the Annual Joint Meeting of the Society for Applied Anthropology, the Society for Medical Anthropology, the Council on Nursing and Anthropology, and the Political Ecology Society, Seattle, Washington, March 6, 1997.

Bing ED. Catch-22 in labor and delivery. *Birth Family J* 1974;1:103.

Biro M, Lumley J. The safety of team midwifery: The first decade of the Monash Birth Centre. *Med J Aust* 1991;155:478–480.

Blais R, Lambert J, Maheux B, Loiselle J, Gauthier N, Framarin A. Controversies in maternity care: Where do physicians, nurses, and midwives stand? *Birth* 1994;21:63–70.

Blanchette H. Comparison of obstetric outcome of a primary-care access clinic staffed by certified nurse-midwives and a private practice group of obstetricians in the same community. *Am J Obstet Gynecol* 1995;172:1864–871.

Booker G. A study of 461 midwife-managed births in California. California Association of Midwives, Sacramento, CA, 1991. (Unpublished study; internally produced and distributed on request.)

Borgatta L, Piening SL, Cohen WR. Association of episiotomy and delivery position with deep perineal laceration during spontaneous delivery in nulliparous women. *Am J Obstet Gynecol* 1989;160:294–297.

Borino J. Personal communication, March 21, 1996. (Jana Borino is the administrative director of the Florida School of Traditional Midwifery in Gainesville, FL.)

Borsellega J. Personal communication, 1993. (Johanna Borsellega was director of the United States Air Force Nurse-Midwifery Education Program from 1985 to 1990.)

Borst CG. Wisconsin's midwives as working women: Immigrant midwives and the limits of a traditional occupation, 1870–1920. *J Am Ethnic History* 1989;8:24–59.

Boston Women's Health Book Collective. Preface/introduction. In *The New Our Bodies, Ourselves.* Simon & Schuster, New York, 1984.

Bottoms SF, Hirsch VJ, Sokal RJ. Medical management of arrest disorders of labor: A current overview. *Am J Obstet Gynecol* 1987;156: 935–939.

Bourgeault IL. Direct entry midwifery in Ontario: Politics, professionalization and the transformation of the model of midwifery education. Paper presented during the Annual Joint Meeting of the Society for Applied Anthropology, the Society for Medical Anthropology, the Council on Nursing and Anthropology, and the Political Ecology Society, Seattle, Washington, March 6, 1997.

Bowland K. Personal communication, December 15, 1993. Kate Bowland was a member of the Birth Center of Santa Cruz.

Boyce JG. Letter to Joseph Lelyveld, executive editor of *The New York Times*, March 10, 1995.

Boylan PC. Active management of labor: Results in Dublin, Houston, London, New Brunswick, Singapore and Valparaiso. *Birth* 1989; 16:114–118.

Bradley L. Personal communication, December 10, 1996. (Lisa Bradley is vice president of Citizens for Midwifery.)

Bradsher K. As 1 million leave ranks of insured, debate heats up. *The New York Times*, August 26, 1995.

Brain M. Quoted in "Midwives want to separate from nurses." *Br Med J* 1990;301:195.

Breckinridge M. *Wide Neighborhoods: A Story of the Frontier Nursing Service*. The University Press of Kentucky, Lexington, 1981.

Brennan P. Using homepathy to turn babies. *Midwifery Today* Winter 1992–93;24:16.

Brenner WE, Edelman DA, Hendricks CH. Characteristics of patients with placenta previa and results of expectant management. *Am J Obstet Gynecol* 1978;132:180–189.

Broach J, Newton N. Food and beverages in labor. Part I: Cross-cultural and historical practices. *Birth* 1988;15:81–85.

Brodie P. Australian team midwives in transition. In *Proceedings of the International Confederation of Midwives 24th Triennial Congress*, Oslo, May 26–31, 1996, International Confederation of Midwives, London, pp. 132–135.

Brodsky A. Personal communication, December 10, 1996. (Archie Brodsky is a former president of Massachusetts Friends of Midwives, co-author of a textbook on home birth, and Research Associate in the Program on Psychiatry and the Law, Harvard Medical School, Cambridge, Massachusetts.)

Brooks T. Personal communication, March 1996. (Tonya Brooks is director of the Association for Childbirth at Home International [ACHI] and the ACHI Institute for Midwifery Studies [AIMS], Glendale, California.)

Brooten D, Roncoli M, Finkler S, Arnold L, Cohen A, Mennuti M. A randomized trial of early hospital discharge and home follow-up of women having cesarean birth. *Obstet Gynecol* 1994;84:832–883.

Brown S, Lumley J. Satisfaction with care in labor and birth: A survey of 790 Australian women. *Birth* 1994;24:4–13.

Brown SA, Grimes DE. A meta-analysis of nurse practitioners and nurse-midwives in primary care. *Nursing Res* 1995;44:332–339.

Brown SS. Drawing women into prenatal care. *Family Planning Perspectives* 1989;21(2):73–80.

Brown SS, Eisenberg L (Eds). *The Best Intentions: Unintended Pregnancy and the Well-being of Children and Families*. National Academy Press, Washington, DC, 1995.

Browne H, Isaacs G. The Frontier Nursing Service: The primary care nurse in the community hospital. *Am J Obstet Gynecol* 1976;124 (1):14–17.

Brozan N. Women gain as technology becomes part of natural birth. *The New York Times*, November 13, 1988.

Brucker MC, Muellner M. Nurse-midwivery care of adolescents. *J Nurse Midwifery* 1985;30(5): 277–279.

Bryce RL, Stanley FJ, Garner JB. Randomized controlled trial of antenatal social support to prevent preterm birth. *Br J Obstet Gynaecol* 1991; 98:1001–1008.

Buescher PA, Ward NI. A comparison of low birth weight among Medicaid patients of public health departments and other providers of prenatal care in North Carolina and Kentucky. *Public Health Reports* 1992;107:54–59.

Buhler L, Glick N, Sheps SB. Prenatal Care: A comparative evaluation of nurse-midwives and family physicians. *Can Med Assoc J* 1988;139:397–403.

Burgin K. Canadian midwifery: Travail and triump. *J Nurse Midwifery* 1994;39:1–4.

Burkhardt P. All the news that's fit? *Quickening*, March/April 1996a, pp. 4–5.

Burkhardt P. Nurse-midwifery: Advanced practice nursing? *Nursing Clin North Am* 1996b;31: 439–448.

Burkhardt P. Tortuous curves and unexpected difficulties. *Quickening*, July/August 1996c, pp. 5–6.

Burnett CA, Jones JA, Rooks J, Chong HC, Tyler C, Miller A. Home delivery and neonatal

mortality in North Carolina. *JAMA* 1980;
244:2741–2745.

Burnett JE Jr. A physician-sponsored community
nurse-midwifery program. *Am J Obstet Gynecol*
1972;40:719–723.

Burns R. New law gives moms 2-day hospital stays.
The Oregonian, September 27, 1996, p. A12.
(Copyright by the Associated Press.)

Burst HV. On the essentiality of professional mid-
wives in any good maternity plan. In Stewart
D, Stewart L (Eds.), *Compulsory Hospitaliza-
tion: Freedom of Choice in Childbirth?* National
Association for Parents & Professionals for
Safe Alternatives in Childbirth, Marble Hill,
MO, 1978, pp. 371–378.

Burst HV. Hospital practice privileges. In Rooks J,
Haas JE (Eds.), *Nurse-Midwifery in America.*
ACNM Foundation, Washington, DC, 1986,
pp. 60–63.

Burst HV. Preliminary report on committee survey regarding hospital practice privileges and
JCAH and DOD regulations. American College of Nurse-Midwives, Washington, DC,
May 5, 1987.

Burst HV. "Real" midwifery. *J Nurse Midwifery*
1990;35:189–191.

Burst HV. An update on the credentialing of midwives by the ACNM. *J Nurse Midwifery*
1995a;40:290–296.

Burst HV. DOA seeks membership response.
Quickening, September/October 1995b,
p. 22.

Burst HV. Memorandum to the ACNM membership from the chair of the Division of Accreditation. *Quickening,* January/February 1996,
p. 19.

Burt RD, Vaughan TL, Daling JR. Evaluating the
risks of cesarean section: Low Apgar score in
repeat C-section and vaginal deliveries. *Am J
Public Health* 1988;78:1312–1314.

Butler J, Abrams B, Parker J, Roberts JM, Laros RK.
Supportive nurse-midwife care is associated
with a reduced incidence of cesarean section.
Am J Obstet Gynecol 1993;168:1407–1413.

Butler NR, Alberman ED. *Perinatal Problems: The
Second Report of the 1958 British Perinatal Mortality Survey.* Churchill Livingstone, Edinburgh, 1969.

Campbell R, MacFarlane A. Place of delivery: A
review. *Br J Obstet Gynaecol* 1986;93:675–683.

Campbell R, MacFarlane A. *Where To Be Born? The
Debate and the Evidence,* 2nd ed. National Perinatal Epidemiology Unit, Oxford, 1994.

Canoodt L. Utilization and economic analysis of
the MCA's Childbearing Center: 1976–1980.
Health Affairs Research. Blue Cross and Blue
Shield of Greater New York, January 1982.

Carberry C, Carey A. Challenging boundaries: A
dynamic midwifery care model. In *Proceedings
of the International Confederation of Midwives
24th Triennial Congress,* Oslo, May 26–31,
1996, ICM, London, pp. 141–146.

Carney JK. Commissioner, State of Vermont Department of Health. Memorandum regarding Vermont non-hospital (home) birth
study, March 8, 1990; memorandum regarding additional data from the home birth
study, July 9, 1990.

Carr KC. Nurse-midwifery and family practice
physicians. In Rooks J, Haas JE (Eds.), *Nurse-
Midwifery in America.* ACNM Foundation,
Washington, DC, 1986, pp. 70–71.

Carrier D, Doray B, Stern L, Usher R. Effect of
neonatal intensive care on mortality rates in
the province of Quebec. *Ped Res* 1972;6:408.

Cawthon L, Kenny F, Schrager L. First Steps database: Characteristics of the expansion group, a
preliminary report. Office of Research & Data
Analysis, Planning, Evaluation and Professional
Development, Washington Department of Social and Health Services, January 31, 1992.

Center for Disease Control. Teenage fertility in
the United States: 1960, 1970, 1974. In *Regional and State Variation and Excess Fertility,*
Author, Atlanta, GA, February 1978.

Center for Health Economics Research. Access to
Health Care: Key Indicators for Policy. The
Robert Wood Johnson Foundation, Prince-
ton, NJ, November 1993.

Centers for Disease Control. Trends in length of
stay for hospital deliveries—United States,
1970–1992. *MMWR* 1995;44:335–337.

Chalmers B. Childbirth and breastfeeding in the
countries of central and eastern Europe. In
*Proceedings of the International Confederation of
Midwives 24th Triennial Congress,* Oslo, May
26–31, 1996, ICM, London, pp. 27–30.

Chalmers I. The perinatal research agenda:
Whose priorities? *Birth* 1991;18(3):137–141.

Chalmers I, Enkin M, Keirse MJNC. *Effective Care
in Pregnancy and Childbirth.* Oxford University
Press, New York, 1989.

Chamberlain G. The place of birth—striking a
balance. *The Practitioner* 1988;232:771–774.

Chambliss LR, Daly C, Medearis AL, Ames M,
Kayne M, Paul R. The role of selection bias in

comparing cesarean birth rates between physician and midwifery management. *Obstet Gynecol* 1992;80:161–15.

Chaney J. Birthing in early America. *J Nurse Midwifery* 1980;25(2):5–13.

Chanis M, O'Donohue N, Stanford A. Adolescent pregnancy. *J Nurse Midwifery* 1979;24(3): 18–22.

Charvet T. Letter to the editor. *J Nurse Midwifery* 1983;28(3).

Chase HC. A study of risks, medical care, and infant mortality. *Am J Public Health* September 1973;63(suppl):41–56.

Cherry J, Foster JC. Comparison of hospital charges generated by certified nurse-midwives and physician clients. *J Nurse Midwifery* 1982;27(1):7–11.

Church L. California nurse-midwives fight attorney general's opinion on episiotomies. *Quickening* September/October 1995;26(5);pp. 1, 11.

Citizens *for* Midwifery. Brochure. Citizens *for* Midwifery, Athens, GA, 1996.

Clark SL, Koonings PP, Phelan JP. Placenta previa/accreta and prior cesarean section. *Obstet Gynecol* 1985;66:89–92.

Clark-Coller T. Letter to the editor in "Mismanaged journalism: Responsible reporting in peril at *The New York Times.*" *J Nurse Midwifery* 1995;40:3009–310.

Clarke SC, Martin JA, Taffel SM. Trends and characteristics of births attended by midwives. *Statistical Bull.* Jan–Mar 1997:9–18.

Coalition for Improving Maternity Services. The mother-friendly childbirth initiative: 10 steps to mother-friendly hospitals and birth centers, 1996. Available from CIMS, c/o ASPO-LAMAZE, 1200 19th St., NW, Suite 300, Washington, DC 20036.

Cogan R, Edmunds E. The unkindest cut? *Contemp Ob/Gyn* 1977;9:55–59.

Cohen RL. A comparative study of women choosing two different childbirth alternatives. *Birth* 1982;9: 13–19.

Cohn S, Cuddihy N, Kraus N, Tom SA. Legislation and nurse-midwifery practice in the USA. *J Nurse Midwifery* 1984;29(2):57–174.

Cohn SD. Professional liability insurance and nurse-midwifery practice. In Rostow, VP, Bulger, RJ (Eds.), *Medical Professional Liability and the Delivery of Obstetrical Care,* Vol. II, *An Interdisciplinary Review,* Institute of Medicine, National Academy Press, Washington, DC, 1989, pp. 104–112.

Colby RN. Modern-day practitioners of magic arts come full circle. *The Oregonian,* October 31, 1996, p. A9.

Cole S. Choosing your lead maternity career. *Kiwi Parent,* June/July, 1996:pp. 18–20.

Collaborative Group on Preterm Birth Prevention. Multicenter randomized, controlled trial of a preterm birth prevention program. *Am J Obstet Gynecol* 1993;169:352–366.

Collea JV, Chein C, Quilligan EJ. The randomized management of term frank breech presentation: A study of 208 cases. *Am J Obstet Gyncol* 1980;137:235–244.

College of Midwives of Ontario. Clinical practice parameters & facility standards for free standing birth centres where only midwives provide primary care. Author, Toronto, Ontario, January 12, 1994.

Collins C. Initiative petition gains wide backing. *Oregon Health Forum,* March 1996, p. 3.

Committee on Perinatal Health. Toward improving the outcome of pregnancy: Recommendations for the regional development of maternal and perinatal health services. National Foundation, March of Dimes, White Plains, NY, 1976.

Commonwealth Fund. The health of American women. Commonwealth Fund survey by Louis Harris and Associates, July 1993.

Commonwealth Fund. Women's health: Choices and challenges. *The Commonwealth Fund Quarterly,* September 1996, pp. 1–2.

Conboy M. South Australia. In McDonald W, Davis JA (Eds.), *History of Midwifery Practice in Australia and the Western Pacific Regions.* Western Australian Branch of the National Midwives Association of Australia, Perth, 1984, pp. 49–60. (Book prepared for the 20th Congress of the International Confederation of Midwives.)

Connelly LM, Keele BS, Kleinbeck SVM, Schneider JK, Cobb AK. A place to be yourself: Empowerment from the client's perspective. *Image: J Nursing Scholarship* 1993;25:297–303.

Conrad PD, Wilkening RB, Rosenberg AA. Safety of newborn discharges in less than 36 hours in an indigent population. *Am J Dis Child* 1989;143:98–101.

Conway-Welch C. Assuring the quality of nurse-midwifery education: The ACNM Division of Accreditation. In Rooks J, Haas JE (Eds.),

Nurse-midwifery in America. ACNM Foundation, Washington, DC, 1986, pp. 10–13.

Corbett MA, Burst HV. Nurse-midwives and adolescents: The South Carolina experience. *J Nurse Midwifery* 1976;21(4):13–17.

Corbett MA, Burst HV, Nutritional intervention in pregnancy. *J Nurse Midwifery* 1983;28(4): 23–29.

Cowan RK, Kinch RA, Ellis B, Anderson R. Trial of labor following cesarean delivery. *Obstet Gynecol* 1994;83:933–936.

Cowper-Smith F. Letter to the editor published in *MANA News* 1985;3(2):11.

Crawford JS. The pre-anesthesia fasting period. Br J Anaesth 1984;56:925–926.

Crotty M, Ramsay AT, Smart R, Chan A. Planned homebirths in South Australia 1976–1987. *Med J Aust* 1990;153:663–671.

Crowell F. The midwives of Chicago. *JAMA* 1908;50:1346–1350.

Cunningham FG, MacDonald PC, Gant NF, Leveno KJ, Gilstrap III LC. *Williams Obstetrics,* 19th ed. Appleton & Lange, Norwalk, CT, 1993.

Curran CR. The future of the academic health center in a cost-driven market. Curran Group, Seattle, WA, 1994.

Curry MA. *Access to Prenatal Care: Key to Preventing Low Birthweight.* American Nurses' Association, Kansas City, KS, 1987.

Curry, MA. Personal communication, October 8, 1996. (Mary Ann Curry is a professor at the Oregon Health Sciences University School of Nursing, Portland, OR.)

Curry MA, Brandon P. Differences among Oregon WIC recipients planning home births. *Birth* 1986;13:91–95.

Cushner I. The health care team: A physician's perspective. *J Nurse Midwifery* 1986a;31:216–218.

Cushner IM. *Relationships between nurse-midwives and obstetricians.* In Rooks J, Haas JE (Eds.), *Nurse-Midwifery in America.* ACNM Foundation, Washington, DC 1986b, pp. 64–69.

Damstra-Wijemga SMI. Home confinement: The positive results in Holland. *J Roy College Gen Pract* 1984;34:425–430.

Danforth DN. Contemporary titans: Joseph Bolivar DeLee and John Whitridge Williams. *Am J Obstet Gynecol* 1974;120:577–588.

Darlington T. The present status of the midwife. *Am J Obstet* 1911;63:870–876.

Davis E. *Heart and Hands: A Midwife's Guide to Pregnancy and Birth,* 2nd ed. Celestial Arts, Berkeley, 1987.

Davis E. Quoted in Schlinger H, *Circle of Midwives,* 1992, pp. 102–103.

Davis LG, Riedmann GL, Sapiro M, Minogue JP, Kazer RR. Cesarean section rates in low-risk private patients managed by certified nurse-midwives and obstetricians. *J Nurse Midwifery* 1994;39:91–97.

Davis-Floyd RE. *Birth as an American Rite of Passage.* University of California Press, Berkeley, CA, 1992.

Davis-Floyd RE. Foreword. In Harper B, *Gentle Birth Choices.* Healing Arts Press, Rochester, VT, 1994.

Davis-Floyd R. In Frye A, Introduction. *Holistic Midwifery: A Comprehensive Textbook for Midwives in Homebirth Practice,* Vol. I, *Care During Pregnancy.* Labrys Press, Portland, OR, 1995.

Davis-Floyd R. Birth of a dream, death of a dream: Direct-entry midwifery in New York. Paper presented during the Annual Joint Meeting of the Society for Applied Anthropology, the Society for Medical Anthropology, the Council on Nursing and Anthropology, and the Political Ecology Society, Seattle, WA. March 6, 1997.

Davis-Floyd R, Davis E. Intuition as authoritative knowledge in midwifery and home birth. *Med Anthropol Quarterly* 1996;237–269.

Davis-Floyd R, St. John G. *From Doctor to Healer: The Paradigm Shift of Holistic Physicians.* Rutgers University Press, New Brunswick, NJ, 1997.

Daviss BA. Regional report, Region 7, Canada. *Midwives' Alliance North Am* Newsletter 1996;XIV(1):9–11.

Daviss, B.A. Personal communication, 1996 and 1997. (Betty-Anne Daviss is a midwife practicing in Ontario and Québec.)

Daviss BA. *Heeding warnings from the canary, the whale, and the Inuit: A Framework for Analyzing Competing Types of Knowledge About Childbirth.* In Davis-Floyd R, Sargent C (Eds.), *Childbirth and Authoritative Knowledge: Cross-Cultural Perspectives.* University of California Press, Berkeley, 1997a.

Daviss BA. Separating the legislation of midwifery from the movement to change childbirth and empower women. Paper presented during the Annual Joint Meeting of the Society for Applied Anthropology, the Society for Medical Anthropology, the Council on Nursing and Anthropology, and the Political Ecology Society, Seattle, Washington, March 6, 1997b.

Daviss BA, Johnson K. Personal communication, 1996. (Betty-Anne Daviss is a direct-entry midwife, and Ken Johnson, her husband, is an epidemiologist. Both are active with the Ontario Midwives Association and in the Statistics and Research Committee of MANA.

Daviss-Putt BA. Quoted in Schlinger H. *Circle of Midwives,* 1992, pp. 91–93.

de Veer AJE, Meijer WJ. Interdisciplinary co-operation in Dutch maternity care. In *Proceedings of the International Confederation of Midwives 24th Triennial Congress,* Oslo, May 26–31, 1996, ICM, London, pp. 193–194.

Dearing RH, Gordon HA, Sohner DM, Weidel LC. *Marketing Women's Health Care.* Aspen Publishers, Rockville, MD, 1987.

Decker B. Implementation of the mastery learning/modular curriculum in nurse-midwifery Education. *J Nurse Midwifery* 1990;35:3–9.

Declercq ER. The transformation of American midwifery: 1975–1988. *Am J Public Health* 1992;82:680–684.

Declercq ER. Where babies are born and who attends their births: Findings from the revised 1989 United States certificate of live birth. *Obstet Gynecol* 1993;81:997–1004.

Declercq ER. Midwifery care and medical complications: The role of risk screening. *Birth* 1995;22:68–73.

Declercq ER, Paine LL, Winter MR. Home birth in the United States, 1989–1992: A longitudinal descriptive report of national birth certificate data. *J Nurse Midwifery* 1995;40: 474–482.

Dejong RN Jr, Shy KK, Carr KC. An out-of-hospital birth center using university referral. *Obstet Gynecol* 1981;58:703–707.

DeLee JB. Progress toward ideal obstetrics. *Trans Am Assoc Study and Prevention of Infant Mortality.* 1915;6:114–138.

DeLee JB. The prophylactic forceps operation. *Am J Obstet Gynecol* 1920;1:34–44.

Department of Health, Education and Welfare. Guidelines concerning the development of health-systems plans and annual implementation plans. Issued under PF 93-641, National Health Planning and Resources Development Act of 1974, December 23, 1977.

Department of Health and Human Services. *Promoting Health/Preventing Disease: Objectives for the Nation.* Public Health Service, Washington, DC, 1980.

Department of Health and Human Services. *Caring for Our Future: The Content of Prenatal Care, a Report of the Public Health Service Expert Panel on the Content of Prenatal Care.* Public Health Service, Washington, DC, 1989.

Department of Health and Human Services. *Healthy People 2000: National Health Promotion and Disease Prevention Objectives.* U.S. Government Printing Office, Washington, DC, 1990.

Devitt N. The statistical case for elimination of the midwife: Fact versus prejudice, 1890–1935 (parts 1 and 2). *Women & Health* 1979;4(1): 81–96 and 4(2):169–183.

DeVries R. *Regulating Birth: Midwives, Medicine & the Law.* Temple University Press, Philadelphia, 1985.

DeVries RG. Barriers to midwifery: An international perspective. *J Perinatal Ed* 1992;1(1): 1–10.

DeWitt PM. The birth business. *Am Demographics* September 1993:44–49.

Dick-Read G. *Childbirth Without Fear,* 2nd ed. Harper & Row, New York, 1959.

Division of Nursing. Advance notes from the national sample survey of registered nurses, March 1996. (Unpublished data available from the Division of Nursing, Bureau of Health Professions, Health Resources and Services Administration, 5600 Fishers Lane, Rockville, MD 20857. E-mail: emoses @hrsa.dhhs.gov.)

Dobie SA, Hart LG, Fordyce M, Rosenblatt RA. Do women choose their obstetric providers based on risks at entry into prenatal care? *Obstet Gynecol* 1994;84:557–564.

Donley J. The New Zealand College of Midwifery (NZCOM). *Birth* 1990;17:53.

Douglas MJ. Commentary: The case against a more liberal food and fluid policy in labor. *Birth* 1988;15:93–94.

Doulas of North America, 1995, 1100 23th Avenue East, Seattle, Washington 98112.

Doyle BM, Widhalm MV. Midwifing the adolescents at Lincoln Hospital's teen-age clinics. *J Nurse Midwifery* 1979;24(4):27–32.

Dunlop W. Commentary on "Changing Childbirth." *Br J Obstet Gynaecol* 1993;100;1072–1074.

Durand AM. The safety of home birth: The Farm study. *Am J Public Health* 1992;82:450–453.

Durant W. *The Story of Civilization: The Age of Faith (part IV)*. Simon & Schuster, New York, 1950.

Eakins PS, O'Reilly WB, May LJ, Hopkins J. Obstetric outcomes at the Birth Place in Menlo Park: The first seven years. *Birth* 1989;16 (3);123–129.

Eakins PS, Richwald GA. Free-standing birth centers in California: Structure, cost, medical outcome and issues. California Department of Health and Human Services, Berkeley, 1986.

Eberts M, Schwartz A, Edney R, Kaufman K. Report of the Task Force on the Implementation of Midwifery in Ontario. Ministry of Health, Government of Ontario, Toronto, 1987.

Eden RD, Seifert LS, Winegar A, Spellacy WN. Perinatal characteristics of uncomplicated post-date pregnancies. *Obstet Gynecol* 1987;69: 296–299.

Ehrenreich B, English D. *Witches, Midwives and Nurses: A History of Women Healers*. The Feminist Press, Old Westbury, NY, 1973.

Eisenberg DM, Kessler RC, Foster C, Norlock FE, Calkins DR, Delbanco TL. Unconventional medicine in the United States: Prevalence, costs, and patterns of use. *N Engl J Med* 1993;328:246–252.

Ellings JM, Newman RB, Hulsy T, Bivins HA, Keenan A. Reduction in very low birth weight deliveries and perinatal mortality in a specialized, multidiscplinary twin clinic. *Obstet Gynecol* 1993;81:387–391.

Engstrom JL, McFarline BL, Sampson MB. Fundal height measurement, part 4: Accuracy of clinicians' identification of the uterine fundus during pregnancy. *I Nurse Midwifery* 1993; 38:318–323.

Engstrom JL, Sittler C, Swift KE. Fundal height measurement, part 5: The effect of clinician bias on fundal height measurements. *J Nurse Midwifery* 1994;39:130–140.

Enkin MW. Risk in pregnancy: The reality, the perception, and the concept. *Birth* 1994;21: 131–134.

Enkin M, Keirse MJNC, Chalmers I. *A Guide to Effective Care in Pregnancy and Childbirth*. Oxford University Press, New York, 1989.

Enkin M, Keirse MNJC, Renfrew MJ, Neilson JP. *A Guide to Effective Care in Pregnancy and Childbirth*, 2nd ed. Oxford University Press, New York, 1995.

Epstein JL, McCartney M. A home birth service that works. *Birth Family J* 1977;4(2):71–75.

Erikson, SL. Personal communication, 1997. (Susan L. Erickson is at the Department of Anthropology, University of Colorado at Boulder.)

Ernst EKM. Tomorrow's child. *J Nurse Midwifery* 1979;24(5):7–12.

Ernst EKM. The future of nurse-midwifery education. In *The Next Fifty Years: Midwifery Education*. Maternity Center Association, New York, 1982, pp. 75–85.

Ernst EKM. NACC presentation at the ICEA/NIN forum in Washington, DC, July 1985. *NACC News* 1985;3:8–10.

Ernst EKM. Nurse-midwifery in the freestanding birth center. In Rook, J., Haas JE (Eds.), *Nurse-Midwifery in America*. ACNM Foundation, Washington, DC, 1986, pp. 32–35.

Ernst EKM. Mainstreaming the freestanding birth center. In Kassabian L (Ed.), *Prelude to Action II*. Maternity Center Association, New York, 1995.

Ernst EM, Gordon KA. 53 years of home birth experience at the Frontier Nursing Service, Kentucky: 1925–1978. In Stewart D, Steward L, (Eds.), *Compulsory Hospitalization: Freedom of Choice in Childbirth?* Vol. II. National Association of Parents & Professionals for Safe Alternatives in Childbirth, Marble Hill, MO, 1979, pp. 505–516.

Estes MN. A home obstetric service with expert consultation and back-up. *Birth Family J* 1978;151–156.

European Midwives Liaison Committee. *Activities, Responsibilities and Independence of Midwives Within the European Union*. Author, 7 Dalestones, West Hunsbury, Northampton NN49UU, UK, 1996.

Ewigman BG, Crane JP, Frigoletto FD, LeFevre ML, Bain RP, McNellis D, and the RADIUS Study Group. Effect of prenatal ultrasound screening on perinatal outcome. *N Engl J Med* 1993;329:821–827.

Expert Maternity Group. *Changing Childbirth, Part I: Report of the Expert Maternity Group*. Her Majesty's Stationery Office, London, 1993.

Faison JB, Pisani BJ, Douglas RG, Cranch GS, Lubic RW. The Childbearing Center: An alternative birth setting. *Obstet Gynecol* 1979;54: 527–532.

Farr MM, Funches JM. A successful pilot off-campus nurse-midwifery program. *J Nurse Midwifery* 1982;27(3):31–36.

Feinbloom RI. A proposed alliance of midwives and family practitioners in the care of low-risk pregnant women. *Birth* 1986;13(2): 109–116.

Feldman E, Hurst M. Outcomes and Procedures in low risk birth: A comparison of hospital and birth center settings. *Birth* 1987;14: 18–24.

Fennell KS. Prescriptive authority for nurse-midwives: A historical review. *Nursing Clin North Am* 1991;26:511–521.

Fennel KS. Medicare: The golden rule. *Quickening*, July/August 1994, p. 537.

Fiedler DC. Authoritative knowledge and birth territories in contemporary Japan. *Med Anthropol Quarterly* 1996; 10(2):195–212.

Fiscella K. Does prenatal care improve birth outcomes? A critical review. *Obstet Gynecol* 1995;85:468–479.

Flamm B. Personal communication, March 1996. (Bruce Flamm is Research Chair, Department of Obstetrics and Gynecology, Kaiser Permanente, Riverside, California.)

Flamm BL, Goings JR, Liu Y, Wolde-Tsadik G. Elective repeat cesarean delivery versus trial of labor: A prospective multicenter study. *Obstet Gynecol* 1994;83:927–932.

Flanagan J. Direct entry midwifery at North Central Bronx: A policy analysis prepared for Charlotte Elsberry, CNM, Director, Nurse-Midwifery Programs, North Central Bronx Hospital, New York City Health and Hospital Corporation. John F. Kennedy School of Government, Harvard University, 1990.

Fleck AC. Hospital sizes and outcomes of pregnancy. Office of the Assistant Commissioner for Child Health, New York State Department of Public Health, February 23, 1977.

Flexner A. *Medical Education in the United States and Canada: A Report to the Carnegie Foundation for the Advancement of Teaching.* Bulletin 4. Carnegie Foundation for the Advancement of Teaching, New York, 1910.

Forestier R. Midwifery in France. *J Nurse Midwifery* 1983;28(4):37–38.

Forman AM, Cooper EM. Legislation and nurse-midwifery practice in the USA: Report on a survey conducted by the Legislation Committee of the American College of Nurse-Midwives. *J Nurse Midwifery* 1976;21(2):1–52.

Fortney J. Antenatal risk screening and scoring: A new look. *In J Gynecol Obstet* 1995;50(suppl 2):S53–S58.

Fossett J, Perloff SJ, Peterson J, Kletke P. Medicaid in the inner city: The case of maternity care in Chicago. *Milbank Q* 1990:68:111–141.

Foster DC, Guzick DS, Pulliam RP. The impact of prenatal care on fetal and neonatal death rates for uninsured patients: A "natural experiment" in West Virginia. *Obstet Gynecol* 1992;79:40–45.

Foster JC. Ensuring competence of nurse-midwives at entrance into the profession: The national certification examination. In Rooks J, Haas JE (Eds.), *Nurse-Midwifery in America.* ACNM Foundation, Washington, DC, 1986, pp. 14–16.

Franklin Communications. Readership and practice profile of members of the American College of Nurse-Midwives: Findings of a direct mail survey. *J Nurse Midwifery* 1994;39:29–38.

Fraser W. Methodologic issues in assessing the active management of labor. *Birth* 1993; 20:155–156.

Freda MC, Andersen HF, Damus K, Merkatz IR. Are there differences in information given to private and public prenatal patients? *Am J Obstet Gynecol* 1993;169:155–160.

Freed GL, Clark SJ, Sorenson J, Lohr JA, Cefalo R, Curtis P. National assessment of physician's breast-feeding knowledge, attitudes, training and experience. *JAMA* 1995;273: 472–476.

Fremont Women's Clinic Birth Collective. A working lay midwife home birth program, Seattle, Washington: A collective approach. In *21st Century Obstetrics Now!*, Vol. 2. National Association of Parents & Professionals for Safe Alternatives in Childbirth, Chapel Hill, NC, 1977, pp. 507–544.

Freudenheim M. Health costs paid by employers drop for first time in a decade. *The New York Times*, February 14, 1995, pp. A1, C7.

Friedman EA. The graphic analysis of labor. *Am J Obstet Gynecol* 1954;68:1568.

Friedman EA, Sachtleben MR. Dysfunctional labor: A comprehensive program for diagnosis, evaluation, and management. *Obstet Gynecol* 1965;25:844.

Friedrich J. Midwifery in Europe, German speaking countries. In *Proceedings of the International Confederation of Midwives 24th Triennial Congress*, Oslo, May 26–31, 1996, ICM, London, pp. 238–242.

Fries K. Paper on the "Philosophy of the ACNM." Submitted as assignment to the Community-based Nurse-Midwifery Education Program, Frontier School of Midwifery and Family Nursing, Hyden, Kentucky, December 23, 1994.

Frigoletto Jr, FD, Lieberman E, Lang JM, Cohen A, Barss V, Ringer S, Datta S. A clinical trial of active management of labor. *N Engl J Med* 1995;333:745–750.

Fritsch J. New York hospital agency issues new rules for midwife deliveries. *The New York Times,* December 30, 1995, pp. 1, 31.

Fritsch J, Baquet D. Mismanaged care: A health system in peril. *The New York Times,* March 5, 1995, pp. 1, 12–13; March 6, 1995, pp. A1, 12–13; March 7, 1995, pp. A1, 10–11.

Frontier Nursing Service. Summary of the first 10,000 confinement records of the Frontier Nursing service. *Q Bull Frontier Nurs Service* 1958;33:45–55.

Frye A. Quoted in Schlinger H, *Circle of Midwives,* 1992a, pp. 97–98.

Frye A. Report of the Registry Board. *MANA News* 1992b;X(1):6–7.

Frye A. *Understanding Diagnostic Tests in the Childbearing Year.* Labrys Press, Portland, OR, 1993.

Frye A. *Healing Passage: A Midwife's Guide to the Care and Repair of the Tissues Involved in Birth,* 5th ed. Labrys Press, Portland, OR, 1995a.

Frye A. *Holistic Midwifery: A Comprehensive Textbook for Midwives in Homebirth Practice,* Vol. I, *Care During Pregnancy.* Labrys Press, Portland, OR, 1995b.

Frye A. Personal communication, at various times during 1996. (Anne Frye is a direct-entry midwife in Portland, Oregon.)

Fukuzawa. Japan. In McDonald W, Davis JA (Eds.), *History of Midwifery Practice in Australia and the Western Pacific Regions.* Western Australian Branch of the National Midwives Association of Australia, Perth, 1984, pp. 61–64. (Book prepared for the 20th Congress of the International Confederation of Midwives.)

Fullerton JT. 1994 task analysis of American certified nurse-midwifery. *J Nurse Midwifery* 1994;39:348–357.

Fullerton J. Personal communication, 1996. (Judith Fullerton is associate dean for the Graduate Nursing Program, School of Nursing, University of Texas Health Science Center at San Antonio.)

Fullerton JT, Severino R. In-hospital care for low-risk childbirth: Comparison with results from the National Birth Center Study. *J Nurse Midwifery* 1992;37:331–340.

Fullerton JT, Severino R. Factors that predict performance on the National Certification examination. *J Nurse Midwifery* 1995;40:19–25.

Fullerton JT, Greener DL, Gross LJ. Criterion-referenced competency assessment and the National Certification Examination in Nurse-Midwifery. *J Nurse Midwifery* 1989;34(2):71–74.

Fullerton JT, Roberts JE, Valhoff WL. Recent developments in professional midwifery education and credentialing. *J Nurse Midwifery* 1996;41:322–327.

Gabay M, Wolfe SM. Encouraging the use of nurse-midwives: A report for policymakers. Public Citizen Health Research Group, Washington, DC, November 1995.

Gagnon AJ, Waghorn K. Supportive care by maternity nurses: A work sampling study in an intrapartum unit. *Birth* 1996;23:1–6.

Garrison A and co-workers of the Midwives Section. Tasmania. In McDonald W, Davis JA (Eds.), *History of Midwifery Practice in Australia and the Western Pacific Regions.* Western Australian Branch of the National Midwives Association of Australia, Perth, 1984, pp. 45–48. (Book prepared for the 20th Congress of the International Confederation of Midwives.)

Gaskin IM. *Spiritual Midwifery.* The Book Publishing Company, Summertown, TN, 1975.

Gaskin IM. Empirical Midwifery. In Stewart D, Stewart L (Eds.), *Compulsory Hospitalization: Freedom of Choice in Childbirth?* National Association of Parents & Professionals for Safe Alternatives in Childbirth, Marble Hill, MO, 1978, pp. 385–398.

Gaskin IM. Statistics for 1,827 births attended by the Farm midwives, November 1970 to January 1993. Paper distributed at the First Annual Birth Gazette Midwifery Conference, Summertown, Tennessee, August 6–8, 1993.

Gaskin IM. Personal communication, October 1994. (Ina May Gaskin is president of MANA.)

Gaskin IM. Personal communication, July/September 1996. (Ina May Gaskin is president of MANA.)

Gatewood TS. Obstetrician/nurse-midwife private practice: An example from Americus, Georgia. In Rooks J, Haas JE (Eds.), *Nurse-Midwifery in America.* ACNM Foundation, Washington, DC, 1986, pp. 28–29.

Gatewood TS, Stewart RB. Obstetricians and nurse-midwives: The team approach in private practice. *Am J Obstet Gynecol* 1975; 123:35.

Gazette. May 1992;3(1) and January 1993;3(1). (The *Gazette* was a publication of the Ontario Interim Regulatory Council on Midwifery. The articles cited were not authored. All articles were published in Volume 3, No. 1, May 1992, or Volume 3, No. 1, January 1993.)

Gazmararian JA, Adams MM, Saltzman LE, Johnson CH, Bruce FC, Marks J, Zahniser SC, PRAMS Working Group. The relationship between pregnancy intendedness and physical violence in mothers of newborns. *Obstet Gynecol* 1995;85:1031–1038.

General Accounting Office. *Better Management and More Resources Needed to Strengthen Federal Efforts to Improve Pregnancy Outcome.* U.S. Government Printing Office, Washington, DC, 1979.

Gibby NW. Relationship between fetal movement charting and anxiety in low-risk pregnant women. *J Nurse Midwifery* 1988;33(4):185–188.

Gilmore E. Advantages and disadvantages of the apprentice model of midwifery education. Paper prepared for a conference of the National Coalition of Midwifery Educators, Flagstaff, Arizona, June 1990.

Glass GV, McGaw B, Smith ML. *Meta-analysis in Social Research.* Sage, Beverly Hills, CA, 1981.

Glover P. Midwifery education by distance: It can be done. In Proceedings of the International Confederation of Midwives 24th Triennial Congress, Oslo, May 26–31, 1996, ICM, London, pp. 516–519.

GMENAC. *Summary Report of the Graduate Medical Education National Advisory Committee to the Secretary, Department of Health and Human Services, Vol. 1.* Public Health Service, Health Resources Administration, U.S. Department of Health and Human Services, Washington, DC, 1980.

Goer H. *Obstetric Myths Versus Research Realities: A Guide to the Medical Literature.* Bergin & Garvey, Westport, CT, 1995.

Goings JR. Success in a health maintenance organization: Kaiser Permanente of Anaheim, California. In Rooks J, Haas JE (Eds.), *Nurse-Midwifery in America.* ACNM Foundation, Washington, DC, 1986, pp. 36–37.

Golay J, Vedam S, Sorger L. The squatting position for the second stage of labor: Effects on labor and on maternal and fetal well-being. *Birth* 1993;20(2):73–78.

Gold RB, Kenny AM, Singh S. *Blessed Events and the Bottom Line: Financing Maternity Care in the United States.* Alan Guttmacher Institute, New York, 1987.

Goldenberg RL, Andrews WW. Editorial: Intrauterine infection and why preterm prevention programs have failed. *Am J Public Health* 1996;86:832–836.

Goldenberg RL, Davis RO, Copper RL, Corliss DK, Andrews JB, Carpenter AH. The Alabama preterm birth prevention project. *Obstet Gynecol* 1990;75:341–345.

Gordon R. The effects of malpractice insurance on certified nurse-midwives: The case of rural Arizona. *J Nurse Midwifery* 1990;35:99–106.

Gould JB, Davey B, Stafford RS. Socio-economic differences in rates of cesarean section. *N Engl J Med* 1989;321:233–239.

Goyert GL, Bottoms SF, Treadwell MC, Nehra PC. The physician factor in cesarean birth rates. *N Engl J Med* 1989;320:706–709.

Gray AM, Steele R. The economics of specialist and general practitioner maternity units. *J Roy College Gen Pract* 1981;31:586–592.

Gregory S. Man-midwifery exposed and corrected (1848). In Rosenberg, C and Smith-Rosenberg, C (Eds.), *The Male Midwife and the Female Doctor.* Arno Press, New York, 1974.

Greulich B, Paine LL, McClain C, Barger MK, Edwards N, Paul R. Twelve years and more than 30,000 nurse-midwive attended births: The Los Angeles County and University of Southern California Women's Hospital Birth Center experience. *J Nurse Midwifery* 1994;39:185–196.

Guilliland K. Personal communication, 1997. (Karen Guilliland is National Coordinator of the New Zealand College of Midwives.)

Guilliland K, Pairman S. *The Midwifery Partnership: A Model for Practice.* Department of Nursing and Midwifery, Victoria University of Wellington, Wellington, NZ, 1995. Monograph series 95/1.

Gulbransen G, Hilton J, McKay L, Cox A. Home birth in New Zealand 1973–93: Incidence and mortality. *NZ Med J* 1997;110:87–88.

Gullemette J, Fraser W. Differences between obstetricians in cesarean section rate and the management of labour. *Br J Obstet Gynaecol* 1992;99:105–108.

Haadem K, Dahlstrom JA, Ling L, Ohrlandere S. Anal sphincter function after delivery rupture. *Obstet Gynecol* 1987;70(1):53–56.

Haas JE. National Survey of factors contributing to and hindering the successful practice of nurse-midwifery. In Rooks J, Haas JE (Eds.), *Nurse Midwifery in America*. ACNM Foundation, Washington, DC, 1986, pp. 25–27.

Haas JE, Rooks JP. National survey of factors contributing to and hindering the successful practice of nurse-midwifery: Summary of the American College of Nurse-Midwives Foundation Study. *J Nurse-Midwifery* 1986;32(5): 212–215.

Hage D, Black RF. New surgery for health care. *U.S. News & World Report*, February 27, 1995, pp. 68–69.

Haire D. *The Cultural Warping of Childbirth*. International Childbirth Education Association, Hillside, NJ, 1972.

Haire D. Health insurance coverage for nurse-midwifery services: Results of a national survey. *J Nurse Midwifery* 1982;27(6):35–36.

Haire D. Development of direct entry midwifery programs in England. Paper presented at the Seminar on Midwifery Education convened by the Carnegie Foundation for the Advancement of Teaching, Princeton, NJ, July 22, 1990.

Haire DB, Elsberry CC. Maternity care and outcomes in a high-risk service: The North Central Bronx Hospital Experience. *Birth* 1991; 18:33–37.

Hale RW. Women, ob-gyns and primary care: An essential relationship. *J Med Assoc Georgia* 1994;83:559–562.

Handler A, Rosenberg D. Improving pregnancy outcomes: Public versus private care for urban, low-income women. *Birth* 1992;19:123–130.

Hannah EM, Hannah WJ, Helman J, Hewson S, Milner R, Willan A, and the Canadian Multicenter Post-Term Pregnancy Trial Group. Induction of labor as compared with serial antenatal monitoring in post-term pregnancy. A randomized controlled trial. *N Engl J Med* 1992;326:1587–1592.

Harper B. *Gentle Birth Choices*. Healing Arts Press, Rochester, VT, 1994.

Harper, B. Personal communication, 1995. (Barbara Harper is founder of the Global Maternal/Child Health Association, West Linn, OR.

Harris D, Daily EF, Lang DM. Nurse-midwifery in New York City. *Am J Public Health* 1971;61:1.

Hartley C. Helping Hands: The Apprentice Workbook. Ancient Arts Midwifery Institute, Claremont, OK, 1988.

Harvey S, Jarrel J, Brant R, Math M, Stainton C, Rach D. A randomized, controlled trial of nurse-midwivery care. *Birth* 1996;23(3): 128–135.

Hatem-Asmar M, Blais R, Lambert J, Maheux, B. A survey of midwives in Québec: What are their similarities and differences? *Birth* 1996; 23:94–100.

Hauth JC, Goldenberg RL, Andrews WW, DuBard MB, Cooper RL. Reduced incidence of preterm delivery with metronidazole and erythromycin in women with bacterial vaginosis. *N Engl J Med* 1995;333:1732–1736.

Haverkamp AD, Orleans M, Langendoerfer S, McFee J, Murphy J, Thompson HE. A controlled trial of the differential effects of intrapartum fetal monitoring. *Am J Obstet Gynecol* 1979;35:627–642.

Hayes P, Bayliss. New South Wales. In McDonald W, Davis JA (Eds.), *History of Midwifery Practice in Australia and the Western Pacific Regions*. Western Australian Branch of the National Midwives Association of Australia, Perth, 1984, pp. 23–30. (Book prepared for the 20th Congress of the International Confederation of Midwives.)

Haynes de Regt, Minkoff HL, Feldman J, Schwarz RH. Relation of private or clinic care to the cesarean birth rate. *N Engl J Med* 1986;315: 619–624.

Hays KE. Satisfaction with midwifery care among women who choose home birth: The development of a questionnaire. June 5, 1996. (Scholarly project for master's in nursing degree, University of Washington.)

Hedegaard M, Henriksen TB, Sabroe S, Secher NJ. Psychological distress in pregnancy and preterm delivery. *Br Med J* 1993;307:234–239.

Heilmann MR. Childbirth as personal growth for women. In *Proceedings of the International Confederation of Midwives 24th Triennial Congress*, Oslo, May 26–31, 1996, ICM, London, pp. 260–263.

Heins HC, Nance NW, McCarthy BJ, Efird CM. A randomized trial of nurse-midwifery prenatal care to reduce low birth weight. *Obstet Gynecol* 1990;75:341–345.

Hellman, L. Personal communication, 1975. (Louis Hellman was deputy assistant secretary for Population Affairs, Department of Health, Education and Welfare, now deceased.)

Hellman L, Pritchard JA. *Williams Obstetrics,* 14th ed. Appleton-Century-Crofts, New York, 1971.

Hemminki E. Pregnancy and birth after cesarean section: A survey based on the Swedish birth register. *Birth* 1987;14:12–17.

Hemminki E, Simukka R. The timing of hospital admission and progress of labor. *Eur J Obstet Gynecol Reprod Biol* 1986;22:85–94.

Hemschemeyer H. Our 30th Anniversary—A tribute. *Bull Nurse-Midwifery* 1962:5–10.

Herman S. Personal communication, December 12, 1996. (Sarah Herman is with the Oregon Center for Health Statistics.)

Herron MA, Katz M, Creasy RK. Evaluation of a preterm birth prevention program: Preliminary report. *Obstet Gynecol* 1982;59:452–456.

Hiddinga A. Dutch obstetric science: Emergence, growth, and present situation. In Abraham-Van der Mark E (Ed.), *Successful Home Birth and Midwifery: The Dutch Model.* Bergin & Garvey, London, 1993, pp. 45–77.

Hillier SL, Nugent RP, Eschenbach DA, Krohn MA, Gibbs RS, Martin DH, Cotch MF, Edelman R, Pastorek JG, Rao V, McNellis D, Regan JA, Carey C, Klebanoff MA. Association between bacterial vaginosis and preterm delivery of a low-birth-weight infant. *N Engl J Med* 1995;333:1737–1742.

Hinds MW, Bergeisen GH, Allen DT. Neonatal outcome in planned *v* unplanned out-of-hospital births in Kentucky. *JAMA* 1985; 253:1578–1582.

Hingstman L. Primary care obstetrics and perinatal health in the Netherlands. *J Nurse Midwifery* 1994;39:379–386.

Hobbs V. Quoted in Schlinger H, *Circle of Midwives,* 1992, pp. 31–32.

Hodges D. Midwifery education. *MANA News* 1992;X(1):12.

Hodges, S. Personal communication, April 24, 1997. (Susan Hodges is president of Citizens for Midwifery.)

Hodnett E, Osborn R. Effects of continuous intrapartum professional support on childbirth outcomes. *Res Nurs Health* 1989;12: 289–297.

Hofmeyr GJ, Nikodem VC, Wolman W-L, Chalmers BE, Kramer T. Companionship to modify the clinical birth environment: Effects of progress and perceptions of labour and breastfeeding. *Br J Obstet Gynaecol* 1991; 98:756–764.

Hogan A. A tribute to the pioneers. *J Nurse Midwifery* 1975;20(Summer):6–11.

Holley M, Cameron J. The American College of Nurse-Midwives National Certification Examination: A report to the governing board of the ACNM Division of Examiners. ACNM, Washington, DC, April 1978.

Hon EH. Apparatus for continuous monitoring of the fetal heart rate. *Yale J Biol Med* 1960;32: 397–399.

Hoope-Bender, P. Personal communication, 1997. (Petra Hoope-Bender is a midwife in private practice with three other midwives in Rotterdam, the Netherlands.)

Horoschak MJ. Letter from the assistant director of the Federal Trade Commission to Joseph A. Parker, president of the Georgia Hospital Association, May 28, 1993.

Horton JA, Cruess DF, Pearse WH. Primary and preventive care services provided by obstetrician–gynecologists. *Obstet Gynecol* 1993;82: 723–726.

Hoúd, S. Personal communication, April and May 1997. (Suzanne Hoúd is Director of Diploma Courses for Midwives, The School of Advanced Nursing, Aarhus University, Arhus, Denmark.)

House Committee on Interstate and Foreign Commerce. Nurse-Midwifery: Consumers' freedom of choice. 96th Congress, 2nd Session, December 18, 1980.

House of Commons Health Committee. *Health Committee Report on the Maternity Services,* Vol. 1. Her Majesty's Stationery Office, London, 1992.

Howe C. Personal communication, December 1995. (Carol Howe is director of Nurse-midwifery Education Program, Oregon Health Sciences University, Portland, OR.)

Howe KA. Home births in southwest Australia. *Med J Aust* 1088;149:296–302.

Howie PW, Forsyth JS, Ogston SA, Clark A, Florey C. Protective effect of breastfeeding against infection. *Br Med J* 1990;300:11–16.

Hsia L. Fifty years of nurse-midwivery education: Reflections and perspectives. *J Nurse Midwifery* 1982;27(4):1–3.

Hsia L. Nursing and nurse-midwifery: Reflections and dilemmas. *J Nurse Midwifery* 1984;29(3): 175–176.

Hueston WJ, Murry M. A three-tier model for the delivery of rural obstetrical care using a nurse midwife and family physician copractice. *J Rural Health* 1992;8:283–290.

Hueston WJ, Applegate JA, Mansfield CJ, King DE, McClaflin RR. Practice variations between family physicians and obstetricians in the management of low-risk pregnancies. *J Fam Pract* 1995;40(4):345–351.

Huffman S, Labbock M, Coly S. *Breastfeeding Saves Lives*. Institute for Reproductive Health, Washington, DC, 1996.

Husk LL. Of prime concern: Obstetricians and gynecologists tooling up for primary care. *Views*, Spring 1996, pp. 12–13. (*Views* is a publication of the Oregon Health Sciences University, Portland, OR.)

Inside Ambulatory Care. Volume up, costs down as nurse midwives take on new roles. *Inside Ambulatory Care* 1995;1(12):2,7.

Institute of Medicine. *Research Issues in the Assessment of Birth Settings: Report of a Study*. National Academy Press, Washington, DC, 1982.

Institute of Medicine. *Preventing Low Birthweight*. National Academy Press, Washington, DC, 1985.

Institute of Medicine. *Prenatal Care: Reaching Mothers, Reaching Infants*. National Academy Press, Washington, DC, 1987.

Institute of Medicine. *The Effect of Medical Professional Liability on the Delivery of Obstetric Care*. National Academy Press, Washington, DC, 1989.

Institute of Medicine. *Defining Primary Care: An Interim Report*. National Academy Press, Washington, DC, 1994.

International Confederation of Midwives. Mission Statement. Author, London, 1996.

Ito K. Issei: A history of Japanese immigrants in North America. *Birth*, Spring 1987:13.

Jackson B, Jensen J. Home care tops consumer's list. *Modern Health Care*, May 1, 1984.

Jacobson PH. Hospital care and the vanishing midwife. *Millbank Memorial Fund Quarterly* 1956;34:1735–1744.

James S. Personal communication, January 15, 1997. (Susan James is a midwife in Edmonton, Alberta.)

Janssen PA, Holt VL, Myers SJ. Licensed midwife-attended, out-of-hospital births in Washington State: Are they safe? *Birth* 1994;21:141–148.

Jenkins SM. The myth of vicarious liability: Impact on barriers to nurse-midwifery practice. *J Nurse Midwifery* 1994;39:98–106.

Jenkins S. New practice laws and regulations enacted in Arkansas, D.C., Indiana, and Vermont. *Quickening*, May/June 1995a, pp. 25–26.

Jenkins S. *State Legislative Handbook*, 1995 Ed. ACNM, Washington, DC, 1995b.

Jenkins SM, Fennell KS. Medicaid managed care. *Quickening*, November/December 1994, pp. 4–5.

Johnson K, Daviss BA. Personal communication, 1996. (Kenneth Johnson is a Canadian epidemiologist working in Ottawa. Betty-Anne Daviss is chair of MANA's Statistics and Research Committee.)

Johnston E. Personal communication, July 15, 1996. (Edward Johnston is vital records registrar for the State of Oregon.)

Jolly H. Personal communication, March 1996. (Helen Jolly runs the Family Birth Services Midwifery Course in Grand Prairie, TX.)

Kahn NB, Garner JG, Schmittling GT, Ostergaard DJ, Graham R. Results of the 1996 National Resident Matching Program: Family practice. *Fam Med* 1996a;28:548–552.

Kahn NB, Schmittling GT, Garner JG, Graham R. Entry of US medical school graduates into family practice residencies: 1995–1996 and 3-Year Summary. *Fam Med* 1996b;28:539–547.

Kaiser Commission on the Future of Medicaid. Health Needs and Medicaid Financing: State Facts. Kaiser Commission on the Future of Medicaid, Washington, DC, 1995.

Kalisch PA, Scobey M, Kalisch BJ. Louyse Bourgeois and the emergence of modern midwifery. *J Nurse Midwifery* 1981;26(4):3–17.

Kaminski HM, Stafl A, Aiman J. The effect of epidural analgesia on the frequency of instrumental obstetric delivery. *Obstet Gynecol* 1987;69:770–773.

Kanne K. Alaskan legislative update. *Birth Gazette* 1992;8(4):21–22.

Kassirer JP. Our ailing public hospitals: Cure them or close them? *N Engl J Med* 1995;333:1348–1349.

Katz ME, Holmes MD, Power KL, Wise PH. Mortality rates among 15- to 44-year old women in Boston: Looking beyond reproductive status. *Am J Public Health* 1995;85:1135–1138.

Katz-Rothman B. Quoted in Schlinger H, *Circle of Midwives*, 1992, pp. 131–133.

Kaufman K. Developments in Canadian midwifery. Presented at an international conference entitled "How should maternal and child health services be delivered in the 21st century?" The conference was convened by the University of South Florida Health Sciences Center and the French–American Foundation in Tampa, FL, April 20–22, 1997a.

Kaufman K. Personal communication, April and May, 1997b. (Karyn Kaufman is Chair of the Midwifery Education Programme at McMaster University in Hamilton, Ontario.)

Kaufman KJ. The introduction of midwifery in Ontario, Canada. *Birth* 1991;18:100–106.

Kaye B. Today's nurse-midwife: A model for solo practice. *Midwifery Today* 1991;18:12–13,47.

Keeler EB, Brodie MA. Economic incentives in the choice between vaginal delivery and cesarean section. *Milbank Q* 1993;71(3):365–404.

Keenan R, Joske P, Denny RJ. Western Australia. In McDonald W, Davis JA (Eds.), *The History of Midwifery Practice in Australia and the Western Pacific Regions.* Western Australian Branch of the National Midwives Association of Australia, Perth, 1984, pp. 1–10. (Book prepared for the 20th Congress of the International Confederation of Midwives.)

Keirse MJNC. A final comment . . . managing the uterus, the woman, or whom? *Birth* 1993;20(3):159–162.

Kennell J, Klaus M, McGrath S, Robertson S, Hinkley C. Continuous emotional support during labor in a US Hospital. *JAMA* 1991;265:2197–2201.

Kennell JH. The time has come to reassess delivery room routines. *Birth* 1994;21(1):49–50.

Kent J, MacKeith N, Maggs C. Direct but different: An evaluation of the implementation of pre-registration midwifery education in England. (A research project for the Department of Health, Executive Summary.) Maggs Research Associates, Bath, England, 1994.

King T. Personal communication, December 1995. (Tekoa King is a CNM at the University of California at San Francisco Medical Center.)

Kingsepp J. Quoted in Schlinger H, *Circle of Midwives,* 1992, p. 24.

Kitzinger S. *The Complete Book of Pregnancy and Childbirth.* Alfred A. Knopf, New York, 1983.

Kitzinger S. Sheila Kitzinger's letter from England: Birth in a fresh climate? *Birth* 1995;22:43–44.

Kizer E, Ellis A. C-section rate related to payment source. *Am J Public Health* 1988;78:96–97.

Klaus MH. Commentary: The early hours and days of life: An opportune time. *Birth* 1995;22(4):201–203.

Klaus MH, Kennell JH, Robertson SS, Sosa R. Effects of social support during parturition on maternal and infant morbidity. *Br Med J* 1986;293:585–587.

Klee L. Home away from home: The alternative birth center. *Social Sci Med* 1986;23:9–16.

Klein M. Commentary: Midwifery—A family doctor's view from Quebec. *Birth* 1991;18:103–106.

Klein MC, Gauthier RJ, Jorgensen SH, *et al.* Does episiotomy prevent perineal trauma and pelvic floor relaxation? *Online J Curr Clin Trials* 1992;July 1 (Document 10).

Klein RPD, Girt NF, Nicholson J, Standleyu K. A study of father and nurse support during labor. *Birth* 1981;10(3):161–164.

Klerman LV, Jekel JF. School Age Mothers: Problems, Programs & Policy. The Shoe String Press, Hamden, CT, 1973.

Kloosterman JG. Why midwifery? *The Practicing Midwife,* Spring 1985, pp. 5–10.

Knowles M. *The Modern Practice of Adult Education.* Cambridge Adult Education, Englewood Cliffs, NJ, 1980.

Knox L. Midwifery in Canada: A new beginning or echoes from the past? Keynote address given by the president of the Midwives Association of British Columbia during the opening session of the Triennial Congress of the International Confederation of Midwives, Vancouver, BC, 1993.

Koehler NU, Soloman DA, Murphy M. Outcomes of a rural Sonoma County home birth practice: 1976–1982. *Birth* 1984;11(3);165–169.

Kondo J. Personal communication, April and May, 1997. (Junko Kondo is director of the nursing department, Tenshi Women's College, Sapporo, Japan, and vice president of the Japanese Midwives' Association.)

Kolimaga JT, Osborne D, Ricketts TC. Registered nurses and nurse practitioners. In *Rural Health Professionals Facts: Supply and Distribution of Health Professionals in Rural America.* North Carolina Rural Health Research Program, Cecil G. Sheps Center for Health Services Research, Chapel Hill, NC, 1992.

Konner M. *Childhood.* Little, Brown and Company, Boston, 1991.

Konner M. *Dear America: A Concerned Doctor Wants You to Know the Truth About Health Reform.* Addison-Wesley, Reading, MA, 1993.

Koons C. The lay midwife: A current perspective. In Steward D, Stewart S (Eds.), *21st Century Obstetrics Now!* National Association of Parents & Professionals for Safe Alternatives in Childbirth, Chapel Hill, NC, 1977, pp. 552–556.

Kost K, Forrest JD. Intention status of U.S. births in 1988: Differences by mothers' socioeconomic and demographic characteristics. *Family Planning Perspectives* 1995;27(1):11–17.

Kotelchuck M, Schwartz JB, Anderka MT, Finison KS. WIC participation and pregnancy outcomes: Massachusetts statewide evaluation project. *Am J Public Health* 1984;74:1086–1092.

Kozak LJ. Surgical and nonsurgical procedures associated with hospital delivery in the United States: 1980–1987. *Birth* 1989;16:209–213.

KPMG Peat Marwick. Health benefits in 1993. Kaiser Permanente Medical Group, Oakland, CA, 1993.

Kraus N. Malpractice litigation: A painful lesson in professional responsibility. *J Nurse Midwifery* 1990;35:125–126.

Krumlauf J, Oakley D, Mayes F, Wranesh B, Springer N, Burke M. Certified nurse-midwives and physicians: Perinatal care charges. *Nursing Economic$* 1988;6(1):27–30.

Kruse J, Phillips D, Wesley RM. Factors influencing changes in obstetric care provided by family physicians. *J Fam Pract* 1989;28:597–603.

Kurokawa JS. Rural midwifery and electronic communications. *J Nurse Midwifery* 1996;41:263–264.

Kusserow RP. A survey of certified nurse-midwives. Office of Inspector General, Department of Health and Human Services, Washington, DC, March 1992.

Laird M. Report of the Maternity Center Association Clinic, New York, 1931–1951. *Am J Obstet Gynecol* 1955;69:178–184.

Land D. Personal communication, 1995. (Dorthea Land is director of Midwifery Programs for the Maternity, Infant Care—Family Planning Projects, Medical & Health Research Association of New York City.)

Lang R. *The Birth Book.* Genesis Press, Palo Alto, CA, 1972.

Larimore WL, Davis A. Relationship of infant mortality to availability of care in rural Florida. *J Am Board Fam Pract* 1995;8:392–399.

Larsson P, Platz-Christensen J, Bergman B, Wallstersson G. Advantage or disadvantage of episotomy compared with spontaneous perineal laceration. *Gynecol Obstet Invest* 1991;31:213–216.

Leavitt J. Science enters the birthing room: Obstetrics in America since the 18th century. *J Am History* 1983;70(2):281–304.

Leavitt JW. *Brought to Bed: Childbearing in America, 1750–1950.* Oxford University Press, New York, 1986.

Leavitt JW. Joseph B. DeLee and the practice of preventive obstetrics. *Am J Public Health* 1988;78:1353–1360.

Lederman R, Lederman E, Work B, McCann D. The relationship of maternal anxiety, plasma catecholamines, and plasma cortisol to progress in labor. *Am J Obstet Gynecol* 1978;132:459–499.

Lee FE, Glasser JH. Role of lay midwifery in maternity care in a large metropolitan area. *Public Health Reports* 1974;89(6);537–54.

Leeman L. Letter to the editor. *Birth* 1995;22:236.

Lehmann DK, Mabie WC, Miller JM Jr, Pernoll ML. The epidemiology and pathology of maternal mortality: Charity Hospital of Louisiana in New Orleans, 1965–1984. *Obstet Gynecol* 1987;69:833–840.

Lehrman EJ. Findings of the 1990 annual American College of Nurse-Midwives membership survey. *J Nurse Midwifery* 1992;37:33–47.

Lehrman EJ. Nurse-midwifery practice: A descriptive study of prenatal care. *J Nurse Midwifery* 1981;26:27–41.

Lehrman EJ, Paine LL. Trends in nurse-midwifery: Results of the 1988 ACNM Division of Research Mini-Survey. *J Nurse Midwifery* 1990;35:192–203.

Leonard C. Quoted in Schlinger H, *Circle of Midwives,* 1992, pp. 28–29.

Leppert PC. An analysis of the reasons for Japan's low infant mortality rate. *J Nurse Midwifery* 1993;38:353–356.

Leveno KJ, Cunningham FG, Nelson S, Roark M, Williams ML, Guzick D, Dowling S, Rosenfeld, CR, Buckley A. A prospective comparison of selective and universal electronic fetal monitoring in 34,995 pregnancies. *N Engl J Med* 1986;315:615–619.

Levitt C, Hanvey L, Avard D, Chance G, Kaczorowski J. *Survey of Routine Maternity Care and Practices in Canadian Hospitals.* Health Canada and Canadian Institute of Child Health, Ottawa, 1995.

Levy BS, Wilkinson FS, Marine WM. Reducing neonatal mortality rates with nurse-midwives. *Am J Obstet Gynecol* 1971;109:50–58.

Lewin ME. The quest for health care reform: Some notes on the endgame. *J Med Pract Manage* November 1995.

Lewit E, Monheit A. Expenditure on health care for children and pregnant women. Agency for Health Care Policy and Research, Department of Health and Human Services, Washington, DC, December 1992. AHCPR Publication 93–0022.

Lieberman E, Lang JM, Frigoletto F, Richardson DK, Ringer SA, Cohen A. Epidural analgesia, intrapartum fever, and neonatal sepsis evaluation. *Pediatrics* 1997;99:415–419.

Lindell SG, Rossi MA. Compliance with childbirth education classes in second stage labor. *Birth* 1986;13(2):96–99.

Lindmark G, Nyberg K. The Swedish experience. Presented at an international conference entitled "How should maternal and child health services be delivered in the 21st Century?" The conference was convened by the University of South Florida Health Sciences Center and the French–American Foundation in Tampa, FL, April 20–22, 1997.

Linden AD, Urang S. "Mismanaged Care." A Response from midwives. The NY State Chapters of the ACNM, New York, May 15, 1995.

Litoff JB. The midwife throughout history. *J Nurse Midwifery* 1982;27(6):3–11.

Litoff JB. *The American Midwife Debate: A Sourcebook on Its Modern Origins.* Greenwood Press, New York, 1986.

Long SH, Marquis MS, Harrison ER. The costs and financing of perinatal care in the United States. *Am J Public Health* 1994;84: 1473–1478.

Lonsdale L, Murdaugh A, Stiles D. Su Clinica Familiar—Georgetown University pilot project. *J Nurse Midwifery* 1982;27(5):25–33.

López-Zeno JA, Peacement AM, Adashek JA, Socol ML. A controlled trial of a program for the active management of labor. *N Engl J Med* 1992;326:450–454.

Lops VR. Midwifery: Past to present. *J Prof Nursing* 1988;4(6):402–407.

Lops VR, Dixon L, Hunter LP. The evolving practice of nurse-midwifery. *Adv Pract Nurs Q* 1995;1(1):29–36.

Loudon I. *Death in Childbirth: An International Study of Maternal Care and Maternal Mortality, 1800–1950.* Clarendon Press, Oxford, 1992.

Lubic RW. The impact of technology on health care—the Childbearing Center: A case for technology's appropriate use. *J Nurse Midwifery* 1979;24(1):6–10.

Lubic R. Evaluation of an out-of-hospital maternity center for low-risk patients. In Aiken L (Ed.), *Health Policy and Nursing Practice,* McGraw-Hill, New York, 1981.

Lubic R. Birth centers: Delivering more for less. *Am J Nursing.* 1983;83:1053–1056.

Lubic RW. Some comments on the Chicago Maternity Center and on the NYC Maternity Center Association. *Am J Public Health* 1988; 78:1360.

Lubic RW, Ernst EKM. The Childbearing Center: An alternative to conventional care. *Nursing Outlook* 1978;26(12):754–760.

Lumley J, Small R, Yelland J. *Having a Baby in Victoria: Final Report of the Ministerial Review of Birthing Services in Victoria.* Health Department, Victoria, Australia, 1990.

Lyall S. British mothers' hospital time is cut. *The New York Times,* December 3, 1995.

Lydon-Rochelle M, Albers L. Research trends in the *Journal of Nurse-Midwifery* 1987–1992. *J Nurse Midwifery* 1993;38:343–348.

Lydon-Rochelle M, Albers L, Gorwoda J, Craig E, Qualls C. Accuracy of Leopold maneuvers in screening for malpresentation: A prospective study. *Birth* 1993;20:122–135.

MacDonald D. Cerebral palsy and intrapartum fetal monitoring. *N Engl J Med* 1996;334: 659–660.

MacDonald D, Grant A, Sheridan-Pereira M, Boylan P, Chalmers I. The Dublin randomized controlled trial of intrapartum fetal heart monitoring. *Am J Obstet Gynecol* 1985;152: 524–539.

MacDonald M. Midwives in Ontario: Representation and identity. Paper presented during the Annual Joint Meeting of the Society for Applied Anthropology, the Society for Medical Anthropology, the Council on Nursing and Anthropology, and the Political Ecology Society, Seattle, Washington, March 6, 1997.

MacDonald SE, Voaklander K, Birtwhistle RV. A comparison of family physicians' and obstetricians' intrapartum management of low-risk pregnancies. *J Fam Pract* 1993;37(5): 457–462.

Madrona MM, Madrona LM. The future of midwifery in the United States. *NAPSAC News* 1993;18(3–4):1,3–32.

Magill-Cuerden J. Not such a "common market" for midwives. *Midwives Chronicle & Nursing Notes,* April 1977, pp. 76–78.

Maine, D. *Safe Motherhood Programs: Options and Issues.* Columbia University, New York, 1991.

Main DM, Gabbe SG, Richardson D, Strong S. Can preterm deliveries be prevented? *Am J Obstet Gynecol* 1985;151:829–898.

Main DM, Richardson DK, Hadley CB, Gabbe SG. Controlled trial of a preterm labor detection program: Efficacy and costs. *Obstet Gynecol* 1989;74:873–877.

MANA. State midwifery associations, newsletters & certification processes. Author, 1993.

MANA Legislative Committee. State legal status as of December 1994.

MANA News, 1987; IV(4).

March of Dimes Birth Defects Foundation. *Toward Improving the Outcome of Pregnancy: The 90s and Beyond.* Author, White Plains, NY, 1993.

Martinez G, Nalezienski J. 1980 update: The Recent trend in breastfeeding. *Pediatrics* 1981; 67:686–692.

Matsuoka J, Hirasawa M, Kumazawa M, Sasaki K, Kiura C. Evaluation of hospital midwives' work and the development of burnout syndrome. *Proceedings of the International Confederation of Midwives 24th Triennial Congress,* Oslo, May 26–31, 1996, ICM, London, pp. 274–275.

Matyac HG. Personal communication, 1996. (Helen Gordon Matyac is Nurse-Midwifery Program Specialist for the North Carolina Office of Rural Health and Resource Development, Raleigh, NC.)

Mayfield JA, Rosenblatt RA, Baldwin LM, Chu L, Logerfo JP: The relation of obstetrical volume and nursery level to perinatal mortality. *Am J Public Health* 1990;80:819–823.

McAnarney ER, Roghmann KJ, Adams BN, Tatelbaum RC, Kash C, Coulter M, Plume M, Charney E. Obstetric, neonatal and psychosocial outcome of pregnant adolescents. *Pediatrics* 1978;61:199–205.

McCallum WT. The maternity center at El Paso. *Birth Family J* 1979;6:259–266.

McClain CS. Perceived risk and choice of childbirth service. *Social Sci Med* 1983;17:1857–1865.

McCool W, McCool S. Feminism and nurse-midwifery: Historical overview and current issues. *J Nurse Midwifery* 1989;34:323–334.

McCormick MC. The contribution of low birth weight to infant mortality and childhood mortality. *N Engl J Med* 1985;312:82–90.

McCormick MC, Shapiro S, and Starfield BH: The regionalization of perinatal services. *JAMA* 1985;253:799–804.

McCreary A. The quiet crisis—Kathryn Barnard examines the plight of America's youngest children. *Connections,* Spring 1996, pp. 3–4. (Published by University of Washington School of Nursing, Seattle.).

McDonald TP, Coburn AF. Predictors of prenatal care utilization. Soc Sci Med 1988; 27: 167–172.

McDonald W, Davis JA. *History of Midwifery Practice in Australia and the Western Pacific Regions.* Western Australian Branch of the National Midwives Association of Australia, Perth, 1984. (Book prepared for the 20th Congress of the International Confederation of Midwives.)

McGinnis JM, Lee PR. Healthy people 2000 at mid decade. *JAMA* 1995;273:1123–1129.

McIntyre J. "The calling": Lay midwives' pursuit of livelihood. Paper presented at the Southwestern Anthropologic Association Annual Meeting, April 8, 1982.

McKay S. Models of midwifery care: Denmark, Sweden, and the Netherlands. *J Nurse Midwifery* 1993;38:114–120.

McKee K, Adams E. Nurse midwives' attitudes toward abortion performance and related procedures. *J Nurse Midwifery* 1994;39:300–311.

McLaughlin FJ, Altemeier WA, Christensen MJ, Sherrod KB, Dietrich MS, Sterm DT. Randomized trial of comprehensive prenatal care for low-income women: Effect on infant birth weight. *Pediatrics* 1992;89:128–132.

McNiven P, Hodnett E, O'Brien-Pallas LL. Supporting women in labor: A work sampling study of the activities of labor and delivery nurses. *Birth* 1992;19:3–8.

Meckler L. Doctors suffer cut in income. *The Oregonian,* August 24, 1996, pp. C1, C6.

Medical World News. Pain-killers in labor: "Caution flag is up." February 5, 1979, pp. 23–24.

Meglen M. Personal communication, 1993. (Marie Meglan is director of the Bureau of Maternal and Child Health, South Carolina Department of Health and Environmental Control.)

Meglen M, Burst H. Nurse-midwives make a difference. *Nursing Outlook* 1974;22(6):386–389.

Mehl LE. Research on alternatives in childbirth: What can it tell us about hospital practice? *21st Century Obstetrics Now!*, Vol. 1. National Association of Parents & Professionals for Safe Alternatives in Childbirth, Marble Hill, MO, 1977, pp. 171–207.

Mehl LE, Peterson GH, Shaw, NS, Creevy DC. Complications of home birth. *Birth Family J* 1975;2(4):123–131.

Mehl LE, Peterson GH, Whitt M, Hayes WE. Outcomes of elective home births: A series of 1,146 cases. *J Reprod Med* 1977;19:281–290.

Mehl LE, Ramiel JR, Leininger B, Hoff B, Kroenthal K, Peterson G. Evaluation of outcomes of non-nurse midwives: Matched comparisons with physicians. *Women & Health* 1980;5:17–29.

Mehl-Madrona L. Personal communication, 1996/1997. (Lewis Mehl-Madrona, MD, is at the Native American Research and Training Center, University of Arizona College of Medicine, Tuscon, Arizona.)

Mehl-Madrona L, Madrona MM. Physician- and midwife-attended home births: Effects of breech, twin, and post-dates outcome data on mortality rates. *J Nurse Midwifery* 1997;42:91–98.

Meigs GL. A survey of the problems of childbirth, 1911–16. *Am J Public Health* 1985;75:546.

Meijer WJ, Veer AJE de, Groenewegen PP. Obstetric co-operation, risk selection and outcome. In *Proceedings of the International Confederation of Midwives 24th Triennial Congress*, Oslo, May 26–31, 1996, ICM, London, pp. 176–178.

Meikle SF, Orleans M, Leff M, Shain R, Gibbs RS. Women's reasons for not seeking prenatal care: Racial and ethnic factors. *Birth* 1995;22:81–86.

Melber R, Malone P. Georgia midwifery from granny to nurse. Georgia Department of Human Resources, Atlanta, May 1987. (An unpublished historical overview prepared by the Family Health Section, Division of Public Health, Georgia Department of Human Resources.)

Mendelson DL. The aspiration of stomach contents into the lungs during obstetric anesthesia. *Am J Obstet Gynecol* 1949;52:191–205.

Merkatz I, Fanaroff A. The regional perinatal network. In Sweeney WJ, Caplan RM (Eds.), *Advances in Obstetrics and Gynecology*. Williams and Wilkins, Baltimore, 1978.

Merkatz IR, Thompson JB. *New Perspectives on Prenatal Care*. Elsevier Science Publishing, New York, 1990.

Merz T. A working lay midwife birth center, Madison, Wisconsin. In Steward D, Stewart S (Eds.) *21st Century Obstetrics Now!* National Association of Parents & Professionals for Safe Alternatives in Childbirth, Chapel Hill, NC, pp. 545–551.

Metropolitan Life Insurance Company. Summary of the tenth thousand confinement records of the Frontier Nursing service. *FNS Quarterly Bull* 1958;33(4):44–55.

Meyer HBP, Wagner L, Dorsen WJ. A regional system for the transport of sick neonates in Arizona. *Ped. Res.* 1971;5:376. (Abstract.)

Meyer Memorial Trust. *Report for 1995–1996*. Author, Portland, OR, 1997.

Middleton JP. Private nurse-midwifery practice with hospital deliveries. In Rooks J, Haas, JE (Eds.), *Nurse-Midwifery in America*. ACNM Foundation, Washington, DC, 1986, pp. 30–31.

Miller CA. *Maternal Health and Infant Survival*. National Center for Clinical Infant Programs, Washington, DC. 1987.

Miller CA. Personal communication, October 1996. (C. Arden Miller is Chair of the Department of Maternal and Child Health, School of Public Health, University of North Carolina at Chapel Hill.)

Miller JM Jr. Maternal and neonatal morbidity and mortality in cesarean section. *Obstet Gynecol Clin North Am* 1988;15:629–638.

Milligan C. Personal communication, 1995. (Carol Milligan was chief of the Branch of Nurse-Midwifery, Indian Health Service, 1977–1994.)

Milliken N. In *The Obstetrician/Gynecologist in the Twenty-First Century: Meeting Society's Needs*. Josiah Macy, Jr. Foundation, New York, 1993, pp. 11–31.

Mitchell MD, Flint APF, Bibby J, Brunt J, Arnold JM, Anderson ABM, Turnbull AC. Rapid increases in plasma prostaglandin concentrations after vaginal examination and amniotomy. *Br Med J* 1977;2:1183–1185.

Mitford J. *The American Way of Birth*. Dutton/Penguin Books, New York, 1992.

Mittendorf R, Williams MA, Berkey CS, Cotter PF. The length of uncomplicated human gestation. *Obstet Gynecol* 1990;75(6):929–932.

Monroe LR. Who should pay for graduate medical education? *Oregon Health Forum,* March 1996, pp. 10–11.

Montagu A. Social impacts of unnecessary intervention and unnatural surroundings in childbirth. In Steward D, Stewart S (Eds.), *21st Century Obstetrics Now!,* Vol. 2. National Association of Parents & Professionals for Safe Alternatives in Childbirth, Chapel Hill, NC, 1977, pp. 589–610.

Moon BJ. Prescriptive authority and nurse-midwives. *J Nurse Midwifery* 1990;35:50–52.

Morales E. Personal communication, 1996. (Elisa Morales is a certified nurse-midwife with a home birth practice in Portland, OR.)

Moreau R. Mission to Toronto and Seattle concerning course work and ongoing training in midwifery. Attachment to a letter from René Moreau, Responsable de planification de la mise à jour des connaissances des candidates sages-femmes, Service de planification des resources humaines, Gouvernement du Québec, Ministére de la Santé et des Services Sociaux, Direction générale des relations de travall, to Jo Anne Myers-Ciecko, Seattle Midwifery School, September 14, 1992.

Morningstar SK. Midwives, myths, medicine, miracles and maybe babies. *MANA Newsletter* 1994;12(1):30–31.

Morten A, Kohl M, O'Mahoney P, Pelosi K. Certified nurse-midwifery care of the postpartum client: A descriptive study. *J Nurse Midwifery* 1991;36(5):276–284.

Morton SC, Williams, MS, Keeler EB, Gambone JC, Kahn KL. Effect of epidural analgesia for labor on the cesarean delivery rate. *Obstet Gynecol* 1994;83:1045–1052.

Munster K, Schmidt L, Helm P. Length and variation in the menstrual cycle—a cross-sectional study from a Danish county. *Br J Obstet Gynaecol* 1992;99:422–429.

Murdaugh A. Experiences of a new migrant health clinic. *Women & Health* 1976;1(6):25–28.

Murdaugh A. Quoted in Schlinger H, *Circle of Midwives,* 1992, pp. 14–15.

Murphy PA. Preterm birth prevention programs: A critique of current literature. *J Nurse Midwifery* 1993;38:324–335.

Murphy PA. Primary care for women: Health assessment, health promotion, and disease prevention services. *J Nurse Midwifery* 1996;41:83–91.

Murphy PA. Personal communication, 1996. (Patricia Aikins Murphy is a nurse-midwife epidemiologist and assistant professor at Columbia University Nurse-Midwifery Education Program and co-investigator for the ACNM Home Birth Study.)

Myers RE, Williams MV. Lost opportunities for the prevention of fetal asphyxia: Sedation, analgesia, and general anesthesia. *Clin Obstet Gynaecol* 1982;9(2):369–414.

Myers S. Midwifery in the United States: How regulations affect the profession. December 1986. (This unpublished paper is available from the Seattle Midwifery School, 2524 16th Avenue, South, Suite 300, Seattle, WA 98144-5014.)

Myers SA, Gleicher N. A successful program to lower cesarean-section rates. *N Engl J Med* 1988;319:1511–1516.

Myers-Ciecko JA. Direct-entry midwifery in the USA. In Kitzinger S (Ed.), *The Midwife Challenge.* Pandora Press, London, 1988, pp. 61–84.

Myers-Ciecko JA. Personal communication, 1994–1997. (Jo Anne Myers-Ciecko is executive director of the Seattle Midwifery School.)

Myers-Ciecko JA, Stallings T. Personal communication, 1994. (Jo Anne Myers-Ciecko and Therese Stallings are on the faculty of the Seattle Midwifery School.).

National Association of Childbearing Centers. Report of the 1994 NACC survey of birth center experience. Author, Perkiomenville, PA, 1995.

National Center for Health Statistics. Health Manpower and Health Facilities, 1976–77. *Health Resources Statistics.* U.S. Government Printing Office, Washington, DC, 1997. DHEW Publication 79–1509.

National Center for Health Statistics. Office visits by women: The national ambulatory medical care survey. Prepared by BK Cypress. *Vital and Health Statistics,* Series 13, No. 45. Public Health Service. U.S. Government Printing Office, Washington, DC, March 1980. DHHS Publication 80-1976.

National Center for Health Statistics. Advance report of final natality statistics, 1980. *Monthly Vital Statistics Report,* Vol. 31, No. 8, suppl. Public Health Service, Hyattsville, MD, November 1982. DHHS Publication 83-1120.

National Center for Health Statistics. Advance report of final natality statistics, 1989. *Monthly*

Vital Statistics Report, Vol. 40, No. 8, suppl. Public Health Service, Hyattsville, MD, 1991.

National Center for Health Statistics. Advance report of new data from the 1989 birth certificate. *Monthly Vital Statistics Report,* Vol. 40, No. 12, suppl. Public Health Service, Hyattsville, MD, 1992.

National Center for Health Statistics. Advance report of final natality statistics, 1990. *Monthly Vital Statistics Report,* Vol. 41, No. 9, suppl. Public Health Service, Hyattsville, MD, 1993a.

National Center for Health Statistics. Advance report of maternal and infant health data from the birth certificate, 1990. *Monthly Vital Statistics Report* Vol 42, No. 2, suppl. Public Health Service, Hyattsville, MD, 1993b.

National Center for Health Statistics. Advance report of final natality statistics, 1991. *Monthly Vital Statistics Report,* Vol. 42, No. 3, suppl. Public Health Service, Hyattsville, MD, 1993c.

National Center for Health Statistics. Advance report of maternal and infant health data from the birth certificate, 1991. *Monthly Vital Statistics Report,* Vol. 42, No. 11, suppl. Public Health Service, Hyattsville, MD, 1994a.

National Center for Health Statistics. *Health, United States, 1993.* Public Health Service, Hyattsville, MD, 1994b.

National Center for Health Statistics. *Healthy People 2000 Review, 1993.* Public Health Service, Hyattsville, MD, 1994c.

National Center for Health Statistics. *Health, United States, 1994 Chartbook.* Public Health Service, Hyattsville, MD, 1995.

National Center for Health Statistics. *Healthy People 2000 Review, 1995–96.* Public Health Service, Hyattsville, MD, 1996a.

National Center for Health Statistics. *Health, United States, 1995.* Public Health Service, Hyattsville, MD, 1996b.

National Coalition of Midwifery Educators. Conference report and statement of support for national accreditation of midwifery education, Flagstaff, Arizona, June 1990.

National Commission on Nurse-Midwifery Education. *Educating Nurse-Midwives: A Strategy for Achieving Affordable, High-Quality Maternity Care, Executive Summary.* ACNM, Washington, DC, 1993.

National Commission to Prevent Infant Mortality. *Death Before Life: The Tragedy of Infant Mortality.* Author, Washington, DC, August 1988.

National Institute of Neurological Disease and Stroke. *The Women and Their Pregnancies: The Collaborative Perinatal Study of the National Institute of Neurological Disease and Stroke.* Author, Bethesda, MD, 1972, pp. 363–388. DHEW Publication 73–79.

National Institutes of Health. *Cesarean Childbirth: Report of a Consensus Development Conference.* Sponsored by the National Institute of Child Health and Human Development in Conjunction with the National Center for Health Care Technology and assisted by the Office for Medical Application of Research, October 1981, NIH Publication 82-2067.

National League for Nursing. *Nursing Datasource,* Vol. 1, *Trends in Contemporary Nursing Education.* NLN Research, New York, 1995.

Nation's Health. From horseback to four-wheel drive: 'Frontier nurses' mark 50 years' service. American Public Health Association, Washington, DC, May 1976, p. 5.

Nation's Health. American Public Health Association, Washington, DC, November 1978, p. 8.

Nation's Health. Lack of primary care physicians could scuttle health care reform. American Public Health Association, Washington, DC, August 1993, p. 14.

Nation's Health. More Medicaid patients in managed care plans in 1994. American Public Health Association, Washington, DC, January 1995, p. 5.

Nation's Health. States turning more to managed care for Medicaid. American Public Health Association, Washington, DC, March 1995, p. 11.

Nation's Health. Budget slashing puts public health services at risk. American Public Health Association, Washington, DC, September 1995, pp. 1, 6.

Nation's Health. Managed care and public health struggling to coexist. American Public Health Association, Washington, DC, May/June 1996, p 1.

Nation's Health. States take health care reform down many different roads. American Public Health Association, Washington, DC, August 1996, p. 8.

Neilson I. Nurse-midwifery in an alternative birth center. *Birth Family J* 1977;4:24–27.

Nelson KB, Dambrosia JM, Ting TY, Grether JK. Uncertain value of electronic fetal monitoring in predicting cerebral palsy. *N Engl J Med* 1996;334:613–618.

Nesbitt TS. Rural maternity care: New models of access. *Birth* 1996;23:161–165.

Nesbitt TS, Connell FA, Hart LG, Rosenblatt RA. Access to obstetrical care in rural areas: Effect on birth outcomes. *Am J Public Health* 1990;80:814–818.

Nestel S. A new profession to the white population in Canada: Ontario midwifery and the politics of race. Paper presented during the Annual Joint Meeting of the Society for Applied Anthropology, the Society for Medical Anthropology, the Council on Nursing and Anthropology, and the Political Ecology Society, Seattle, Washington, March 6, 1997. (Subsequent to hearing Dr. Nestel's presentation at this meeting, I have had personal communication with her regarding her research. She is on the faculty of the Department of Sociology at the University of Toronto.)

Neutra RR, Fienberg SE, Greenland S, Friedman EA. Effect of fetal monitoring on neonatal death rates. *N Engl J Med 1978;299:324–326.*

Newton N. Special issues in nurse-midwifery: A look at the past and future. *J Nurse Midwifery* 1986;31(5):232–239.

Newton N, Foshee D, Newton M. Parturient mice: Effects of environment on labor. *Science* 1966;151(717):1560–1561.

Newton N, Peeler D, Newton M. Effect of disturbance on labor: Experiment using one hundred mice with dated pregnancies. *Am J Obstet Gynecol* 1968;101(8):1096–1102.

Newton RW, Hunt IP. Psychosocial stress in pregnancy and its relation to low birthweight. *Br Med J* 1984;288:1191–1194.

Nichols M. Personal communication in response to his review of Chapters 9 and 11, 1996. (Mark Nichols is on the faculty of the Department of Obstetrics and Gynecology, Oregon Health Sciences University, Portland, OR.)

Nickel S, Gesse T, MacLaren A. Ernestine Wiedenback: Her professional legacy. *J Nurse Midwifery* 1992;37:161–167.

North American Registry of Midwives. Entry level midwifery skills/task analysis report. January 26, 1994. Copies of this document can be obtained from Schroeder Measurement Technologies Inc., 2536 Countryside Blvd., Clearwater, FL 34623. 1-800-556-0484.

North American Registry of Midwives. *NARM 1995 Job Analysis.* Author, 1996. Copies of this document can be obtained from Schroeder

Measurement Technologies, Inc., 2536 Countryside Blvd., Clearwater, FL 34623. 1-800-556-0484.

Notzon FC. International differences in the use of obstetric interventions. *JAMA* 1990;263 (24):3286–3291.

Novy MJ, McGregor JA, Iams JD. New perspectives on the prevention of extreme prematurity. *Clin Obstet Gynecol* 1995;38(4);790–808.

Nursing Progress. Anonymously authored article reporting an interview with Mary Ann Curry, a professor at the Oregon Health Sciences University. Spring 1996;7(3):6–7. (*Nursing Progress* is published by the Oregon Health Sciences University School of Nursing, Portland, OR.)

Oakley D. Personal communication, May 3, 1996. (Deborah Oakley is a professor at the Center for Nursing Research, University of Michigan School of Nursing, Ann Arbor, MI.)

Oakley D, Murtland T, Mayes F, Hayashi R, Petersen BA, Rorie C, Andersen F. Processes of Care: Comparisons of certified nurse-midwives and obstetricians. *J Nurse Midwifery* 1995;40:399–409.

Oakley D, Murray ME, Murtland T, Hayashi R, Andersen F, Mayes F, Rooks J. Comparisons of outcomes of maternity care by obstetricians and certified nurse-midwives. *Obstet Gynecol* 1996;88:823–829.

O'Brien B, Naber S. Nausea and vomiting during pregnancy: Effects on the quality of women's lives. *Birth* 1992;19(3):138–143.

O'Brien B, Zhou Q. Variables related to nausea and vomiting during pregnancy. *Birth* 1995;22(2):93–100.

O'Brien J, Green S. Northern Territory. In McDonald W, Davis JA. (Eds.), *History of Midwifery Practice in Australia and the Western Pacific Regions.* Western Australian Branch of the National Midwives Association of Australia, Perth, 1984, pp. 11–22. (Book prepared for the 20th Congress of the International Confederation of Midwives.)

O'Brien M. Home and hospital confinement: A comparison of the experiences of mothers having home and hospital confinements. *J Roy College Gen Pract* 1978;28:460–466.

O'Conner B. The home birth movement in the United States. *J Med Philosophy* 1992;18: 147–174.

O'Connor S, Vietze PM, Sherrod KB, Sandler HM, Altemeier III WA. Reduced incidence of parenting inadequacy following rooming-in. *Pediatrics* 1980;66(2):176–182.

Odent M. *Birth Reborn,* 2nd ed. Birth Works Press, London, 1994.

O'Driscoll K, Foley M, MacDonald D. Active management of labor as an alternative to cesarean section for dystocia. *Obstet Gynecol* 1984; 63:485–490.

Offenbacher S, Katz V, Fertik G, Collins J, Boyd D, Maynor G, McKaig R, Beck J. Periodontal infection as a possible risk factor for preterm low birth weight. *J Periodontology* 1996;67(10, suppl S):1103–1113.

Office of Disease Prevention and Health Promotion. *The 1990 Health Objectives for the Nation: A Midcourse Review.* Public Health Service, U.S. Department of Health and Human Services, Washington, DC, November 1986.

Office of Inspector General. A survey of certified nurse-midwives. Department of Health and Human Services, Washington, DC, March 1992.

Office of Technology Assessment. U.S. Congress. *Nurse Practitioners, Physicians Assistants, and Certified Nurse-Midwives: A Policy Analysis.* U.S. Government Printing Office, Washington, DC, 1986.

Office of Technology Assessment, U.S. Congress. *Healthy Children: Investing in the Future.* U.S. Government Printing Office, Washington, DC, 1988.

Official Journal of the European Communities. Legislation. English Edition, February 11, 1980, pp. 2–3.

Olds DL, Henderson CR, Tatelbaum R, Chamberline R. Improving the delivery of prenatal care and outcomes of pregnancy. A randomized trial of nurse home visitation. *Pediatrics* 1986;77:16–18.

Oliver DR. Eleventh annual report on physician assistant educational programs in the United States, 1994–1995. Association of Physician Assistant Programs. Arlington, VA, June 1995.

O'Neil J, Kaufert PA. The politics of obstetric care: The Inuit experience. In Handwerker WP (Ed.), *Births and Power: Social Change and the Politics of Reproduction.* Westview Press, San Francisco, 1990.

O'Neill P. A women's specialty. *The Oregonian,* June 25, 1995, pp. B1, B4.

Oregon Department of Human Resources. *Oregon Vital Statistics Annual Report 1991.* Health Division, Center for Disease Prevention and Epidemiology, Center for Health Statistics, Portland, Oregon, July 1993.

Oregon Department of Justice. Opinion No. 7468, June 17, 1977, Salem, OR.

Oregon Health Sciences University. Medical staff bylaws, 1994–95. Author, Portland, OR.

Osborn A, Esty L. Standardized education: Does it prepare better midwives and birth educators? What are the shortcomings and strengths of your own preparation? A collection of responses from practicing midwives. In *Getting an Education.* Midwifery Today, Eugene, OR, 1995, pp. 3–4.

Oski FA. Editorial: By the numbers. *Contemporary Pediatrics,* November 1993. p. 9.

Oudshoorn C. A new curriculum in the Netherlands. *Midwives Chronicle & Nursing Notes,* August 1993, pp. 290–291.

Owens A. Where do you fit in? *Med Economics* 1982:246–259.

Paine LL, Tinker DD. The effect of maternal bearing-down efforts on the arterial umbilical cord pH and length of the second stage of labor. *J Nurse Midwifery* 1992;37:61–63.

Paine LL, Payton RG, Johnson TR. Auscultated fetal heart rate accelerations, part I: Accuracy and documentation. *J Nurse Midwifery* 1986;31:68–72.

Paine LL, Johnson TRB, Turner MH, Payton RG. Auscultated fetal heart rate accelerations, part II: An alternative to the nonstress test. *J Nurse Midwifery* 1986;31:73–77.

Pairman S. Midwifery: A partnership between the woman and the midwife. In *Proceedings of the International Confederation of Midwives 24th Triennial Congress,* Oslo, May, 26–31, ICM, London, pp. 297–301.

Papiernik E. An effective approach to prenatal care: Goals, methods and results of the French system. Presented at an international conference entitled "How should maternal and child health services be delivered in the 21st century?" The conference was convened by the University of South Florida Health Sciences Center and the French-American Foundation in Tampa, FL, April 20–22, 1997.

Papiernik-Berkuauer E. Prediction of the preterm baby. *Clin Obstet Gynecol* 1980;11:315–319.

Parker B, McFarlane J, Soeken K. Abuse during pregnancy: Effects on maternal complications and birth weight in adult and teenage women. *Obstet Gynecol* 1994;84:323–328.

Parker JD. Ethnic differences in midwife-attended US births. *Am J Public Health* 1994; 84:1139–1141.

Parra A. Thoughts on the apprentice's path. In *Getting an Education*. Midwifery Today. Eugene, OR, 1995, pp. 3–4.

Patamia KJP. ACNM marks milestone with 50 education programs. *Quickening* 1996;27(6):1, 16, 21.

Patch RB, Holaday SD. Effects of changes in professional liability insurance on certified nurse-midwives. *J Nurse Midwifery* 1989; 34:131–136.

Patkelly M. Quoted in Schlinger H, *Circle of Midwives*, 1992, p. 45.

Payton R. Personal communication, 1993. (Ruth Payton was director of the United States Air Force Nurse-Midwifery Education Program from 1980 to 1985.)

Pearse WH. Defining the obstetrician–gynecologist of the future. In *The Obstetrician/Gynecologist in the Twenty-First Century: Meeting Society's Needs*. Josiah Macy, Jr. Foundation, New York, 1993, pp. 59–91.

Pearse W, quoted in *OB-Gyn News* 1980;15(11):1.

Pearse WH. The home birth crisis. *Bull ACOG*, July 1977.

Peoples-Sheps MD, Hogan VK, Ng'andu N. Content of prenatal care during the initial workup. *Am J Obstet Gynecol* 1996;174:220–226.

Perry DS. The early midwives of Missouri. *J Nurse Midwifery* 1983; 28(6):15–22.

Peters MH. Midwives and the achievement of safer motherhood. *Int J Gynecol Obstet* 1995;50(suppl 2):S89–S92.

Petitti DB, Cefalo RC, Shapiro S, Whalley P. In-hospital maternal mortality in the United States: Time trends and relation to method of delivery. *Obstet Gynecol* 1982;59:6–12.

Pew Health Professions Commission. *Critical Challenges: Revitalizing the Health Professions for the Twenty-First Century*. Center for the Health Professions, University of California at San Francisco, San Francisco, 1995.

Pfost KS, Stevens MJ, Matejcak AJ. A counselor's primer on postpartum depression. *J Counseling Dev* 1990;69:148–151.

Philipps LHC, O'Hara MW. Prospective study of postpartum depression: 4½-year follow-up of women and children. *J Abnorm Psychol* 1991;100:151–155.

Piechnik SL, Corbett MA. Reducing low birth weight among socioeconomically high-risk adolescent pregnancies: Successful intervention with certified nurse-midwife-managed care and a multidisciplinary team. *J Nurse Midwifery* 1985;30(2):88–98.

Piper JM, Ray WA, Griffin MR. Effects of Medicaid eligibility expansion of prenatal care and pregnancy outcomes in Tennessee. *JAMA* 1990;264:2219–2223.

Piper JM, Mitchel EF, Snowden M, Hall C, Adams M, Taylor P. Validation of 1989 Tennessee birth certificates using maternal and newborn hospital records. *Am J Epidemiol* 1993; 137:758–768.

Piper JM, Mitchel EF, Ray WA. Presumptive eligibility for pregnant Medicaid enrollees: Its effects on prenatal care and perinatal outcome. *Am J Public Health* 1994;84:1626–1630.

Piper S, Parks PL. Predicting the duration of lactation: Evidence from a national survey. *Birth* 1996;23:7–12.

Pittard WB 3d, Geddes KM. Newborn hospitalization: A closer look. *J Pediatr* 1988;112:257–261.

Placek PH, Taffel SM. Recent patterns in cesarean delivery in the United States. *Obstet Gynecol Clin North Am* 1988;15:607–627.

Placksin S. New moms get a world of different treatments. *The Oregonian*, May 5, 1996.

Platt LD, Angeline DJ, Paul RH, Quilligan EJ. Nurse-midwifery in a large teaching hospital. *Obstet Gynecol* 1985;66:816–820.

Porreco RP. High cesarean section rate: A new perspective. *Obstet Gynecol* 1985;65:307–311.

Porreco RP. Meeting the challenge of the rising cesarean birth rate. *Obstet Gynecol* 1990;75: 133–136.

Porter, Novelli and Associates. Professional liability insurance and its effects: Report of a survey of ACOG's membership. ACOG, Washington, DC, 1983.

Prodromidis M, Field T, Arendt R, Singer L, Yando R, Bendell D. Mothers touching newborns: A comparison of rooming-in versus minimal contact. *Birth* 1995;22:196–200.

Public Health Service. *Caring for Our Future: The Content of Prenatal Care*. U.S. Department of Health and Human Services, Washington, DC, 1989.

Quickening. Midwifery gains in Canada. American College of Nurse-Midwives, Washington, DC, March/April, 1993, pp. 21–22.

Quickening. State news. American College of Nurse-Midwives, Washington, DC, November/December 1995, p. 16.

Quilligan E. Cesarean section: Modern perspective. In Queenan JT (Ed.), *Management of the High Risk Pregnancy,* 2nd ed. Medical Economics, Oradell, NJ, 1985, pp. 594–600.

Radin TG, Harmon JS, Hanson DA. Nurses' care during labor: Its effect on the cesarean birth rate of healthy, nulliparous women. *Birth* 1993;20:14–21.

Raisler J. Interview with a rural midwife. *J Nurse Midwifery* 1978;22(4):36–38.

Raisler J. Nurse-midwifery education: Issues for survival and growth. *J Nurse Midwifery* 1987; 32(1):1–3.

Raisler J. The International Confederation of Midwives: Past history, present activities, and future challenges. *J Nurse Midwifery* 1994;39: 326–328.

Record J, Cohen H. The introduction of midwifery in a prepaid group practice. *Am J Public Health* 1972;62:354–360.

Reeves N, Potempa K, Gallo A. Fatigue in early pregnancy: An exploratory study. *J Nurse Midwifery* 1991;36:303–308.

Reid AF, Carroll JC, Ruderman J, Murray MA. Differences in intrapartum obstetric care provided to women at low risk by family physicians and obstetricians. *Can Med Assoc J* 1989;140:625–633.

Reid M. Apprenticeship into midwifery: An American example. *Midwifery* 1986;2:126–134.

Reid ML, Morris JB. Perinatal care and cost effectiveness: Changes in health expenditure and birth outcome following the establishment of a nurse-midwife program. *Med Care* 1979; 17(5):491–500.

Reinke C. Outcomes of the first 527 births at the Birthplace in Seattle. *Birth* 1982;9:231–238.

Renfrew, M. Personal communication, 1997. (Mary Renfrew is Professor and Head of the Division of Midwifery in the School of Healthcare Studies, University of Leeds, Leeds, United Kingdom.)

Reynolds JL. The final fatal blow to routine episiotomy. *Birth* 1993;20:162–163.

Richardson T. Personal communication, March 1996. (Terra Richardson is founder of Resourcing Birth, Boulder, Colorado.)

Richter A. Personal communication, September/October 1996. (Anne Richter is deputy director of the Florida Midwifery Resource Center, Tampa, FL.)

Righard L. How do newborns find their mother's breast? *Birth* 1995;22(3):174–175.

Righard L, Alade MO. Sucking technique and its effects on success of breastfeeding. *Birth* 1992;19(4):185–189.

Rivo ML, Saultz JW, Wartman SA, DeWitt TG. Defining the generalist physician's training. *JAMA* 1994;271:1499–1511.

Robert Wood Johnson Foundation. *Special Report: Regionalized Perinatal Services.* Robert Wood Johnson Foundation, Princeton, NJ, 1978.

Roberts J. ACOG guidelines promote "closer ties" with nurse-midwives. *Quickening,* November/December 1995a, p. 3.

Roberts J. The role of graduate education in midwifery in the USA. In (Murphy-Black T (Ed.), *Issues in Midwifery,* Vol. I. Churchill Livingstone, New York, 1995b, pp. 119–161.

Roberts J. Dictating the content of nurse-midwifery care. *Quickening,* January/February 1996a, p. 3.

Roberts J. The certification of non-nurse midwives by the American College of Nurse-Midwives. *J Nurse Midwifery* 1996b;41:1–2.

Roberts J. The switch to managed care: What it means for nurse-midwives. *Quickening,* May/June 1996c, pp. 3, 7.

Roberts JE, Goldstein SA, Gruener JS, Maggio M, Mendez-Bauer C. A descriptive analysis of involuntary bearing-down efforts during the expulsive phase of labor. *J Obstet Gynecol Neonatal Nurs* 1987;Jan/Feb:48–55.

Robinson K. Emerging midwifery: The importance of creating unity among midwives. Paper presented during the Annual Joint Meeting of the Society for Applied Anthropology, the Society for Medical Anthropology, the Council on Nursing and Anthropology, and the Political Ecology Society, Seattle, Washington, March 6, 1997.

Robinson S. Career intentions of newly qualified midwives. *Midwifery* 1986;2:25–36.

Robinson S, Thompson AM. *Midwives, Research and Childbirth, Volume 1.* Chapman and Hall, London, 1989.

Robinson S, Golden J, Bradley S. A study of the role and responsibilities of the midwife. Department of Health and Social Security, London, 1983.

Robinson SA. A historical development of midwifery in the black community: 1600–1940. *J Nurse Midwifery* 1984;29(4):247–250.

Rooks JB. Estrogen treatment of teenage girls in the United States: Description of the treated population. *Pediatrics* 1978; 62: 1098–1103.

Rooks JP. The context of nurse-midwifery in the 1980s: Our relationships with medicine, nursing, lay-midwives, consumers and health care economists. *J Nurse Midwifery* 1983;28 (5):3–8.

Rooks JP, Carr KC. Criteria for accreditation of direct-entry midwifery education. *J Nurse Midwifery* 1995;40:297–303.

Rooks JB, Fischman SH. American nurse-midwifery practice in 1976–1977: Reflections of 50 years of growth and development. *Am J Public Health* 1980;70:990–996.

Rooks JB, Schmidt MA. Hospital privileges: Experience of the certified-nurse midwife. *Clin Psychologist* 1980;33:10–11.

Rooks J, Winikoff B (Eds.). *A Reassessment of the Concept of Reproductive Risk in Maternity Care and Family Planning Services.* The Population Council, New York, 1992.

Rooks J, Fischman S, Kaplan E, Lescynski P, Morgan G, Witek J. *Nurse-Midwifery in the United States: 1976–1977.* ACNM, Washington, DC, 1978.

Rooks JP, Weatherby NL, Ernst EKM, Stapleton S, Rosen D, Rosenfield A. Outcomes of care in birth centers: The National Birth Center Study. *N Engl J Med* 1989;321:1804–1811.

Rooks JP, Carr KC, Sandvold I. The importance of non-master's degree options in nurse-midwifery education. *J Nurse Midwifery* 1991; 36:124–130.

Rooks JP, Weatherby NL, Ernst EKM. The National Birth Center Study, part I: Methodology and prenatal care and referrals. *J Nurse Midwifery* 1992a;37:222–253.

Rooks JP, Weatherby NL, Ernst EKM. The National Birth Center Study, part II: Intrapartum and immediate postpartum and neonatal care. *J Nurse Midwifery* 1992b; 37:301–330.

Rooks JP, Weatherby NL, Ernst EKM. The National Birth Center Study Part III: Intrapartum and immediate postpartum and neonatal complications and transfers, postpartum and neonatal care, outcomes, and client satisfaction. *J Nurse Midwifery* 1992c;37:361–397.

Rosen MG. A message from the chairman. In Department of Health and Human Services, *Caring for Our Future: The Content of Prenatal Care, A Report of the Public Health Service Expert Panel on the Content of Prenatal Care.* Public Health Service, Department of Health and Human Services, Washington, DC, 1989.

Rosen MG, Dickinson JC. The paradox of electronic fetal monitoring: More data may not enable us to predict or prevent infant neurologic morbidity. *Am J Obstet Gynecol* 1993;168: 745–751.

Rosenbaum S. Nurse-midwives and care of the poor. In Rooks J, Haas JE (Eds.), *Nurse-Midwifery in America.* ACNM Foundation, Washington, DC, 1986, pp. 54–56.

Rosenberg EE, Klein M. Is maternity care different in family practice? A pilot matched pair study. *J Fam Pract* 1987;25:237–240.

Rosenberg HM, Ventura SJ, Maurer JD, Heuser RL, Freedman MA. Births and deaths: United States, 1995. Monthly Vital Statistics Report, Vol. 45, No. 3, suppl 2. National Center for Health Statistics, Hyattsville, MD, 1996.

Rosenblatt RA. The future of obstetrics in family practice. *J Fam Pract* 1988; 26:127–129.

Rosenblatt R. New Zealand's regionalized perinatal system. In Rooks J, Winikoff B (Eds.), *Reassessment of the Concept of Reproductive Risk in Maternity Care and Family Planning Services.* The Population Council, New York, 1992.

Rosenblatt RA, Detering A. Changing patterns of obstetric practice in Washington State: The impact of tort reform. *Family Med* 1988; 20:100–107.

Rosenblatt RA, Cherkin DC, Schneeweiss R, Hart LG, Greenwald H, Kirkwood CR, Perkoff GT. The structure and content of family medicine: Current status and future trends. *J Fam Pract* 1982;15:681–722.

Rosenblatt RA, Reinken J, Shoemack P. Is obstetrics safe in small hospitals? Evidence from New Zealand's regionalized perinatal system. *The Lancet* 1985;2(8452):429–432.

Rosenblatt RA, Hart LG, Gamliel G, Goldstein B, McClendon BJ. Identifying primary care disciplines by analyzing the diagnostic content of ambulatory care. *J Am Board Fam Pract* 1995;8:34–45.

Rosenblatt RA, Dobie SA, Hart LG, Baldwin LM, Schneeweiss R, Gould D, Raine TR, Jenkins L, Benedetti TJ, Fordyce M, Pirani MK, Perrin EB. Interspecialty differences in obstetric care. *Am J Public Health* 1997;87:344–351.

Ross MG. Health impact of a nurse-midwife program. *Nursing Res* 1981;30:353–355.

Rothman BK. Awake & aware, or false consciousness: The cooptation of childbirth reform in America. In Romalis S (Ed.), *Childbirth Alter-*

native to Medical Control. University of Texas Press, Austin, 1981.

Rothman BK. Anatomy of a compromise: Nurse-midwifery and the rise of the birth center. *J Nurse Midwifery* 1983;28(4):3–7.

Rothman BK. Childbirth management and medical monopoly: Midwifery as (almost) a profession. *J Nurse Midwifery* 1984;29(5): 300–306.

Roush RE. The development of midwifery—male and female, yesterday and today. *J Nurse Midwifery* 1979;24(3):27–37.

Rowley M, Hensley M, Grinsmead M, Wlodarczyk J. Continuity of care by a midwife team versus routine care during pregnancy and birth: A randomized trial. *Med J Aust* 1995;163: 289–293.

Roy WR. The changing social contract of the obstetrician–gynecologist. In *The Obstetrician/ Gynecologist in the Twenty-First Century: Meeting Society's Needs.* Josiah Macy, Jr. Foundation, New York, 1993, pp. 43–58.

Runnerstrom L, Cramer B, Fischman S, Matousek I, Nissen C. *Descriptive Data: Nurse-Midwives, USA.* American College of Nurse-Midwives, New York, 1971.

Routledge C. Personal communication, 1997. (Carolyn Routledge directs the nurse-midwifery education program operated collaboratively by The University of Texas at El Paso and Texas Tech University.)

Ryan A, Martinez G. Breast-feeding and the working mother: A profile. *Pediatrics* 1989;83: 524–531.

Ryan KJ. Giving birth in America, 1988. *Family Planning Perspectives* 1988;20:298–301.

Sachs BP, Yeh J, Acker D, Driscoll S, Brown DAJ, Jewett JF. Cesarean section-related maternal mortality in Massachusetts, 1954–1985. *Obstet Gynecol* 1987;71:385–388.

Safriet B. Health care dollars and regulatory senses: The role of advanced practice nursing. *Yale J Regulation* 1992;9(2):417–488.

Sakala C. Content of care by independent midwives: Assistance with pain in labor and birth. *Soc Sci Med* 1988;26:1141–1158.

Sakala C. Midwifery care and out-of-hospital birth settings: How do they reduce unnecessary cesarean section births? *Soc Sci Med* 1993;37: 1233–1250.

Sakala C. Personal communication, 1996. (Carol Sakala is adjunct assistant professor, Boston University School of Public Health.)

Sallomi P, Pallow A, O'Mara P. *Midwifery and the Law.* Mothering Publications, Albuquerque, NM.

Sammon A. Personal communication, 1996. (Alice Sammon is treasurer of NARM.)

Sampselle CM, Petersen BA, Murtland TL, Oakley DJ. Prevalence of abuse among pregnant women choosing certified nurse-midwife or physician providers. *J Nurse Midwifery* 1992; 37:269–273.

Sanchez-Ramos L, Kaunitz AM, Peterson HB, Martines-Schell B, Thompson RJ. Reducing cesarean sections at a teaching hospital. *Am J Obstet Gynecol* 1990;163:1081–1088.

Sanchez-Ramos L, Moorhead RI, Kaunitz AM. Cesarean section rates in teaching hospitals: A natural survey. *Birth* 1994;21(4):194–196.

Sandall J. Professionalisation of midwifery in Britain: A feminist paradigm of practice? In *Proceedings of the International Confederation of Midwives 24th Triennial Congress,* Oslo, May, 26–31, ICM, London, pp. 198–201.

Savage DG. Births decline as boomers' babies mature. *LA Times-Washington Post Service,* August 1, 1995.

Scherjon S. A comparison between the organization of obstetrics in Denmark and the Netherlands. *Br J Obstet Gynaecol* 1986;93: 684–689.

Scheuermann K. Midwifery in Germany: Its past and present. *J Nurse Midwifery* 1995;40:438–447.

Schimmel LM, Lee KA, Benner PE, Schimmel LD. A comparison of outcomes between joint and physician-only obstetric practice. *Birth* 1994;21:197–205.

Schlinger H. *Circle of Midwives,* 1992.

Schneider G, Soderstrom B. Analysis of 275 planned home births and 10 unplanned home births. *Can Fam Phys* 1987;33:1163–1171.

Schön D. *Educating the Reflective Practitioner.* Jossey-Bass, San Francisco, 1987.

Schorn MN, McAllister JL, Blanco JD. Water immersion and the effect on labor. *J Nurse Midwifery* 1993;38:336–342.

Schramm WF, Barnes DE, Bakewell J. Neonatal mortality in Missouri home births, 1978–84. *Am J Public Health* 1987;77(8):1–5.

Scupholme A. Nurse-midwives and physicians: A team approach to obstetrical care in a perinatal center. *J Nurse Midwifery* 1982;27(1): 21–27.

Scupholme A, Carr KC. CNMs and primary care: Practice models and types of service. *Quickening*, November/December 1993, p. 14.

Scupholme A, Kamons AS. Are outcomes compromised when mothers are assigned to birth centers for care? *J Nurse Midwifery* 1987; 32(4):211–215.

Scupholme A, Walsh L. Home-based services by nurse-midwives: Sample data from phase II of Nurse-Midwifery Care to Vulnerable Populations in the United States. *J Nurse Midwifery* 1994;39:358–362.

Scupholme A, McLeod AGW, Robertson EG: A birth center affiliated with the tertiary care center: Comparison of outcome. *Obstet Gynecol* 1986;67:598–603.

Scupholme A, DeJoseph J, Strobino DM, Paine LL. Nurse-midwifery care to vulnerable populations, phase I: Demographic characteristics of the national CNM sample. *J Nurse Midwifery* 1992;37:341–348.

Scupholme A, Paine LL, Lang JM, Kumar S, DeJoseph JF. Time associated with components of clinical services rendered by nurse-midwives: Sample data from phase II of Nurse-Midwifery Care to Vulnerable Populations in the United States. *J Nurse Midwifery* 1994; 39:5–12.

Seattle Midwifery School Bulletin. BC's first College of Midwives established. May/June 1995.

Shah MA. Editorial. *J Nurse Midwifery* 1975;20 (Summer):4.

Shah MA. The unification of midwives: A time for dialogue. *J Nurse Midwifery* 1982;27(5):1–2.

Shah MA. Personal communication, December 1996. (Mary Ann Shah is special projects coordinator for the direct-entry midwifery education program at the State University of New York Health Science Center at Brooklyn in partnership with the North Central Bronx Hospital.)

Shah MA, Hsia L. Direct-entry midwifery education: History in the making. *J Nurse Midwifery* 1996;41:351–353.

Sharp ES. Interdependence reexamined. *J Nurse Midwifery* 1980;25(5):1–3.

Sharp ES. Nurse-midwifery education: Its successes, failures, and future. *J Nurse Midwifery* 1983;28(2):17–23.

Sharp ES. Personal communication, November 1995. (Elizabeth S. Sharp is Director, Nurse–Midwifery, Emory University, Atlanta, GA.)

Sharp ES, Lewis LE. A decade of nurse-midwifery practice in a tertiary university-affiliated hospital. *J Nurse Midwifery* 1984;29(6):353–365.

Sheehan KH. Caesarean section for dystocia: A comparison of practices in two countries. *The Lancet* 1987;1(8532):548–551.

Sherwood M. The midwives of Baltimore. *JAMA* 1909;52:2009–2011.

Shoemaker HT. Nurse-midwifery. *The Catholic Nurse* 1953;1:23.

Sholles H. Personal communication, March 1996, (Holly Sholles is director of Birthingway Midwifery School, Portland, OR.)

Shryock RH. *Medical Licensing in America.* Johns Hopkins Press, Baltimore, 1967.

Silver GA. In *The Midwife in the United States: Report of a Macy Conference.* Josiah Macy, Jr Foundation, New York, 1968, pp. 3–14.

Simkin P. *Pregnancy, Childbirth and the Newborn.* Meadowbrook Books, Deephaven, MN, 1984.

Simkin P. Stress, pain, and catecholamines in labor: Part 1. A review. *Birth* 1986a;13;227–233.

Simkin P. Stress, pain and catecholamines in labor: Part 2. Stress associated with childbirth events: A pilot survey of new mothers. *Birth* 1986b;13:234–240.

Simkin P. Just another day in a woman's life? Women's long-term perceptions of their first birth experience. Part I. *Birth* 1991; 18:203–210.

Simkin P. Reducing pain and enhancing progress in labor: A guide to nonpharmacologic methods for maternity caregivers. *Birth* 1996; 23:161–171.

Singh S, Gold RB, Frost JJ. Impact of the Medicaid eligibility expansions on coverage of deliveries. *Family Planning Perspectives* 1994;26 (1):31–33.

Sinquefield G. Technology: A reality and an issue for nurse-midwives. *J Nurse Midwifery* 1993; 38:1S.

Skubi D. Personal communication, February 1994. (Desmond Skubi is a nurse-midwife practicing in Washington State.)

Slattery LE, Burst HV. ACNM accredited and preaccredited nurse-midwifery education programs. *J Nurse Midwifery* 1995;40:349–364.

Slattery LE, Burst HV. ACNM accredited and preaccredited nurse-midwifery education programs: Program information. *J Nurse Midwifery* 1996;41:305–321.

Slome C, Wetherbee H, Daly M, Christensen K, Meglen M, Thiede H. Effectiveness of certified nurse-midwives: A prospective evaluative study. *Am J Obstet Gynecol* 1976;124: 177–182.

Smith MC, Holmes LJ. *Listen to Me Good: The Life Story of an Alabama Midwife*. Ohio State University Press, Columbus, OH, 1996.

Smucker DR. Obstetrics in family practice in the state of Ohio. *J Fam Med* 1988;26:165–168.

Socal ML, Garcia PM, Peaceman AM, Dooley SL. Reducing cesarean births at a primarily private university hospital. *Am J Obstet Gynecol* 1993;168:1748–1758.

Soderstrom B, Chamberlain M, Kaitell C, Steward PJ. Midwifery in Ontario: A survey of interest in services. *Birth* 1990;17: 139–143.

Soloway B, Calman N, Miller E, Swartz J, Weiser J, Sacco J, Roethel L. Letter to the Editor. *J Nurse Midwifery* 1995;40:305–306.

Sosa R, Kennell J, Klaus M, Robertson S, Urrutia J. The effect of a supportive companion on perinatal problems, length of labor, and mother–infant interactions. *N Engl J Med* 1980;303:597–600.

Speert, H. Midwives, nurses, and nurse-midwives. In *Obstetrics and Gynecology in America: A History*. American College of Obstetricians and Gynecologists, Chicago, 1980.

Spencer N. Personal communication, April 1, 1996. (Nancy Spencer is a licensed midwife in Washington State and a member of the Group Health Cooperative Licensed Midwifery and Home Birth Task Force, Seattle, WA.)

Spencer T, Thomas H, Morris J. A randomized controlled trial of the provision of a social support service during pregnancy: The South Manchester Family Worker Project. *Br J Obstet Gynaecol* 1989;96:281–288.

Spindel P. Quoted in Schlinger H, *Circle of Midwives*, 1992, pp. 100–101.

Spitzer MC. Birth centers: Economy, safety, and empowerment. *J Nurse Midwifery* 1995;40: 371–375.

Stafford RS. Cesarean section use and source of payment: An analysis of California hospital discharge abstracts. *Am J Public Health* 1990;80:313–315.

Stafford RS, Sullivan SD, Gardner LB. Trends in cesarean section use in California, 1983 to 1990. *Am J Obstet Gynecol* 1993;168:1297–1302.

Stallings T. Quoted in Schlinger H, *Circle of Midwives*, 1992, pp. 16–17, 46.

Stallings T. Personal communication, 1994. (Therese Stallings is a member of the faculty of the Seattle Midwifery School.)

Stallings T. International midwifery issues. *MANA Newsletter* 1995;XIII(1):14–15.

Stark R, Mann R, DeJoseph JF, Emery M. The Women's Health Care Training Project: An alternative for training midwives. *J Nurse Midwifery* 1984;29(3):191–196.

Starr P. *The Social Transformation of American Medicine: The Rise of a Sovereign Profession and the Making of a Vast Industry*. Basic Books, New York, 1982.

Steele E. Report on the fourth thousand confinements of the Frontier Nursing service. *Q Bull Frontier Nurse Service* 1941;16:4–13.

Steiger C. *Becoming a Midwife*. Hoogin House Publishing, Portland, OR, 1987.

Stein E. Peer review in a New York chapter of the ACNM, 1987–1994. *J Nurse Midwifery* 1996; 41:401–404.

Stern TL. A landmark in interspecialty cooperation. *J Fam Pract* 1977; 5:523–524.

Stewart D. The limits of science in childbirth. In *21st Century Obstetrics Now!* Vol. 2. National Association of Parents & Professionals for Safe Alternatives in Childbirth, Chapel Hill, NC, 1978, pp. 281–309.

Stewart PJ, Beresford JM. Opinions of physicians assisting births in Ottawa-Carleton about the licensing of midwives. *Can Med Assoc J* 1988;139:393–397.

Stewart PJ, Dulberg C, Arnill AC, Elmslie T, Hall PF. Diagnosis of dystocia and management with cesarean section among primiparous women in Ottawa-Carleton. *Can Med Assoc J* 1990;142:459–463.

Stewart RB, Clark L. Nurse-midwifery practice in an in-hospital birthing center: 2050 births. *J Nurse Midwifery* 1982;27(3):21–26.

Stimpson GE. Independent midwifery practice in New Zealand. In *Proceedings of the International Confederation of Midwives 24th Triennial Congress*, Oslo, May 26–31, 1996, ICM, London, pp. 167–170.

Stone PW, Walker PH. Cost-effectiveness analysis: Birth center vs. hospital care. *Nursing Economic$* 1995;13:299–308.

Stone SE, Brown MP, Westcott JP. Nurse-midwifery service in a rural setting. *J Nurse Midwifery* 1996;41:377–382.

Suarez SH. Midwifery is not the practice of medicine. *Yale J Law Feminism* 1993;5(3):315–365.

Sullivan DA. *Labor Pains*. Yale University Press, New Haven, CT, 1988.

Sullivan DA, Beeman R. Four years' experience with home birth by licensed midwives in Arizona. *Am J Public Health* 1983;73: 641–645.

Sullivan ME. North American Registry Exam for Midwives: Technical documentation, January 1994. P.O. Box 15, Linn, WV 26384.

Sullivan N. Personal communication, 1996. (Nancy Sullivan is a certified nurse-midwife at the Oregon Health Sciences University, Portland, OR.)

Sullivan P. Midwives not needed: CMA. *Can Med Assoc J* 1987;136:648.

Summers L. The genesis of the ACNM 1971 statement on abortion. *J Nurse Midwifery* 1992;37:168–174.

Swartz DP. In *The Midwife in the United States: Report of a Macy Conference.* Josiah Macy, Jr Foundation, New York, 1968, pp. 44–57.

Taffel SM. Characteristics of American Indian and Alaska native births: United States, 1984. *Monthly Vital Statistics Report,* Vol. 36, No. 3, suppl, Public Health Service, Hyattsville, MD, June 19, 1987. DHHS Publication 87–1120.

Taylor DH, Ricketts TC. Helping nurse-midwives provide obstetrical care in rural North Carolina. *Am J Public Health* 1993;83:904–905.

Taylor M, Yohalem M. *Medical practice in the 1980s: Physicians look at their changing profession.* Louis Harris and Associates, 1981.

Tew M. Landmark decision for British homebirth and midwifery. *The Birth Gazette* 1992;8(3): 3840.

Tew M, Damstra-Wijmenga SMI. The safest birth attendants: Recent Dutch evidence. *Midwifery* 1991;7:55–65.

Thacker SB, Banta HB. Benefits and risks of episiotomy: An interpretive review of the English language literature, 1860–1980. *Obstet Gynecol Surv* 1983;38:322–338.

Thacker SB, Stroup DF, Peterson HB. Efficacy and safety of intrapartum electronic fetal monitoring: An update. *Obstet Gynecol* 1995; 86:613–620.

Thomas MW. *The Practice of Nurse-Midwifery in the United States.* Children's Bureau, Department of Health, Education and Welfare, Washington, DC, 1965.

Thompson J. Peer review in an American College of Nurse-Midwives local chapter. *J Nurse Midwifery* 1986;31:289–295.

Thompson JB. Safety and effectiveness of nurse-midwifery care: Research review. In Rooks J, Haas JE (Eds.), *Nurse-Midwifery in America.* ACNM Foundation, Washington, DC, 1986, pp. 40–44.

Thompson JE. Nurse-midwifery care: 1925–1984. In Wenley HH, Fitzpatrick JT, Taunton RL (Eds.), *Ann Rev Nursing Res* 1986;4:153–173.

Thorp JA, Breedlove G. Epidural analgesia in labor: An evaluation of risks and benefits. *Birth* 1996;23:63–83.

Thorp JA, Hu DH, Albin RM, McNitt J, Meyer BA, Cohen GR, Yeast JD. The effect of intrapartum epidural analgesia on nulliparous labor: A randomized, controlled, prospective trial. *Am J Obstet Gynecol* 1993;169:851–858.

Thorpe K. Changes in the growth in health spending: Implications for consumers. Medical Center Institute for Health Services Research, New Orleans, LA, April 1997. (Report prepared by health economist Kenneth E. Thorpe of Tulane University.)

Tom SA. Agnes Shoemaker Reinders: A biographical tribute. *J Nurse Midwifery* 1980; 25(5):9–12.

Tom SA. Nurse-midwifery: A developing profession. *Law, Medicine & Health Care,* December 1982a, pp. 262–282.

Tom SA. The evolution of nurse-midwifery: 1900–1960. *J Nurse Midwifery* 1982b;27(4): 4–13.

Tom SA. Personal communication, 1993. (At the time of this communication, Sally A. Tom was the ACNM's government affairs liaison.)

Treffers PE. Selection as the basis of obstetric care in the Netherlands. In Abraham-Van der Mark E (Ed.), *Successful Home Birth and Midwifery: The Dutch Model.* Bergin & Garvey, London, 1993, pp. 97–114.

Treffers PE, Laan R. Regional perinatal mortality and regional hospitalization at delivery in the Netherlands. *Br J Obstet Gynaecol* 1986;93: 690–693.

Treistman JM, Carr KC, McHugh MK. Community-based nurse-midwifery education program: Distance learning in nurse-midwifery education. *J Nurse Midwifery* 1993;38: 358–365.

Trepiccione A. Twins can be born naturally. *The Birth Gazette* 1994;10(2):22–23.

Tritten J. What does it take to become a midwife? *Midwifery Today* 1992;21:33.

Tritten J. Personal communication, May 10, 1996. (Jan Tritten is editor of *Midwifery Today.*)

Tully G. A perspective on home breech birth. Unpublished paper available from Gail Tully, 2220 West 98th Street, Bloomington, MN 55431, 1993.

Turnbull D, Holmes A, Shields N, Cheyne H, Twaddle S, Gilmour WH, McGinley M, Reid M, Johnstone R, Geer I, McIlwaine G, Lunan CB. Randomized, controlled trial of efficacy of midwife-managed care. *The Lancet* 1996; 348(9022):213–218.

Tymstra T. The impact of medical-technological developments on midwifery in the Netherlands. In Abraham-Van der Mark E (Ed.), *Successful Home Birth and Midwifery: The Dutch Model.* Bergin & Garvey, London, 1993, pp. 129–137.

Tyson H. Outcomes of 1001 midwife-attended home births in Toronto, 1983–1988. *Birth* 1991;18:14–19.

University of Washington School of Public Health and Community Medicine. Midwifery outside of the nursing profession: The current debate in Washington. Author, Seattle, October 1980. Document of the Health Policy Analysis Program, RD-37.

Uzodinma M. Personal communication, 1995. (Minta Uzodinma is chief nurse consultant in the Mississippi State Department of Health.)

Vadeboncoeur H. Why did Québec decide to experiment with the practice of midwifery while Ontario legalized the profession? Paper presented during the Annual Joint Meeting of the Society for Applied Anthropology, the Society for Medical Anthropology, the Council on Nursing and Anthropology, and the Political Ecology Society, Seattle, Washington, March 6, 1997. (This paper was published in French in the journal *Rutures— Revue Transdisciplinaire en Santé* 1996;3(2): 224–242.)

Vadeboncoeur H. Personal communication, 1997. (Hélène Vadeboncoeur is pursuing a doctorate in public health at the University of Montreal.)

Vallardi RH, Orter J, Winberg J. Does the newborn find the nipple by smell? *The Lancet* 1990;344:989–990.

Van Alten, Eskes M, Treffers PE. Midwifery in the Netherlands. The Wormerveer study: Selection, mode of delivery, perinatal mortality and infant morbidity. *Br J Obstet Gynaecol* 1989;96:656–662.

van Blarcom CC. Midwives in America. *Am J Pub Health* 1914;8(4):197–207.

van Daalen R. Family change and continuity in the Netherlands: Birth and childbed in text and art. In Abraham-Van der Mark E (Ed.), *Successful Home Birth and Midwifery: The Dutch Model.* Bergin & Garvey, London, 1993, pp. 77–94.

van Heijst M-L, van Roosmalen G, Keirse MJNC. Classifying meconium-stained liquor: Is it feasible? *Birth* 1995;22(4):191–195.

van Lier D, Manteuffel B, Dilorio C, Stalcup M. Nausea and fatigue during early pregnancy. *Birth* 1993;20(4):193–197.

Van Teijlingen ER. The profession of maternity home care assistant and its significance for the Dutch midwifery profession. *Int J Nurse Stud* 1990;27:355–366.

Van Teijlingen ER, McCaffery P. The profession of midwife in the Netherlands. *Midwifery* 1987;3:178–186.

Varney H. *Nurse-Midwifery,* 1st ed. Blackwell Scientific Publications, Boston, 1980.

Varney H. *Nurse-Midwifery,* 2nd ed. Blackwell Scientific Publications, Boston, 1987.

Ventre F. Quoted in Schlinger H, *Circle of Midwives,* 1992, pp. 4–5.

Ventre R, Leonard C. The future of midwifery: An alliance. *J Nurse Midwifery* 1982;27(5):23–24.

Ventura SJ, Martin JA, Taffel SM, Mathews MS, Clarke SC. Advance report of final natality statistics, 1992. *Monthly Vital Statistics Report,* Vol. 43, No. 5, suppl. National Center for Health Statistics, Hyattsville, MD, 1994.

Ventura SJ, Martin JA, Taffel SM, Mathews MS, Clarke SC. Advance report of final natality statistics, 1993. *Monthly Vital Statistics Report,* Vol. 44, No. 3, suppl. National Center for Health Statistics, Hyattsville, MD, 1995.

Ventura SJ. Martin JA, Mathews TJ, Clarke SC. Advance report of final natality statistics, 1994. *Monthly Vital Statistics Report,* Vol. 44, No. 11, suppl. National Center for Health Statistics, Hyattsville, MD, 1996.

Vermont Vital Statistics System. Data provided by Mike Nyland-Funk, biostatistician with the Vermont Vital Statistic System, Burlington, Vermont, June 28, 1996.

Vogler C. Quoted in Schlinger H, *Circle of Midwives,* 1992, pp. 96–97.

Wagner M. Letter to the editor: Don't blame midwives in maternity care crisis. *The New York Times,* March 13, 1995.

Wagner M. Personal communication in response to review of a draft of Chapter 13, 1996a. (Marsden Wagner is an American physician who served as Regional Officer for Women's and Children's Health, World Health Organization, Regional Office for Europe, from 1978 through 1991.)

Wagner MG. Infant mortality in Europe: Implications for the United States, Statement to the National Commission to Prevent Infant Mortality. *J Pub Health Pol* 1988; 9:473–481.

Wagner MG. Midwife-managed care. *The Lancet* 1996b:348:208.

Waldenström U. Personal communication, November 15, 1993. (Ulla Waldenström was a midwife at the Alternative Birth Center Unit, Department of Obstetrics and Gynecology, Southern Hospital, and Department of Obstetrics and Gynecology, Karolinska Hospital, Stockholm, Sweden.)

Waldenström U. Personal communication, 1996 and 1997. (Ulla Waldenström is professor of midwifery, Graduate Clinical School of Midwifery and Women's Health, La Trobe University, Carlton, Victoria, Australia.)

Waldenström U. Challenges and issues for midwifery. *J Aust College Midwives* 1997;10(3):in press.

Waldenström U, Gottvall K. A randomized trial of birthing stool or conventional semirecumbent position for second-stage labor. *Birth* 1991;18(1):5–10.

Waldenstöm U, Nilsson CA. Women's satisfaction with birth care center: A randomized, controlled study. *Birth* 1993:20:3–13.

Wallace AM, Boyer DB, Dan A. Holm K. Aerobic exercise, maternal self-esteem, and physical discomforts during pregnancy. *J Nurse Midwifery* 1986;31(6):255–261.

Wallach EE. Introduction. In *The Obstetrician/Gynecologist in the Twenty-First Century: Meeting Society's Needs.* Josiah Macy, Jr. Foundation, New York, 1993, pp. 7–9.

Wallach HR, Matlin MW. College women's expectations about pregnancy, childbirth, and infant care: A prospective study. *Birth* 1992; 19:202–207.

Walsh LV. Midwife means with woman: An historical perspective. ACNM, Washington, DC, 1991. (A brochure to accompany an exhibition on the history of midwifery at the National Library of Medicine, September 16, 1991–January 15, 1992.)

Walsh LV. "A special vocation"—Philadelphia midwives, 1910–1940. A dissertation in nursing presented to the facilities of the University of Pennsylvania in partial fulfillment of the requirements for the degree of doctor of philosophy, 1992.

Walsh LV, Boggess JH. Findings of the American College of Nurse-Midwives annual membership surveys, 1993 and 1994. *J Nurse Midwifery* 1996;41:230–236.

Walsh LV, DeJoseph J. Findings of the 1991 annual American College of Nurse-Midwives membership survey. *J Nurse Midwifery* 1993; 38:35–41.

Washington Department of Licensing. An assessment of childbirth outcomes in Washington: Report to the legislature. Authors, Olympia, WA, 1987.

Washington Post, February 24, 1992.

Waters MA, Lee KA. Differences between primigravidae and multigravidae mothers in sleep disturbances, fatigue, and functional status. *J Nurse Midwifery* 1996;41:364–367.

Wegman ME. Annual summary of vital statistics—1990. *Pediatrics* 1991;88:1081–1092.

Weig M. Audit of independent midwifery, 1987–1991. Royal College of Midwives, London, 1993.

Weiner CP. Vaginal breech delivery in the 1990. *Clin Obstet Gynecol* 1992;35:559–569.

Weitz R. English midwives and the association of radical midwives. *Women & Health* 1987;12 (1):79–89.

Weitz R, Sullivan D. Licensed lay midwifery and the medical model of childbirth. *Sociology Health Illness* 1985;7(1):36–54.

Weitz R, Sullivan D. Midwife licensing. In Rothman BK (Ed.), *Encyclopedia of Childbearing: Critical Perspectives.* ORYZ, Phoenix, AZ, 1993, pp. 245–247.

Welt SI, Cole JS, Myers MS, Sholes DM Jr, Jelovsek FR. Feasibility of postpartum rapid hospital discharge: A study from a community hospital population. *Am J Perinatal* 1993;10:384–387.

Wente S. Nurse-midwifery practices in hospitals for the indigent. In Rooks J, Haas JE (Eds.), *Nurse-Midwifery in America.* ACNM Foundation, Washington, DC, 1986, p: 25–27.

Wertz DC. What birth has done for doctors: A historical view. *Women & Health* 1983;8(1):7–24.

Whelan A. Centering birth: A prospective cohort study of birth centres and labour wards. Thesis submitted in fulfillment of the requirements for the degree of doctor of philosophy, Department of Public Health, University of Sydney, August 1994.

White House Conference on Child Health and Protection. Midwives. *Obstetric Education.* Appleton-Century, New York, 1932.

Widström AM. Short-term effects of early sucking and touch of the nipple on maternal behavior. *Early Hum Dev* 1990;21:153–163.

Wilcox A. Quoted in "Conceptual shift," *Discover,* 1996, p. 12.

Williams DR. Credentialing certified nurse-midwives. *J Nurse Midwifery* 1994a;39:471–477.

Williams D. Physician supervision of nurse-midwifery practice. *Quickening,* July/August 1994b, p. 10.

Williams DR. Primary care for women: The nurse-midwifery legacy. *J Nurse Midwifery* 1995; 40:57–58.

Williams JW. Medical education and the midwife problem in the United States. *JAMA* 1912; 2:180–204.

Williamson HA, LeFebre M, Hector, Jr M. Association between life stress and serious perinatal complications. *J Fam Pract* 1989;29: 489–496.

Wilner S, Schoenbarum SC, Monson RR, Winickorr RN. A comparison of the quality of maternity care between a health-maintenance organization and fee-for-service practices. *N Engl J Med* 1981;304:784–787.

Winikoff B. Breastfeeding. *Cur Opin Obstet Gynecol* 1990;2:548–555.

Winship EJ. Midwifery in Europe—Valuing the European Union Midwives Directives. In *Proceedings of the International Confederation of Midwives 24th Triennial Congress,* Oslo, May, 26–31, ICM, London, pp. 187–190.

Withers M. Agnodike: The first midwife/obstetrician. *J Nurse Midwifery* 1979;24(3):4.

Wolf S, Gabay M. Unnecessary cesarean sections: Curing a national epidemic. Public Citizen Health Research Group, Washington, DC, 1994.

Women's Institute for Childbearing Policy. *Childbearing Policy Within a National Health Program: An Evolving Consensus for New Directions.* Author, Roxbury, VT, 1994.

Woodcock HC, Read AW, Moore DJ, Stanley FJ, Bower C. Planned homebirths in Western Australia, 1981–1987: A descriptive study. *J Med Austr* 1990;151:672–687.

Woodcock HC, Read AW, Bower C, Stanley FJ, Moore DJ. A matched cohort study of planned home and hospital births in Western Australia, 1981–1987. *Midwifery* 1994;10: 125–135.

Woodville L. Historical background on International Confederation of Midwives. *Bull ACNM* 1971;16(2):37–38.

World Health Organization. Traditional birth attendants: A joint WHO/UNFPA/UNICEF statement. Author, Geneva, 1992.

World Health Organization. *Care in Normal Birth: A Practical Guide.* Author, Geneva, 1996.

World Health Organization, Regional Office for Europe. *Having a Baby in Europe: Report on a Study.* Author, Copenhagen, 1985.

Wrigley EA, Hutchinson SA. Long-term breastfeeding: The secret bond. *J Nurse Midwifery* 1990;35:35–41.

Wykes SL. Midwife cleared of wrong-doing. *San Jose Mercury News,* April 30, 1993.

Yanco J. Letter to David Mulligan, commissioner of health, Massachusetts Department of Public Health, on behalf of the Boston Women's Health Book Collective, March 6, 1996.

Yates SA. A refresher program for nurse-midwives: The Booth experience. *J Nurse Midwifery* 1983;28(3):11–17.

Yeates DA, Roberts JE. A comparison of two bearing-down techniques during the second stage of labor. *J Nurse Midwifery* 1984;29:3–11.

Young D. Family-centered maternity care: Is the central nursery obsolete? *Birth* 1992;19: 183–184.

Young D. The midwifery revolution in New Zealand: What can we learn? *Birth* 1993;23: 125–127.

Young G. Safety and the place of birth. *Practitioner* 1993;237:736–738.

Zabrek E, Simon P, Benrubi GI. Nurse-midwifery prototypes: Clinical practice and education. The alternative birth center in Jacksonville, Florida: The first two years. *J Nurse Midwifery* 1983;28(4):31–36.

Zahniser SC, Kendrick JS, Franks AL, Saftlas AF. Trends in obstetric operative procedures, 1980 to 1987. *Am J Public Health* 1991;82: 1340–1344.

Zaldivar RZ. Debate clouds full health care story. Knight-Ridder News Service, February 2, 1993.

Zeidenstein L. JNM's 1994 home study program: Nurse-midwifery management of obstetric complications. *J Nurse Midwifery* 1994;39 (suppl):1S–2S.

Index

DATE DUE

JAN 22 '98		
MR 21 '98		
OCT 2 8 1998		
MY 15 '01		
DE 0 7 '02		
MY 29 '03		

GAYLORD   PRINTED IN U.S.A